The Advanced Handbook of
METHODS IN EVIDENCE BASED HEALTHCARE

The Advanced Handbook of
METHODS IN EVIDENCE BASED HEALTHCARE

Edited by

ANDREW STEVENS
KEITH ABRAMS
JOHN BRAZIER
RAY FITZPATRICK
and RICHARD LILFORD

SAGE Publications
London • Thousand Oaks • New Delhi

Editorial arrangement, Introduction and Part Introductions
© Andrew Stevens, Keith R. Abrams, John Brazier,
Ray Fitzpatrick and Richard J. Lilford 2001
Chapters 1–27 © the contributors 2001

First published 2001

 SAGE Publications Ltd
6 Bonhill Street
London EC2A 4PU

SAGE Publications Inc
2455 Teller Road
Thousand Oaks, California 91320

SAGE Publications India Pvt Ltd
32, M-Block Market
Greater Kailash – I
New Delhi 110 048

British Library Cataloguing in Publication data

A catalogue record for this book is available from
the British Library

ISBN 0 7619 6144 5

Library of Congress catalog record available

Typeset by Photoprint, Torquay, Devon
Printed in Great Britain by The Cromwell Press Ltd,
Trowbridge, Wiltshire

Contents

Part II   OBSERVATIONAL AND QUALITATIVE METHODS

Part III   MEASUREMENT OF BENEFIT AND COST

Part IV ANALYTICAL METHODS

Part V CONSENSUS, REVIEWS AND META-ANALYSIS

Contributors

Keith Abrams (editor) is Reader in Medical Statistics, in the Department of Epidemiology and Public Health, at the University of Leicester, having previously held posts at King's College School of Medicine and Dentistry and the London School of Hygiene and Tropical Medicine. He has gained degrees from the Universities of Warwick, Leicester and Liverpool. His research interests include: the development and application of Bayesian methods in Health Services Research (HSR)/Health Technology Assessment (HTA), systematic reviews and meta-analysis, and analysis of time to event data. He is a fellow of the Royal Statistical Society and a Chartered Statistician.

Richard Ashcroft is Lecturer in Medical Ethics at Imperial College School of Medicine. He trained as an undergraduate in mathematics and philosophy at Cambridge University, before completing a PhD in ethics and philosophy of science, also at Cambridge. The chapter in this volume is based on work carried out as a postdoctoral research fellow in the Philosophy Department at Liverpool University, funded by the NHS Health Technology Assessment programme, grant 93/41/4, held by Dr Jane Hutton with Prof. David Chadwick, Prof. Stephen Clark, Prof. Richard Edwards, and Ms. Lucy Frith. He is currently working on ethical issues in medical research and technology assessment.

Janet Askham is Professor of Gerontology and Director of the Age Concern Institute of Gerontology at King's College London. She is a sociologist whose research career has covered topics spanning the life course: fertility behaviour, marriage and family relationships, chronic illness and disability, care in old age. She has particular interests in family life and care for people with dementia, late-life marriage and inter-generational relationships.

Chris Bain is Reader in Social and Preventive Medicine at the University of Queensland. Whilst much of his research is in cancer epidemiology, he has maintained an interest in health services research which was happily fanned into life during a sabbatical spent with his co-authors.

Claire Bamford graduated in Psychology from the University of London and also has an MSc in social research methods from the University of Surrey.

Her research interests include provision of services and informal care to older people with dementia, and the measurement of outcomes of community care. She is currently a research fellow at the Social Policy Research Unit at the University of York working on a Department of Health-funded programme of research into ways of collecting and using information on the outcomes of community care in routine practice.

Cindy Billingham currently works at the Cancer Research Campaign Trials Unit at the University of Birmingham as a Senior Biostatistician. Her area of special interest is the analysis of quality of life data, and she is registered for a part-time PhD at Leicester University researching into joint modelling of quality of life and survival data.

Andrew Black was educated in Pakistan, Scotland and Oxford. He did his Postgraduate clinical training in Oxford, Gloucester, Sydney and Auckland. He was a Lecturer in Anaesthesia at the University of Oxford from 1977–1982. Since then he has been a Consultant Senior Lecturer in Anaesthesia at the University of Bristol. His academic interests are in pulmonary gas exchange, control of breathing, postoperative analgesia, clinical applications of classification approaches including statistical multi-variable and multi-variate modelling and neural networks, applications of medical simulation and role play in medical undergraduate education.

Nick Black is Professor of Health Services Research (since 1995) and Head of the Department of Public Health and Policy at the London School of Hygiene and Tropical Medicine (since May 1998). After qualifying in medicine from Birmingham University in 1974, he worked in NHS hospitals for two-and-a-half years before joining Save the Children Fund and running a child health programme in Nepal for 18 months. He then underwent postgraduate training in public health at Oxford including a doctorate on reasons for the epidemic in surgery for glue ear in the UK. The next three years were spent half time as a lecturer at the Open University writing a new distance-learning course 'Health and Disease' with a biologist, sociologist and economist, and half time as a Consultant in Public Health for Oxfordshire Health Authority. In 1985 he moved to a Senior Lectureship at the LSHTM. His main research interests are the evaluation and audit of health services (particularly in the field of surgery), non-randomised methods of evaluation, R&D policy, and organisational research. He is involved in several aspects of the NHS R&D programme at national and regional levels. In 1996, together with Nick Mays (a Visiting Professor in PHP), he founded the *Journal of Health Services Research & Policy*. He was promoted to a Readership in 1993 and to his current Chair in 1995.

Andrew Boddy is an Honorary Senior Research Fellow in the Department of Public Health, University of Glasgow and was formerly Director of the University's Public Health Research Unit. He has a long-standing interest in the uses of routinely assembled data for health services planning and evaluation, including methods of their analysis and interpretation.

John Bond is a Sociologist with a special interest in social gerontology and health services research. He is currently Professor of Health Services Research at the Centre for Health Services Research at the University of Newcastle upon Tyne and Associate Director at the Institute for the Health of the Elderly, University of Newcastle upon Tyne. His research interests are health policy and older people, in particular looking at social protection policy for dependency in old age; health services research and older people with dementia; health services research and older people who fall; disability and older people; and Health Technology Assessment with particular reference to older people. He is a Member of the Health Technology Assessment, Primary and Community Care Panel and the Health Technology Assessment Commissioning Board.

D. Jane Bower currently holds a Chair in the Department of Economics and Enterprise at Glasgow Caledonian University. She graduated with a PhD in Molecular Genetics from Edinburgh University and worked initially for 15 years as a biomedical scientist at Stanford Medical School, Edinburgh University and the MRC Human Genetics Unit. Since 1989 her research has focused on issues surrounding the development of new technologies into useful application. In the course of this research she has worked with public and private sector organisations in Europe, the USA and Japan.

David Braunholtz is currently Senior Research Fellow in Medical Statistics in the Department of Public Health and Epidemiology at the University of Birmingham, having worked previously in medical schools in Leeds and Managua, at the Greater London Council, and in the Scottish Office. He graduated in Maths and Physics. Interests include research ethics, clinical trials and Bayesian methods.

John Brazier (editor) is Professor of Health Economics and Director of the Sheffield Health Economics Group (which includes 14 health economists) in the School of Health and Related Research at the University of Sheffield. His main interests have been in the measurement and valuation of health services outcomes and economic evaluation, including the development of a preference-based measure from the SF-36 for use in economic evaluation. He continues to be actively involved in the design, analysis and interpretation of economic evaluations conducted alongside clinical trials and modelling.

John Brebner is a Senior Lecturer in the Department of General Practice and Primary Care at the University of Aberdeen; Director of the Remote Health Care Unit/Telemedicine Laboratory and Visiting Professor at the United Arab Emirates University. His main research interests and projects are the human resource implications for the nursing profession in developing telemedicine within the NHS; when and how to assess fast-changing technology; an evaluation of the feasibility and diagnostic acceptability of tele-ultrasonography for rural areas and telemedicine in Primary Care.

Andrew Briggs is a Joint MRC/South East Region Training Fellow in Health Services Research at the Health Economics Research Centre, University of Oxford. Andrew joined the Health Economics Research Centre in 1996. He is particularly interested in statistical issues associated with economic evaluation alongside clinical trials, and currently holds a joint MRC/South East Region Training Fellowship to study statistical methods in cost–effectiveness analysis. He also has a general interest in decision analysis and modelling techniques applied to the economic evaluation of healthcare interventions, and has been involved with economic evaluations of interferon treatment for hepatitis, total hip replacement, and various screening programmes.

Annie Britton is a lecturer at the London School of Hygiene and Tropical Medicine. She has worked in public health research for several years, and her study interests include trial methodology, health promotion evaluation, and most recently an epidemiological assessment of alcohol consumption in Europe. She has published over 20 articles in peer-reviewed journals.

Peter Burney is Professor of Public Health Medicine and Chairman of the Division of Primary Care and Public Health Sciences at King's College London. He is the Honorary Director of the Department of Health's Social Medicine and Health Services Research Unit. His current work is focused on the aetiology and management of allergic and respiratory conditions.

Martin Buxton is Director of the Health Economics Research Group (HERG) at Brunel University. He has been concerned with the economics of healthcare and with health service policy for over 20 years. Martin has been responsible for a number of major projects for the UK Department of Health, including the early evaluation of the costs and benefits of the UK heart transplant programmes. HERG's recent work for the Department includes research on liver transplantation, an evaluation of picture archiving and communication systems, on screening programmes, and a project devising a methodology to assess the payback on Health Services Research. He is involved in many clinical trials, particularly of cardiac interventions. Professor Buxton currently sits on a number of advisory groups: he is a member of the NHS Standing Group on Health Technology, Chair of the NHS R&D Methodology Group and a member of the HEFCE RAE 2001 Panel for Community-Based Clinical Subjects.

John Cairns is an economist who has specialised in the area of health economics for the past ten years. He is currently acting director of the Health Economics Research Unit at the University of Aberdeen.

Michael Campbell is Professor of Medical Statistics with an interest in Primary Care at the University of Sheffield. He is interested in the design and analysis of trials, particularly in primary care. He is interested in sample size calculations and analysis of quality of life data. He is a co-author with David Machin of *Statistical Tables for the Design of Clinical Trials* (Blackwells) and *Medical Statistics: A Common Sense Approach* (Wiley).

Susan Chinn is a Reader in Medical Statistics at the Department of Public Health Sciences, King's College, London. Her current work is mainly in respiratory epidemiology, especially asthma, and she has been involved in child growth surveillance for many years. She is interested in all applications of statistics that further excellence in medical research, of which the design of cluster randomised trials is a good example.

Iain Colthart is currently employed as a research and information officer at the British Medical Association in Edinburgh. He contributed to the chapter in this volume when he was employed as a research associate in the Medical Statistics Unit at the Department of Public Health, University of Edinburgh. His qualifications are B.Com. (Hons) and M.A.

Deborah Cook is an Associate Professor at McMaster University, and a general internist, intensivist and epidemiologist. She is Director of the Academic General Internal Medicine Fellowship at McMaster, Chair of the Canadian Critical Care Trials Group and Consulting Editor for *Journal of the American Medical Association*. Her research interests are in pneumonia, gastrointestinal bleeding, end-of-life decisions and evidence based medicine.

Carl Counsell is a Specialist Registrar in neurology at the Western General Hospital in Edinburgh with research interests in stroke, movement disorders and epidemiology, particularly clinical trials and systematic reviews. He has an MSc in epidemiology, and was involved in setting up the Cochrane Stroke Group.

Rosemary Crow is Professor of Nursing Science in the European Institute of Health and Medical Sciences at the University of Surrey. She trained as a nurse before reading psychology at the University of Edinburgh. Her research interests lie in clinical judgement within the field of medical and surgical nursing.

Claire Davey obtained her Bachelor of Applied Science at the University of Victoria, Australia. She worked in health promotion for three years before moving to the University of Oxford, England in 1992 to work on research into measurement of patient-assessed outcomes and methods of providing information for cancer screening programmes. She is the co-author with Ray Fitzpatrick, Martin Buxton and David Jones of a monograph published by the Health Technology Assessment (HTA) Programme, *Evaluating patient-based* *outcome measures for use in clinical trials*, HTA Programme, University of Southampton, 1998.

Mark Deverill is a research fellow in the Sheffield Health Economics Group at the University of Sheffield. His main research interest lies in the use of quality of life instruments in the economic evaluation of health technologies. With colleagues he has worked on the SF-6D, the generation of utility values from the SF-36.

Robert Dingwall is Professor of Sociology and Director of the Genetics and Society Unit at the University of Nottingham. His career has spanned both medical sociology, the field of his PhD from the University of Aberdeen, and law and society studies, through work at the University of Oxford. These are united by the application of qualitative research methods to questions about professions, work, organisations and social interaction. He is currently developing a new research and graduate programme for the study of social, legal and ethical aspects of new genetic science and technologies as applied to humans, plants and animals.

Allan Donner is Professor and Chair in the Department of Epidemiology and Biostatistics at the University of Western Ontario. His methodologic research has contributed to the design and analysis of clinical trials, with publications over the past ten years appearing in *Biometrics*, *Statistics in Medicine* and the *Journal of Clinical Epidemiology*. Dr Donner served on the Editorial Board of the *American Journal of Epidemiology* from 1991–1999, and is a Fellow of the American Statistical Association.

Lelia Duley is an Obstetric Epidemiologist and MRC Senior Clinical Research Fellow in the Resource Centre for Randomised Trials at the Institute of Health Sciences, Oxford. Her areas of work interest include the design and conduct of randomised trials, systematic reviews, perinatal epidemiology and maternal mortality.

Alison Eastwood is currently a senior research fellow at the NHS Centre for Reviews and Dissemination. Her background is in statistics and economics, and throughout her career she has been involved in health services research. Prior to joining the Centre over five years ago, she was a biostatistician on the myocardial infarction Patient Outcomes Research Team at Harvard Medical School in the US.

Sarah Edwards is Lecturer in Ethics in Medicine at the Centre for Ethics in Medicine, Bristol. Her research interests major on ethics and medical research, but include other methods and types of research besides Randomised Controlled Trials (RCTs). In particular, she is interested in the use of patient records for epidemiologial studies that don't 'use' the patients personally or directly at all. In her previous post in the Department of Public

Health and Epidemiology she completed a review of ethics and RCTs for the NCCHTA.

Ray Fitzpatrick (editor) is Professor of Public Health and Primary Care, Institute of Health Sciences, University of Oxford and Fellow and Dean, Nuffield College, Oxford. He is currently chair of the MRC Health Services and Public Health Research Board. His research interests focus on measurement of outcomes of healthcare, such as health status, quality of life and patient satisfaction and their use in clinical trials and evaluative research. With Gary Albrecht he edited *Quality of Life in Health Care* (JAI Press, Greenwich, Connecticut, 1994). With Stan Newman and other colleagues he wrote *Understanding Rheumatoid Arthritis* (Routledge, London 1995). He co-edited with Nick Black, John Brazier and Barnaby Reeves *Health Service Research Methods: A Guide to Best Practice* (BMJ Books, London 1988). With Gary Albrecht and Susan Scrimshaw he co-edited *The Handbook of Social Studies in Health and Medicine* (Sage, London 2000).

John Gabbay qualified in medicine at Manchester in 1974. After seven years at the University of Cambridge working on the social origins of medical knowledge, he trained in public health. His early research included working on the Templeton Study of NHS managers, and the development and critical evaluation of audit methods. Since 1992, he has directed the Wessex Institute of Health R&D, which now houses the National Co-ordinating Centre for Health Technology Assessment, which runs the HTA programme for the NHS. His recent research includes evaluations of several national pilot schemes to implement clinical effectiveness in the NHS.

Heather Gage is a Senior Lecturer in Economics at the University of Surrey. Her research interests focus on various aspects of health service delivery, including the development of patient-centred outcome measures, international comparisons of healthcare systems, and evaluations of new healthcare technologies. Recent publications have appeared in *The European Journal of Cancer Prevention*, *The Journal of Medical Screening*, *Archives of Neurology* and *Health Technology Assessment*.

Andrew Garratt is co-director of the National Centre for Health Outcomes Development at the Institute of Health Sciences in Oxford. His research interest is in patient-assessed health outcome measures.

Steve George is Senior Lecturer in Public Health Medicine at the University of Southampton. In 1997 he formed and became the first Director of the University of Southampton Health Care Research Unit (HCRU). He has published widely in health services research, and his research grants total over £4,000,000. He is an epidemiologist, and his interests include both the application of epidemiological methods to the evaluation of medical care, and the development and use of outcome measures. A particular interest is the rising demand for healthcare, and the evaluation of attempts to meet it. In 1998 he published the SWOOP study, the first ever randomised controlled trial of a nurse telephone consultation system in primary care, which formed the evidence base for the new NHS Direct telephone service. He was also one of the developers of the EORTC PAN-26, a questionnaire for measuring outcomes in people with carcinoma of the pancreas and, with Professor Mike Campbell, has published on sample size calculations and analysis of quality of life data.

Simon Gilbody has first degrees in medicine and psychology and is a member of the Royal College of Psychiatrists. He currently holds an MRC Special Training Fellowship in Health Services Research at the University of York and is an editor of the Cochrane Schizophrenia Group.

William J. Gillespie is Dean of the Dunedin School of Medicine of the University of Otago in New Zealand. His recent work interests have been in systematic reviews, and in clinical trials in orthopaedic surgery.

Paul P. Glasziou is a general practitioner and Associate Professor in Clinical Epidemiology at the Department of Social and Preventive Medicine, University of Queensland. He is co-editor of the *Journal of Evidence-Based Medicine*, a member of the editorial board of the *British Medical Journal*, and co-chair of the Cochrane Collaboration Methods Group on Applicability and Recommendations.

Adrian Grant is Director of the Health Services Research Unit, a 50-strong Scottish Executive core funded research group within the University of Aberdeen, UK. He leads the Unit's programme on 'Health Care Evaluation'. His work has centred around the place and conduct of pragmatic trials in health technology assessment, and he has a special interest in the evaluation of non-drug technologies, particularly those, such as minimal access surgery, whose evaluation is complicated by learning, skill and preference issues.

Alastair Gray is Reader in Health Economics at the University of Oxford and Director of the Health Economics Research Centre, Institute of Health Sciences, Oxford. He has previously held posts in health economics at Aberdeen University, the Open University and the London School of Hygiene and Tropical Medicine. His main research interests are the methodology and application of economic evaluation in healthcare, priority setting methods, the economics of ageing and the economics of medical negligence.

Colin Green is a Research Fellow in Health Economics at the School of Health and Related Research at the University of Sheffield. His research interests include the measurement and valuation of health outcomes, the application of economic theory to NHS decision-making, and the societal valuation of health and healthcare.

Martin Gulliford is Senior Lecturer in Public Health Medicine at GKT School of Medicine, King's College London. His research interests are in epidemiology as applied to health services research, and Caribbean health.

Sarah E. Hampson is Professor of Psychology and Health at the University of Surrey, Guildford. Her research examines personality and beliefs as determinants of health behaviours.

Gareth Harper is currently a Senior Research Officer in the Policing and Reducing Crime Unit (PRCU), which is part of the Research, Development and Statistics (RDS) Directorate of the Home Office. Prior to this, he was a Research Health Economist at the University of Hertfordshire, where he worked for Professor Joy Townsend in the Centre for Research in Primary and Community Care (CRIPACC). His work was primarily on the methods of Preliminary Economic Evaluation of Health Technologies. Prior to this, Gareth had undertaken postgraduate research on modelling the costs of acute care hospitals, and the efficiency measurement of hospitals.

Jo Hart is currently conducting doctoral research in health psychology at the University of St Andrews. She has considerable experience working on systematic literature reviews.

Emma Harvey graduated with a degree in Psychology in 1991, and spent several years working in the NHS evaluating the provision of local services. In 1995 she moved to the University of York, where she works in the field of evidence based healthcare. She has developed interests in systematic reviewing, multi-centre trials, the implementation of healthcare research findings and effective professional practice. She is currently working on a national trial of physical treatments for back pain, and has recently completed a PhD on health professionals' views and practice in relation to obesity.

Ian Harvey is Professor of Epidemiology and Public Health at the University of East Anglia, Norwich. His research interests include pragmatic randomised trials of non-pharmaceutical interventions in primary and secondary healthcare and social care; and the use of observational studies in the assessment of health technologies.

David Henry is Professor of Clinical Pharmacology at the University of Newcastle, Waratah, Australia. His interests span pharmaco-epidemiology, pharmaco-economics, evidence based practice and health technology assessment. He is a member of the Pharmaceutical Benefits Advisory Committee, and the Health Advisory Committee of NHMRC, and chairs the Economics Sub-Committee of PBAC. Invitations to make presentations on topics listed above include US Congressional advisors, the shadow Ministry of Health in the UK, the Cochrane Colloquium, The American Society of Clinical Pharmacology and Therapeutics, International Society of Technology Assessment in Health Care, the International Society of Pharmaco-Epidemiology, and the International Society for Outcomes Research.

Jenny Hewison is a Senior Lecturer in the School of Psychology at the University of Leeds, specialising in the psychology of health and healthcare. She has particular research interests in mother and child health and in genetics, and more general methodological interests in the evaluation and assessment of health technologies.

Suzanne Hill is Senior Lecturer in Clinical Pharmacology at the University of Newcastle. Her research interests are in pharmaco-economics, the use of evidence in public policy and decision-making, and in applying the results of clinical trials in these settings as well as in clinical practice.

Jennifer Jackson is Senior Lecturer in Philosophy and Director of the Centre for Business and Professional Ethics at the University of Leeds. She has published in academic journals articles on abortion, euthanasia, competence, surrogacy and consent. She has a book forthcoming on Truth, Trust and Medicine (Routledge). She runs a postgraduate MA course on Health Care Ethics.

Ann Jacoby is Professor of Medical Sociology in the Department of Primary Care at the University of Liverpool. Prior to this she was a Reader in Health Services Research at the Centre for Health Services Research at the University of Newcastle. Her areas of work interest include assessment of quality of life in chronic illness, particularly neurological (epilepsy, stroke); patient based outcomes in the context of clinical trials; patient satisfaction and research methods.

Alejandro Jadad is Chief at the Health Information Research Unit; Director, McMaster Evidence-based Practice Center (designated by the US Agency for Health Care Policy and Research); Co-Director, Canadian Cochrane Network and Centre Investigator, Supportive Cancer Care Research Unit; Professor, Departments of Clinical Epidemiology & Biostatistics, McMaster University, Canada; and Associate Medical Director, Program in Evidence-based Care, Cancer Care, Ontario. His current research interests focus on pain and palliative care; the study of the information needs of different decision-makers and their barriers to the use of best available research evidence; the development of strategies to promote interaction and communication amongst decision makers operating at different levels in the healthcare system; the role of the Internet as a source of information for providers and consumers during healthcare decisions; the design and execution of empirical methodological studies to improve the design, conduct, reporting and dissemination of individual studies and systematic reviews; the use of systematic reviews and randomised trials as tools to gather new knowledge in healthcare; and the development of strategies (with members of the public as co-investigators) to transfer health research information to clinicians, patients, managers, policy-makers, journalists and other lay decision-makers, and its use in conjunction with their values and circumstances. He is Chair, Consumers and Health

Informatics Working Group, American Medical Informatics Association; Editor, Cochrane Consumers and Communication Review Group; Associate Editor, *Health Expectations*, a new peer-reviewed journal that focuses on patient participation in healthcare decisions. In 1997, Dr Jadad received the 'National Health Research Scholars Award', by Health Canada, to support his program 'Knowledge synthesis and transfer, consumers and evidence-based health care'. In 1999, he received one of 'Canada's Top 40 Under 40' awards and one of the 'Premier's Research Excellence Awards' in recognition for the achievements and leadership in his multiple areas of interest, and his contributions to society.

Katharine Johnston is a Research Fellow at the Health Economics Research Centre, University of Oxford. She has previously held appointments at Brunel University, the NHS Executive in Edinburgh and the University of Aberdeen. Her research interests include methodological issues in economic evaluation; the economics of screening (particularly breast screening); and the innovation and diffusion of health technologies.

Alison Jones is based at the Thomas C. Chalmers Centre for Systematic Reviews in Ontario. She co-ordinates a series of studies pertaining to the effects of language publication of included randomised controlled trials on the benefits of treatment interventions. She is also involved with the evaluation of the CONSORT statement which was designed to improve the quality of reports of randomised trials.

David Jones completed an MSc and PhD in mathematics before taking up a series of posts in medical statistics and epidemiology in the NHS and several universities. In 1991, he was appointed to the new Chair in Medical Statistics at the University of Leicester. His research interests in the methodology of health services research and clinical trials include meta-analysis, quality of life assessment, and applications of Bayesian methods.

Steven Julious graduated in 1991 from the University of Reading with an MSc in Biometry and took up a post as a medical statistician in the medical school of the University of Southampton. Here he developed an interest in the methodology of clinical trial design, in particular the aspect of sample size estimation, and the statistical methodologies underpinning quality of life assessment. In 1996, Steven left academia to take up a post at Glaxo-Wellcome, and now works in the department of Clinical Pharmacology Statistics, SmithKline Beecham.

Sandra Kiauka is currently working as a staff Epidemiologist at the Institute for Health Care Systems Research in Germany. Previous to this she has worked as a research fellow at the Medical Statistics Unit at the University of Edinburgh and a clinical co-ordinator at Shared Care Informatics in Halifax, Nova Scotia, Canada. Her areas of work interest include health service research, healthcare reforms, service packages, public health, epidemiology and information technology in public health research. She has a B.Sc. in Health Information Sciences and an M.Sc. in Epidemiology.

Alan Kimber is Head of the Department of Mathematics and Statistics at the University of Surrey. He has been a Fellow of the Royal Statistical Society since 1979 and is a Chartered Statistician. His research interests include survival analysis and reliability, statistical modelling and applications of statistics to the medical and health sciences.

Terry Klassen is currently professor and chair of the Department of Pediatrics, University of Alberta in Edmonton, Alberta, Canada. He is the co-ordinator for the Child Health Field for the Cochrane Collaboration. His research interests are in the use of clinical trials and systematic reviews for assessing the effectiveness of interventions in child health.

Donna Lamping is Senior Lecturer and Head of the Health Services Research Unit at the London School of Hygiene and Tropical Medicine. She trained as a research psychologist (specialisation in health psychology, psychometrics/measurement, personality) and worked at universities in Canada (McMaster, McGill) and the USA (Harvard, Fordham) before coming to LSHTM in January 1992. Her research is in two main areas: (i) methodological work on developing and validating patient-based measures of outcome in several areas of medicine and surgery (e.g. prostatectomy, gynaecological surgery, maternity services, HIV/AIDS, renal dialysis, back pain, venous diseases of the leg, multiple sclerosis, ocular disease, neuro-rehabilitation, cardiothoracic surgery, plastic surgery); and (ii) substantive work on quality of life and psychosocial aspects of chronic illness (e.g. elderly people on dialysis, HIV+ women, children at risk for hyperlipidaemia, CABG patients randomised to conventional versus community care, dialysis patients being treated in satellite units, arthritis patients).

James Lewsey is a Research Fellow in the Biostatistics Unit of the Eastman Dental Institute, UCL. His current areas of interest include multilevel modelling and Bayesian analysis in oral health services research, meta-analysis, and generalised linear modelling.

Alastair Leyland is a Research Scientist in the MRC Social and Public Health Sciences Unit at the University of Glasgow. He is head of a programme concerned with measuring health, variations in health and the determinants of health in Scotland, and his current areas of interest include applications of multilevel modelling to health data and the spatial modelling of disease.

Richard Lilford (editor) was born in Cape Town in 1950, received his schooling in Johannesburg, and became a doctor in that city. He moved to

Cape Town where he specialised in obstetrics and gynaecology at the Groote Schuur Hospital, before coming to work in London, first as a registrar and then a senior registrar. He was appointed as a consultant at Queen Charlotte Hospital in 1982, and was then made a professor in Leeds in 1984, where he ran a department for seven years. He then headed the Institute of Epidemiology and Health Service Research at the University of Leeds for a further four years before coming to his present job where he directs the government's programme of research in the West Midlands, directs the central programme of methodological research, and advises the government on trials. He is also a part-time Professor in the Department of Public Health and Epidemiology at the University of Birmingham.

Julia Lowe completed her medical training in the UK and then moved to Australia. She worked part-time in private practice while her children were small, completing a masters degree in clinical epidemiology in her spare time. She moved back to the public sector in 1991 and became Director of General Medicine at John Hunter teaching hospital in 1996. She has established research programmes in diabetes and cardiac failure as well as maintaining an interest in health services research. She is criticism editor for the Cochrane Heart Group.

David Machin is currently Professor of Clinical Trials Research at the University of Sheffield, former Director of the National Medical Research Council, Clinical Trials and Epidemiology Research Unit, Singapore (1996–9) and Chief Medical Statistician MRC Cancer Trials Office, Cambridge (1988–98). His degrees include a MSc from the University of Newcastle upon Tyne, and PhD from the University of Southampton. He is an honorary Member of the Royal College of Radiologists. He has published more than 200 articles and several books on a wide variety of topics in statistics and medicine. His earlier experience included teaching at the Universities of Wales, Leeds, Stirling and Southampton, a period with the European Organisation for Research and Treatment of Cancer, Brussels, Belgium and at the World Health Organization in Geneva, Switzerland working on contraceptive trials. He is an editor of *Statistics in Medicine* and member of the Editorial Board of the *British Journal of Cancer*.

Rachel MacLehose is currently working as a Public Health Epidemiologist at South Essex Health Authority. Previous posts include working as an environmental epidemiologist at the Chemical Incident Response Service at Guy's and St. Thomas' Hospital Trust and as research associate at the University of Bristol. Rachel holds an MSc in Environmental Epidemiology and Policy from the London School of Hygiene and Tropical Medicine.

Theresa Marteau is Professor of Health Psychology and Director of the Psychology and Genetics Research Group at King's College, London. Over the past 15 years she has been conducting research on psychological aspects of health risk assessment. The work has covered genetic testing in pregnancy, adulthood and childhood, as well as population based screening programmes. The conditions studied include heart disease, cervical, breast and bowel cancer and cystic fibrosis. The aim of this research is to understand responses as a first step towards evaluating different methods of communicating information to promote understanding, reduce emotional distress and enhance health-promoting behaviours. She has published over 100 peer-reviewed articles in this and related areas and is co-editor of *The Troubled Helix* (1996; paperback edition: 1999), a book reviewing the psychological implications of the new human genetics.

Elaine McColl has a first degree in Geography and Economics and an MSc in Applied Statistics. She is a native of Dublin and worked for several years in the Department of Statistics, Trinity College, Dublin, where she taught formal courses and provided informal advice on survey design and analysis. Since 1987, she has been a member of the Centre for Health Services Research, University of Newcastle upon Tyne, where she currently holds the post of Senior Research Associate. Her main research interests are in the assessment of health-related quality of life and in survey methodology. She has recently been awarded an NHS Primary Care Career Scientist award, to develop a programme of research into quality of life in chronic disease. Elaine was principal investigator for a recently completed literature review *Designing and using patient and staff questionnaires* which was funded by the NHS Health Technology Assessment Programme and upon which the findings reported here are based.

Lorna McKee is Director of Research at the Department of Management Studies, University of Aberdeen and was previously principal researcher at the Centre for Corporate Strategy and Change, University of Warwick. She is joint author of *Shaping Strategic Change* (1992) with Andrew Pettigrew and Ewan Ferlie, and has published in an extensive range of academic and professional journals. She has recently investigated medical leadership, primary care management and biomedical innovation transfer processes in research projects funded by the ESRC, CSO and NHS. She regularly acts as a consultant to healthcare organisations across the United Kingdom, and jointly co-ordinates the Multi-Disciplinary Primary Care Leadership Pro-gramme leading the module on *Developing and Leading Effective Teams*.

Martin McKee is Professor of European Public Health at the London School of Hygiene and Tropical Medicine and co-director of the School's European Centre on Health of Societies in Transition. His main research interest is health and healthcare in central and eastern Europe and the former Soviet Union, but he also has a more general interest in the interpretation and use of evidence in policy-making.

Klim McPherson is Professor of Public Health Epidemiology in the Cancer and Public Health Unit at the London School of Hygiene and Tropical

Medicine. He has written over 300 refereed papers during his 30-year career in epidemiology. His particular interests include the relationship between breast cancer and hormone supplements such as HRT and oral contraceptives, the incidence of coronary heart disease, the effects of tobacco and alcohol and the widening of public health training to include those who do not come from a conventional and traditional medical background. He is a member of the editorial board of various refereed journals, including the *Journal of Epidemiology and Community Health*, and his membership of different organisations includes the Board of the Faculty of Public Health Medicine and the Council of the UK Public Health Association. He has been the author and co-author of many books and book chapters such as *Hormones and Cancer*, ed. by O'Brien and MacLean, published by the RCOG Press (Chapter 16), a chapter in *Health issues related to consumption*, ed. by Ian MacDonald, published by Blackwell Science, and with Prakash Shetty, he edited *Diet Nutrition and Chronic Disease, Lessons from Contrasting Worlds*, published by John Wiley & Sons.

David Moher is an Assistant Professor in the Departments of Pediatrics, Epidemiology and Community Medicine and Medicine, Faculty of Medicine, University of Ottawa, and Director, Thomas C. Chalmers Centre for Systematic Reviews at the Children's Hospital of Eastern Ontario Research Institute. During the past ten years his interests have focused on how randomised trials and meta-analyses of these studies are conducted and reported. He has been particularly interested in how biases individually and collectively influence estimates of treatment efficacy.

Michael Moher is currently a GP and Research Fellow at the Department of Primary Health Care at the University of Oxford. He is currently involved as medical co-ordinator, in research on the evidence based secondary prevention of coronary heart disease in primary care. This research is comparing, in a randomised controlled trial, three methods of promoting secondary prevention of heart disease in primary care: audit and feedback, the introduction of structure of records, registers and recall, and the introduction of nurse-run clinics.

Graham Mowatt has, since April 1997, been Review Group Co-ordinator for the Cochrane Effective Practice and Organisation of Care Group (EPOC). The focus of EPOC is on producing systematic reviews of interventions designed to improve health professional practice and the delivery of effective health services. This includes various forms of continuing education, quality assurance, informatics, financial, organisational and regulatory interventions that can affect the ability of health professionals to deliver services more effectively and efficiently. Prior to working on the NHS Health Technology Assessment Programme project on assessing fast-changing technologies he was employed by Grampian Health Board for four years on a health service project which was concerned with primary care technological innovation. He also possesses a Master of Business Administration (MBA) degree.

Elizabeth Murphy is a senior lecturer in Sociology and Social Policy at the University of Nottingham. Before moving to Nottingham, she was a research fellow in the Department of Primary Medical Care at the University of Southampton. Her major research interests lie in the medical sociology and the sociology of food. Her doctoral work was concerned with the lay health concepts held by people with non-insulin-dependent diabetes and their implications for their response to medical advice about lifestyle. This interest in responses to behavioural advice has been extended in more recent studies of patients with other chronic disorders and, most recently, a study of the decisions mothers make in relation to infant feeding. While she has used both qualitative and quantitative methods in her research, she has a particular interest in the rigorous application of qualitative methods to policy and practice-related issues.

Maggie Murphy is a lecturer in Social Psychology in the School of Humanities and Social Sciences, University of Glamorgan. Her research interests include social psychological aspects of healthcare provision and social psychological determinants of health behaviours.

Gordon Murray is Professor of Medical Statistics at the University of Edinburgh, having previously worked at the University of Glasgow where he was Director of the Robertson Centre for Biostatistics. A mathematician by training, Professor Murray was recently elected to Fellowship of the Royal College of Physicians of Edinburgh. His main interest is in multicentre clinical trials, particularly in the cardiovascular and cerebrovascular areas. He has also worked extensively in prognostic modelling, and in the application of such methodology to permit casemix adjustment in clinical audit.

Jonathan Myles is a statistician at the MRC Biostatistics Unit. His interests include the application of Bayesian statistics to medicine including the use of Markov Chain Monte Carlo for complex models in epidemiology and population genetics, the assessment of breast cancer screening effectiveness, and problems in AIDS epidemiology.

Dianne O'Connell is a biostatistician with a strong interest in evidence based medicine. She was a Senior Brawn Research Fellow for two years (1997–99), and is now a Senior Research Academic in the Discipline of Clinical Pharmacology, Faculty of Medicine and Health Sciences, University of Newcastle, Australia. Her research interests are in methods for conducting systematic reviews and methods for translating the results of medical research (in particular randomised controlled trials and systematic reviews) into information that can readily be used in clinical decision-making and policy formulation. This work includes developing methods for identifying in which individuals an intervention is more likely to do good than harm (the topic of Chapter 4) and the effects of information framing (how the data about an intervention's effectiveness are presented) on clinical decision-making.

Ba' Pham is a biostatistician with the Thomas C. Chalmers Centre for Systematic Reviews and an associate member of the Children's Hospital of Eastern Ontario Research Institute. His main research interest is to perform empirical studies evaluating statistical methods used to estimate the risks and benefits of healthcare interventions.

Robin Prescott is Director of the Medical Statistics Unit at the University of Edinburgh and has research interests in clinical trials stretching back for 30 years. He has particular interests in the application of mixed models in medicine and in the methodology associated with cross-over trials.

James Raftery is Director of Health Economics Facility and Professor of Health Economics at the Health Services Management Centre (HSMC), University of Birmingham. He joined HSMC to become director of the Health Economics Facility in 1996. Before moving to HSMC, James worked at the Wessex Institute for Research and Development and for Wandsworth Health Authority. He has also worked on secondment as an economic adviser to the Department of Health and to the National Casemix Office. James' current projects include: involvement in several health technology evaluations (anti-coagulation clinics, chondrocyte implantation, stroke services); analysis of the public expenditure impact of new health technologies; the use of routine data in health technology assessment (a national R&D project); and methods of costing diseases, interventions and programmes. He has also edited a series on economic evaluation for the *British Medical Journal*. Other recent publications include the three volume series: Health care needs assessment: the epidemiologically based needs assessment reviews. First and second series, which were edited by Andrew Stevens and James Raftery.

Barnaby Reeves is Senior Lecturer in Epidemiology and Director of the Clinical Effectiveness Unit at the Royal College of Surgeons. Following a doctorate in Experimental Psychology, he worked on the development and evaluation of psychophysical tests in ophthalmology for several years. His interest in healthcare evaluation led him to study epidemiology, following which he was appointed as a senior lecturer in health services research at the University of Bristol. In this post, he designed and set up a wide range of evaluations, including surgical procedures, physiotherapy, nursing, rehabilitation and educational interventions. His main interests are: use of non-randomised or hybrid designs for evaluating interventions, especially surgery, the measurement of the quality of healthcare provision and evaluations of diagnostic accuracy.

Glenn Robert is currently Research Fellow at the Health Services Management Centre, University of Birmingham. Previous to this he was a Research Fellow in the Health Economics Research Group at Brunel University and a researcher at the National Co-ordinating Centre for Health Technology Assessment at the University of Southampton. His recently submitted PhD thesis examines the use of different sources for identifying new healthcare technologies prior to their widespread adoption by the NHS, and makes recommendations regarding the establishment and operation of an early warning system in the United Kingdom.

Paul Roderick trained in general medicine and then public health medicine. He has been senior lecturer in Public Health Medicine at Southampton University since 1993. His main research interests are in evaluating the equity and effectiveness of healthcare delivery, and in defining the epidemiology of chronic renal failure. He is a member of the Steering Committee of the UK Renal Registry.

Sue Ross co-ordinated/edited Chapter 3, 'Factors That Limit the Number, Progress and Quality of Randomized Controlled Trials: a Systematic Review' on behalf of a large group of authors. Sue has worked as a health services researcher for 12 years. She is currently Co-ordinator of Clinical Research at Mount Sinai Hospital, Toronto. At the time the review was carried out, she was Trials Programme Co-ordinator in the Health Services Research Unit at the University of Aberdeen, managing a programme of health technology evaluation trials, mainly in surgery and orthopaedics. Prior to that she had been involved in surgical and primary care trials.

Daphne Russell is a biostatistician based in North Yorkshire. She was educated at the Universities of Cambridge (graduating in Mathematics and Mathematical Statistics) and Aberdeen (Public Health). She has held academic appointments in the Universities of Essex, Newcastle upon Tyne, Aberdeen and Hull (as Director of the University Statistical Support Unit).

Ian Russell has been Founding Professor of Health Sciences at the University of York since 1995. He was educated at the Universities of Cambridge (graduating in Mathematics), Birmingham (Statistics) and Essex (Health Services Research). He has held academic appointments in the Universities of Newcastle upon Tyne, North Carolina, Aberdeen (as Director of the Scottish Health Services Research Unit) and Wales (while Director of R&D for NHS Wales).

Colin Sanderson is Reader is Health Services Research (HSR) at the London School of Hygiene and Tropical Medicine. He has a background in operational research and epidemiology, and has been involved in HSR for over 15 years. His research interests include monitoring quality of care, quantitative modelling for policy evaluation, equitable allocation of healthcare resources and needs assessment.

Jasminka Sarunac obtained a Bachelor of Pharmacy at the University of Belgrade. He went on to be a pharmacist and subsequently Director of the Pharmacy Department at Clinical Centre Dr Lj. D. Kraljevo in Yugoslavia. He has completed a postgraduate course of Clinical Pharmacy Practice and has a Master of Medical Science in Pharmaco-epidemiology Studies from the University of Newcastle, NSW, Australia. He has published work on "GPs' beliefs regarding benefits and risks of Hormone Replacement Therapy: Does framing of information affect enthusiasm for prescribing HRT". He is currently employed by the Pharmacy Department at John Hunter Hospital, Newcastle, Australia in the capacity of Hospital Pharmacist. His areas of research interest include prescribing practices and evidence based medicine.

Trevor Sheldon is Professor and Head of the Department of Health Studies at the University of York and co-director of the York Health Policy Group. He trained in medicine, economics and medical statistics. His main research interests are in resource allocation, healthcare quality, the organisation and delivery of healthcare, and the evaluation of healthcare interventions. He was director of the NHS Centre for Reviews and Dissemination at the University of York from 1993–1998 and manager of the *Effective Health Care* bulletins.

Sue Shepherd is currently a Specialist Registrar in Public Health Medicine, and her special interests are Communicable Disease and Health Needs Assessments. Prior to this she was a Clinical Lecturer in Epidemiology. She has been involved with large epidemiological studies and is presently a co-grant holder in a randomised controlled trial looking at radiotherapy in older women with early breast cancer.

Fujian Song has an MD in public health medicine (China) and a PhD in health services studies (Leeds). He is a senior research fellow at the NHS Centre for Reviews and Dissemination at the University of York. Current areas of work interests include methodology of systematic reviews and evaluation of healthcare interventions.

Jennifer Soutter has a first degree in English and Psychology; her PhD is titled 'Archetypal Elements in the Poetry of Sylvia Plath'. Returning to work after completing six years of higher education, she has worked in health services research for the past ten years, over six of these years being at the Centre for Health Services Research at the University of Newcastle upon Tyne. Her current post is as research associate at the Department of Child Health at the Royal Victoria Infirmary working on a project with children diagnosed with Duchenne muscular dystrophy. This links with work carried out with children with life-limiting illnesses some six years ago.

David Spiegelhalter is a Senior Scientist at the MRC Biostatistics Unit in Cambridge. His current interests include the development and dissemination of Bayesian methods in biostatistics, including applications in health technology assessment and the analysis of performance indicators. He has published widely on Bayesian theory and applications, and has been instrumental in the development of the BUGS and WinBUGS software for Bayesian analysis using graphical models and Markov Chain Monte Carlo methods.

Nick Steen is a medical statistician based at the Centre for Health Services Research at the University of Newcastle upon Tyne with special interests in the design and analysis of cluster randomised trials and the development of health outcome measures. He is currently involved with a number of trials involving the assessment of health technology.

Jonathan Sterne is a Senior Lecturer in Medical Statistics in the Department of Social Medicine at the University of Bristol. His research interests include methods to detect bias in meta-analysis and systematic reviews, the use of statistical methods for the analysis of clustered and longitudinal data, and the epidemiology of asthma and allergic diseases.

Andrew Stevens (editor) is Professor of Public Health and Head of Department in the Department of Public Health and Epidemiology at the University of Birmingham, England. His interests concern health technology assessment, evidence based healthcare, and needs assessment. He is (co-)director of the National Horizon Scanning Centre, providing advance notice of new medical innovations to government; and a founder member of Euro-Scan, a collaborative healthcare horizon scanning group across Europe and Canada. He edits a series of publications on Health Care Needs Assessment and has established a Health Care Evaluation Service which reviews, models cost–utility and appraises the evidence on new and existing health technologies. He was formerly the first Director of the National Co-ordinating Centre for Health Technology Assessment at Southampton University.

Alex Sutton is a Lecturer in Medical Statistics at the University of Leicester. His research interests encompass several aspects of systematic review methodology, including the use of Bayesian methods; methods for addressing publication bias; and methods for the synthesis of results from studies with different designs. He is an active member of the Cochrane Collaboration, contributing to both the statistical and non-randomised studies methods groups.

Hilary Thomas is a Lecturer in the Department of Sociology, University of Surrey. She is President of the European Society of Health and Medical Sociology (1999–2003). Her research interests include the sociology of health and illness, reproduction and women's health, and the sociology of time.

Lois Thomas is a Senior Research Associate at the Centre for Health Services Research and the Department of Epidemiology and Public Health at the University of Newcastle upon Tyne. A nurse by background, her research interests are in stroke, user satisfaction and evidence based practice.

Roger Thomas is a Research Director in the Survey Methods Centre of the National Centre for Social Research (formerly SCPR) and also Director of the ESRC-funded Centre for Applied Social Surveys (CASS). He has more than

30 years' experience as a quantitative social survey project designer and manager in many different topic areas. Much of this was in Social Survey and Census Divisions of the Office for National Statistics, where he was assistant director responsible for survey methodology and also for the design and conduct of major government suveys. In the Survey Methods Centre he acts as consultant on survey design problems, works on methodological research projects and writes on survey methods. As Director of CASS he teaches survey methods courses at postgraduate level and heads a team which develops and disseminates a Social Survey Question Bank, containing examples and commentary on questionnaire design, on the World Wide Web.

Jim Thornton is Reader in Obstetrics and Gynaecology at Leeds University, and honorary consultant at Leeds General Infirmary. He qualified in medicine in Leeds in 1977, and worked for four years in Africa before training as a specialist. He has organised and participated in trials of many pregnancy interventions, and is currently principal investigator of the MRC Growth Restriction Intervention Trial (GRIT). Since 1997 he has been Chairman of Northern and Yorkshire Multicentre Research Ethics Committee. He is an advocate of free-market solutions to healthcare problems, and was in the news in 1999 for suggesting that much NHS health screening would be better done privately!

Joy Townsend is a health economist and statistician, director of the Centre for Research in Primary and Community Care and Professor of Primary Healthcare. For many years she was senior scientist with the Medical Research Council. Her major interests are in prioritisation of research using ex ante modelling of health benefits and costs, randomised controlled trials of new health services and economics of tobacco control.

Peter Tugwell joined the University of Ottawa as Chairman of the Department of Medicine and as Physician-in-Chief at the Ottawa General Hospital (now the Ottawa Hospital) in July 1991. He is the author/co-author of over 170 published articles, which focus principally on technology assessment and the clinical epidemiology of the rheumatic diseases. He is actively involved in several international organisations. He is the editor of the Musculoskeletal review group within the International Cochrane Collaboration Centre. His research interests are in the areas of clinical epidemiology, quality of life, economic evaluation, and technology assessment both within the context of industrialised countries as well as developing countries.

Obioha C. Ukoumunne obtained an MSc in Social Research Methods and Statistics from City University in 1994. He has worked as a Research Statistician at the Department of Medical Statistics and Evaluation, within Imperial College School of Medicine since 1997. His chief research interest is in methods appropriate for the design and analysis of cluster randomised trials. His experience of applied medical statistics is mainly in the fields of psychiatry and general practice. His previous research posts were at the Department of General Practice and the Department of Public Health Sciences, both within GKT School of Medicine. Work on Chapter 17 was completed whilst based at the Department of Public Health Sciences.

Marjon van der Pol is an economist who works for the Health Economics Research Unit at the University of Aberdeen.

Sarah Walker is currently a Research Officer at the Office for National Statistics where she is working with others on improving the coverage of the next UK Population Census. She was a Research Assistant in the Medical Statistics and Computing Department at the University of Southampton and undertook a years' research into 'Sample size determination for quality of life measures'. She investigated QoL measures commonly used with cancer patients which generated categorical responses. She also worked on a variety of clinical trials and survival analyses. Her research interests are still in medical analysis, particularly in the field of disability and housing which, at present, she undertakes on a consultancy or voluntary basis.

INTRODUCTION

Methods in Evidence Based Healthcare and Health Technology Assessment: An Overview

ANDREW STEVENS, RAY FITZPATRICK,
KEITH ABRAMS, JOHN BRAZIER
and RICHARD LILFORD

EVIDENCE BASED MEDICINE, EVIDENCE BASED HEALTHCARE AND HEALTH TECHNOLOGY ASSESSMENT

Evidence based medicine, evidence based healthcare and health technology assessment are terms representing a number of important recent developments in healthcare. The phrase 'health technology assessment' was coined by the United States Office of Technology Assessment in 1972 as part of a wide-ranging interest on the part of Congress in the evaluation of new technologies across not just healthcare, but all major sectors of importance to the US economy.[1] Elsewhere, the term was picked up a decade or so later, such that by 1985, there was an International Society for Health Technology Assessment, an international organisation aiming to promote scientifically based assessment of technologies in healthcare, including drugs, devices, medical and surgical procedures, as well as organisational and administrative systems. The UK adopted the term 'health technology assessment' with the funding in 1993 of a specific programme under that name as part of its National Health Service Research and Development strategy.[2]

'Evidence based medicine' has its roots in clinical epidemiology, owing much to Cochrane's (1972) critique of the effectiveness and efficiency of health services.[3] Cochrane argued that many commonly used treatments and investigations in contemporary healthcare systems have not been shown to be effective in terms of clear and convincing evidence. A growing literature on geographical variations, including Wennberg's notable studies in New England, has underlined how diverse are health professionals' ways of managing similar health problems and how great is the deficit of, and the gap between scientific evidence and clinical practice.[4]

Sackett (1996) describes evidence based medicine as 'the conscientious, explicit, and judicious use of current best evidence in making decisions about the care of individual patients'.[5] The term 'evidence based healthcare' extends the scope to those making decisions about not just patients but also populations. By widening the audience, it has also widened the scope of the subject matter to include not only the evidence for the effectiveness of elements of healthcare, but also its costs and other ramifications. Furthermore, it is acknowledged in both health technology assessment and evidence based healthcare, that the health 'technologies' of interest are very wide, concerning not only pharmaceuticals and healthcare devices, but also procedures, settings, healthcare personnel and more diffuse innovations including, for example, managerial, IT and policy changes in general. In short, evidence based healthcare and health technology assessment have converged to cover an interest in the costs and benefits of all activities within the healthcare system, and indeed even those for which responsibility lies outside the boundaries of the healthcare service.

THE HEALTH TECHNOLOGY ASSESSMENT REVOLUTION

The growth of health technology assessment and evidence based healthcare has lately become something of a revolution. There has been an explosion of journals, conferences, books and research expenditure on health technology assessment. In almost every OECD country, it has become clear that the health services cannot endlessly sustain an acceptance of all innovations, whether they have been evaluated or not, and whether they are affordable or not. Health Technology Assessment (HTA) has become an important part of a strategy to contain costs and maximise value from available healthcare resources. This has led to some countries developing guidelines for the reporting of economic evaluations of pharmaceuticals and other technologies, such as in Canada,[6] Australia[7] and the UK.[8] A single new pharmaceutical, beta-interferon – for multiple sclerosis – has the capacity to cost the UK National Health Service the GDP of many small countries, and cost the United States Health Services the GDP of a number of large ones. A similar story is true of an increasing armoury of new pharmaceuticals.

The effectiveness of not just new technologies, but also of many established ones, has been widely questioned. The problem has been one of both ineffective healthcare being promulgated into health services, and of therapeutically advantageous techniques long being ignored. Antman et al. (1992) demonstrate examples of both, with huge time lags between the arrival of conclusive evidence against antidysrrhythmics, and supportive of thrombolytics in myocardial infarction, and the recognition of these facts in medical text books, quite apart from clinical practice.[9]

So there has been a sea change in thinking about health care, both clinically and at a policy level. There has been a proliferation of attempts to satisfy the demand for evidence based healthcare, covering the growth and scope of interest of funding bodies, the development of networking and co-ordinating bodies, the development of multiple new publications and dissemination media (from new journals to electronic databases to compendia of electronic databases), and systems for developing skills in interpreting evidence. Most importantly, there have been a number of innovations in the development of the research base.

FEATURES OF THE RESEARCH BASE

It is now widely recognised that research for health technology assessment includes not just *primary* research (data gathering), but also *secondary* research (a systematic review of primary research evidence). Indeed, as the latter becomes more formalised, disciplined and by consequence narrow, *tertiary* research synthesising and making accessible multiple primary and secondary research products is also developing. The critical features of good primary research are being increasingly recognised as indispensable: appropriately posed questions, studies designed to reduce bias, and with patient-relevant outcomes, conducted without bias, ethically, and with suitable quality control, drawing conclusions which flow from results, and published regardless of the outcome.

In the same way the critical features of secondary and tertiary research in HTA are agreed: systematic and reproducible reviews using clear search strategies, formal critical appraisal of contributory studies, grading of the evidence from these studies according to their quality and size, selection of relevant outcomes from primary research, and valid methods for integrating the evidence.[10]

THE METHODOLOGY OF HEALTH TECHNOLOGY ASSESSMENT

The growth of demand for health technology assessment does not of itself guarantee the appropriateness and validity of the material it generates. An interest in methods employed to ensure the quality of evidence has emerged. This is manifest, for example, in the number of different professions associated with HTA, including epidemiologists, health economists, sociologists, statisticians, clinicians and others. Each is in a position to supplement – and to some extent confront – the methods used by the others. And the fertile mix of ideas is becoming increasingly apparent. A particular manifestation of the interest in the methods of HTA was the United Kingdom's decision specifically to have a programme of research on the methodology of HTA. It posed a series of questions which fit into the following broad categories:

1   Methods in clinical trials,
2   The place of observational and qualitative research,
3   The measurement of benefits and costs,
4   Analytical (statistical) methods which quantify the uncertainty of the findings,

5 Methods of reviewing, synthesising, and modelling findings, and

6 Methods for identifying gaps in the evidence and selecting priorities.

The chapters of this book are arranged in this logical way. By bringing together the current state of art of knowledge on the methods for health technology assessment, they offer answers to a wide range of methodological questions fundamental to HTA as follows:

> How do we identify potential areas of concern? (Chapter 25, Horizon Scanning)

> Which of these topics is most urgent? (Chapter 27, Preliminary evaluation)

> When does the question need to be tackled? (Chapter 26, Timing)

Having chosen the technologies and questions of interest, and before gathering data afresh, we must ask how much data/evidence is there already?

> Can we be sure we have all relevant evidence? (Chapter 21, Publication bias)

> Having gathered the existing evidence, how can we synthesise it? (Chapter 22, Meta-analysis)

> Can we rely on the syntheses? (Chapter 23, Assessing the quality of randomised controlled trials in meta-analysis)

If the existing data are unsuitable or inadequate, it follows that new data need to be collected.

> What measurements are most useful to make? (Chapter 11, Patient-based outcome measures)

> How should questionnaires be used to generate these data? (Chapter 15, Questionnaires)

> Can these data be combined to generate comparable measures of health status? (Chapter 12, Health Status Measures)

> And how can we measure costs as well as outcomes? (Chapter 13, Collecting resource data)

> How do these costs and benefits become of less immediate value as they are further in the future? (Chapter 14, Discounting)

> And how can we ensure that we have made the best of the cost data? (Chapter 18, Handling uncertainty in cost data)

> How should new data be collected – through new randomised controlled trials, or by collecting data on observed activity? (Chapters 6 and 7, Observational methods)

> If observational methods are deemed adequate, will routine data do? (Chapters 8 and 9, Routine data)

> Or might qualitative methods suffice in some circumstances? (Chapter 10, Qualitative methods)

> Or not using new data at all, but making the best of consensus in some instances? (Chapter 24, Consensus methods)

> If new trials are decided upon – how generalisable are they? (Chapter 4, Generalisability)

> What are the limiting factors in trial design? (Chapter 3, Limiting factors in trial design)

> For example, are they limited by the ethics of undertaking trials? (Chapters 1 and 2)

↓

> Should general account be taken of the placebo effect? (Chapter 5, Placebo effect)

↓

> Whatever the methods used for gathering data, how can we best analyse and interpret it? (Chapter 16, Bayesian methods)

↓

> When data have been collected on both quality and length of life how should they be analysed? (Chapter 20, Quality of life and survival analysis)

↓

> How large should the sample sizes be of the newly collected data? (Chapter 19, Sample size issues)

↓

> Are there special study designs required when the population receiving an intervention is clustered into schools, practices or other units (Chapter 17, Area-wide interventions)

It can be seen that this sequence, in order to follow a logic of asking what the question is and whether it has yet been answered, disrupts the contents order of the book. In the main volume we have stayed with the familiar logic of trials first, horizons last, but either order would be sustainable.

METHODS FOR UNDERTAKING METHODOLOGICAL RESEARCH

All of the contributions in this volume have had to select methods to generate their suggestions for methodology in HTA. Principally these have been those of synthesising the evidence from other pieces of work. This can take the form of either synthesising primary research (e.g. a review of studies seeking to compare consent rates for clinical trials by method of invitation) or synthesising arguments (e.g. arguments over whether a fixed or random effects statistical model is more appropriate for meta-analysis). In some cases authors have also sought to collect

new data themselves (e.g. Leyland's use of routine data), or indeed have triangulated their evidence by drawing on a variety of different methods (e.g. Roberts getting clues on how to horizon scan).

CONCLUSION

The contributions to this volume, and indeed the editorial collaboration in collating the volume, have distinctive origins that are worth underlining. The UK National Health Service established a national Research and Development (NHS R&D) initiative of which the Health Technology Assessment (HTA) Programme has been a major component.[2] It is hoped that several features make this an important development in international, as well as national, terms. In the first place, an elaborate process was established for inviting ideas for research from the widest range of health professionals, researchers, consumer interest groups and others. Secondly, expert panels were asked carefully to develop and prioritise research ideas submitted. Thirdly, research that has been prioritised for funding is commissioned by advertising to researchers throughout the world to submit tenders, with extensive peer review to determine research groups to take forward projects. Great emphasis has been placed on the need for inter-disciplinary strengths for research groups to be commissioned to undertake work for the HTA programme. The methodology programme of research has been a distinctive strand of the HTA programme as a whole. Because of the extensive process of consultation to identify methodological questions and of selecting investigators, and because of the thorough peer-reviewing of outputs, we are confident that the contributions reported here can be considered an authoritative summary of current methodological issues in HTA. Every chapter is a summary of a more extensive study that has gone through many steps of evaluation before emerging to form a monograph for the NHS R&D programme. Efforts were also made to achieve coherence to this body of methodological work by workshops and other forms of communication to share experiences and results.

This volume has not set out to provide readers with a basic introduction to the elementary aspects of topics such as the design of randomised controlled trials or cost–benefit analysis that can be found elsewhere. It does, however, attempt to tackle the frontiers of health technology assessment. The book brings together a unique collection of contributions that will guide the reader through current thinking and debates about the state and direction of research methods in health technology assessment. If the volume stimulates further debate as how to improve our methods of health services research, it will have achieved its goal.

REFERENCES

1. US Congress Office of Technology Assessment. Identifying Health Technologies That Work: Searching For the Evidence. Washington: US Government Printing Office, 1994.
2. Department of Health NHS Executive. Research and Development In the New NHS: Functions and Responsibilities. London: Department of Health, 1994.
3. Cochrane A. *Effectiveness and Efficiency Random Reflections on the Health Service*, Leeds: Nuffield Provincial Hospitals Trust, 1972.
4. Wennberg JE, Freeman JL, Culp WJ. Are hospital services rationed in New Haven or over-utilised in Boston? *Lancet* 1987; **i**: 1185–9.
5. Sackett D, Rosenberg W, Gray J, Haynes R, Richardson W. Evidence based medicine: what it is and what it isn't. *Br. Med. J.* 1996; **312**: 71–2.
6. Canadian Coordinating Office for Health Technology Assessment. *Guidelines for economic evaluation of pharmaceuticals: Canada*. 2nd ed. Ottawa: Canadian Coordinating Office for Health Technology Assessment (CCOHTA); 1997.
7. Commonwealth Department of Health, Housing and Community Service. *Guidelines for the pharmaceuticals industry on the submission to the Pharmaceutical Benefits Advisory Committee*. Canberra: Australian Government Publishing Service, 1992.
8. National Institute for Clinical Effectiveness: Appraisal of new and existing technologies: Interim guidelines for manufacturers and sponsors. December 1999, London: NICE http://www.nice.org.uk/appraisals/appraisals.htm.
9. Antman E, Lau J, Kupelnick B, Mosteller F, Chalmers T. A comparison of results of meta-analyses of randomised control trials and recommendations of experts. *JAMA* 1992; **268**: 240–8.
10. Chalmers I, Altman D. *Systematic Reviews*. London: BMJ Publishing, 1995.

Part I
CLINICAL TRIALS

INTRODUCTION by RICHARD J. LILFORD
and ANDREW STEVENS

The concept of control groups is mentioned as early as the book of Daniel and was formalised by Sir Francis Bacon in the 17th century. James Lind conducted a famous trial of different methods of prophylaxis against scurvy, and discovered the benefits of fruit for sailors.[1] This was not a randomised experiment, and although the idea of allocation of therapy by 'lot' is an old one, practical application is really a 20th century phenomenon. The statistics were worked out by Ronald Fisher in an agricultural context, and a landmark randomised trial in humans was Sir Austin Bradford Hills' study of streptomycin treatment for tuberculosis, conducted during the Second World War.[2]

The Randomised Controlled Trial (RCT) is the archetypal primary research method of Health Technology Assessment (HTA). About a third of a million RCTs are registered on the Cochrane database of controlled clinical trials, and this list falls far short of covering the entire literature base on RCT methodology.[3] RCTs have given some very clear pointers to practice: clot busting and antiplatelet drugs are effective in heart attack, multi-agent chemotherapy delays the onset of AIDS among carriers of HIV virus, and antibiotics are effective in surgery where a contaminated viscus is breached. Some treatments have such spectacular effects that their effectiveness can be established without the need for RCTs – volume replacement for massive haemorrhage, anti-D to prevent rhesus sensitisation in newborns, and use of the supine position to prevent 'cot death'. However, most advances in medicine are less spectacular –

moderate gains which collectively contribute to major overall improvements in welfare. These modest but worthwhile gains cannot be detected easily – unlike the few massive breakthroughs. Moderate biases may obscure or exaggerate such gains or even create the impression of benefit in the face of harm. RCTs, blinded when possible, provide protection against these moderate but relatively important biases.[4] Randomisation provides protection against selection bias – inaccuracy that occurs if patients in treatment and control groups have different capacities to benefit. Randomisation, provided that the allocation is fully concealed, ensures that confounding variables are distributed by chance alone. Blinding prevents the possibility of performance bias (augmented or impaired outcome resulting from administration of different treatments, apart from the treatment of interest, to study or control patients) and outcome bias (distorted outcome, involvement or interpretation in the light of hope and expectation).

It has been shown empirically that randomised controlled trials in general produce more modest estimates of treatment effects than historically controlled studies. Good RCTs – studies which obey the established scientific criteria – produce different results from poorly conducted studies. Well-conducted RCTs are, it is widely agreed, the most reliable method for comparing most health technologies.[5] There may be questions about their external validity (generalisability) and about their practicability in various contexts, but they remain the bedrock of much HTA.

Randomisation is a simple concept, but RCTs have spawned a wide range of complex issues that challenge those who commission and conduct applied research. Large simple trials have led to some very important discoveries such as the value of magnesium in the treatment for eclampsia. However, the range of possible interactions (and hence of potential interactions between interventions) is rising exponentially, and it will not be possible to answer all research questions using the large simple philosophy. Factorial designed studies (where patients are re-randomised to different therapies), families of trials (where patients are offered different trials at different stages of their disease according to eligibility), and trials nested within prospective frameworks for collection of routine data, will all be necessary. Some therapies are given to groups of people, not individuals, and this calls for cluster trials while at the other end of the scale, patients may act as their own controls in $n = 1$ trials. Some interventions are complex 'packages' made up of many components, where measurement of 'fidelity' to the intended package is useful to those who may wish to adopt the results. Trials of rapidly evolving technologies are an increasing concern given the pace of technological development – the question is when to start such studies, and one approach is to offer randomisation at an early stage, accepting that the technology might continue to improve for some time after the start of the study. Another (often related) problem arises from interventions whose effects are critically dependent on practitioner skill or organisational factors – one approach is to ensure recruitment from a very broad sample, and another is to randomise both patient and practitioner. All these refinements have cost implications, and a compromise may be necessary between the ideal and the achievable, in this as in other aspects of life. In short, the study of trial design is still evolving.

This section deals firstly in the ethics of RCTs. A general review and discussion of the ethics of RCTs, by Lilford and colleagues considers the main philosophical positions and shows that from two points of view – utilitarian and deontological – the essential requirements are that the treatments being compared should be an equal bet in prospect, the situation of patient equipoise where the expected utilities of each treatment on offer are equivalent.[6] Clearly the competent patient is in the best position to make this decision, given available 'prior' probabilities; hence there is no conflict between maximising welfare and respecting autonomy, in this area of ethics at least. In the subsequent chapter, Ashcroft shows how these principles may be interpreted in different moral traditions

and considers whether the doctrine of informed consent – so crucial in the West – may be viewed somewhat differently in cultures where an egalitarian relationship between professional and patient is less widely accepted.

Ross and colleagues then discuss the quality of trials. The factors impeding recruitment are classified as those affecting clinicians' willingness to collaborate in a study, their willingness to offer patients entry and patients' willingness to participate, given the offer. Patients seem less willing to participate in trials where the comparator treatments are very different in their nature and immediate effects – surgery versus radiotherapy for prostate cancer is a recent example. The importance of separating the 'business' of running trials from their conception and instigation is stressed. This ensures that those who may have an emotional or pecuniary interest in the results of a trial are kept at arm's length from the processes and analyses which may bias the results – for example, interference in the randomisation sequence is prevented.

However, a strong recommendation from the authors is that trials should be kept simple so that logistic difficulties do not act as a strong disincentive to participation. Reporting of results, so that the link between outcome and allocated treatment is clear, is also discussed in this chapter and the agreed methodology for reporting studies (CONSORT) is emphasised.[7]

O'Connell and colleagues then consider the problem of relating results from randomised trials to patients in another time and place. Most authors address these issues by describing the inclusion and exclusion criteria, subgroup analysis and (less often) comparison of trial participants with those not in the trial. However, there are strong arguments for more individualised assessment of benefits and harms. Clinical trials can be thought of as a method to produce good empirical data with which to populate risk/benefit models, in which probabilities of good and bad outcomes, and the values attached to these outcomes are made explicit. There is also a great need for more empirical work on the transferability of results from one group of patients to another, especially in situations where there is no obvious reason why they might differ. For example, there may be no prior reason to expect results to vary by sex, race or age. It is difficult to know what to do when statistically significant subgroup effects arise. An essential principle, however, is that even if relative risks are fixed across different subgroups, absolute risks may vary. This is where modelling comes into its own, since it enables results to be extrapolated to those with a different base-line prognosis.[8]

Lastly, those who think they understand the 'placebo effect' should read the section by Crowe and Colleagues. Placebo effects result largely from *expectation* and are psychologically mediated. Placebos, however, are not merely inert substances, but include many other aspects of treatment such as practitioners themselves, operations, injections, and so on. An important conclusion to derive from their study is that the placebo effect, as described above, is an important and ineluctable component of many therapies. It follows, therefore, that placebo effects should be controlled out only when they are an artefact of the research design, and not when they would continue to operate in everyday practice. Our current concern is that although the placebo effect is very real in non-trial practice, when patients have no reason to doubt that they are receiving the putative active 'ingredient', this is less certain in the context of the trial, where there is only a say, 50%, chance that the active ingredient is included. The role of the placebo both inside and outwith trials continues to be intriguing and more research is still needed.

REFERENCES

1. Bull JP. The historical development of clinical therapeutic trials. *J. Chron. Dis.* 1959; **10**(3): 218–48.
2. Hill AB. *Statistical Methods in Clinical and Preventive Medicine*, London: Oxford University Press 1962.
3. Cochrane Controlled Trials Register, The Cochrane Library, 1999, Oxford: Update Software Ltd.
4. Chalmers I, Sinclair JC. Promoting perinatal health: is it time for a change of emphasis in research? *Early Human Development* 1985; **10**: 171–91.
5. Peto R, Collins R, Gray R. Large-scale randomized evidence: large, simple trials and overviews of trials. *Ann. N. Y. Acad. Sci.* 1993; **703**: 314–40.
6. Lilford RJ, Jackson JC. Equipoise and the ethics of randomisation. *J. R. Soc. Med.* 1995; **88**: 552–9.
7. Altman D. Better reporting of randomised controlled trials: the CONSORT statement. *Br. Med. J.* 1996; **313**: 570–1.
8. Lilford RJ, Pauker SG, Braunholtz D, Chard J. Decision analysis and the implementation of research findings. *Br. Med. J.* 1998; **317**: 405–9.

1

Ethical Issues in the Design and Conduct of Randomised Controlled Trials

RICHARD J. LILFORD, SARAH J.L. EDWARDS,
DAVID A. BRAUNHOLTZ, JENNIFER JACKSON,
JIM THORNTON and JENNY HEWISON

SUMMARY

We have reviewed the literature on the ethics of clinical trials, and found that there is little agreement about what constitutes moral justification for trials. However, a widely held and defensible view, distilled from both utilitarian and Kantian ethics, is as follows: randomised trials are ethical, from the doctor's and patient's point of view, when competent patients have been fully consulted so that their values determine what is in their best interests and they have consented to trial entry. Decision theory tells us that, in the more usual situation where trial treatments are freely available, patients must be in a state of equipoise (alternative and available treatments have equal expected utilities) before they consent to randomisation. Patients may expect to increase their expected utility by being altruistic, making altruism a discrete factor in its own right.

The interests of patients who cannot give their consent (because of incompetence, say) should be protected, and so altruism should not be assumed. A surrogate, perhaps appointed by the patient themself, must provide the values, using average values for example or, in the case of advance directives, previously elicited values.

In the less usual situation where a treatment is only available in a clinical trial, then randomisation is ethical, provided that patients are in equipoise or better, i.e. provided the restricted treatment is expected to be at least as good as what is available routinely.

Equipoise is a more exacting requirement for the ethical conduct of clinical trials than is 'uncertainty'. It is important that participants are not deceived by doctors equivocating on the term, as this limits their capacity to give an informed choice.

The offer of entry into a clinical trial is not itself psychologically upsetting for the majority of patients. Patients cope best with the invitation to join the clinical trial when they have good overall understanding of the consent material. A number of deliberate experiments have compared different methods for inviting people to participate in clinical trials, and these have shown that giving more information tends to result in greater understanding, although fewer patients then accept randomisation.

There may be some clinical benefit from participating in a clinical trial, even when the trial itself produces a null result. In particular, when there is a pre-existing effective treatment whose effectiveness is enhanced in the trial by the use of protocol or by a Hawthorne effect. Since the Helsinki declaration seeks specifically to reassure patients that their care will not be affected in a detrimental sense if they do not take part in a clinical study, this putative trial effect cannot be used as any form of inducement.

The requirement of equipoise (or better) has a number of implications for RCT practice and design.

1   Under-powered trials are not necessarily unethical in their 'use' of patients.
2   Interim analyses are desirable, although the current practice of keeping preliminary data secret is suspect, especially when trial treatments are widely available.
3   Adaptive designs do not solve the problem of failing to avoid reduced expected utilities for each participant when interim evidence favours a treatment which could be selected outside the trial.
4   Placebo-controlled trials generally are not usually appropriate when proven effective treatments are routine, and those using 'active' placebos with adverse effects to mimic the intervention for the preservation of blinding should be used with caution, if at all.
5   Cluster RCTs can be categorised into cluster–cluster and individual–cluster trials, depending on the type of intervention under study. Guardians should consent to randomisation in both types of trial. The best interests of the cluster is of paramount concern in the former type, while individuals can consent to any intervention in the latter type of trial.
6   Many behavioural interventions may contaminate controls, either directly through fully informed consent or indirectly through close contact with and communication between experimental and control individuals. Zelen randomisation, where consent is typically sought only from the intervention group after randomisation, may be a good compromise in such cases.

Randomised controlled trials have always provoked debate and discussion about ethical concerns because of a variety of issues regarding possible conflicts of interest between society and the individual patient. This chapter sets out these various ethical concerns. We first carried out a systematic search of the literature, relating to the ethics of conducting clinical trials, which included empirical studies to inform and possibly substantiate such discussion. Full details of our search strategy can be found in a recent Health Technology Assessment monograph.[1] We then abstracted the main issues and arguments, together with any informative empirical data. This material was synthesised using an intellectual framework, a product of which is the following narrative focusing on the issue of epistemological uncertainty as justification for entering patients in trials. The idea of uncertainty or, less ambiguously, equipoise was then applied to a number of different methodological and practical situations, and conclusions are offered based on this analysis.

EPISTEMOLOGICAL UNCERTAINTY AS JUSTIFICATION FOR RECRUITING PATIENTS

Introduction

During this century, the medical profession has acquired a growing capacity to distinguish between what they know and what they do not, thereby changing the professional emphasis from demanding public trust without sound epistemological basis to an 'evidence based' approach to medical practice. This is typically contrasted with practice based on simple intuition. Although the two approaches may lead to the same answer in the end, scientific knowledge provides *explicit justification* for belief. The Randomised Controlled Trial (RCT) is deemed the most reliable scientific method in medicine today by virtue of its unique capacity to eliminate selection bias. However, there is an apparent moral tension between serving the interests of society at large, and those of individual participants.

Societal interests

The main reason for using the RCT design is a scientific one, for properly conducted RCTs produce the most valid data from which society can benefit.[2] Medical research advances medical practice and hence goes some way towards alleviating suffering and avoiding harm. The RCT is not always scientifically necessary or desirable, but it is most useful when expected treatment effects are small, yet worthwhile.

It is often thought that any RCT rests exclusively – and some would say precariously – on classical utilitarian justification for its moral acceptability.[3] Society needs the good quality evidence which RCTs offer. However, utilitarianism is not the only moral theory from which the use of RCTs in medical research can draw support. Indeed, Kantians see individuals as having tacit obligations to society at large, too.

Not all RCTs are morally justified, however valuable to society they may seem, and this chapter is concerned with the need to advance medical knowledge, whilst protecting those individuals who are recruited at the same time. Indeed, failure to protect individual's interests and their rights is unlikely to increase social value in the long term, and patients may lose trust in the profession and then reject trials altogether, the burden of involuntary and perpetual altruism being too great to bear.

Individual interests

Perhaps the most common criticism to be levelled at RCTs is that they are insensitive to the best interests of current patients who participate in them and this insensitivity is at odds with the model doctor–patient relationship.[4–6] We will see that, under certain conditions, the societal interest can be promoted without threat to the individual's own best interests.

In this chapter, we will analyse the idea that the tension between societal and individual interests can be resolved by making recourse to the epistemological 'uncertainty' principle.[7] Put simply, if the clinician does not *know* which treatment is *best*, then the patient is not disadvantaged in prospect by being randomised and society benefits from the knowledge gained. However, it is necessary to clarify what 'knowledge' and 'best interests' mean before they can be properly lodged with ethical theory and then operationalised by applying them to practical difficulties with trials and their design.

Knowledge

Dealing first with 'knowledge', consider first two treatments (A and B) with equivalent (or no) side-effects. Knowing can have two meanings: firstly, that there is no preference between two treatments, since they have identical side-effects and A is as likely to be better than B or vice versa. Secondly, that there is some preference in the sense that one of the treatments is more likely to be superior, but this is uncertain; treatment A has not been 'proven' to be more effective than B. Indeed, Gifford observes that most arguments which use uncertainty as justification for RCTs equivocate on the term 'know', sometimes giving the first interpretation above, and sometimes the second.[8] Uncertainty as the opposite of certainty, allows a clinical trial to proceed in the face of considerable preference. However, if there is 'absolute' uncertainty, the decision-maker is 'agnostic' or 'in equipoise' – that is, the benefits in prospect for both treatments are equal, and the outlook for the patient is the same, whether or not a trial is conducted.[9] For those familiar with Bayesian thinking, this situation would arise where the point of balance of the 'prior' for the difference A − B was zero.

Best Interests

We need to clarify the meaning of 'best' in the context of the clinician's obligation to give patients the 'best' treatment. Two situations apply. Firstly, the above situation where treatments A and B (two treatments are discussed here for convenience) have equal side-effects in prospect, and the major outcomes are binary (e.g. live or die). In this situation, A is preferred to B, provided it is more effective (a situation

often referred to as 'probabilistic dominance') because all values are equal to unity. Under these circumstances, equipoise exists if the expected effectiveness of A and B are equal, or, more formally (and in Bayesian notation) if the 'priors' balance on the same point.

However, we must acknowledge that treatments typically have unequal side-effects a priori.[9] A, for example, might be mutilating surgery, while B is a smaller operation or an inexpensive drug with few side-effects. In order for the treatments to be equally desirable under these conditions (i.e. for equipoise to exist), A must be better than B, in prospect, on the major outcome so that superior effectiveness can be traded off against worse side-effects. In decision analytic language, the expected utilities of A and B should be the same; the expected advantages of A on the main outcome measure are precisely offset by the lower side-effects of B. Equipoise under these circumstances occurs when A is expected to be superior (on the main outcome measure) to B. If the expected difference in outcome equals, but does not exceed the trade-off that individual patients require, then the patient is in individual equipoise. Of course, there may be many outcomes where the relative effects of the treatment are uncertain. However, this does not change the fundamental point, that a decision analysis can be constructed around certain effects (such as the mutilation of surgery), uncertain effects (for which 'prior' probabilities exist, albeit within wider credible intervals), and the values that might be ascribed to these various outcomes. If we leave aside, just for a moment, any potential negative or positive effects that the trial itself might have, we may argue that the patient is not disadvantaged relative to routine care, provided the expected utilities of the comparative treatments are equivalent. The subject of decision analysis – or expected utility theory – is fully described elsewhere.[10]

Equipoise: Collective or Individual?

The term equipoise was made popular by Freedman in a landmark article in the *New England Journal of Medicine*,[7] and we argue that its theoretical meaning can be made explicit within a Bayesian and decision analytic framework. Freedman distinguished between two kinds of equipoise – collective and individual. By collective equipoise, he meant that a society of experts (say clinicians contemplating a particular trial) do not know which of two or more treatments is best, although clinicians within the community may have different 'hunches'. By individual equipoise, he meant that a particular clinician was equipoised, or that he had no hunch whatsoever. Using our definition would mean that this clinician regards the treatments as having equal expected utilities. Freedman goes on to argue that ethically collective equipoise is a sufficient condition for recruiting patients to trials, with the proviso that they consent, irrespective of whether the individual clinician in question does or does not have a preference. He starts by pointing out that individual equipoise is a fragile state which might be very hard to find, given the exacting requirement for the interaction between 'prior' probabilities and values to produce precisely equal expected utilities across the comparator treatments. Because individual equipoise is such an elusive state in practice, Freedman argues, it can be discounted as too stringent a moral basis for trial entry. When individuals are equipoised, this is simply a bonus, not a requirement. As scientists, we would like to go along with Freedman, but we are conscious of serious flaws in his argument.

Problems with Freedman's Argument

The first point that Freedman ignores is that collective equipoise is seldom evenly balanced. It, too, is a fragile state, only now among a group of people. Typically, the numbers of clinicians who might have preferences (hunches) for one treatment or another will be unequal in a ratio of, say, 30 to 70. Freedman does not say how widespread a hunch can be before collective equipoise collapses into consensus over which treatment is best. Just how many clinicians need to prefer the trial treatment before a trial of it becomes unethical? This was investigated by Johnson and colleagues,[11] who conducted an ethnometric study to identify the threshold of collective preference beyond which a trial would be unacceptable by members of the public, and showed that, once the ratio of number of clinicians for the trial treatment to the number of clinicians against it went beyond 70:30, the great majority of respondents would regard a trial of a potentially life-saving intervention as unethical.

However, there are yet further problems with Freedman's argument, i.e. that where collective equipoise and individual equipoise do not coincide, collective equipoise is a sufficient moral basis upon which to recruit patients. He argues that the obligation of a doctor to a patient is different from those which, say, a parent has towards a child – Freedman thus argues that clinicians need not adhere to the 'gold standard', whereby one should not randomise a patient unless one was prepared to do the same for a beloved family member. Freedman defends his position on the grounds that doctors are judged by, and should behave according to, collective norms.

However, this does not say how the doctor is supposed to operationalise the concept of collective versus individual equipoise – is the doctor to tell the patient only that there is collective uncertainty about the best treatment while keeping any personal preference under wraps?

Besides, couching consent only in terms of collective uncertainty and not individual equipoise leaves open the very real possibility that the patient will interpret this to mean that the clinician is personally equipoised, whereas the clinician might mean only that the usual statistical conventions of 'certainty' have not been fulfilled. Equivocation can lead to deception.[12] Failure to offer to disclose any such preference at a minimum is an economy with the truth, and tantamount to deception. Deception, intentional or otherwise, is a limit to autonomous decision-making[13,14] and so Freedman's allegiance to collective equipoise does not sit well with his position on autonomy: like most modern authors he strongly asserts the need to respect individual choices. Such autonomy is exerted through different people manifesting their own personal – and often very different – value systems. In Western cultures, it is a reasonable assumption that individuals are likely to have different values, perhaps as a result of their freedom to choose how to live. People may make very different trade-offs. Given this, it follows that there can be no such thing as collective equipoise in any decision involving a trade-off – how can it simultaneously be argued that collective equipoise provides sufficient moral cover for clinical trials and that autonomy is a fundamental principle, when the latter implies that two different people, confronted with exactly the same scenario, may make very different choices! On the basis of the best 'prior' probability estimates, one person may choose treatment A, another treatment B, while a third might be equipoised between A and B and hence willing (or eager) to be randomised. Therefore, we think that anybody who holds autonomy as a central principle must also regard equipoise as the property of the patient. It arises when prior probability estimates and an individual patient's values interact in such a way as to produce equal expected utilities.

There is near-universal agreement that the 'competent' patient should be the source of these values.[1,15,16] Probabilities are normally the province of the care provider who has a moral obligation to bring as much knowledge and experience to bear on the problem as possible under the constraints of practice. In some cases, patients may wish to make their own judgement on probability, and clinicians, in fully respecting autonomy, should be prepared to engage in a discussion of probabilities with patients who wish to do so. It is also worth noting that a null 'prior' does not produce equipoise in a situation where a priori trade-offs are evident, and seems to challenge statistical convention of using such an hypothesis as a basis for data analysis.

Sometimes, a patient who is terminally ill may wish to buy time and may accept some expected short-term losses that otherwise they would not. A new treatment may give long-term gains if it turns out to be beneficial and any losses will be short-lived. So, the probability distribution of the expected benefits of the two trial arms need not always be symmetrical.[9]

How Robust is Personal Equipoise?

Given that patients should not lose out by taking part in a clinical trial, it could be argued that, since equipoise does not normally exist, clinical trials are *necessarily* unethical.[17] This argument is predicated either on a mathematical or pragmatic argument. The mathematical argument concerns itself with the extremely low likelihood that values and 'prior' probabilities may interact in such a way as to provide precisely equal expected utilities. The pragmatic argument is that in ordinary clinical practice, clinicians and patients do come off the fence and decide one way or the other – hence, the argument goes – equipoise is a theoretical concept with no practical application. Alderson and colleagues, for example, reported that 75% of physicians thought they were *never* in equipoise.[18] However, people may only come off the fence because they have to – in which case randomisation may provide a convenient and useful method to unblock an otherwise blocked decision. The first argument, concerning the likelihood of finding a situation of exactly equal expected utilities, is one that we have analysed in more detail elsewhere.[19] In brief, equipoise might not be as rare as the requirement for a mathematical dead hit between expected utilities would at first imply. It has been argued that it is unrealistic to regard prior probabilities and value trade-offs as exact and precise numerical values, given that they are constructed in the mind. There may be *zones* of indifference where the patient cannot distinguish between the benefits of one treatment or another (or over which a clinician could not say that one probability is more likely than another). This argument is predicated in part on the hypothesis that in assigning probabilities or values, people are often able to articulate numerical values which are *not* the most likely

or desirable, but are not able to say exactly where the most likely or desirable 'point' estimate lies. A clinician might say that the most likely prior effect of a new operation on cancer mortality lies between 4 and 6 percentage points, and a patient might say that a gain between 2% and 5% would justify the effects of surgery. In this case, it could be argued, overlap between 'prior' probabilities and values is a sufficient basis for trial entry. Empirical investigation is needed on this point.

The Altruistic Patient

The argument hitherto has presupposed that patients wish to maximise their personal expected utilities, but patients might wish to enter a study for altruistic reasons.[20] The empirical evidence on this point suggests that patients participate slightly more out of self-interest than out of altruism, although it is difficult to draw any solid conclusions from the data.[21] We would argue that altruism should not be assumed, but any altruism should be voluntarily given, otherwise the burden of expectation on patients could erode their trust in the core aims and objectives of the profession, especially in life and death situations. Moreover, acknowledging that patients may include an element of altruism in their decisions to enter trials is very different from saying that doctors should request such a gesture, still less couch their invitation to participate in such ambiguous terms as to elicit unwitting self-sacrifice. Furthermore, recognising that patients may wish to forego some advantage for the good of others, does not change the fundamental nature of equipoise, as it simply means that the utility the patient gains in making such an altruistic gesture, could be factored into the expected utility equation.

It is disturbing to note, however, that many patients suspect that their clinicians may enter them in trials, even when equipoise is not present, implying that a degree of altruism might have been assumed by the use of collective uncertainty.[21] The proportion of patients/members of the public, who thought it likely that doctors put people in trials even when physician equipoise was not present, ranged from 26% to 70% across two studies, both of which used hypothetical trial scenarios.[22,23] Such variation might be explained in part by the populations sampled: the general public and an exclusively African American population respectively.

This fear is not unfounded, as a substantial proportion of clinicians (in many countries) still seem to put their scientific duties ahead of their obligations to do their best for each individual patient. Alderson and colleagues, for example, reported that 75% of physicians thought they were *never* in equipoise, at the same time as 53% of the same sample being prepared to enter their patients in a placebo-controlled trial of taxomifen.[18] Likewise, 73% of responding surgeons, in another study, thought a trial would be ethical, even though only 28% were 'uncertain' about whether HRT could cause a recurrence of cancer.[24] It is possible, however, that they thought equipoise could exist notwithstanding, as some patients may be prepared to trade-off some survival advantage against the relief of symptoms. Taylor explored this issue in more detail, reporting that 36% of respondents would be prepared to enter their patients in a trial, even when out of equipoise.[25]

Competent Decisions: Patient's Understanding prior to Assigning Values

Before patients can assign values to an array of possible outcomes, clinical and psychological, they must be able to understand what these outcomes mean. They also need to appreciate that trial entry means that their treatment will be allocated by lot, and not selected according to preference. Patients might find it difficult to understand the information prior to consent because of the nature of the information itself, or because of the way in which it is relayed.[26]

A great many descriptive studies show that the conceptual nature of clinical trials (for example, the importance of controls or the need for randomisation) is much less readily understood than technical details, such as the side-effects of various treatments.[27–51] The true situation might be still worse, since the quantitative literature seems to overestimate the extent to which patients understood trial details in the above studies, and a qualitative study by Snowdon and colleagues has shown that many people completely failed to grasp that they had been assigned to a control group in a study of neonatal extra-corporeal oxygen therapy.[52] A further qualitative study concluded that the concepts of equipoise and of randomisation proved most difficult for patients to understand.[53] This suggests that the amount and quality of communication is often inadequate. On the whole patients, however, seemed satisfied with their lot,[27,54,55] although this could just mean that they do not appreciate what they are missing.

The findings from studies comparing different methods of obtaining consent on patients' understanding and on consent rate are not easy to interpret, but the following results stand out.[26]

1   Giving people more information increases their knowledge up to a point, after which confusion seems to set in.[33,36,51,56–58]
2   Consent rates to trials are reduced by further information, and giving a patient more time to consider his or her response may also reduce willingness to participate.[33,51,58,59]

Incompetent Patients: Whose Values?

When patients are incompetent, either temporarily or permanently, they are unable to give their consent and so it may be unclear whose values should be used in the decision-making process. When a situation of incompetence has been foreseen and the patient has made voluntary advance directives for the specific situation in hand, the doctor may take heed of the values, documented in such directives. A recent comparative study suggests that practitioners' attitudes to advance directives generally are less favourable than the patients' own attitudes, which viewed such directives as a bona fide expression of their autonomy.[60] However, there is no literature on the validity of advance directives when it comes to entering RCTs, and we should be cautious about generalising the above data, taken in the context of routine practice, to trials.

Sometimes the help of a relative or proxy will be enlisted. Such people may have further insight into what the patient may have wanted. In the absence of such a person or in an emergency, some have argued that randomisation should be avoided, notwithstanding the large societal costs of doing so.[61] Some Kantians would object to the use of proxies in such circumstances, unless they have been nominated in advance by the patients themselves or if the patient is over 16 years. Others, including the MRC,[62] the Royal College of Physicians,[63] and the FDA,[64] have argued that, since routine practice must proceed on the basis of 'assumed' preferences, i.e. those of the 'average' patient, or 'implied consent', randomisation may still be ethical. If a clinician thinks, that on this point at least, his or her own views are 'typical', then all they have to do is follow the gold standard, and treat the patient as they would themselves wish to be treated. We believe, however, that it is necessary to add one further caveat – under these circumstances, no altruism whatever should be assumed – to act otherwise, on such vulnerable patients (children, people with severe mental illness, or the unconscious) would be tantamount to exploiting the vulnerable, and this would find little support in the moral literature.

A somewhat different situation arises when a fully conscious and technically 'competent' patient seeks to delegate the decision to the clinician. This is arguably a valid expression of autonomy.[14] Here, it seems appropriate to respect the patient's wish not to have to decide and to accept delegated decision-making responsibility – again assuming that the patient has a 'typical' value system. Again, how we deal with trial situations mirrors how we deal with non-trial practice.

Could the Offer of Trial Entry be Distressing?

Trials, the above argument suggests, are ethical when a patient has been fully consulted, such that his or her values are brought into play alongside prior probabilities and equipoise has resulted. However, all of this assumes that the offer of trial entry is itself neutral, that expected utilities are not affected (either way) simply by making the offer to participate. For example, if patients' experience of their care were systematically and significantly degraded by the offer of trial entry, then we would have to think seriously about continuing advocacy of trials.

Comparative studies of different methods of obtaining consent have shown that anxiety is increased by enhanced levels of information,[58] albeit for a short period only.[33] There also seems to be an interaction between good overall understanding at consent and low anxiety.[51]

Are Trials on Average a Better Bet than Routine Practice?

As well as the offer of trial entry, we must consider the effect of the whole trial itself on participants. Much is often made about putative beneficial effects of clinical trials on physical well-being. We have reviewed this topic and found that, although the evidence is weak, there seems to be a tendency for patients entered in clinical trials to have better clinical outcomes, even when the trial itself produced a null result.[65–79] However, further analysis of this data, suggests that this effect occurs when there is a pre-existing effective treatment whose effectiveness could be enhanced in a trial by the use of protocol or by a Hawthorne effect.[1] It therefore seems that any trial effect, if true (and of course these results are observational, not experimental), may be contingent upon careful use of existing treatments. Since we should aspire to apply this standard to all patients, it seems egregious to argue for more liberal entry into clinical trials on the basis of a 'trial effect'. Moreover, it is a specific tenet of the Helsinki accord, that a patient's care should be *unaffected*

by whether or not they agree to participate in a clinical study. We conclude that the relevance of any trial effect should not be oversold and that, while any such effect is broadly reassuring at the societal level, it cannot be used as an inducement for an individual patient to participate.

Restrictions on Trial Treatments

So far, we have considered the situation which arises when the treatments in question are normally freely available – the patient may choose treatment A, treatment B, or randomisation between these alternatives. However, the situation can arise in which a type of treatment – we will call it treatment A – is not available outside the trial, say, because a government has restricted its use. Under these circumstances, we argue that the requirement of equipoise between A and B need not apply, it is necessary only that B is not superior to A. If the patient is indeed equipoised between treatments A and B, then all the above arguments apply. If, however, the patient prefers A, then the likelihood of receiving the preferred treatment is maximised by participating in the trial.

Restrictions on access are part of a broader issue of distributive justice, the allocation of benefits and disbenefits across society. Distributive justice implies that discrimination without good reason is wrong and, in the medical context, this usually means that individuals who are in need of treatments should be given an equal chance of getting them. Doctors should at least offer trial entry in such cases. There could still be an issue, however, over what to do once the trial has come to term. Should randomisation continue in order that some people at least get the preferred treatment? The issue is particularly pertinent in Third World trials where the local economics do not always permit widespread use of the treatments used in the trials after the trial has finished.[17] Should all participants be offered the beneficial treatment after the trial? And who should pay for the continued use of such treatments?

Some authors have questioned whether policy-makers should contrive a situation, where treatments are restricted to trial patients, in the first place. Is it ethical to mount such a trial? Space precludes detailed consideration of this issue, but here we simply observe that individual clinicians have very different obligations from policy-makers. The latter are quite properly concerned with the common welfare, while the former, it seems reasonable to argue, have a primary duty to maximise the welfare of individual patients (exceptions arise where patients' unfettered actions may seriously threaten others, as occurs when people with poorly controlled epilepsy continue to drive). If we start from the (reasonable) assumption that resources are limited, and that policy-makers are charged with getting the best value for the public purse, and if we make the further assumption that the chances of doing so are maximised by obtaining good trials evidence, then a compelling argument could be made for a policy whereby new treatments are restricted to patients in clinical trials, even though individual patients acting only in self interest might prefer the new method. Moreover, if our earlier argument is accepted (that the requirement for a clinical trial is more exacting than had hitherto been assumed since it must be based on equipoise rather than just uncertainty), then it would seem that the argument to restrict access is strengthened – tying the hands of clinicians and then patients seems to provide the best way to enhance the common good, while enshrining the concept of the sanctity of the doctor/patient relationship.

It has been argued that simply restricting preferred treatments to trials does not *necessarily* impinge on a patient's autonomy, since it merely limits the options open to the patient and is not coercive in the sense that it forces patients to enter trials.[80] Other ethicists have argued, however, that it is unethical to restrict new treatments to trials when those treatments are potentially life-saving and when there is no effective standard outside. They argue that, in such cases, individuals are so desperate that they are, to all intents and purposes, coerced into participating.[81,82] The ECMO and AIDS trials are just two examples. An extreme view is that doctors should not be coerced into accepting the unethical policy of restricting access to new treatments. What do the patients think? Interestingly, a large proportion (79%) of responding AIDS patients across two studies,[41,83] and parents of very ill children in a further one[52] thought that such medications should be available to sufferers outside the trial, notwithstanding the scientific need for proper evaluation and notwithstanding the resource pressures that general availability would pose. However, it is not easy to interpret these data, for respondents could have been making a general point about prioritising health care or rationing rather than the specific point about restricting some new treatments to RCTs.

Sometimes, however, there does seem to be a real risk of exploitation by restricting strongly preferred treatments to trials when the control arm is expected to be worse than routine or standard care, but the net expected utility of the trial is greater than that of routine care. This could be construed as bribery. Patients may understandably be tempted by a restricted treatment, but those who land up in the control group will be used solely for the sake of science by drawing the very short straw and receiving substandard care. However, if, after randomisation, controls were to guess correctly or be told that they were in fact getting worse care than they would be getting outside the trial, they could simply withdraw and select a better treatment outside the trial. If patients were to refuse trial entry, they would just be offered routine care, but they would have no chance of getting their preferred treatment. For example, some placebo-controlled trials, which do not include an existing standard treatment, yet are compatible with it, are contrived to get patients to forgo the standard in exchange for a chance of getting the preferred treatment which they can only obtain by accepting the chance of receiving a placebo.[84] Placebo-controlled trials in the face of standard treatments which could be, but are not, offered as part of the trial would be using individuals solely for the sake of estimating 'absolute' effectiveness of the treatment under evaluation, as opposed to its effectiveness relative to the current standard.

Applying the Constraint of Equipoise to RCT Design

A clear understanding of equipoise – by which we mean patient equipoise – has many practical and methodological corollaries.

Underpowered Trials

It has been argued elsewhere that the widely promulgated notion that 'underpowered' clinical trials are unethical in terms of their use of patients, is not as authoritative as it sounds; as long as patients are equipoised, they are not losing out in prospect by taking part, and therefore the ethics of 'underpowered' studies turns on the opportunity costs – that is, value for money – not on obligations to individuals.[85] It follows that if the amount of transferable resource used in carrying out such a study is minimal, then such trials are not unethical, although their scientific value must not be oversold so that any altruism is in proportion to their true scientific value. In assessing the latter, it should be borne in mind that some unbiased information is better than none,[86] and that most trials are replicated at some time or another, so that individually underpowered studies – provided they are carried out to a high-quality standard – can contribute to a precise overall estimate of effects.[87–89]

Interim Analysis

The sample size – and hence recruitment period – for studies is typically designed around a power calculation. Such power calculations have been shown frequently to be based on arbitrary parameters, and in particular have been criticised for setting different false-positive and false-negative rates.[90] The point at which the trial should stop recruiting is set in advance. However, because treatments may have bigger positive or negative effects than originally anticipated, it has become popular to examine the data at certain fixed points, prior to the proposed end point, with a view to early stopping of the trial if strong positive or negative effects are detectable.[91–96] However, it is widely believed that general dissemination of accumulating evidence would result in clinicians/patients reaching premature conclusions. For this reason, interim results are sequested, and made available only to a Data Monitoring and Ethics Committee.[97,98] This committee is then left with an extremely onerous decision, in which the broader societal interests have to be balanced against those of future study patients. But such potential study patients remain in a state of ignorance rather than equipoise. It could, however, be argued that this practice is ethical; a veil of ignorance allows doctors and patients to take part in the trial, while society obtains the kind of firm evidence needed to assist future patients. We, however, are not convinced that clinicians and their patients would, in fact, all move out of equipoise, forcing a premature end to the trial, on the basis of publicly accessible interim data.[99] Since different people have different 'priors' and different values, the *meaning* of a given set of results will be very different from different doctor/patient pairs. As a result, some people might become willing to enter a clinical trial, even as others, previously so disposed, move out of equipoise.[100] It seems unacceptable to delegate such a crucial decision to a small group of people who must act without any clear guidelines and with no democratic mandate whatsoever. Lastly, the rising acceptability of Bayesian statistics, which allow multiple looks at the data to be made without any complex statistical adjustment, renders the practice of disclosure of internal results acceptable from a statistical point of view, so that the only point to keeping the data secret would be to promote experimentation on people, who, if they saw the data, would refuse randomisation. The first and fifth authors are, in fact, conducting a Medical Research Council-funded trial of early versus delayed intervention for growth retarded fetuses, entirely on the above lines.

Adaptive Designs

Adaptive designs seek to redress the balance between individual and collective interests by changing the ratio of randomisation over time.[101] The design could start by randomising patients to the trial arms in the ratio 50:50, assuming only two trial arms, perhaps on the basis of widespread equipoise, and then this ratio will change in line with accumulating data showing evidence of a difference in treatment effectiveness. That is to say, the ratio of the number of patients getting the treatment showing the most promise of the moment to the number of patients getting the inferior treatment in prospect will be dictated by the strength of any preliminary data and the size of the then observed difference in efficacy. More patients will receive the more promising treatment than the less promising one, and so the tension between individual and collective interests during the course of the trial is allegedly minimised. However, it is crucial to keep in mind the pragmatic distinction between a trial treatment being routinely and freely available and it being restricted to a trial. Indeed, in the context of the former, Lilford and Jackson point out that adaptive designs still mean that no one can be sure that the next patient will definitely get the preferred treatment, and so it is still not a perfect solution from the individual participant's point of view.[9] Given knowledge of preliminary data, a patient already in the trial could simply withdraw from it and select his or her preferred treatment outside.[9] In brief, adaptive designs do not appear to avoid reduced expected utilities for individual trial patients relative to routine care when trial treatments are freely and routinely available anyway. However, this may not be as bad as the current practice of randomising in equal ratios throughout until the DMC halts the trial and makes the data public.

Adaptive designs do seem to be a respectable compromise, whether or not current practice of keeping interim data secret persists, when a preferred treatment (now increasingly promising) is restricted to the trial. But it is still necessary to decide how often the randomisation ratio should be changed and by how much.

Placebo-Controlled Trials

Placebo-controlled trials are typically unethical when a known effective treatment is available,[84] unless patients are altruistic. However, given that the practice of informed consent is imperfect and patients often have false expectations of benefit from participating in trials,[21] such trials may be questionable notwithstanding.

Sometimes, there is a scientific desire to preserve blinding by using active placebos (placebos, such as sham operations, which mimic the adverse effects of a new intervention).[102] However, their use is almost always unethical and may rely solely on altruism for recruitment when the intervention is an otherwise freely available treatment.[103] Arguably, this is implausible when the active placebo is highly invasive. There may be less scientific need to use active placebos anyway when minor adverse effects do not give the intervention away.

Cluster RCTs and Behavioural Interventions

Cluster trials are of two sorts – those where the treatment is indivisible at the individual level (such as advertising campaigns on local radio), and those where the intervention in question may be accepted or refused by individuals. In the first type of study, we cannot consider individuals in isolation for the purposes of 'consent', and one person's choice will impinge on another's. We have argued elsewhere that to preclude all such studies on this basis would be unjustifiable; this would be tantamount to saying that alterations in service delivery were acceptable, as long as they were uncontrolled and hence not part of a formal prospective evaluation.[104] Therefore, we argue that the same conditions should apply as do for conventional trials – the more risky or controversial the intervention, the greater the safeguards that should be required, so that a relatively uncontroversial measure, such as an advertising campaign advocating a low-fat diet, would require little consultation, while a more intrusive measure (such as fluoridating the water supply) might require extensive local consultation or even a referendum.

Cluster trials at the individual level are usually done in order to promote beneficial herd effects or to avoid 'contamination', where the effect of the intervention on one person affects others in a locality (such as a form of educational therapy to prevent substance misuse). The problem with these latter types of intervention arises from the fact that it is very hard to separate consent for the intervention from the intervention itself, and this poses a particular difficulty for controls. Zelen randomisation has been advocated in these circumstances, whereby consent is obtained only from the intervention patients, but not from controls.[105] This is highly controversial, and has been debated extensively elsewhere in the context of individual trials.[106–109] Proponents of this method argue that consent would not be sought in non-trial practice, and

since the controls get exactly the same form of care as people elsewhere who are not involved in the trial, there is no need to obtain their consent specifically for participating in research, but consent is sought for any routine treatments on offer.[110] Others argue that to carry out randomisation and follow-up without a person's consent amounts to a form of deception.[15] There seems to be no way to resolve fully these arguments, but we make two points here. Firstly, in the case of behavioural interventions, we suggest that 'assent' to take part in the study may be sought from controls, whereby they understand that they are the controls for an educational intervention, and consent to follow-up, but to remain, at least temporarily, ignorant of further details. Secondly, that surveys have shown that some individuals find the Zelen method deeply unpopular, when used as a method to avoid distressing controls in trials of potentially effective interventions.[111] It is not clear, however, from this study, whether these people are objecting to being kept in the dark *per se*, or whether restricted access to a promising new treatment is the real problem. Whether the intervention is individual or not, we have argued that individual(s) who 'deliver' clusters into a trial should sign a consent form.[104] Such individuals or 'guardians' could look after the best interests of their cluster.

We have discussed how a patient's best interests can be reconciled with the societal need to advance medical knowledge through RCTs. We have argued that Freedman is wrong in thinking that collective uncertainty is a sufficient condition for mounting a trial and then recruiting patients, and we have clarified what best interests mean for patients in terms of what we know about a treatment's effectiveness and of what values might determine best treatment. Competent patients, provided that they understand all material information, can use their own values to decide whether any particular trial would be a good bet. In the case of incompetent patients, average values or advance directives, perhaps nominating a proxy or foreseeing a specific situation, must be used to protect them. When trial treatments are freely available, patients must be in a state of personal equipoise.

This requirement has a number of implications for RCT practice and design.

1   Underpowered trials are not necessarily unethical in their 'use' of patients.
2   Interim analyses are desirable, although the current practice of keeping preliminary data

secret is suspect, especially when trial treatments are widely available.

3 Adaptive designs do not solve the problem of reducing expected utilities for participants when trial treatments are widely available.

4 Placebo-controlled trials generally are not usually appropriate when standard treatments exist, and those using 'active' placebos with adverse effects should be used with caution if at all.

5 Cluster RCTs can be categorised into cluster–cluster and individual–cluster trials, depending on the type of intervention under study. Guardians should consent to randomisation in both types of trial. The best interests of the cluster is of paramount concern in the former type and individuals can consent to interventions in the latter type of trial.

6 Many behavioural interventions may contaminate controls, either directly through fully informed consent or indirectly through close contact of individuals. Cluster trials may be used, but it may be necessary to withhold information about the intervention from controls.

REFERENCES

1. Edwards SJL, Lilford RJ, Braunholtz DA, Thornton J, Jackson J, Hewison J. *Ethical issues in the design and conduct of Randomised Clinical Trials*. HTA, 1998.
2. Gillon R. Recruitment for clinical trials: the need for public professional cooperation. *J. Med. Ethics* 1994; **20**: 3–4.
3. Fox TF. The ethics of clinical trials. *Medico-legal J.* 1960; **28**: 132–41.
4. Pringle M, Churchill R. Randomised controlled trials in general practice [editorial] [see comments]. *Br. Med. J.* 1995; **311**: 1382–3.
5. Schafer A. The ethics of the randomized clinical trial. *N. Eng. J. Med.* 1982; **307**: 719–24.
6. Vere DW. Controlled clinical trials – the current ethical debate. *Proc. R. Soc. Med.* 1981; **74**: 85–7.
7. Freedman B. Equipoise and ethics of clinical research. *N. Eng. J. Med.* 1987; **317**: 141–5.
8. Gifford F. The conflict between randomized clinical trials and the therapeutic obligation. *J. Med. Phil.* 1986; **11**: 347–66.
9. Lilford RJ, Jackson J. Equipoise and the ethics of randomization. *J. R. Soc. Med.* 1995; **88**: 552–9.
10. French S. *Decision theory: an introduction to the mathematics of rationality*. New York: John Wiley and Sons, 1986.
11. Johnson N, Lilford RJ, Brazier W. At what level of collective equipoise does a clinical trial become ethical? *J. Med. Ethics* 1991; **17**: 30–4.
12. Jackson J. Telling the truth. *J. Med. Ethics* 1991; **17**: 5–9.
13. Mill John Stuart. *Utilitarianism*. London: Longmans, Green, Reader and Dyer, 1874.
14. Dworkin G. *The theory and practice of autonomy*. Cambridge University Press, 1988.
15. Ashcroft RE, Chadwick DW, Clark SRL, Edwards RHT, Frith L, Hutton JL. Implications of socio-cultural contexts for the ethics of clinical trials. *Health Technology Assessment* 1997; **1**(9).
16. CIOMS and WHO. International guidelines for biomedical research involving human subjects. 1993.
17. Lockwood M, Anscombe GEM. Sins of omission? The non-treatment of controls in clinical trials. *Aristotelian Society* 1983; **57**: 222.
18. Alderson P, Madden M, Oakley A, Wilkins R. Women's knowledge and experience of breast cancer treatment and research. Social Science Research Unit, 1994.
19. Chard JA, Lilford RJ. The use of equipoise in clinical trials. *Soc. Sci. Med.* 1998; **47**: 891–8.
20. Nagel T. *The possibility of altruism*. Princetown: Princetown University Press, 1970.
21. Edwards SJL, Lilford RJ, Hewison J. The ethics of RCTs from the perspectives of patients, the public and health care professionals. *Br. Med. J.* 1998; **317**: 1209–12.
22. Millon-Underwood S. Determinants of participation in state-of-the-art cancer prevention, early detection, screening, and treatment trials. *Cancer Nursing* 1993; **16**: 25–33.
23. Cassileth BR, Lusk EJ, Miller DS, Hurtwitz S. Attitudes toward clinical trials among patients and the public. *JAMA* 1982; **248**: 968–70.
24. Marsden J, Sacks NPD, Baum M, Whitehead MI, Crook D. *A pilot study investigating the feasibility of conducting a randomised trial of HRT use in women with a history of breast cancer – preliminary report of findings*. 1999; Unpublished report.
25. Taylor KM. Informed consent: the physicians' perspective. *Soc. Sci. Med.* 1987; **24**: 135–43.
26. Edwards SJL, Lilford RJ, Thornton J, Hewison J. Informed consent for clinical trials: in search of the best method. *Social Science and Medicine* 1998; **47**(11): 1825–40.
27. Hassar M, Weintraub M. 'Uninformed' consent and the wealthy volunteer: an analysis of patient volunteers in a clinical trial of a new anti-flammatory drug. *Clin. Pharmacol. Ther.* 1976; **20**: 379–86.
28. Marini SB. An evaluation of informed consent with volunteer prisoner subjects. *Yale Journal of Biology and Medicine* 1976; **427**: 434.

29. Bergler JH, Pennington AC, Metcalfe M, Freis ED. Informed consent: how much does the patient understand? *Clin. Pharmacol. Ther.* 1980; **27**: 425–40.

30. Howard JM, Demets D, BHAT Research Group. How informed is informed consent? The BHAT experience. *Controlled Clinical Trials* 1981; **2**: 287–304.

31. Penman DT, Demets D, BHAT Research Group. Informed consent for investigational chemotherapy: Patients' and physicians' perceptions. *J. Clin. Oncol.* 1984; **2**: 849–55.

32. Rodenhuis S, van den Heuvel WJ, Annyas AA, et al. Patient motivation and informed consent in a phase I study of anticancer agent. *Euro. J. Cancer Clin. Oncol.* 1984; **20**: 457–62.

33. Simes RJ, Tattersall MH, Coates AS, Raghavan D, Solomon HJ, Smartt H. Randomised comparison of procedures for obtaining informed consent in clinical trials of treatment for cancer. *Br. Med. J. (Clin. Res. Ed.)* 1986; **293**: 1065–8.

34. DCCT Research Group. Implementation of a multicomponent process to obtain informed consent in a diabetes control and complications trial. *Controlled Clinical Trials* 1998; **10**: 96.

35. Rennie D, Yank V. Disclosure to the reader of institutional review board approval and informed consent. *JAMA* 1997; **277**: 922–3.

36. Davis S, Seay J, Stone J, et al. *Does knowing about clinical trials increase participation?* Unpublished report.

37. Lynoe N, Sandlund M, Dalqvist G, Jacobsson L. Informed consent: study of the quality of information given to participants in a clinical trial. *Br. Med. J.* 1991; **303**: 613.

38. Oddens BJ, Oddens BJ, Algra A, van Gijn J. How much information is retained by participants in clinical trials? *Ned. Tijdschr. Geneeskd.* 1992; **136**: 2272–6.

39. Jensen AB, Madsen B, Anderson P, Rose C. Information for cancer patients entering a clinical trial: evaluation of an information strategy. *Eur. J. Cancer* 1999; **29**: 2235–8.

40. Gallet M, Aupetit JF, Servan E, Lestaevel M, Lopez M, Chassoux G. Informed consent, what information is left after a therapeutic trial? *Arch. Mal. Coeur Vaiss.* 1994; **87**: 39–45.

41. Tindall B, Forde S, Ross MW, et al. Effects of two formats of informed consent on knowledge amongst persons with advanced HIV disease in a clinical trial of didanosine. *Patient Education and Counselling* 1994; **24**: 266.

42. Maslin A. A survey of the opinions on 'informed consent' of women currently involved in clinical trials within a breast unit. *Eur. J. Cancer Care* 1994; **3**: 153–62.

43. Miller C, Searight HR, Grable D, Schwartz R, Sowell C, Barbarash RA. Comprehension and recall of the informational content of the informed consent document: An evaluation of 168 patients in a controlled clinical trial. *J. Clin. Res. Drug Dev.* 1994; **8**: 237–48.

44. Daugherty C, Ratain, MJ, Grochowski E, et al. Perceptions of cancer patients and their physicians involved in phase I trials. *J. Clin. Oncol.* 1995; **13**: 1062–72.

45. DeLuca SA, Korcuska LA, Oberstar BH, et al. Are we promoting true informed consent in cardiovascular clinical trials? *J. Cardiovasc. Nursing* 1995; **9**: 54–61.

46. Harth SC, Thong YH. Parental perceptions and attitudes about informed consent in clinical research involving children. *Soc. Sci. Med.* 1995; **40**: 1573–7.

47. Harrison K, Vlahov D, Jones K, Charron K, Clements ML. Medical eligibility, comprehension of the consent process, and retention of injection drug users recruited for an HIV vaccine trial. *J. Acquired Immune Deficiency Syndr. Hum. Retrovirol.* 1995; **10**: 386–90.

48. Olver I, Buchanan L, Laidlaw C, Poulton G. The adequacy of consent forms for informing patients entering oncological clinical trials. *Ann. Oncol.* 1995; **6**: 867–70.

49. Postlethwaite RJ, Reynolds JM, Wood AJ, Evans JH, Lewis MA. Recruiting patients to clinical trials: lessons from studies of growth hormone treatment in renal failure. *Arch. Dis. Child* 1995; **73**: 30–5.

50. Tomamichel M, Sessa C, Herzig S, de Jong J, Pagani O, Willems Y, Cavalli F. Informed consent for phase I studies: evaluation of quantity and quality of information provided to patients. *Ann. Oncol.* 1995; **6**: 363–9.

51. Aaronson NK, Visserpol E, Leenhouts GHMW, Muller MV, Vanderschot ACM, Vandam FSAM, Keus RB, Koning CCE, Huinink WWT. Telephone-based nursing and intervention improves the effectiveness of the informed consent process in cancer clinical trials. *J. Clin. Oncol.* 1996; **14**: 984–96.

52. Snowdon C, Garcia J, Elbourne D. Making sense of randomisation: responses of parents of critically ill babies to random allocation of treatment in a clinical trial. *Soc. Sci. Med.* 1997; **45**: 1337–55.

53. Featherstone K, Donovan JL. Random allocation or allocation at random? Patients' perspectives of participation in a randomised controlled trial [see comments]. *Br. Med. J.* 1998; **317**: 1177–80.

54. Wilcox M, Schroer S. The perspective of patients with vascular disease on participation in clinical trials. *J. Vasc. Nurs.* 1994; **12**: 112–16.

55. Bevan EG, Chee LC, McGhee SM, McInnes GT. Patients' attitudes to participation in clinical trials. *Br. J. Clin. Pharmacol.* 1993; **35**: 204–7.

56. Davis S., Seay J., Stone J. et al. Does knowing about clinical trials increase participation?

[Abstract]. *Proc. Am. Soc. Clin. Oncol.* 1990; **9**: A232 (Abstract).

57. White DR, Muss HB, Michielutte R, et al. Informed consent: patient information forms in chemotherapy trials. *Am. J. Clin. Oncol.* 1984; **7**: 183–90.

58. Epstein LC, Lasagna L. Obtaining informed consent. Form or substance. *Arch. Intern. Med.* 1969; **123**: 682–8.

59. Dal-Re R. [Clinical trial of drugs: a study of the influence of information on adverse reactions on obtaining of informed consent] Investigacion clinica con farmacos: estudio de la influencia de la informacion sobre reacciones adversas en la obtencion del consentimiento informado. *Med. Clin. (Barc.)* 1991; **96**: 566–9.

60. Blondeau D, Valois P, Keyserlingk EW, Hebert M, Lavoie M. Comparison of patients' and health care professionals' attitudes towards advance directives. *J. Med. Ethics* 1998; **24**: 328–35.

61. Kapp MB. Proxy decision-making in Alzheimer disease research. *Alzheimer Disease Association* 1994; **8**: 28–37.

62. Working Party on Research on the Mentally Incapacitated. *The ethical conduct of research on the mentally incapacitated*. London: MRC, 1991.

63. The Royal College of Physicians, London. A Report to the Royal College of Physicians. Guidelines on the practice of Ethics Committees in medical research involving human subjects. 2nd ed., 1990.

64. Hastings Center Report. Symposium on Informed Consent. In case of emergency: no need for consent. *Hastings Center Report* 1997; **27**(1): 7–12.

65. Mahon J, Laupacis A, Donner A, Wood T. Randomised study of *n* of 1 trials versus standard practice [see comments] [published erratum appears in *Br. Med. J.* 1996 Jun 1; 312(7043): 1392]. *Br. Med. J.* 1996; **312**: 1069–74.

66. Reiser J, Warner JO. The value of participating in an asthma trial. *Lancet* 1985; **1**: 206–7.

67. Antman K. A comparison of randomized vs concurrent controls. *Proc. Am. Assoc. Cancer Res.* 1983; **24**: 146.

68. Bertelsen K. Protocol allocation and exclusion in two Danish randomised trials in ovarian cancer. *Br. J. Cancer* 1991; **64**: 1172–6.

69. Anonymous Coronary artery surgery study (CASS): a randomized trial of coronary artery bypass surgery. Comparability of entry characteristics and survival in randomized patients and nonrandomized patients meeting randomization criteria. *J. Am. Coll. Cardiol.* 1984; **3**: 114–28.

70. Davis S, Wright PW, Schulman SF, Hill LD, Pinkham RD, Johnson LP, Jones TW, Kellogg HB, Radke HM, Sikkema WW, Jolly PC, Hammar SP. Participants in a prospective, randomized clinical trial for resected non-small cell lung cancer have improved survival compared with nonparticipants in such trials. *Cancer* 1985; **56**: 1710–18.

71. Jha P, Deboer D, Sykora K, Naylor CD. Characteristics and mortality outcomes of thrombolysis trial participants and non-participants: a population-based comparison. *J. Am. Coll. Cardiol.* 1996; **27**: 1335–42.

72. Karjalainen S, Palva I. Do treatment protocols improve end results? A study of survival of patients with multiple myeloma in Finland [see comments]. *Br. Med. J.* 1989; **299**: 1069–72.

73. Lennox EL, Stiller CA, Jones PH, Wilson LM. Nephroblastoma: treatment during 1970–3 and the effect on survival of inclusion in the first MRC trial. *Br. Med. J.* 1979; **2**: 567–9.

74. Duration of survival of children with acute leukaemia. Report to the Medical Research Council from the Committee on Leukaemia and the Working Party on Leukaemia in Childhood. *Br. Med. J.* 1971; **4**: 7–9.

75. Schmoor C, Olschewski M, Schumacher M. Randomised and non-randomised patients in clinical trials: experiences with comprehensive cohort studies. *Stat. Med.* 1996; **15**: 263–71.

76. Stiller CA, Draper GJ. Treatment centre size, entry to trials, and survival in acute lymphoblastic leukemia. *Arch. Dis. Child.* 1989; **64**: 657–61.

77. Stiller CA, Eatock EM. Survival from acute non-lymphocytic leukaemia, 1971–88: a population based study. *Arch. Dis. Child* 1994; **70**: 219–23.

78. Ward LC, Fielding JW, Dunn JA, Kelly KA. The selection of cases for randomised trials: a registry survey of concurrent trial and non-trial patients. The British Stomach Cancer Group. *Br. J. Cancer* 1992; **66**: 943–50.

79. Williford WO, Krol WF, Buzby GP. Comparison of eligible randomized patients with two groups of ineligible patients: can the results of the VA Total Parenteral Nutrition clinical trial be generalized? *J. Clin. Epidemiol.* 1993; **46**: 1025–34.

80. Logue G, Wear S. A desperate solution: individual autonomy and the double-blind controlled experiment. *J. Med. Philos.* 1995; **20**: 57–64.

81. Minogue BP, Palmer-Fernandez G, Udell L, Waller BN. Individual autonomy and the double-blind controlled experiment: the case of desperate volunteers. *J. Med. Philos.* 1995; **20**: 43–55.

82. Truog RD. Randomized control trials: lessons from ECMO. *Clin. Res.* 1992; **40**: 519–27.

83. Twomey JG. Investigating pediatric HIV research ethics in the field. *West. J. Nurs. Res.* 1994; **16**: 413.

84. Rothman KJ, Michels KB. The continuing unethical use of placebo controls. *N. Eng. J. Med.* 1994; **331**: 394–8.

85. Edwards SJ, Lilford RJ, Braunholtz D, Jackson J. Why 'underpowered' trials are not necessarily unethical [see comments]. *Lancet* 1997; **350**: 804–7.

86. Lilford RJ, Braunholtz D. The statistical basis of public policy: a paradigm shift is overdue [see comments]. *Br. Med. J.* 1996; **313**: 603–7.

87. Fayers PM, Machin D. Sample size: how many patients are necessary? [editorial]. *Br. J. Cancer* 1995; **72**: 1–9.

88. Barnard GA. Must clinical trials be large? The interpretation of p-values and the combination of test results. *Stat. Med.* 1990; **9**: 601–14.

89. Laupacis A. Research by collaboration [see comments]. *Lancet* 1995; **345**: 938.

90. Lilford RJ, Johnson N. The alpha and beta errors in randomized trials [letter]. *N. Eng. J. Med.* 1990; **322**: 780–1.

91. Armitage P. Interim analysis in clinical trials. *Stat. Med.* 1991; **10**: 925–35.

92. Ashby D, Machin D. Stopping rules, interim analyses and data monitoring committees [editorial]. *Br. J. Cancer* 1993; **68**: 1047–50.

93. Berry DA. Interim analyses in clinical research. *Cancer Invest.* 1987; **5**: 469–77.

94. Berry DA. Interim analyses in clinical trials: classical vs. Bayesian approaches. *Stat. Med.* 1985; **4**: 521–6.

95. Freedman LS, Spiegelhalter DJ. Comparison of Bayesian with group sequential methods for monitoring clinical trials [see comments]. *Control. Clin. Trials* 1989; **10**: 357–67.

96. Pocock SJ. The role of external evidence in data monitoring of a clinical trial. [Review] *Stat. Med.* 1996; **15**: 1285–93.

97. Clayton D. Ethically optimized designs. *Br. J. Clin. Pharmacol.* 1982; **13**: 469–80.

98. Royall RM. Ethics and statistics in randomized clinical trials, with discussion. *Stat. Sci.* 1991; **6**: 52–88.

99. Prescott RJ. Feedback of data to participants during clinical trials. In: Tagnon HJ, Staquet MJ. *Anonymous Controversies in cancer: Design of trials and Treatment.* New York, 1979; 55–61.

100. Thornton JG, Lilford RJ. Preterm breech babies and randomised trials of rare conditions [comment]. [Review] *Br. J. Obstet. Gynaecol.* 1996; **103**: 611–13.

101. Simon R. Adaptive treatment assignment methods and clinical trials. *Biometrics* 1977; **33**: 743–9.

102. Shapiro AK, Shapiro E. *The Powerful Placebo.* The Johns Hopkins University Press, 1997.

103. Edwards SJL, Braunholtz DA, Stevens AJ, Lilford RJ. *Are some placebo-controlled trials unethical?* Unpublished report.

104. Edwards SJL, Braunholtz DA, Lilford RJ, Stevens AJ. Ethical issues in the design and conduct of cluster RCTs. *Br. Med. J.* 1999; **318**: 1407–9.

105. Donner A. Some aspects of the design and analysis of cluster randomized trials. *Appl. Statist.* 1998; **47**: 95–113.

106. Horwitz RI, Feinstein AR. Advantages and drawbacks of the Zelen design for randomized clinical trials. *J. Clin. Pharmacol.* 1980; **20**: 425–7.

107. Gore SM. Zelen randomisation [letter]. *Lancet* 1984; **2**: 226–7.

108. Taube A. [n or more in clinical trials? Zelen's models for randomization] n eller flera vid kliniska provningar? Zelens modeller för randomisering. *Lakartidningen.* 1994; **91**: 977–82.

109. Torgerson DJ, Roland M. What is Zelen's design? *Br. Med. J.* 1998; **316**: 606.

110. House A, Knapp P. Informed consent. Trials that use Zelen's procedure should be acceptable [letter; comment]. *Br. Med. J.* 1997; **315**: 251.

111. Snowdon C, Elbourne D, Garcia J. Zelen randomization: attitudes of parents participating in a neonatal clinical trial. *Control. Clin. Trials* 1999; **20**: 149–71.

2

Ethics of Clinical Trials: Social, Cultural and Economic Factors

RICHARD E. ASHCROFT

SUMMARY

It is now generally agreed that drug therapies cannot be licensed and adopted without thorough testing on human patients in properly designed and managed clinical trials. This methodology is now also widely applied in assessment of other healthcare interventions ('health technologies'). The ethical debate about the rights and responsibilities of subjects and researchers is arguably as old as clinical trials methodology itself.[1,2] Traditionally this debate has focussed upon subjects' autonomy and informed consent, and upon balancing the risks and benefits of the research to the individuals and to society.[3] Typically, debate has used the Beauchamp and Childress 'Four Principles' approach as a method for analysing the ethical issues.[4] These are the principles of Beneficence, Non-maleficence, respect for Autonomy, and Justice. Until recently, little attention has been paid to issues of justice. Typical questions of justice include: the fairness of recruitment or non-recruitment into clinical trials; the fairness of randomisation; continued access to treatment after the trial; research into rare conditions; and the legitimacy of incentive payments to participating doctors or patients. Since these questions have often been pertinent not only to individuals but also to definable groups in society (social, economic, national or cultural), awareness has grown of the possibility that particular groups may be systematically, but unwittingly, discriminated against on ostensibly scientific grounds.[5,6] However, there is also a more general question: are the ethical standards typically used by Ethics Committees and others to evaluate research shared by all social groups? Are there alternative ethical codes and systems of belief, held by particular social or cultural groups which dissent from the common consensus regarding research ethics? Does this lead to actual or potential conflict or injustice?

The aim of this review was to collate, assess and analyse the available evidence on these two main areas of development in research ethics: justice in access to, and participation in, trials, and whether current research ethics represent a culturally universal standard. The methods used for research were adapted from standard systematic review techniques. The evidence used was drawn from medical, social science and philosophical literature. The chief conclusions are that injustice in various forms is a serious concern, but that it arises mainly in healthcare systems where the patient (or their private insurer) is responsible for paying for treatments, and when research is 'exported' from rich to poor countries. Injustice can also arise from spurious interpretations of the importance of risk to particular groups, which results in the exclusion of these groups. There is very little evidence for or against cultural factors producing dissenting views on research ethics.

CONTEXT

It is widely accepted that the assessment of technologies in healthcare cannot be made on the basis of animal and in-vitro experiments alone, but also requires experimentation on human patients. It is now generally accepted that experimentation on patients involves ethical issues. Even where there is an ethical consensus about what these issues are, and what the particular ethical requirements are in respect of the proposed experiment, this consensus needs to be underwritten by sound argument. The principal requirement of any experiment is that it should be scientifically useful. This requirement is a necessary condition, although it is not sufficient on its own. Most health researchers agree that the most scientifically rigorous method for treatment evaluation is the randomised, controlled clinical trial (RCT).[7-10] This is not accepted by all writers, and there is evidence to suggest that randomisation and control are concepts not well understood by many patients, and that many patients are unhappy with being assigned randomly to a treatment, or with being assigned to the control group.[11-15] As a consequence, an important body of opinion has formed which argues against particular elements of the RCT methodology on ethical grounds, and which has proposed a number of modifications, or alternatives, to the RCT.

Our hypothesis was that some of the objections to the RCT on methodological or ethical grounds might have a systematic basis, not solely attributable to misunderstanding of the aims, premises and methods of the RCT, in some particular cases or in general. These objections, if they are systematic, may reflect the beliefs (political, philosophical, religious or cultural) of particular groups within society. Should this be the case, these systematic beliefs would require Local Research Ethics Committees or Institutional Review Boards to pay special attention to the interests of such groups in assessing RCTs for their ethical adequacy.[16] More than this, these objections might be such that alternatives to the RCT should be considered more sympathetically, as health assessment technologies more widely acceptable to the ethical beliefs of *all* groups in society. But this would also require showing that alternatives to the RCT did meet the first requirement of human experimentation, which is scientific adequacy and efficiency. Finally, then, objections to the RCT might necessitate a negotiated compromise between the need for validated health technologies and the requirements of objecting groups' ethical principles.

In the course of the research, we quickly became aware that there was a second kind of problem for ethical research. Groups' objections to RCTs, and low recruiting of members of some groups were sometimes due to issues of actual or perceived injustice in trial recruitment and process.[17] In some cases the perception of injustice was due to historical factors: past and present discrimination against the group in medical and other contexts.[18,19] In other cases there is concern that some injustice is brought about by features of trial methodology.[20,21] Further, there is concern that some groups are over- or under-represented due to economic factors influencing the delivery of healthcare inside or outside clinical trials.[22] It is difficult to disentangle the cultural and the economic here, because often the poor happen to be members of groups that are discriminated against (or feel themselves to be so). These considerations once again lead us to consider whether there could be methods to recruit more fairly, for instance, without compromising the scientific integrity of the trial.

METHODS USED IN THE REVIEW

The report was commissioned as a systematic review of the literature on ethics, clinical trials, and relevant socio-cultural factors. It was not intended that the study should undertake any new research beyond the critical philosophical analysis of the literature surveyed. The aim of a systematic review is to determine what work has been done, and with what quality; to indicate the current state of knowledge for practical application; and to guide future research and practice. The survey concentrated on the British context, using American and other developed countries for comparison and, where appropriate, amplification. The literature survey was restricted, for reasons of convenience, to literature published or abstracted in English.

The questions framed in our hypothesis were partly philosophical and partly empirical. We needed to know whether there were in fact any common objections to the RCT methodology (or to particular trials); and we needed to assemble the interpretative and philosophical resources to make sense of them. We used a modified systematic reviewing strategy to assemble a database of articles and book chapters. Systematic searches on Medline, Psychlit and Sociofile CD ROM databases, together with hand-searches on the most important relevant medical, bioethics and philosophy journals, were used to assemble as wide a range of empirical and analytic material as possible and useful. Objections were sought of both direct and indirect kinds. Direct objections comprise explicit statements by patients and healthcare workers of worries, objections, and problems to do with recruitment to particular trials, compliance with protocols, and methodology of trials. Indirect objections were limited proactive attempts on the part of the project team to extrapolate and infer objections that particular groups might make to trials, on the basis of explicit statements about topics analogous to features of trial methodology, but not directly connected to it. For instance, many religious groups object on principle to any form of gambling, whence it might be inferred that they should also object to random assignment. The absence of any objection along these lines as yet, may perhaps indicate only that this is a pitfall-in-waiting. A wide remit was adopted, on the grounds that careful foresight would benefit from moderate speculation.

Searches for analytic material were, of necessity, much broader in scope, because the kinds of objections that might arise could have quite broad significance, for example economic, social, political, religious or cultural. Such objections might reflect aspects of philosophical arguments which are not normally canvassed in contemporary medical ethics, narrowly defined. Particular care was taken to discover relevant books, as these are often less well represented in electronic databases than are abstracted articles.[1,23]

EVIDENCE: QUALITY AND DEPTH

Electronic database searches were conducted on Medline (1990–September 1996), Psychlit (1990–September 1996), Sociofile (1974–June 1996) and Life Sciences (1990–June 1996). Hand searches were performed on the *British Medical Journal*, *The Lancet*, the *New England Journal of Medicine*, the *Journal of the American Medical Association* (all 1995–November 1996), the *Hastings Center Report*, the *Journal of Medical Ethics*, and *Statistics in Medicine* (all complete runs). Some websites of interest were identified, but they generated little evidence.

In the electronic searching, nearly 7000 items were identified by use of defined search terms; however, the relevance of most of these articles (determined by reading abstracts) was low, and 1134 articles were collected. In the final report just over 300 of these articles were referenced.

The searching process uncovered no studies directly concerned with the attitudes and beliefs of different cultural groups to clinical trial methodology. There is a lot of research, using the whole range of experimental methodology, into the effectiveness of different methods of obtaining informed consent, and into methods for recruitment generally. Some of this material was relevant to the issues in hand – particularly those studies which looked at trials with poor recruitment rates. However, much of the best of this research is hard to generalise, either because it was linked to particular trials, or because it is linked to particular local social circumstances. Much American evidence does not apply to the UK or European health services. However, this paints too black a picture. In our study, where we were interested in the quality of the arguments used as much as in the evidence used in their support (if any), we were able to use evidence from a variety of sources as illustrations of more general rational arguments.

Conversely, we would argue that much evidence in ethics research can *only* be used in this illustrative way. For example, quantitative research about methods of obtaining consent may show that some methods lead to higher recruitment rates than others; however it is not clear what to conclude from this alone about the relative ethical statuses of the methods under trial. Likewise, quantitative methods are good at identifying patterns of patients' preferences, and degrees of preference satisfaction; but satisfaction of preference and moral rightness are by no means always equivalent.

It is, however, true that ethical debate about trials does often turn on matters of fact, and when this is so, it is crucial that the facts be determined reliably and accurately. Much that has been published overlooks the role of evidence in argument.[24] The relative dearth of useable factual evidence forced us to adopt a theoretical and analytical approach to this topic, but we also recommend further research to improve our knowledge and policy-making in this area.[1,23]

KEY ISSUES AND CONTROVERSIES

The following issues can be identified: RCT methodology in principle; RCT methods in particular cases; recruitment and representation; consent in principle; and consent in practice.

RCT Methodology in Principle

Much of the debate about clinical trials arises in particular cases, especially when the trial involves treatments for high-profile diseases (for example cancer and HIV/AIDS), or when the trial involves a particular population who are identified medically by suffering from or susceptibility to some given condition but who are also identified socially by some socio-cultural marker (for example gender, ethnic group or social class). There are usually two levels to debates framed in this way – a debate about the features of RCTs in general (control groups, randomisation, comparison of therapies, blinding, risk–benefit calculus and placebo-control), and a debate about the appropriateness of applying this methodology to this given group at this particular time.

Randomisation is very poorly understood by most people, and generates much controversy. There is sometimes a demand for people to be allowed to choose which arm they are assigned to, or – more honestly – a demand that people should be able to insist on the experimental therapy.[25–28] They can insist on *not* getting it by withholding their consent to enter the trial. The debate here breaks down into two parts – a debate about the scientific necessity for randomisation and controlled comparison, and a debate about whether there is something simply wrong and immoral about this methodology, regardless of its scientific merits. The reasoning strategy in the first debate is 'consequentialist', and in the second is 'deontological'.[29] Consequentialism holds that an act is right when it has the best consequences. In contrast, deontological reasoning holds that acts are right in virtue of their conforming to certain fixed principles, and so an act can be wrong even where it has the best consequences (for example, lying is just wrong, even where it protects a third party). In the first debate an RCT is acceptable only if it has the best outcome for the participants and society. 'Best' is defined with reference to the alternatives – not testing at all, obtaining other kinds or grades of evidence, allowing patient choice, and so on. However, in the second debate, consequences are trumped by considerations about the rights of subjects, the duties of triallists, or theological considerations. For an example, it is conceivable that randomisation might be thought wrong in the same way that gambling is thought wrong by many religions.

The consequentialist debate is very well known, and most of the language and techniques we have for discussing RCT ethics are drawn from this debate, particularly the concept of proportionality of risk and benefit. This debate has a socio-cultural dimension – perception of risk and benefit can be linked to social and cultural factors; and the definition of risk and benefit and their chances can be contested. To some extent this is a technical matter, but acceptance of this fact, and of what it indicates in a given trial, rests on a relationship of trust between population, participants and triallists.[30] This relationship is sometimes very strained, for a variety of reasons. This debate also encompasses issues of distributive justice relating to recruitment: a fair distribution of the chances of access to the trial and of risks and benefit within it, together with wider issues about the chances of exposure to trials as part of one's healthcare and about overall access to healthcare of a given quality.[31,32]

The deontological debate is less developed, save in one particular area – consent – and this will be discussed separately. One of our chief concerns in this study was to uncover evidence about religious contributions to this deontological debate, particularly from the non-Christian religions. The rights-based debate is not well developed, partly because consent gives rights theorists most of what they want, and partly because few rights theorists in practice use consequentialist reasoning to determine what the rights in question involve in the given case. Similarly, duty-based reasoning is very familiar (the Declaration of Helsinki specifies a set of duties that bind researchers), but in practice can be weak, because of ambiguity, exceptions and hard cases for interpreting what the principle in question actually requires.[33–35]

RCT Methodology in Particular Cases

In particular situations, it may be argued that a full RCT is inappropriate or unfair, either because the disease is serious or rare and it might be invidious to recruit some but not all of the affected population, or to assign some members of the population the new therapy, but not all. Another argument may be that this trial is unjust because it draws on a population which has already been used as a trial population many more times than average, or is at increased risk of other discriminatory or risky practices. Arguments of this type have become familiar from AIDS research, research on rare diseases and, on the world stage, the 'exporting' of clinical research to poor or developing countries.[36,37] Recruitment and randomisation are sometimes seen as unjust because they replicate, or even magnify, existing injustices against disadvantaged social, cultural or economic groups. Some cultural groups have succeeded in establishing the necessity of a group consent prior to individual consent as a mechanism for protecting their group's interests.[38–40]

One important controversial issue is the use of placebo control in trials. It is now generally agreed that placebo control is ethical only when no 'standard' (that is, non-experimental) therapy is available, or if there is evidence that this therapy is actually ineffective or harmful.[41–43] This consensus arises from the conviction that a trial is ethical only if it represents a fair choice for the patient. This is the case if equipoise obtains, but the concept of equipoise is not entirely straightforward.[44–46] Also, in extremis, patients' desires can be strong for a treatment not yet known to be (in)effective rather than a treatment known to be ineffective (or placebo). It is not at all clear that this desire is irrational or unethical.

If the intervention being tested is for a rare disease or condition, comparative trials are somewhat controversial, because of the difficulty in enrolling 'sufficiently many' patients for a prospective trial. Alternative methods for testing interventions in this case do exist, but they are subject to some technical controversy. Ethically, the main worry is that these difficulties may lead to therapies not being tested in these areas, or being developed very slowly, thus harming the interests of the affected patients.[47]

Recruitment

It is sometimes argued that regulation of clinical trials has unwittingly harmed the interests and the health of some groups by over-representing some groups and under-representing others. For example, some regulations exclude some or all women from some trials which would be beneficial to them, on the grounds of possible harms to future or actual fetuses.[48,49] In the US healthcare funding context, it is thought by some authors that the urban poor are unfairly exposed to the risks of trials, because they are enrolled into trials as a cheap form of treatment.[50,51] Some authors argue that not only are there injustices in trial management which should be addressed through recruitment which is 'socially representative', but that these injustices also bias the studies, making their results ungeneralisable. For instance, if a drug whose main users will be women is not tested on women, then it could be that the results of the study regarding safety or effectiveness may not apply to just the situations the drug will be used in most.[52,53] The same argument is applicable to some paediatric therapies, where recruitment may be difficult or impossible.

Consent in Principle

While informed consent has been a cornerstone of medical research ethics since the seminal Nuremberg Code, and while the obligation to seek consent is very widely established in law, the status of consent has been controversial in the past, and occasionally continues to be so.[54] Most writers argue that the moral foundation of the importance of informed consent is two-fold: it protects the subject from exploitation and harm, and ensures respect for the patient's autonomy. The status of autonomy as a moral cultural universal is not clear, however, and there is evidence that autonomy is less prized in some cultures than in the West.[55–57] It is arguable that some cultures treat women, for instance, as incompetent to give full consent, in the same way that we regard children or the mentally ill as incompetent. Also, autonomy might imply individualism, but it is well known that many cultures regard decision-making as hard, or impossible, without consultation with the family or other social grouping.[58,59] So there is some debate about whether informed consent is not a universal human right at all. In fact, we regard this argument as misleading because although autonomy may be more or less important than it is widely believed to be, the role of consent as a protective test remains unchallenged as a principle.

Informed Consent in Practice

In practice, however, informed consent continues to be challenged – the number of situations where it can be set aside for some reason is growing. The old argument that patients cannot consent because they do not know any medicine still attracts some attention.[60,61] Much more significant are arguments that patients are not able to give *free* consent due to lack of understanding (of language, or of the explanation given), due to the power relations implicit in the medical situation, or due to their own anxiety or desperation.[62,63] The argument that the requirement to obtain consent harms patients, by creating anxiety, is often raised, as is the argument that patients have a right to know only as much as they want to know.[64,65] In some branches of medicine it is claimed that the consent requirement holds up valuable research or even prevents it (in emergency medicine, perhaps). Finally, there is the argument that consent is at best a pious fiction because it implies a real choice where in fact the patient may have – or believe themselves to have – no real alternatives.[66,67]

IMPLICATIONS FOR METHODOLOGISTS

The area of RCT ethics is controversial, and it can sometimes be difficult to disentangle arguments of different kinds, and to distinguish arguments, which are susceptible to evidence, from prejudices which, generally, are not. In the previous sections these arguments were briefly stated. These arguments are now critically examined, and we draw out the consequences for good practice in RCT methodology.

RCT Methodology in Principle and Practice

There is a literature debating the necessity of randomisation and comparison for the testing and evaluation of therapies. Does randomisation defeat the influence of known and unknown 'confounders'? The importance of this debate is that a trial involving human subjects, and exposing them to some degree (even if tiny) of risk, can only be ethical if it has a good prospect of reaching its goal: knowledge. Unscientific or unsound experimentation is unethical. The debate about the necessity for randomisation under a Bayesian philosophy of inference is continuing, but it is worth noting that most practising Bayesian statisticians use randomisation.[68,69] It is safe to say, then, that the weight of scientific opinion supports randomisation, and so that the RCT remains the method of choice. However what is not clear is the *degree* to which alternative methodologies are less reliable, and the usual rhetoric of 'gold standard' methods is not helpful.[70,71]

A second strand of the controversy concerns the degree to which RCT methodology relies on a philosophy of inference which makes impossible early termination of trials when there is clear evidence of benefit or harm. This is a technical issue, beyond the scope of this article, but which has clear ethical relevance. In this area, the controversy is resolved just by constructing reliable stopping rules.[72]

So randomisation as such presents some scientific issues, out of which ethical issues grow. Yet most ethical worries about randomisation and controlled comparison arise through failure of understanding of the way the method works, and of the initial requirements of cognitive equipoise and proportionality of risk and benefit within each arm of the trial.

We can distinguish consequentialist and deontological approaches to the ethics of RCTs. Consequentialists will usually be satisfied by the arguments just rehearsed to the effect that the RCT method is reliable and superior to the alternatives; once it is granted that drugs and other interventions require testing in the interests of improving treatment and ensuring safety, it is clear that one should use the best available method. Consequentialists will then concentrate their attention on particular features of the trial in question, rather than on the methodology as such.

The open question which remains is whether the superiority of the RCT method is irrelevant because it breaches some prima facie duty, right, or theological imperative. The chief difficulty which RCT ethics presents in the light of this question is the apparent conflict between duties to (and rights of) present patients and the needs of society. Patients might have a duty to society, especially if society shares the cost of treatment.[73,74] The combined rights of future patients might deserve consideration.[75] Giving one group of patients something which no one else can have, even if blinding means we cannot know which group this is, is apparently unfair either to the recipient group because it is in fact less good than the alternative, or to everyone else because it is better. This apparent problem collapses when one considers that we have no reliable knowledge of harm or benefit unless and until we have a trial to find out. However, this non-problem can be a difficult political issue. It has sometimes been argued that patients should be able to choose which treatment they receive. Various methods which honour patient preferences have been tried. It is not clear that patient preferences can be honoured without introducing bias. In addition, whether patients have a right to specify which treatment they shall receive is still debated.[25–28] Of course they have a right to refuse treatment, and a right to refuse to enter a trial without incurring any penalty, such as less good treatment than is standard.[76]

This area is difficult, and one strategy for responding to patient preferences may be to help patients to understand why clinical equipoise exists regarding the treatments in the trial, and therefore why there is a trial at all. Another strategy may be to help patients define their own end points – what they want to get out of the trial.[77,78] Either of these techniques may overcome the initial difference of perception and interest. Whether it is right to seek to change people's preferences in the interests of successful trial management remains a difficult question.

Finally, evidence about the attitudes of particular religious or cultural groups to the RCT methodology as such was considered. We discovered some evidence that certain groups have an objection to human experimentation, but that the nature of this objection is of lack of trust in the experimenters, and so if this trust can be remade, the objection would disappear.[19,30] Contrary to our initial hypothesis, we found no evidence that any religion has an objection to randomisation. Some cultural groups have difficulty in accepting equipoise, because they have difficulty respecting the doctor who claims ignorance on some important medical matter.[55,56] This objection surfaces more visibly in the context of consent in particular trials.

Representation and Recruitment

By far the bulk of the evidence for the importance of socio-cultural factors in RCTs concerns
problems of recruitment. This is not surprising.
It would be surprising if there were well-defined
cultural or religious responses to the RCT methodology, which is both relatively new and (for
most people) rather a recherché topic. Instead,
objections usually arise and are defined, when
individuals first face recruitment into a trial (or
if they have had – or their community has had –
bad experiences in the past).[6,18]

Recruitment problems originate in the selection criteria of the study, so it is crucial that
these be scientifically sound. These are defined
in the first instance with reference to a population of possible research subjects, which will be
the same as a subset of the population of possible such patients. When it is necessary to
define the research population as a proper subset
of the defined patient population, it is crucial
that this subset be identified by relevant and
specific biomedical characters. Subjects should
not be excluded on grounds which are irrelevant
to the testing of the intervention – for instance,
social grounds. In most cases, exclusion of
adults on the basis of age, nationality or ethnicity, or gender cannot be justified, as these
have no biomedical correlate which is relevant
to the trial's validity.[79]

It is sometimes argued that drawing patients
at random from this defined population is insufficient to protect against overt, covert, or unintended discrimination, and so it is necessary to
have an active policy for ensuring a socially
representative sample. It should be noted that
sometimes whole social groups are excluded
from the population of research subjects on
spurious grounds (for example women of child-
bearing age). This should certainly attract the
attention of Research Ethics Committees, who
should want to know the justification for the
inclusion and exclusion criteria of the study. But
beyond this, the approach to preventing discrimination in therapeutic drug trials through sample
construction on 'social' criteria rather than on
medically well-founded principles is most unreliable and cannot be justified. Instead, proper
care should be taken to ensure that the recruitment mechanism is free of sampling bias, and
that it does not erect artificially discriminating
barriers to recruitment. For example, it may be
that certain disadvantaged groups have difficulty
in accessing relevant trials because of transport
costs. This can be addressed by trial managers.
The complementary worry would be that this
would result in 'over-recruitment' of the socially

vulnerable, and the question of when overcoming 'inconvenience' turns into 'inducement'
is hard to answer.[20,80,81]

While all of these concerns about recruitment
and representativeness are important, in practice
most of the methodological aspects of recruitment should be picked up at the peer review
stage, and at the Research Ethics Committee
stage. Fairness in assignment to arms of the trial
is achieved through adequately concealed randomisation; provided that the population is
fairly and scientifically defined, and provided
that the recruitment process is unbiased, then
inside the trial discrimination is prevented. The
reason why representativeness is an issue at all
is in part historical and in part geographical.
Historically, studies have been done which have
not had sound and fair definitions of the population: this has created some distrust: this can be
addressed by researchers improving their public
profile and being explicit about the criteria used
to construct studies.[18,19,50] The geographical factor is harder to address. All research takes place
somewhere, so necessarily will draw on the
population near to its centre or centres.[31,32] This
can mean that some populations are habitually
exposed to more research recruitment exercises
than others. Unfair exclusion or inclusion can
arise – unfair access to 'state-of-the-art treatment' or unfair exposure to 'experimental risks'.
This is true on all scales, from the most local to
the geopolitical. Globally, some populations are
targeted because of lower administrative costs,
or laxer views on the need for consent.[36,37]

Similarly, there is a question of equity in the
setting of research priorities. Where does the
money go in healthcare and medical research?
There is a widespread worry that it goes toward
the diseases widespread in well-off populations,
and toward cures that involve high technology
and long courses of treatment. This worry is
hard to substantiate (and is beyond the scope of
this chapter), but it is certainly plausible. In
AIDS research, it is clear that the demand for
treatment is very high in Africa, so that Africa
makes an excellent context for experimental
testing. However, the expense of the treatment is
very high, and so the purchasers of the licensed
treatments will be not Africans, but the wealthy
West. Justice insists that subjects in these
studies should continue to receive the treatment,
if they wish, after the completion of the trial.
But the majority still will have no access to
treatment during or after the trial. Arguably,
African populations take on much of the risk of
this research, while receiving very little of the
benefit.

This last issue is clearly political, rather than
methodological. But methodologists need to
keep issues of justice in mind, as well as their

more familiar constraints (time, money, and complexity), when they define research populations. A clear threat to the viability of research is presented by the possibility that a whole population may decide that it is being treated as a population of guinea pigs used for others' benefit.

Consent

The issues surrounding recruitment to trials bite at the point where potential subjects are asked to consent to their participation in the trial. There is an enormous literature on consent. Most of it is highly repetitive; we found 340 hits, but could use only 43 articles as contributing new material. Much of the literature addressed difficulties in obtaining consent; modifications, or exceptions, to the consent test; a lot concerns difficulties in obtaining consent; some concerns methods for obtaining consent; the psychological mechanisms and effects of consent; and whether consent is a culturally variable phenomenon are also considered. It was found helpful to distinguish among the barriers to consent in practice, before identifying whether there were 'in principle' culturally based objections to the consent test, because there is much more evidence concerning the former.

Barriers to consent in practice

The principal barrier to consent is – of course – not asking for it! From time to time studies do come to light where consent was not sought. Generally this occurs where for some reason it is believed that seeking consent would be 'harmful' to patients, or where seeking consent is pragmatically difficult or impossible.[60,82] Occasionally, consent is not sought for research (although it is sought for the intervention), because the difference between research and ordinary practice (especially between research and audit) may not be clear, even to the investigators themselves.[83] However, informed consent remains the paramount requirement for ethical research. So the main barriers to consent lie in the nature of 'informing' the patient. These barriers to consent depend on failures of understanding. The patient may fail to understand that they have a choice; and that they have a right to be treated well, even if they refuse consent. They may not understand the concepts in the research, such as the concept of the trial method, or of the therapies under test. And they may not understand the language used to seek consent. Linguistic barriers (for instance, access to translators) are easiest to resolve. Research Ethics Committees are now well practised in ensuring that patient information sheets are clearly and simply written. So the major worry and barrier to true informed consent remains the 'social distortions' present in the medical situation.[63]

A conversation between a patient and a doctor may be very unequal, because of the vulnerability of the patient due to illness, because of the belief that the doctor knows best (or at any rate more than the patient) about diagnosis and treatment, and – commonly – because there is a difference in education and social status.[62] This can make the seeking of consent a complex and unreliable process, because of the different expectations the parties bring to the consent procedure. This difference in expectation can be greatly increased when cultural differences in expectation about medicine and the role of the doctor are present. There is good evidence that in many non-Western societies a greater degree of authority or frank paternalism is expected by both patient and doctor. In trials, this can mean that the requirement of equipoise can be understood as an admission of ignorance, and hence of incompetence.[55,56] In practice, this misunderstanding must be overcome, because consent must be insisted on in the interests of protecting patients.

Consent as a cultural principle

As noted, there is evidence that consent is not universally accepted as a primary component of the medical relationship. But is this a matter of ethical principle, or more a matter of cultural convention? In other words, does any culture have explicit objections to consent, either in general, or for particular classes of subjects? Note that the legal and conceptual identification of competence and capacity to give consent underpins Western 'commonsense' exceptions to the consent principle of young children, the mentally ill or disabled, and (sometimes) prisoners, and even students and employees of the researcher. Do other cultures have the same exclusion classes? Historically, it would appear so – prisoners were once thought ideal 'volunteers' for human subjects research.[6] It is also rumoured occasionally that some cultures hold women to be incompetent to give consent to their own treatment, though we found no evidence for this, and in practice this belief – in the absence of firm evidence to support it – is flatly racist.

One cultural factor which has an impact on consent is the existence of certain groups (such as the Maori of New Zealand) which have a strong collectivist ethos, and which have historically been harmed by the dominance of other groups' interests. In New Zealand, any research which involves Maoris as subjects must be scrutinised by the Maori community, and the community as a whole must give its consent before individuals' consent can be sought. Philosophically, the force of a 'group consent' is rather controversial, but politically it is a necessity in that cultural and historical context, and is widely accepted.[84-86]

Another important cultural factor is the family. In many societies, individuals will always consult with their family before making a decision, and may in fact be unable to make a decision with which they feel happy unless they can so consult. Individuals may even reverse their own judgement if their family disagrees with them. Autonomy-centred cultures (like those of Northern Europe) may find this peculiar or suspicious. Families can be as coercive as any other institution,[87] but most recent research indicates that the role of the family is beneficial, in that it helps the patient to decide what their best interests actually are.[58]

In sum, it appears from the evidence we have on consent that no culture actually disputes or disregards its importance. But we could distinguish between broader and narrower understandings of what consent involves. On the narrow understanding, all that matters is voluntary agreement to the suggested intervention, and this is what is envisaged in the Nuremberg Code. On the broad understanding, what matters is autonomous, that is, self-determining, choice of the intervention: a decision that this is what I want, rather than the more passive agreement to do what you recommend. The broad understanding is not culturally universal, and different understandings involving family, community, priest or expert authority take its place. What is universal is the importance of the narrow understanding of consent. Difficulties exist in establishing that the decision is voluntary (that is, that it does not rest on a misunderstanding or on implied coercion). However, a voluntary decision is required and, except in extreme situations (clearly specified in advance) it is not to be negotiated away.[88,89]

Implications for Health Service Staff and Practitioners

All of the above remarks, which are aimed at triallists and methodologists involved in the design of research, apply equally to health service staff and practitioners. For instance, ways to incorporate families into the decision-making process, for example, by allowing the patient several days to consider trial entry, while maintaining that the final decision is the patient's, must be borne in mind. Sensitivity to cultural variation and its impact on patients' needs,

wants and attitudes must be encouraged.[90] Most of all, good practice must recognise that refusals and consents are similar in nature: both involve a similar mixture of reflection on evidence, judgement of interests, cultural background, socio-economic situation and past (individual or community) experience. Some 'consents' may be more worrying than some refusals, if what the 'consent' rests on is a misunderstanding of the recruitment proposal. The main finding of this study is that it is not possible simply to separate out a 'cultural factor' in ethics of clinical trials which can be dealt with, or ignored, simply and apart from addressing educational, communication and political 'barriers to participation'.

Justice must be the main area of concern. There is little convincing evidence of any systematic cultural objection to the RCT in general, or to particular RCTs in practice. Naturally it is good practice to be sensitive to cultural differences when implementing health services and providing healthcare, though many of the relevant differences do not apply specifically to clinical trials, but rather to scientific medicine as such. Certain cultures have long-established, and significantly different, philosophies of medicine. To the extent that individuals from this cultural background choose Western methods of care, this is an indication of at least a provisional acceptance of the methods used for applying and establishing the relevant medical techniques. Moreover, individuals are increasingly sophisticated in deciding which types of medicine they will use and in which circumstances they will use them.[91] This applies to members of all cultures who live in contemporary multicultural society. Given all of this, the objections to trial methodology and to particular trials, and the ethical sensibilities that such objections express, which must receive most attention in healthcare practice, are those which are social and economic in nature.

Issues of justice in healthcare are now at the top of most agendas, both in academic medical ethics and in health services practice. A large literature now exists on rationing and resource allocation. However, very little attention has been focussed on priority setting for research and health technology assessment. It is clearly important for health services planning and priority setting that fair resource allocation should keep one eye on the medium term, as well as on this year's issues. Research should be targeted to address present and future need trends. This would directly address the worry that much clinical research may unjustly focus on highest visibility conditions, rather than on highest need conditions. The 'Health of the Nation' and 'Our

Healthier Nation' initiatives in the United Kingdom are examples of how research could be prioritised. But there is also the complementary worry that the utilitarian focus on greatest need may lead to 'rare conditions' receiving too little attention.

Related to this issue of justice in targeting trials, is the issue of justice to participants after the trial. Many triallists arrange for participants to continue to receive the treatment free after the completion of the trial, and patients may receive treatments on a 'named patient' basis if the treatment seems to do them good, even if the trial indicates that in general the treatment is unsafe or ineffective. These are only fair. Just governance of trials may require this in general, where at present this is only an occasional practice.

The main area where justice considerations apply is in the definition of population and in selection of subjects. This is primarily an issue for triallists, but health service managers and referring physicians not directly participating in trials should also be aware of the concerns raised above.

While the main onus of ethical trial practice falls on the triallists, the burden of ensuring that ethical standards are established and maintained belongs to Local and Multi-centre Research Ethics Committees (or Institutional Review Boards). Research Ethics Committees are very experienced in considering whether proper mechanisms exist for obtaining informed consent, in obtaining assessments of the scientific validity of the trial, and in scrutinising the risks and benefits of the trial to participants. Two areas where they are less sure-footed are the assessment of inclusion and exclusion criteria for fairness and statistical soundness, and awareness of the relevance of socio-cultural factors to their deliberations. The first issue could usefully be addressed by ensuring that Committees either have a statistician member or ready access to statistical support. Such support may need to be independent of the Research and Development Support Units often used by researchers in designing their studies. Both issues can be addressed by appropriate training, and by contact (perhaps through the Community Health Councils or their equivalents) with community groups in their area. It is worth noting that one of the few reasons a Local Research Ethics Committee can withhold approval from a study approved by a Multi-centre Research Ethics Committee is the existence of particular local factors. These local factors will in practice be precisely the social and cultural issues discussed in this chapter, because it is these factors (rather than general ethical issues) which are *local*.

SUGGESTIONS FOR FUTURE RESEARCH

As we have made clear throughout, the evidence in this area is patchy, and all conclusions have had to be tentative. So there is a clear need for good-quality research into all the areas raised in this chapter. The present state of academic knowledge of non-Western ethical traditions regarding medicine is weak. Research into these traditions is needed, but in principle little such research will bear on the topic of this chapter, simply because of the historical novelty of clinical trial methodology. A more appropriate form of research would involve a focussed dialogue with representatives and authorities of these traditions, cultures and communities, to determine their responses to health services research methodology. A second key area for research is the development of tools for just priority setting in research and technology assessment. Additionally, health technology assessments typically acknowledge the need for social and ethical 'impact assessment' of the assessed technology, but there is little consensus on what this is and how it is to be achieved. Finally, existing research into consent should continue: much attention has been given to addressing researchers' problems (poor recruitment rates, lack of understanding by patients, poor recall of the detail of consent after the fact, and so on). Less attention has been paid to why patients join or refuse to join trials, although altruism is often hypothesised, and compliance rates are much studied as part of the trial analysis itself. Because there is little attention to the decision-making of patients it is hard to interpret refusals; and it is refusals which indicate objections, and objections which have been – perforce – our main source of relevant data drawn from the studies reviewed in this chapter. It is too early to say whether there are in fact cultural objections to trials, but it is clear that the social and economic context of a trial has a large impact on its success, and is a major component in the ethical status and public acceptability of the trial.[1]

ACKNOWLEDGEMENTS

This chapter is partly based on work presented in Ashcroft RE, Chadwick DW, Clark SRL, Edwards RHT, Frith L, Hutton JL, 'Implications of Socio-cultural contexts for ethics of clinical trials'. *Health Technology Assessment*, 1997; 1(9).[1] This work was funded by NHS R&D

Health Technology Assessment programme grant 93/41/4. Dr Ashcroft thanks Professors Chadwick, Clark, and Edwards, Ms Frith and Dr Hutton (the lead applicant) for their encouragement and backing.

REFERENCES

1. Ashcroft RE, Chadwick DW, Clark SRL, Edwards RHT, Frith L, Hutton JL. Implications of socio-cultural contexts for ethics of clinical trials. *Health Technology Assessment* 1997; **1**(9).
2. Hill AB. Medical ethics and controlled trials. *Br. Med. J.* 1963; **1**: 1043–9.
3. Levine RJ. *Ethics and regulation of clinical research.* Baltimore: Urban & Schwarzenberg, 1986.
4. Beauchamp TL, Childress JF. *Principles of biomedical ethics*, 4th ed. Oxford: Oxford University Press, 1994.
5. Epstein S. Democratic science? AIDS activism and the contested construction of knowledge. *Socialist Rev.* 1991; **21**: 35–64.
6. Rothman DJ. Ethics and human experimentation: Henry Beecher revisited. *N. Engl. J. Med.* 1987; **317**: 1195–9.
7. Cochrane AL. *Effectiveness and efficiency: random reflections on health services.* London: Nuffield Provincial Hospitals Trust, 1971.
8. Hutton JL. The ethics of randomised controlled trials: a matter of statistical belief? *Health Care Analysis* 1996; **4**: 95–102.
9. Palmer CR. Ethics and statistical methodology in clinical trials. *J. Med. Ethics* 1993; **19**: 219–22.
10. Urbach P. The value of randomisation and control in clinical trials. *Statist. Med.* 1993; **12**: 1421–41.
11. Papineau D. The virtues of randomisation. *Br. J. Philos. Sci.* 1994; **45**: 712–15.
12. Thornton H. Clinical trials – a brave new partnership? *J. Med. Ethics* 1994; **20**: 19–22.
13. Baum M. Clinical trials – a brave new partnership: a response to Mrs Thornton. *J. Med. Ethics* 1994; **20**: 23–5.
14. McPherson K. The best and the enemy of the good: randomised controlled trials, uncertainty and assessing the role of patient choice in medical decision-making. *J. Epidemiol. Community Health* 1994; **48**: 6–15.
15. Llewellyn-Thomas HA, McGreal MJ, Thiel EC, Fine S, Erlichman C. Patients' willingness to enter clinical trials: measuring the association with perceived benefit and preference for decision participation. *Soc. Sci. Med.* 1991; **32**: 35–42.
16. McNeill PM. *The ethics and politics of human experimentation.* Cambridge: Cambridge University Press, 1993.
17. Roberson NL. Clinical trial participation: viewpoints from racial/ethnic groups. *Cancer* 1994; **74**: 2687–91.
18. Dula A. African American suspicion of the healthcare system is justified: what do we do about it? *Cambridge Q. Healthcare Ethics* 1994; **3**: 347–57.
19. Gamble VN. A legacy of distrust: African Americans and medical research. *Am. J. Prevent. Med.* 1993; **9**(suppl. 3): 35–8.
20. Winn RJ. Obstacles to the accrual of patients to clinical trials in the community setting. *Semin. Oncol.* 1994; **21**(suppl. 7): 112–17.
21. Sperber AD, Henkin Y, Shanty S. Methodological issues in conducting a community-based clinical drug trial. *Family Practice Res. J.* 1993; **13**: 311–21.
22. French GR. When manufacturers are unwilling to accept the risks or invest the capital: vaccine production by the Salk Institute to the specification of the US army. *AIDS Research and Human Retroviruses* 1994; **10**(suppl. 2): S309.
23. Hutton JL, Ashcroft RE. What does 'systematic' mean for reviews of methodology? In: Black N, Brazier J, Fitzpatrick R, Reeves B (eds). *Methods for Health Care Research: A Guide to Best Practice.* London: BMJ Books, 1998: 249–54.
24. Mike V. Philosophers assess randomised clinical trials: the need for dialogue. *Controlled Clinical Trials* 1989; **10**: 244–53.
25. Zelen M. Randomised consent designs for clinical trials: an update. *Statist. Med.* 1990; **9**: 645–56.
26. Altman DG, Whitehead J, Parmar MKB, Stenning SP, Fayers PM, Machin D. Randomised consent designs in cancer clinical trials. *Eur. J. Cancer* 1995; **31A**: 1934–44.
27. Logue G, Wear S. A desperate solution: individual autonomy and the double-blind controlled experiment. *J. Med. Philos.* 1995; **20**: 57–64.
28. Angell M. Patients' preferences in randomised clinical trials. *N. Engl. J. Med.* 1984; **310**: 1385–7.
29. Mackie JL. *Ethics: Inventing right and wrong.* Harmondsworth: Penguin, 1977.
30. Alderson P. Trust in informed consent. *IME Bulletin* 1988: 17–19.
31. Lenhard RE Jr. A large private university hospital. *Cancer* 1993; **72**: 2820–3.
32. Freeman HP. The impact of clinical trial protocols on patient care systems in a large city hospital: access for the socially disadvantaged. *Cancer* 1993; **72**: 2834–8.
33. Christakis NA. Ethics are local: engaging cross-cultural variation in the ethics of clinical research. *Soc. Sci. Med.* 1992; **35**: 1079–91.
34. Davis DS. It ain't necessarily so: clinicians, bioethics and religious studies. *J. Clin. Ethics* 1994; **5**: 315–19.

35. Engelhardt HT JR. *The Foundations of Bioethics*, 2nd edn. Oxford: Oxford University Press, 1996.
36. Basch TF. Technology transfer to the developing world: does new technology have any relevance for developing countries? *Tubercle and Lung Disease* 1993; **74**: 353–8.
37. Maier-Lenz H. Implementing multicentre, multinational clinical trials. *Drug Information J.* 1993; **27**: 1077–81.
38. Enquselassie F, Nokes J, Cutts F. Communities' confidentiality should be maintained and community consent sought. *Br. Med. J.* 1996; **312**: 54–5.
39. O'Neil JD. The cultural and political context of patient dissatisfaction in cross-cultural encounters: a Canadian Inuit study. *Medical Anthropology Quarterly* 1989; **3**: 325–44.
40. Carrese JA, Rhodes LA. Western bioethics on the Navajo reservation: benefit or harm? *JAMA* 1996; **274**: 826–9.
41. Lockwood M, Anscombe GEM. Sins of Omission? The non-treatment of controls in clinical trials *Aristotelian Society* 1983; **Suppl. LVII**: 207–27.
42. DeHeyn PP, d'Hooge R. Placebos in clinical practice and research. *J. Med. Ethics* 1996; **22**: 140–6.
43. Rothman KJ, Michels KB. The continuing unethical use of placebo controls. *N. Engl. J. Med.* 1994; **331**: 394–8.
44. Freedman B. Equipoise and the ethics of clinical research. *N. Engl. J. Med.* 1987; **317**: 141–5.
45. Johnson N, Lilford RJ, Brazier W. At what level of collective equipoise does a clinical trial become ethical? *J. Med. Ethics* 1991; **17**: 30–4.
46. Alderson P. Equipoise as a means of managing uncertainty: personal, community and proxy. *J. Med. Ethics* 1996; **22**: 135–9.
47. Lilford RJ, Thornton JG, Braunholtz D. Clinical trials and rare diseases: a way out of a conundrum. *Br. Med. J.* 1995; **311**: 1621–5.
48. Merton V. The exclusion of the pregnant, pregnable and once-pregnable people (a.k.a. women) from biomedical research. *Am. J. Law & Medicine* 1993; **XIX**: 369–451.
49. Merkatz RB, Junod SW. Historical background of changes in FDA policy on the study and evaluation of drugs in women. *Academic Medicine* 1994; **69**: 703–7.
50. McCarthy CR. Historical background of clinical trials involving women and minorities. *Academic Medicine* 1994; **69**: 695–8.
51. Levinsky NG. Social, institutional and economic barriers to the exercise of patients' rights. *N. Engl. J. Med.* 1996; **334**: 532–4.
52. Dresser R. Wanted: single, white male for medical research. *Hastings Center Report* 1992; **22**: 24–9.
53. Mastroianni AC, Faden R, Federman D. Women and health research: a report from the Institute of Medicine. *Kennedy Institute of Ethics J.* 1994; **4**: 55–61.
54. Annas GJ, Grodin MA (eds). *The Nazi doctors and the Nuremberg Code: human rights in human experimentation.* Oxford: Oxford University Press, 1992.
55. Ishiwata R, Sakai A. The physician–patient relationship and medical ethics in Japan. *Cambridge Q. Healthcare Ethics* 1994; **3**: 60–6.
56. Sanwal AK, Kumar S, Sahni P, Nundy P. Informed consent in Indian patients. *J. R. Soc. Med.* 1996; **89**: 196–8.
57. Levine RJ. Informed consent: some challenges to the universal validity of the Western model. *Law, Medicine and Healthcare* 1991; **19**: 207–13.
58. Nelson HL, Nelson JL. *The patient in the family: an ethics of medicine and families.* London: Routledge, 1995.
59. Zion D. Can communities protect autonomy? Ethical dilemmas in HIV preventative drug trials. *Cambridge Q. Healthcare Ethics* 1995; **4**: 516–23.
60. Tobias JS, Souhami RL. Fully informed consent can be needlessly cruel. *Br. Med. J.* 1993; **307**: 1199–201.
61. Thornton H. Many subjects in trial were not asked for consent. *Br. Med. J.* 1996; **312**: 509.
62. Alderson P. Consent and the social context. *Nursing Ethics* 1995; **2**: 347–50.
63. Habermas J. *Communication and the evolution of society.* London: Heinemann Educational, 1979.
64. Silverman WA. The myth of informed consent in daily practice and in clinical trials. *J. Med. Ethics* 1989; **15**: 6–11.
65. Lilleyman JS. Informed consent: how informed and consent to what? *Pediat. Hematol. Oncol.* 1995; **12**(6): xiii–xvi.
66. Burchell HB. Vicissitudes in clinical trial research: subjects, participants, patients. *Controlled Clinical Trials* 1992; **13**: 185–9.
67. Brownlea A. Participation: myths, realities and prognosis. *Soc. Sci. Med.* 1987; **25**: 605–14.
68. Berry DA. A case for Bayesianism in clinical trials. *Statist. Med.* 1993; **12**: 1377–404.
69. Whitehead J. The case for frequentism in clinical trials. *Statist. Med.* 1993; **12**: 1405–19.
70. Schulz KF, Chalmers I, Hayes RJ, Altman DG. Empirical evidence of bias: dimensions of methodological quality associated with estimates of treatment effects in controlled trials. *JAMA* 1995; **273**: 408–12.
71. D'Agostino RB, Kwan H. Measuring effectiveness: what to expect without a randomised control group. *Medical Care* 1995; **33**: AS95–AS105.
72. Berry DA. Interim analyses in clinical trials: classical versus Bayesian approaches. *Statist. Med.* 1985; **4**; 521–6.
73. Caplan AL. Is there a duty to serve as a subject in biomedical research? In: *If I were a rich man,*

could I buy a Pancreas? And other essays on the ethics of healthcare. Bloomington: Indiana University Press, 1992.

74. Emson HE. Rights, duties and responsibilities in healthcare. *J. Appl. Philos.* 1992; **9**: 3–11.

75. Parfit D. *Reasons and Persons.* Oxford: Oxford University Press, 1984.

76. Nuremberg Code and Helsinki Declaration, both reprinted in Annas and Grodin, op. cit. (54).

77. Fox R. What do patients want from medical research? *J. R. Soc. Med.* 1996; **89**: 301–2.

78. Kee F. Patients' prerogatives and perceptions of benefit. *Br. Med. J.* 1996; **312**: 958–60.

79. Ashcroft RE. Human research subjects, selection of. In: Chadwick R (ed.), *Encyclopedia of Applied Ethics.* San Diego: Academic Press, 1997, vol. 2: 627–39.

80. Antman K. Reimbursement issues facing patients, providers and payers. *Cancer* 1993; **72**: 2842–5.

81. Royal College of Physicians. Research involving patients: summary and recommendations. *J. R. Coll. Physicians* 1990; **24**: 10–14.

82. Karlawish JHT, Hall JB. The controversy over emergency research: a review of the issues and suggestions for a resolution. *Am. J. Resp. Crit. Care Med.* 1996; **153**: 499–506.

83. Reiser SJ. Criteria for standard versus experimental care. *Health Affairs* 1994; **13**: 127–36.

84. Campbell AV, Charlesworth M, Gillett G, Jones G. *Medical Ethics,* 2nd edn. Oxford: Oxford University Press, 1997.

85. Verdun-Jones S, Weisstub DN. Consent to human experimentation in Quebec: the application of the civil law principle of personal inviolability to protect special populations. *Int. J. Law Psychiatry* 1995; **18**: 163–82.

86. Kymlicka W. *Liberalism, Community and Culture.* Oxford: Oxford University Press, 1989.

87. Anonymous. The case of the coercive family. *Cambridge Q. Healthcare Ethics* 1995; **5**: 135–42.

88. Jonas H. Philosophical reflections on experimenting with human subjects. *Daedalus* 1969; **98**: 219–47.

89. Fethe C. Beyond voluntary consent: Hans Jonas on the moral requirements of human experimentation. *J. Med. Ethics* 1993; **19**: 99–103.

90. Gostin LO. Informed consent, cultural sensitivity and respect for persons *JAMA* 1995; **274**: 844–5.

91. Bhopal RS. The interrelationship of folk, traditional and western medicine within an Asian community. *Soc. Sci. Med.* 1986; **22**: 99–105.

3

Factors that Limit the Number, Progress and Quality of Randomised Controlled Trials: A Systematic Review

SUE ROSS, CARL E. COUNSELL,
WILLIAM J. GILLESPIE, ADRIAN M. GRANT,
ROBIN J. PRESCOTT, IAN T. RUSSELL,
IAIN R. COLTHART, SANDRA KIAUKA,
DAPHNE RUSSELL and SUE M. SHEPHERD

SUMMARY

Background

The randomised controlled trial (RCT) is widely accepted as the most powerful research method for evaluating health technologies. However, randomised trials have often experienced difficulties in their conduct, meaning that the results have proved less than useful. We therefore carried out a systematic review with the following objectives:

(a) to assemble and classify a comprehensive bibliography of factors limiting the quality, number and progress of RCTs; and
(b) to collate and report the findings, identifying areas where firm conclusions can be drawn and areas where further research is necessary.

Results and Recommendations for Practice

Design issues

Following a systematic review of existing evidence, a well-formulated question should be developed, specifying participants, interventions and outcomes. Wide patient eligibility criteria are generally preferred to give representativeness and good recruitment rates. Outcome measures need to be clinically and socially relevant, well-defined, valid, reliable, sensitive to important change, and measured at appropriate times. The most common design is the simple parallel group design with a fixed sample size. Protection from selection bias is provided by secure random allocation, and by analysis based on the groups as allocated, thus ensuring that the groups being compared differ only by chance. Pre-study sample size calculations should always be made.

Barriers to participation

To overcome barriers to clinician recruitment, the trial should address an important research question, and the protocol and data collection should be as straightforward as possible. The demands on clinicians and patients should be kept to a minimum. Dedicated research staff may be required to support clinical staff and patients. The recruitment aspects of a RCT should be carefully planned and piloted.

Conduct and structure

Many trials fail to start, mainly because of lack of funding or logistical problems. Of those that start, half have difficulty with recruitment, leading to abandonment or reduced size and loss of statistical power. Recruitment problems may be reduced by piloting, using multiple recruitment strategies, making contingency plans in case recruitment is slow, and by using recruitment co-ordinators. Inadequate compliance with the study protocol can lead to false-negative or false-positive results. Some assessment of compliance (clinician and patient) should be made, but it can be difficult to measure. Trials need a good organisational and administrative base, but there is little research evaluating the optimal structure.

Analysis

Study protocols should identify a predetermined primary outcome supplemented by secondary outcomes and a clear statistical plan. Intention-to-treat analysis is the method of choice to provide an unbiased estimate of treatment effects.

Reporting

The introduction of the CONSORT guidelines should improve reporting of randomised trials. The conclusions of reports should be supported by the results. About 10% of trials remain unpublished, whilst many are published only as conference proceedings, particularly if the studies are small and show non-significant treatment effects: prospective registration of all trials is recommended. Multiple publication of the same study is also a problem for those showing significant results.

Costs

Few randomised trials report an economic evaluation, possibly because of difficulties in conducting such evaluations, and the lack of generalisability from one healthcare context to another. The use of statistical tests and confidence intervals can help. Little research has investigated trial costs, but the costs of caring for patients in randomised trials may be perceived as an unaffordable new service, delaying or preventing recruitment in some centres.

Conclusions

There is evidence available to guide many aspects of the design, conduct and analysis of randomised trials. However, the evidence is not always being applied.

The randomised controlled trial (RCT) is widely accepted as the most powerful research method for evaluating health technologies. Its principal strength is that it minimises bias – the misleading effect of systematic errors. Protection from 'selection bias' is provided by random allocation of patients to alternative technologies and analysis based only on those allocations. This ensures that the groups being compared differ only by chance. Assessing patient outcomes in ignorance of their treatment allocation avoids 'ascertainment bias'. RCTs minimise 'co-intervention bias', either by blinding patients and their doctors to their treatments, or by ensuring that the treatment of each group is essentially the same apart from the technology being evaluated.

These principles are generally recognised and understood by policy-makers, clinicians and researchers. Health service decision-makers are increasingly looking for evidence from RCTs. Indeed, many funding agencies now expect that RCTs should be used to compare alternative care regimes unless there is good reason for an alternative approach. Furthermore, systematic searching in electronic bibliographies and key journals has identified tens of thousands of RCTs covering most fields of healthcare. Nevertheless, most therapeutic activities lack enough reliable information from RCTs to draw firm conclusions. Why is this?

Firstly, health services have until recently failed to conduct and use systematic reviews of evidence. Recent initiatives need time to rectify this omission in full. Secondly, neither professionals nor public fully recognise the place of research within healthcare. But it is the quality of the design, conduct, analysis and reporting of RCTs on which this chapter focuses.

Trials often fail to address questions of current importance to healthcare systems, for many reasons. Technological developments may make irrelevant the results of RCTs assessing a previous treatment modality. The choice of comparators in many trials is dictated by the vested interests of funders, either commercial or charitable, or researchers. Generalisability may be limited by the choice of participants, sometimes so tightly defined that the results have little relevance in practice. End-points are often intermediate or surrogate, and of importance to researchers rather than patients.

Most RCTs are too small to identify the size of effect that might plausibly be expected. When there is no significant difference, the resulting estimate of the treatment effect is usually so imprecise that it is impossible to rule out a clinically important difference. There is therefore a high risk of drawing a false conclusion – that there is no difference when one does exist. Furthermore, reported differences may distort the truth as only large effects reach 'statistical significance' in small trials. The pooling of data through meta-analysis sometimes resolves this problem. Nevertheless, it needs great care and considerable effort, and the findings may be distorted by publication bias, inadequate reporting of trial methods, insecure random allocation, losses to follow-up, and failure to base analyses on the randomised groups.

These concerns about the design, conduct, analysis and reporting of RCTs led us to carry out a systematic review of the literature on trials with two main aims:

1 To assemble and classify a comprehensive bibliography of factors limiting the number, progress and quality of RCTs.
2 To collate and report the findings, identifying areas where firm conclusions can be drawn and areas where further research is necessary.

METHODS

We undertook a systematic review of the literature on trials, based on three bibliographic databases, Medline, Embase and CINAHL, covering the period 1986 to 1996. The scope of the review was too broad to be comprehensive in all of the areas covered. Rather, the review attempted to cover the diversity of factors limiting the quality, number and progress of RCTs.

The issues were considered under the following categories: design issues; barriers to participation; conduct; and structure; analysis; reporting; and costs. After initial screening of references identified electronically, all those English language references considered 'possibly relevant' were obtained. From each full text article, data were extracted on category of reference (as above), study methodology (primary research, reviews, other articles), subject area, intervention type, clinical activity (prevention, treatment, screening or diagnosis), and setting (hospital, general practice, or community). A scoring system was used to classify each article from 3, 'highly relevant', to 0, 'irrelevant', for each category. There was considerable overlap in relevant articles between categories, for example relevant articles for 'design' were often relevant for 'conduct'.

All references identified of relevance to individual subject areas were passed to the author responsible for that section of the review for synthesis. Methods of synthesis varied between sections depending on the type of material identified for that part of the review.

THE EVIDENCE AND IMPLICATIONS FOR METHODOLOGISTS

The literature identified for this methodological review differed in a number of important ways from reviews of effectiveness or efficacy. Firstly, theory needed to be given relatively more weight than empirical evidence, largely because there were many areas of the review where it was not possible to carry out empirical research. In other areas where evidence would have been expected, it was rare, and rigorous evidence even rarer. The 'best' method for recruiting patients to randomised trials provides an apt example. Whether we applied the criterion of effectiveness (p. 43) or that of cost effectiveness (p. 48), we were unable to make any clear recommendations based on comparative studies. This can be attributed both to the general lack of rigour in the published comparisons, none of which was experimental, and to the wide range of topics and contexts in which these comparisons were set. The variety of published material ensured that the character of each section of the review differed enormously: an introductory paragraph at the start of each section highlights the main features.

Design Issues

The evidence for this section tended not to be the outcome of empirical research, but rather the result of reviews of research methods and theoretical discussion. In addition, text books on trial design were considered, for example that by Pocock.[1] Using the evidence, various recommendations for trial design are proposed.

Defining participants, interventions and outcomes

We recommend that, following a systematic review of existing evidence, a relevant well-formulated question should be developed, specifying participants, interventions and outcomes. Wide patient eligibility criteria are generally preferred to give representativeness and good recruitment rates.[2,3] However, a more homogeneous group may be preferable when evaluating expensive or hazardous interventions. The choice of treatment and comparator should take into account the results of previous research and the objectives of the trial: the use of a placebo or active comparison treatment, and the need for a run-in phase should be considered. Several review articles considered outcome measures and recommended that they need to be clinically and socially relevant, well-defined, valid, reliable, sensitive to important change, and measured at appropriate times. For example, cancer prevention trials may require longer follow-up than treatment trials.[4] The establishment of a central core of sensitive outcome measures has been suggested for use in trials in rheumatoid arthritis.[5] Data should be collected by appropriately trained individuals on only a small number of outcomes, and complicated or irrelevant outcomes should be avoided.[6] There is evidence that the use of intermediate or surrogate outcomes has been misleading.[7]

Choice of design

The most frequent choice of study design is between a parallel group or a crossover design, although a crossover design is inappropriate if a carry-over effect is possible.[8] The simultaneous investigation of two or more treatments is efficiently approached by the use of a factorial design, although such studies are uncommon, for example, Silagy and Jewell found only 4% of trials published in the *British Journal of General Practice* used a factorial design.[9] The simple parallel group design with a fixed sample size was found to be the most common design in a number of reviews of published trials (for example, references 8 to 10), but other designs should be considered.

Randomisation and minimisation of bias

As discussed in the Introduction of this chapter, random allocation is crucial to minimise selection bias. In evaluating health technologies, randomisation is usually at the patient level, but for some topics may be at a different level, for example at general practice level.[11] (The additional considerations of 'cluster' trials were outwith the scope of this review.) Stratification may be used to ensure balance between treatment groups in respect of key prognostic variables, supplemented if necessary using randomised permuted blocks, or minimisation (a dynamic method of allocation which ensures balance with each possible allocation). Such approaches were advocated by a number of authors including Talley,[8] Taves,[12] and Altman and Dore.[13]

Protection from selection bias is provided by secure random allocation and by analysis based on the groups as allocated, thus ensuring that the groups being compared differ only by chance.[1] Schulz et al. noted that random number lists and sealed envelopes held by the clinician entering patients are not secure, and recommended that assignment codes should be drawn up by someone who has not been involved with patient recruitment.[14] Randomisation by contacting a central office, for example by telephone, is probably the best way to conceal allocation (recommended among others by Schulz et al.[14] and Chalmers et al.[15]). Schulz and co-authors also stressed the need for auditing the process of allocation to ensure adherence.[14] Performance bias can be minimised by blinding treatments (where possible) and by employing clearly described treatment policies. Detection bias may be avoided by blind outcome assessment, and attrition bias by ensuring follow-up of all patients randomised.

Sample size

Pre-study sample size calculations should always be made, based on four elements: the level of statistical significance which is sought; the risk of obtaining a non-significant result when a specified difference exists; the difference which it is important for the trial to be able to detect as significantly significant; and the expected variability of the response variable. Peto et al. noted that large trials are necessary to detect small but useful treatment effects: such effects are particularly important in common conditions.[16] Funding bodies, independent protocol review bodies and journal editors should all require provision of sample size calculations. Sample size calculations should consider a sensitivity analysis and give estimates rather than unrealistically precise numbers.[17] A number of authors, including Fayers and Machin[17] and Edwards and colleagues,[18] support the view that small trials should be reported as hypothesis-forming.

Barriers to Participation

The section on barriers to participation in trials took a different approach to the other sections, concentrating on empirical evidence of barriers. The quality of the material identified was variable. The nature of the issue lends itself to descriptive studies, such as surveys of participants and non-participants, and to qualitative research, such as case studies of failed trials. Such research is often retrospective, with the potential of merely justifying non-participation rather than explaining its causes. Some more 'rigorous' evaluations are included in the review, particularly those investigating different forms of patient information and consent. However, the results of these are of little practical applicability because they were designed to understand patient decision-making rather than to offer solutions for the conduct of research. Furthermore, the majority of papers are from cancer research, from the USA, and are hospital based: extrapolation of the findings to other clinical settings and geographical areas may not be ideal. Despite the limitations of the papers, many barriers to participation were indeed found. Synthesis of the material was into three major categories: barriers to clinician recruitment; barriers to patient recruitment; and the clinician as a barrier to patient recruitment.

Barriers to clinician participation

Lack of time was considered a major barrier in several studies, including the time pressures from usual clinical practice and management duties: such pressures may be increasing for clinicians.[19,20] The time demands of recruitment, the consent process, and follow-up in trials may be a further barrier.[19,21–24] Clinicians participating in clinical trials may be ill-prepared for a research role because of inadequate research experience,[20,25] training,[26] or clinical skills.[27] Lack of support staff, for example clinical trial nurses, has been blamed for poor clinician recruitment.[19,26–28]

Participation in RCTs may alter the doctor–patient relationship and concern about this may act as a barrier. The main issues highlighted by a number of authors were the difficulty for clinicians of admitting that they do not know which treatment is best[21,23,24] and the perceived conflict between the clinician role and research (or scientific) role.[27,29,30] As a result, some clinicians feel that their rapport with patients can be damaged by participation in a trial.[21,23,31]

Concern of the clinician for the patient may affect their decision to take part in a trial or not, including worry about treatment toxicity or side effects,[19,25] the burden of the trial for patients,[19,22,24,28,29] or a reluctance to recruit severely ill patients.[32] Benson and colleagues found that a fear of feeling responsible if the patient did not receive the treatment which turned out to be best deterred surgeons from taking part in a trial.[21]

Loss of clinical autonomy, including loss of decision-making power and independence, being accountable to a third party, and restriction of the ability to individualise patient care, were also causes for concern.[21,23,30,33] Obtaining consent can also be an important barrier to clinician participation.[21,23,24,31]

It is unclear whether lack of financial rewards is a deterrent to clinician participation.[19,28] Schaeffer and colleagues stressed the need for personal encouragement and support to achieve successful participation.[33]

Two studies mentioned the importance of the research question. Scientifically uninteresting trials were felt to be an impediment to recruitment by 17% of respondents in a survey by Ashery and McAuliffe.[19] One reason given for

Tognoni et al. for a failed trial was that the questions to be tested were not of sufficient interest to participating clinicians.[28]

Barriers to patient participation

The review confirmed that the additional demands of a study may cause concern for some patients, influence their decision to participate, and lead to later 'drop-out'. The main causes of concern were additional procedures and appointments which may cause discomfort, inconvenience or additional expense.[34–39] Travel and travel costs were unpopular with participants and were reasons for refusing to take part, for missing appointments and for 'dropping-out'.

A strong preference for, or against, a particular treatment (offered in the trial or outside it) can limit recruitment. Such preferences included a wish not to change medication,[40,41] not to take placebo,[35,42] not to take an 'experimental' medication, or not to take any medication.[41] Some patients requested a specific intervention.[35,38,42–44] Patients may choose not to take part in research at all,[29,37,44,45] or have an aversion to treatment choice by random allocation.[36,38,46]

Patients may find the issues of uncertainty difficult to cope with, particularly if they feel that the efficacy of the treatment on offer is unproven, and may have a distrust of hospital or medicine and fear the unknown.[41,47] Under such circumstances, they find it unpleasant to decide about taking part in a trial[48] and may even prefer the doctor to make the decision.[49]

Information and consent emerged as major concerns. Evidence about the provision of information on trials was conflicting, because patients – both participating and non-participating – wanted more information on trials,[39,40,48,50] although providing information may reduce recruitment and alter the response to treatment.[45,46,51] Many authors have recommended that the information should be simply presented, including Harth and Thong,[38] Bevan et al.,[42] Antman et al.,[47] Roberson[51] and Jensen et al.[52] For a more detailed discussion of trials of strategies for patient recruitment, see Chapter 1.

Clinician as barrier to patient participation

Atwood and colleagues[35] and Sutherland and colleagues[53] found that an 'important person' (e.g. spouse, family member, close friend) had a considerable influence on the decision to participate, with patients unlikely to participate if those close to them were against it. However, the doctor recruiting to the trial has been reported by many authors to have the greatest influence on the decision to enter a trial.[34,49,52] Clinicians themselves may therefore act as a barrier to patient recruitment, even in trials where they have agreed to take part. The protocol itself was blamed for restricting recruitment in several studies,[19,24,37,43,54,55] including incompatibilities of the protocol with usual clinical practice[21,23,29,56,57] or excessive and poorly designed data collection.[24,54]

Clinicians may find giving information difficult, when describing both clinical trials in general and specific trials,[29,57] with particular concerns about assessing the level of information required by patients.[23,27] Even amongst clinicians who have agreed to collaborate in a trial, the level of information and the process of obtaining consent vary.[58]

Recommendations for clinician and patient recruitment

The review set out to identify barriers to participation in trials, rather than strategies to overcome such barriers. The findings confirm results of previous reviews of the subject (for example by Hunninghake et al.[59] and Swanson and Ward[60]) suggesting that even though evidence is available on the topic, solutions have not been implemented. Despite the limitations of our review, it is possible to make recommendations from the findings.

To overcome problems with clinician recruitment, the RCT should address a question that is seen as important. The protocol should be clear and simple, with the minimum required of clinicians, and straightforward data collection. Where possible, dedicated research staff should be available to provide support and encouragement for the clinical staff. Pragmatic trial designs are likely to be more acceptable to clinicians, since this type of design permits more clinical freedom.

To overcome barriers to patient recruitment, the demands of the study should be kept to a minimum consistent with the scientific purpose of the study, with the extent and purpose of the study and investigations clearly explained. Patients should be supported in what may be a difficult decision to take part in a RCT, and should not be placed under pressure to do so. Dedicated research staff may help with providing information and obtaining patient consent, and monitoring the recruitment process. The recruitment aspects of a RCT should be carefully planned and piloted to avoid poor recruitment.

Conduct and Structure

Many of the original articles identified for this section simply reported problems and possible solutions experienced in individual trials, and most review articles were based on anecdotal evidence. Some more rigorous studies, including trials were also identified. From the articles, a number of problems were identified which can arise during the conduct of a trial, to prevent it starting, or limit its progress and quality, along with possible solutions.

Failure to start

There are no good data on the number of randomised trials that fail to start, however one survey by Easterbrook and Matthews of clinical studies which had received ethics approval found that 21% never started largely due to lack of funding, the principal investigator leaving the institution, logistic problems or expected recruitment problems.[20]

Poor recruitment

Recruitment is often a major problem in RCTs. Easterbrook and Matthews estimated that half of all clinical studies fail to reach their planned size.[20] A survey by Coombs and colleagues of recruitment amongst a cohort of 41 trials showed only 34% achieved or surpassed their planned size, whilst a further 34% recruited less than 75% of their planned size.[6] In addition to problems in the design (such as narrow inclusion criteria) and participation (discussed earlier), overestimating the pool of eligible patients or the recruitment rate, using too few recruitment strategies, and lack of active involvement of the staff in recruitment, have also been blamed.[59,61]

Poor recruitment can increase the cost of the study, or lead to its abandonment or reduced size and hence loss of statistical power.[19,20,59] In one trial, Neaton and co-workers found that poor recruitment led to falsification of recruitment.[62] Possible solutions suggested by various authors (for example by Ashery and McAuliffe[19] and Hunninghake et al.[59]) include careful planning and piloting of recruitment, use of multiple research strategies, close monitoring of recruitment (using recruitment logs), the use of recruitment co-ordinators, setting recruitment goals, having contingency plans in case of poor recruitment, and providing training in recruitment.

Early stopping

Trials may stop early because of logistical problems, because of the results of other similar trials, because the intervention being tested is superseded, or because interim analyses demonstrate unequivocal evidence of harm or benefit, or that the trial has little chance of showing a clinically important benefit.[20,63–65] Interim analyses should be planned, be based on good-quality data and use appropriate statistical tests and stopping guidelines to avoid inappropriate conclusions.[63–65] Any decision to stop a trial early should be based on clinical and ethical considerations, as well as statistical ones.[63–66]

Compliance

Poor compliance with a trial protocol either by the investigator or the patient can have important effects on the overall result, although the effects will vary depending on the intervention under study.[67] Investigators may recruit ineligible patients, prescribe prohibited medication, fail to prescribe or carry out the allocated treatment adequately, or transfer the patient from one arm of the trial to another (so-called crossovers).[68,69] Participants may take too much or too little medication, may take it at inappropriate intervals, may fail to attend for follow-up appointments, or fail to undergo certain tests.[68,70–72]

Poor compliance reduces the power of a trial to identify a treatment effect, resulting in the need for increased sample size or an increased risk of a false-negative or false-positive error.[73–75] It is therefore important to measure compliance to assess the risk of false-positive or -negative results and to evaluate acceptability of the treatment to patients.

However, compliance appears to be rarely assessed in trials,[67] perhaps due to difficulties in defining and measuring it.[72,71] Vander Stichele suggested defining patients as compliers, partial compliers, overusers, erratic users, partial drop-outs and drop-outs, but did not give clear definitions.[74] Measuring compliance with pharmacological treatments is possible, although all methods are flawed.[70–72,74,76] Defining and measuring compliance with non-pharmacological treatments is even more difficult.[77,78]

The effort expended on improving compliance depends on the type of trial: in explanatory or efficacy trials, compliance is essential; in pragmatic or clinical management trials, interested in assessing whether the treatment is effective for the average patient under circumstances that reflect real life, compliance should also reflect real life.[72,74] Several solutions have been proposed to improve compliance in trials: education about the trial; assessing compliance during a run-in period to exclude obvious non-compliers; simplifying treatment and follow-up regimens; and maintaining communication with participants by newsletter or telephone calls.[35,56,61] (For further discussion of trials-assessing methods to improve patient compliance with non-trial medications, see the recent review by Cochrane.[79])

Drop-outs and loss to follow-up

The results of a trial may be invalid if a large proportion of those randomised are excluded from analysis because of protocol violation, or are lost to follow-up. Surveys of the reporting of trial results have shown that trials often exclude a significant number of randomised patients from the analysis (for example, surveys by Rossetti et al.,[10] Liberati et al.,[80] Kleijnen et al.,[81] Solomon et al.,[82] Sonis and Joines,[83] Lionetto et al.,[84] Schulz et al.[85]). It is important to collect as many details as possible about the patient at the time of recruitment to help with follow-up, and tagging records in national registers may help.[86] Patients who withdraw from treatment, or who violate the protocol, should still be followed-up to allow an intention-to-treat analysis (see p. 45).

Blinding

During a trial any of the following individuals may be blinded to treatment allocation to reduce the risk of bias: the patient/participant, the healthcare professional, or the outcome assessor. It is not always possible to blind the patient or health professional, for example in surgical trials, but it is usually possible to blind the outcome assessor. In several 'double-blind' trials (where doctors and patients are supposed to have been unaware of treatment allocation), doctors and patients became unblinded during the trial because of treatment effects, side-effects, or the lack of them. Unblinding may lead to bias because the doctor may monitor or treat one group differently, or the patient's knowledge may affect the outcome:[87,88] unblinding the outcome assessor may also lead to bias.[89,90] We therefore suggest that outcome assessment should be blind wherever possible.

Quality assurance

It is extremely important that data collected and processed during a trial should be accurate.[91,92] Good clinical practice guidelines emphasise the need for quality assurance and audit throughout the study to identify fraudulent or careless practice.[91–93] However, high levels of quality assurance increase the administrative cost and workload of trials, and may not always be feasible.[94]

Collaboration and communication

Problems can arise in trials that require collaboration amongst a number of different health professionals and agencies, although these can usually be solved through good communication.[19] Inexperienced trialists should be supported by experienced trialists,[6] and the principal investigator should provide clear leadership through to the completion of the trial.[95] Multicentre trials provide additional problems with requirement for collaborators' meetings, site visits and possibly translation of trial material into appropriate languages.[95,96] Staff turnover at sites can hinder the progress of trials,[97] and the loss of the principal investigator can be particularly disruptive.[20]

Conflict of interest

Van Gijn and Bogousslavsky discussed the problems of conflict of interest.[93,98] Investigators can be involved in several trials simultaneously, and this could lead to conflict of interest, although it may be minimised if the inclusion criteria are clearly different. Commercially sponsored trials where investigators receive a large honorarium for each patient entered are likely to be given preference over unsponsored trials, and this may not be in the public interest. Bogousslavsky and van Gijn suggested that investigators should receive reimbursement only for the extra work involved in entering patients into the trial, and that no additional honoraria should be given. However, calculating the cost of this additional work may be difficult.

Organisational structure

Randomised controlled trials probably need to have a good organisational and administrative base to succeed, but little has been published about this. Large multi-centre trials need a Steering Committee with overall responsibility for the trial, a co-ordinating centre to handle materials, data collection and communication with trialists, a trial co-ordinator to run the co-ordinating centre, and a data monitoring committee.[95] Smaller trials probably need a scaled-down, but similar, structure. Some individuals may be on committees for several trials which could lead to conflicts of interest:[98] we did not identify research relating to this issue, or how members of Steering Committees or Data Monitoring Committees are selected.

The main role of the Data Monitoring Committee is to review planned interim analyses to see if there is accumulating evidence to suggest that the trial should be stopped early, or in some instances prolonged.[66] Data Monitoring Committees should be: independent from the trial and the sponsor, include experts from all necessary disciplines, have explicit terms of reference, have access to the necessary data, collaborate with other similar trials, and have appropriate resources.[64–66] However, Fleming and DeMets,

and Rockhold and Enas have argued that it is not feasible for all trials to have a Data Monitoring Committee due to the cost and lack of experienced statisticians and independent experts.[64,99] They recommend formal Data Monitoring Committees for large 'pivotal' trials, that is those measuring life-threatening end-points and those where there is the potential for serious side-effects. In other trials, interim analyses could be carried out by the trial statistician and principal investigator with the option of forming a Data Monitoring Committee if necessary.[66,99,100] Interim analyses should not be released to other investigators unless there are good reasons: evidence from a study by Green and colleagues suggested that open reporting of interim results was associated with declining recruitment, stopping trials without meeting defined objectives and early publication of results found later to be inconsistent with final results.[101]

The concern that involvement of a commercial sponsor in the design, data collection, analysis and reporting of a trial may lead to bias in favour of their product is difficult to substantiate. However, there are examples where bias has occurred, such as: the reporting of data from only favourable centres; the use of dosage regimens that favour the drug manufactured by the sponsor; and the reporting of conclusions that do not match the data presented.[94,102] This is particularly worrying since a survey from one region of the UK showed that 65% of trials are sponsored by the pharmaceutical industry.[103] Van Gijn recommended that pharmaceutical industry sponsored trials also required independent Steering Committees and Data Monitoring Committees.[93]

Analysis

Because of the variety of trial designs and types of data, discussion of analysis is limited to those areas which have attracted criticism in the literature, where empirical evidence leads us to make recommendations for practice. Hence important areas, such as discussion of the Bayesian and frequentist philosophies, are excluded. (For a full discussion of Bayesian and frequentist philosophies, see Chapter 16.)

Intention-to-treat analysis

The principle of 'intention-to-treat' analysis arises from randomised trials where, for a number of reasons, the treatment to which a patient is randomised might not be received, in full or part, by that patient. In these circumstances, there is a concern that those patients who do not receive the allocated treatment may well differ in some way from those who do receive it, and that the selection processes may differ between treatment groups. An analysis based on only those patients who received the treatment as randomised would therefore give a biased estimate of treatment differences. This bias can be mitigated by analysing according to the groups into which patients were randomised. If outcome observations are available on all patients, treatment comparisons are potentially unbiased (though of course bias may arise from some other aspect of the trial's design or conduct). Another advantage of intention-to-treat is that it mimics 'real life' with respect to errors in treatment and poor adherence to treatment, and gives a more realistic assessment of treatment policy.

The majority of papers dealing with general issues in the analysis of RCTs emphasise the importance of intention-to-treat analysis.[65,104] Studies by Peduzzi and colleagues, and Lee and colleagues which compared the use of intention-to-treat analysis to alternative strategies, concluded that only intention-to-treat is recommended.[105,106] However, in systematic reviews reporting the proportion of trials presenting intention-to-treat analysis, adherence to the principle is not widely demonstrated.[9,10,83,107,108]

Concerns about intention-to-treat analysis include the possible need for a larger sample size than the 'true' treatment difference would suggest, concerns about trials where large numbers of patients have crossed over to the alternative management option, concern about ignoring compliance, reduction in power, and loss of analysis of a treatment's efficacy (see for example, Rabeneck et al.[109] and Sheiner and Rubin[110]). An alternative approach to intention-to-treat analysis is the 'per protocol' analysis, in which only subjects conforming to the protocol are subject to analysis. In addition to the concerns about selection bias outlined above, Lee and colleagues highlight the danger inherent in this approach of its susceptibility to manipulation and data dredging.[106]

Comprehensive cohort follow-up study design

One criticism which is made of RCTs is that they often lack generalisability. This may arise because only a small proportion of the available population may be successfully randomised into a trial. An alternative approach is the 'comprehensive cohort follow-up approach', described by Olschewski et al. and Schmoor et al., in which everybody eligible for entry into a trial should be followed-up in a similar manner, irrespective of whether they accepted randomisation.[111,112] The treatment difference between the randomised treatments will be estimated in those accepting randomisation (the approach normally taken in randomised trials). A separate estimate of the treatment difference will also be obtained from those patients rejecting randomisation but selecting one of the treatments under investigation. Analysis of the results focuses on inferences about the difference between the size of the treatment effects in the randomised and non-randomised subgroups, with formal significance testing being based on a 'treatment by randomisation' interaction. The main disadvantage of such an approach is an increased workload for trialists, and its routine use is not recommended.[112,113]

Multiple end-points

Multiple end-points are one of several ways in which the interpretation of significance tests can be affected by a multiplicity of tests being performed. A systematic review by Pocock and colleagues of 45 RCTs in prestigious journals found a median of six end-points being reported, with a median of four significance tests being reported.[114] They highlighted the particular multiple testing problem of analysis of repeated measures over time, seriously increasing the risk of finding a difference where one does not exist.

Subgroup analysis

An understandable objective of trialists can be to identify subgroups of patients who respond particularly well to a particular treatment. Statistical considerations highlight the dangers of multiple testing arising from this approach, such that chance alone will be responsible for enhanced treatment differences within some subgroups. The review cited above found that 51% of trials reported subgroup analyses.[114] Another systematic review by Gøtzsche et al. found that results from subgroup analyses were stressed in four trials where the main analysis had not favoured the new drug.[115] Freedman and colleagues recommended that the goals of analysis should be to test the primary question posed by the trial over the total set of subjects, with the conduct of secondary analyses to identify questions with sufficient scientific basis to be tested as primary questions in future trials.[116]

Significance levels

Criticisms of the use of significance levels identified by this review have been focussed on the interrelationship between statistical significance and clinical significance. As such, it is as much a design issue as an issue for analysis. Analyses often focus on statistical significance rather than clinical significance,[117,118] although they may not necessarily be the same.[104] In a systematic review of respiratory trials, 22% mentioned sample size, although only 5% discussed power.[118] A well-designed trial will have a high power to detect as statistically significant a difference which is clinically significant.

Reporting

The evidence for this section is largely based on surveys of the quality of reporting of trials.

Quality of reporting

There have been many articles highlighting the poor reporting of RCTs, but many fail to differentiate between poor reporting and poor conduct. There may well be a correlation between the quality of the design and conduct of a trial and its reporting – good quality trials might be expected to be better reported – but there is little evidence to support this. One study by Liberati and co-workers,[80] where authors were contacted to find out further details of published trials, found that if an item of conduct was not reported it did not occur, and that some trials were actually of worse quality than appeared from the publication.

Many surveys of the quality of trials were found by this review, and only a few of those that assessed ten or more trials are discussed here. The surveys were not consistent in their views of adequacy of reporting. For some items, many surveys simply assessed whether trials reported any details at all, and it is likely that the details given were often inappropriate or inadequate. For other items, the reliability of the results is questionable. For example, several surveys[10,83,84,107,108,119] assessed whether intention-to-treat analyses were performed. However, Schulz and colleagues found that even statisticians had difficulty in agreeing whether trials had been analysed by intention-to-treat, and so decided not to collect these data.[14] Despite the limitations, an overview of the surveys shows that no features were consistently well reported, and some items were very poorly reported (for example, sample size, method of randomisation). Some studies have shown that the quality of reporting has improved over time, whilst others have not.

Reporting of conclusions

The conclusions of a trial should be supported by the data presented. We identified only one study that assessed this issue: Rochon and colleagues assessed the results and conclusions of 61 published trials in a blinded fashion and then compared them to see if the conclusion matched the data.[102] Most of the trials were sponsored by pharmaceutical companies. Only 88% of positive conclusions were supported by the data (conclusions always favoured the sponsor's agent). Similarly, only 45% of reports of reduced toxicity were supported by the data. However, Julian points out that even in trials without commercial sponsorship there may also be pressure to produce positive results to secure future funding and status.[94]

The results of a trial should be put into context by comparing it with similar trials to give a balanced authoritative discussion. This is best done by quoting or performing relevant systematic reviews, but this is rarely done. A survey by Clarke and Chalmers of 26 trials published in five major journals showed that only two presented their results in the context of an updated systematic review.[120] Other surveys by Gøtzsche and Ravnskov have shown that positive trials tend to cite other positive trials rather than co-existing negative ones.[115,121] Thus, it appears that the discussion sections of many trial reports may be biased.

Guidelines for reporting

Due to the deficiencies in the reporting of trials demonstrated above, several groups of experts have developed guidelines to improve reporting. The most widely accepted is the CONSORT guidelines.[122] This guideline consists of 21 items to be included in the reports of RCTs, along with a flow chart to document patient selection and follow-up, and recommendations about the title, abstract, introduction and discussion. However, it has been argued that the items relating to data collection on those not randomised are unnecessary, and it has been suggested that some important items relating to data quality have been omitted. The CONSORT guidelines do not cover the statistical aspects of trials, and so should be used in conjunction with existing statistical guidelines.[123]

Failure to report

Failure to publish the results of completed trials may be considered scientific misconduct because it deprives clinicians and patients of information they need to make rational decisions.[124] There are a number of reasons for failure to publish. Publication bias is the tendency to publish studies based on the 'direction or strength of study findings': trials showing large statistically significant treatment effects tend to be published more frequently than those showing small, non-significant effects. The effect of publication bias was demonstrated in studies by Easterbrook et al. and Dickersin and Min who found that a significantly greater proportion of trials with statistically significant results were published compared to those with non-significant results, and those with external funding were also more likely to be published.[103,125] However, trials sponsored by pharmaceutical companies are less likely to be published, often because the sponsors had control of the data. The main reason identified by Dickersin and Min for trials being unpublished was that the authors did not write them up: no trial remained unpublished because of rejection by a journal, although this does occur.[125] Another survey by Davidson of trials published in major journals found that the majority of trials supported by pharmaceutical companies reported results that favoured the company's product.[126] By comparison, fewer trials which did not acknowledge commercial support reported results in favour of a new therapy over traditional therapy.

Many studies including RCTs are only published in abstract form and therefore may be difficult to identify. A systematic review by Scherer et al. showed that about 35% of RCTs initially presented as abstracts were never published in full, and this was more likely if they were small and had non-significant results.[127] As a result of publication bias, world-wide prospective registration of randomised trials has been called for, since retrospective identification of unpublished trials is unsatisfactory.[128]

Multiple publication of the same trial

Failure to publish trial results causes problems but, paradoxically, so too does multiple publication of the same trial. Again, this is more common for trials showing statistically significant results.[103] Multiple reports can cause confusion, since it may be unclear that they all relate to the same trial and there may be discrepancies in the results and conclusions of different reports.

Costs

Consideration of costs related to two issues: the need for economic evaluation as part of a health technology assessment; and the costs of undertaking the research itself. The papers reviewed for this section were based on methodological or theoretical papers, reviews, and case studies or surveys.

Economic evaluation

Few randomised trials have reported an economic evaluation, possibly because of difficulties in conducting such evaluations and the lack of generalisability from one healthcare context to another. The recommendations from this section are those suggested by Drummond and Davies[129] endorsed by others, as follows:

(a) Treatments to be compared should be those likely to be considered by future decision makers.[130,131]

(b) Because resource use may be more or less variable than patient outcomes, sample size calculations should consider economically important effect sizes, notably in costs and patient utilities, as well as clinically important effect sizes.[131-133]

(c) The estimation of treatment costs should exclude all trial costs, though this is rarely easy.[131,134]

(d) The reporting of treatment costs should separate the quantities of resources used from the prices paid.[135,136]

(e) Patient outcome measures should be rigorously chosen and should generally include clinical measures, disease-specific measures of quality of life, and generic measures of patient utility.[137,138]

(f) If the economic value of different technologies is to be compared across trials, findings about resources and outcomes should be reported in standard form, for example net direct costs (that is, direct costs minus direct financial benefits) and net gain in 'quality-adjusted life years'.[137,139]

(g) Extrapolating the findings of the trial to other settings should generally be based on economic modelling that takes account of differences between trial centres and uses data from other centres, for example on treatment costs.[23,136,137]

In addition, we recommended that clinicians considering the inclusion of an economic evaluation should work closely with health economists.[131,133,135,139]

Trial costs

The absence of resources to undertake trials is certain to reduce their number, and shortage of resources is likely to limit their progress or general quality, or both.[23] Additional costs to patients of taking part in trials (particularly of consideration in the US medical system) can act as a deterrent to recruitment,[60,140,141] particularly if the additional treatment costs will be passed on to the patient,[22,142] or the insurer who may refuse to reimburse such costs.[140,142]

Many authors advocate that patients should be fully reimbursed for all their resulting costs and some even propose fees for participants.[60,143] The costs could be either covered by research funds[60,141] or national initiatives.[22,142] It has been suggested that unproven treatments should be funded only for patients in peer-reviewed trials.[23]

The cost of conducting the research itself was also considered in a number of American studies. For example, several studies (including those by Silagy et al.,[144] BjornsonBenson et al.[145] and King et al.[146]), compared the effectiveness or cost effectiveness of different methods of recruiting patients, without identifying consistent results. Little work has been carried out on other aspects of research conduct, for example, the costs of tests and investigations, clinician time or quality assurance processes.

IMPLICATIONS FOR THE HEALTH SERVICE

The main implication of this review – and one which will be difficult to implement – is to try and change the culture of the health service. The value of evidence provided by RCTs is increasingly understood. However, the need to carry out such research within the health service is less widely accepted: it is considered an additional function over and above clinical and administrative efforts. There needs to be recognition that for results of trials to be of most relevance, they should be carried out under usual clinical conditions within the health service. We therefore believe that research should be encouraged as a core activity of clinicians.

The 1998 changes in funding arrangements within the UK National Health Service, implementing the recommendations of the Research and Development Task Force (the 'Culyer Report'[147]), should go some way towards changing the culture, and should overcome some of the previous financial barriers to trials. These changes ensure that both treatment costs and 'service support costs' of peer-reviewed trials are met by the NHS. We believe that the new arrangements may also help in eliminating research that is not worth supporting in the UK.

To ensure that new technologies are not adopted into widespread use before they are fully evaluated, we suggest that guidelines should be developed for the evaluation of new technologies in the UK. The health service should be actively involved in developing these guidelines and in setting the wider UK research agenda, not only for the NHS Research and Development Programme.

SUGGESTIONS FOR FURTHER RESEARCH

In common with much research, this review has identified more questions than answers. The most general need is for prospective studies to identify features that cause trials to be successful or unsuccessful. Which trials fail to start or to make progress? It is possible that it is the weaker trials that fail, through weak designs or lack of clinical support for the question. If so, they need to be strengthened or stopped. However, many specific issues also require more research to be carried out.

Design

Research is required to identify the most appropriate and cost-effective designs of trials: for example, when would it be most appropriate to use the comprehensive cohort design? It would appear sensible to measure core outcome variables in trials within specific clinical areas, such that comparisons could be made between trials, but further research is needed to identify the most valuable sets of measures. Further work is needed to distinguish the best types of analysis, in particular for the use of repeated measures and subgroup analyses.

Structure and Administration

The structure and organisational features of a trial may be the key to its success or failure. However, little is known of the impact of such organisational structures such as: the setting of the research; the role of individuals within the research team, for example the principal investigator, the clinical collaborators and the research co-ordinator; the appropriate levels of quality control; the measurement of compliance; the function of Steering Committees and Data Monitoring Committees. In addition, the ideal structure for small trials and large trials may differ significantly, as may the structures of commercially sponsored trials. A particularly under-researched area is that of the costs of conducting trials.

Recruitment

Recruitment was identified by the review as probably the greatest problem affecting all trials. Further research is needed to identify the types of research designs which least interfere with clinical practice and cause least disruption to patients. We need a better understanding of clinician and patient motivation for taking part in trials, so that we can identify the best methods to approach potential participants in order to obtain their fully informed participation, whilst minimising anxiety. The role of rewards for clinicians and patients requires further investigation.

Reporting

The introduction of the CONSORT guidelines for reporting trials was believed to herald an improvement in the standards of reporting, but further work is needed to find out if this was the outcome. There is a particular need to investigate the reporting of commercially sponsored research.

CONCLUSIONS

This review was designed to identify factors that limit the number, progress and quality of RCTs. Indeed, we have identified so many factors that our admiration for the trials that are successful is even greater. These successful trials, and the evidence of this chapter, provide an excellent yardstick for all trialists, both new and existing. We exhort them all to continue to enhance the number and quality of randomised trials. Only thus can we all improve the quality of the evidence base for healthcare, and thus the quality of healthcare itself.

REFERENCES

1. Pocock SJ. *Clinical Trials – A Practical Approach*. John Wiley: Chichester, 1983.
2. Yusuf S, Held P, Teo KK, Toretsky ER. Selection of patients for randomized controlled trials: implications of wide or narrow eligibility criteria. *Statist. Med.* 1990; **9**: 73–83.
3. Collins R, Peto R, Gray R, Parish S. Large-scale randomized evidence: trials and overviews. *Oxford Textbook of Medicine*, 3rd edn, 1996; **1**: 21–32.
4. Nixon DW. Special aspects of cancer prevention trials. *Cancer* 1994; **74**(9 Suppl.): 2683–6.
5. Blair PS, Silman AJ. Can clinical trials in rheumatology be improved? *Curr. Opin. Rheumatol.* 1991; **3**(2): 272–9.
6. Coombs DW, Dimick A, Bronstein JM, Potts LH, Bowens B. Conceptual and methodologic problems in the evaluation of a new burn treatment modality. *J. Burn Care Rehabilitation* 1993; **14**: 568–71.
7. Fleming TR, DeMets DL. Surrogate end points in clinical trials: are we being misled? *Ann. Intern. Med.* 1996; **125**: 605–13.
8. Talley NJ. A critique of therapeutic trials in *Helicobacter pylori*-positive functional dyspepsia. *Gastroenterology* 1994; **106**: 1174–83.
9. Silagy CA, Jewell D. Review of 39 years of randomized controlled trials in the *British Journal of General Practice. Br. J. Gen. Pract.* 1994; **44**(385): 359–63.
10. Rossetti L, Marchetti I, Orzalesi N, Scorpiglione N, Torri V, Liberati A. Randomized clinical trials on medical treatment of glaucoma. Are they appropriate to guide clinical practice? *Arch. Ophthalmol.* 1993; **111**: 96–103.
11. Balas EA, Austin SM, Ewigman BG, Brown GD, Mitchell JA. Methods of randomized controlled clinical trials in health services research. *Medical Care* 1995; **33**: 687–99.
12. Taves RR. Minimization: a new method of assigning patients to treatment and control groups. *Clin. Pharmacol. Ther.* 1974; **15**: 443–53.
13. Altman DG, Dore CJ. Randomisation and baseline comparisons in clinical trials. *Lancet* 1990; **335**: 149–53.
14. Schulz KF, Chalmers I, Hayes RJ, Altman DG. Empirical evidence of bias. Dimensions of methodological quality associated with estimates of treatment effects in controlled trials. *JAMA* 1995; **273**: 408–12.
15. Chalmers TC, Celano P, Sacks HS, Smith H. Bias in treatment assignment in controlled clinical trials. *N. Engl. J. Med.* 1983; **309**: 1358–61.
16. Peto R, Collins R, Gray R. Large-scale randomized evidence: large, simple trials and overviews of trials. *J. Clin. Epidemiol.* 1995; **48**: 23–40.
17. Fayers PM, Machin D. Sample size: how many patients are necessary? *Br. J. Cancer* 1995; **72**: 1–9.
18. Edwards SJL, Lilford RJ, Braunholtz D, Jackson J. Why 'underpowered' trials are not necessarily unethical. *Lancet* 1997; **350**: 804–7.
19. Ashery RS, McAuliffe WE. Implementation issues and techniques in randomized trials of outpatient psychosocial treatments for drug abusers: recruitment of subjects. *Am. J. Drug Alcohol Abuse* 1992; **18**: 305–29.
20. Easterbrook PJ, Matthews DR. Fate of research studies. *J. R. Soc. Med.* 1992; **85**: 71–6.
21. Benson AB, Pregler JP, Bean JA, Rademaker AW, Eshler B, Anderson, K. Oncologists' reluctance to accrue patients onto clinical trials: an Illinois Cancer Center study. *J. Clin. Oncol.* 1991; **9**: 2067–75.
22. Foley JF, Moertel CG. Improving accrual into cancer clinical trials. *J. Cancer Education* 1991; **6**: 165–73.
23. Smyth JF, Mossman J, Hall R, Hepburn S, Pinkerton R, Richards M, Thatcher N, Box J. Conducting clinical research in the new NHS: the model of cancer. United Kingdom Co-ordinating Committee on Cancer Research. *Br. Med. J.* 1994; **309**: 457–61.
24. Aaronson NK, VisserPol E, Leenhouts GHMW et al. Telephone-based nursing intervention

improves the effectiveness of the informed consent process in cancer clinical trials. *J. Clin. Oncol.* 1996; **14**: 984–96.

25. Taylor KM, Kelner M. Interpreting physician participation in randomized clinical trials: the physician orientation profile. *J. Health Soc. Behav.* 1987; **28**: 389–400.

26. Taylor KM, Feldstein ML, Skeel RT, Pandya KJ, Ng P, Carbone PP. Fundamental dilemmas of the randomized clinical trial process: results of a survey of the 1,737 Eastern Cooperative Oncology Group investigators. *J. Clin. Oncol.* 1994; **12**(9): 1796–805.

27. Winn RJ, Miransky J, Kerner JF, Kennelly L, Michaelson RA, Sturgeon, SR. An evaluation of physician determinants in the referral of patients for cancer clinical trials in the community setting. *Prog. Clin. Biol. Res.* 1984; **156**: 63–73.

28. Tognoni G, Alli C, Avanzini F, Bettelli G, Colombo F, Corso R, Marchioli R, Zussino A. Randomized clinical trials in general practice: lessons from a failure. *Br. Med. J.* 1991; **303**: 969–71.

29. Penn ZJ, Steer PJ. Reasons for declining participation in a prospective randomized trial to determine the optimum mode of delivery of the preterm breech. *Controlled Clinical Trials* 1990; **11**: 226–31.

30. Shea S, Bigger JT, Campion J, Fleiss JL, Rolnitzky LM, Schron E, Gorkin L, Handshaw K, Kinney MR, Branyon M. Enrolment in clinical trials: institutional factors affecting enrollment in the cardiac arrhythmia suppression trial (CAST). *Controlled Clinical Trials* 1992; **13**: 466–86.

31. Henzlova MJ, Blackburn BH, Bradley EJ, Rogers WJ. Patient perception of a long-term clinical trial: Experience using a close-out questionnaire in the Studies of Left Ventricular Dysfunction (SOLVD) trial. *Controlled Clinical Trials* 1994; **15**: 284–93.

32. Siminoff LA, Fetting JH, Abeloff MD. Doctor-patient communication about breast cancer adjuvant therapy. *J. Clin. Oncol.* 1989; **7**: 1192–200.

33. Schaeffer MH, Krantz DS, Wichman A, Masur H, Reed E, Vinicky JK. The impact of disease severity on the informed consent process in clinical research. *Am. J. Med.* 1996; **100**: 261–8.

34. Wadland WC, Hughes JR, SeckerWalker RH, Bronson DL Fenwick J. Recruitment in a primary care trial on smoking cessation. *Family Medicine* 1990; **22**: 201–4.

35. Atwood JR, Haase J, Rees-McGee S et al. Reasons related to adherence in community-based field studies. *Patient Education & Counselling* 1992; **19**: 251–9.

36. Bowen J, Hirsch S. Recruitment rates and factors affecting recruitment for a clinical trial of a putative anti-psychotic agent in the treatment of acute schizophrenia. *Human Psychopharmacol.* 1992; **7**: 337–41.

37. Autret E, Dutertre JP, Barbier P, Jonville AP, Pierre F, Berger C. Parental opinions about biomedical research in children in Tours, France. *Dev. Pharmacol. Ther.* 1993; **20**: 64–71.

38. Harth SC, Thong YH. Parental perceptions and attitudes about informed consent in clinical research involving children. *Soc. Sci. Med.* 1995; **40**: 1573–7.

39. Schwartz CE, Fox BH. Who says yes? Identifying selection biases in a psychosocial intervention study of multiple sclerosis. *Soc. Sci. Med.* 1995; **40**: 359–70.

40. Newburg SM, Holland AE, Pearce LA. Motivation of subjects to participate in a research trial. *Applied Nursing Research* 1992; **5**: 89–93.

41. Plaisier PW, Berger MY, van der Hul RL, Nijs HG, den Toom R, Terpstra, OT, Bruining HA. Unexpected difficulties in randomizing patients in a surgical trial: a prospective study comparing extracorporeal shock wave lithotripsy with open cholecystectomy. *World J. Surg.* 1994; **18**: 769–72.

42. Bevan EG, Chee LC, McInnes GT. Patients' attitudes to participation in clinical trials. *Br. J. Clin. Pharmacol.* 1992; **34**: 156P–7P.

43. Langley GR, Sutherland HJ, Wong S, Minkin S, Llewellyn-Thomas HA, Till JE. Why are (or are not) patients given the option to enter clinical trials? *Controlled Clinical Trials* 1987; **8**: 49–59.

44. Slevin M, Mossman J, Bowling A, Leonard R, Steward W, Harper P, McIllmurray M, Thatcher N. Volunteers or victims: patients' views of randomized cancer clinical trials. *Br. J. Cancer* 1995; **71**: 1270–4.

45. Bergmann JF, Chassany O, Gandiol J, Deblois P, Kanis JA, Segrestaa JM, Caulin C, Dahan R. A randomized clinical trial of the effect of informed consent on the analgesic activity of placebo and naproxen in cancer pain. *Clinical Trials and Meta-Analysis* 1994; **29**: 41–7.

46. Dahan R, Caulin C, Figea L, Kanis JA, Caulin F, Segrestaa JM. Does informed consent influence therapeutic outcome? A clinical trial of the hypnotic activity of placebo in patients admitted to hospital. *Br. Med. J.* 1986; **293**: 363–4.

47. Antman K, Amato D, Wood W, Carson J, Suit H, Proppe K, Carey R, Greenberger J, Wilson R, Frei E. Selection bias in clinical trials. *J. Clin. Oncol.* 1985; **3**: 1142–7.

48. Stone JM, Page FJ, Laidlaw CR, Cooper I. Selection of patients for randomized trials: a

study based on the MACOP-B vs CHOP in NHL study. *Aust. N. Z. J. Med.* 1994; **24**: 536–40.

49. Lynoe N, Sandlund M, Dahlqvist G, Jacobsson L. Informed consent: study of quality of information given to participants in a clinical trial. *Br. Med. J.* 1991; **303**: 610–13.

50. Llewellyn-Thomas HA, McGreal MJ, Thiel EC, Fine S, Erlichman C. Patients' willingness to enter clinical trials: measuring the association with perceived benefit and preference for decision participation. *Soc. Sci. Med.* 1991; **32**: 35–42.

51. Roberson NL. Clinical trial participation. Viewpoints from racial/ethnic groups. *Cancer* 1994; **74**(9 Suppl.): 2687–91.

52. Jensen AB, Madsen B, Andersen P, Rose C. Information for cancer patients entering a clinical trial – an evaluation of an information strategy. *Eur. J. Cancer* 1993; **29A**: 2235–8.

53. Sutherland HJ, Carlin K, Harper W, Martin LJ, Greenberg CV, Till JE, Boyd NF. A study of diet and breast cancer prevention in Canada: why healthy women participate in controlled trials. *Cancer Causes Control* 1993; **4**: 521–8.

54. Miller C, Searight HR, Grable D, Schwartz R, Sowell C, Barbarash RA. Comprehension and recall of the informational content of the informed consent document: An evaluation of 168 patients in a controlled clinical trial. *J. Clin. Res. Drug Dev.* 1994; **8**: 237–48.

55. Gallo C, Perrone F, De Placido S, Giusti C. Informed versus randomized consent to clinical trials. *Lancet* 1995; **346**: 1060–4.

56. Dunbar J, Cleary PA, Siebert C, Baker L, Brink S, Nathan DM. Implementation of a multi-component process to obtain informed consent in the diabetes control and complications trial. *Controlled Clinical Trials* 1989; **10**: 83–96.

57. Dickinson CJ. Clinical research in the NHS today. *J. R. Coll. Phys. (Lond.)* 1994; **28**: 460–3.

58. Chang RW, Falconer J, Stulberg SD, Arnold WJ, Dyer AR. Prerandomization: an alternative to classic randomization. The effects on recruitment in a controlled trial of arthroscopy for osteoarthrosis of the knee. *J. Bone Joint Surg.* 1990; **72**: 1451–5.

59. Hunninghake DB, Darby CA, Probstfield JL. Recruitment experience in clinical trials: literature summary and annotated bibliography. *Controlled Clinical Trials* 1987; **8**(4 Suppl.): 6S–30S.

60. Swanson GM, Ward AJ. Recruiting minorities into clinical trials: toward a participant-friendly system. *J. Nat. Cancer Inst.* 1995; **87**: 1747–59.

61. Diekmann JM, Smith JM. Strategies for accessment and recruitment of subjects for nursing research. *West. J. Nursing Res.* 1989; **11**: 418–30.

62. Neaton JD, Grimm RH, Jr., Cutler JA. Recruitment of participants for the multiple risk factor intervention trial (MRFIT). *Controlled Clinical Trials* 1987; **8**(4 Suppl.): 41S–53S.

63. Pocock SJ. When to stop a clinical trial. *Br. Med. J.* 1992; **305**: 235–40.

64. Fleming TR, DeMets DL. Monitoring of clinical trials: issues and recommendations. *Controlled Clinical Trials* 1993; **14**: 183–97.

65. Anonymous. The early termination of clinical trials: causes, consequences, and control. With special reference to trials in the field of arrhythmias and sudden death. Task Force of the Working Group on Arrhythmias of the European Society of Cardiology. *Eur. Heart J.* 1994; **15**: 721–38.

66. Buyse M. Interim analyses, stopping rules and data monitoring in clinical trials in Europe. *Statist. Med.* 1993; **12**: 509–20.

67. Urquhart J. Role of patient compliance in clinical pharmacokinetics. A review of recent research. *Clin. Pharmacokinet.* 1994; **27**: 202–15.

68. Besch CL. Compliance in clinical trials. *AIDS* 1995; **9**: 1–10.

69. Klein MC, Kaczorowski J, Robbins JM, Gauthier RJ, Jorgensen SH, Joshi AK. Physicians' beliefs and behaviour during a radomized controlled trial of episiotomy: Consequences for women in their care. *Can. Med. Assoc. J.* 1995; **153**: 769–79.

70. Rudd P, Ahmed S, Zachary V, Barton C, Bonduelle D. Improved compliance measures: applications in an ambulatory hypertensive drug trial. *Clin. Pharmacol. Ther.* 1990; **48**: 676–85.

71. Urquhart J. Ascertaining how much compliance is enough with outpatient antibiotic regimens. *Postgrad. Med. J.* 1992; **68**(Suppl. 3): S49–58.

72. Melnikow J, Kiefe C. Patient compliance and medical research: Issues in methodology. *J. Gen. Intern. Med.* 1994; **9**: 96–105.

73. Pledger GW. Compliance in clinical trials: impact on design, analysis and interpretation. *Epilepsy Research* 1988; **1**(Supplement): 125–33.

74. Vander Stichele R. Measurement of patient compliance and the interpretation of randomized clinical trials. *Eur. J. Clin. Pharmacol.* 1991; **41**: 27–35.

75. Schechtman KB, Gordon ME. A comprehensive algorithm for determining whether a run-in strategy will be a cost-effective design modification in a randomized clinical trial. *Statist. Med.* 1993; **12**: 111–28.

76. Stephenson BJ, Rowe BH, Haynes RB, Macharia WM, Leon G. Is this patient taking the treatment as prescribed? *JAMA* 1993; **269**: 2779–81.

77. Lawrence W. Some problems with clinical trials. (James Ewing lecture) *Arch. Surg.* 1991; **126**: 370–8.
78. Richmond RL, Anderson P. Research in general practice for smokers and excessive drinkers in Australia and the UK. II: representativeness of the results. *Addiction* 1994; **89**: 41–7.
79. Haynes RB, McKibbon KA, Kanani R. Systematic review of randomized controlled trials of the effects of patient adherence and outcomes of interventions to assist patients to follow prescriptions for medications. Collaboration on Effective Professional Practice Module of The Cochrane Database on Systematic Reviews 1996; **1**.
80. Liberati A, Himel HN, Chalmers TC. A quality assessment of randomized control trials of primary treatment of breast cancer. *J. Clin. Oncol.* 1986; **4**: 942–51.
81. Kleijnen J, ter Riet G, Knipschild P. Acupuncture and asthma: a review of controlled trials. *Thorax* 1991; **46**: 799–802.
82. Solomon MJ, Laxamana A, Devore L, McLeod RS. Randomized controlled trials in surgery. *Surgery* 1994; **115**: 707–12.
83. Sonis J, Joines J. The quality of clinical trials published in *The Journal of Family Practice*, 1974–1991. *J. Family Practice* 1994; **39**: 225–35.
84. Lionetto R, Pugliese V, Bruzzi P, Rosso R. No standard treatment is available for advanced pancreatic cancer. *Eur. J. Cancer* 1995; **31A**: 882–7.
85. Schulz KF, Grimes DA, Altman DG, Hayes RJ. Blinding and exclusions after allocation in randomized controlled trials: survey of published parallel group trials in obstetrics and gynaecology. *Br. Med. J.* 1996; **312**: 742–4.
86. Stewart LA, Clarke MJ. Practical methodology of meta-analyses (overviews) using updated individual patient data. Cochrane Working Group. *Statist. Med.* 1995; **14**: 2057–79.
87. Fisher S, Greenberg RP. How sound is the double-blind design for evaluating psychotropic drugs? *J. Nervous Mental Dis.* 1993; **181**: 345–50.
88. Kirsch I, Rosadino MJ. Do double-blind studies with informed consent yield externally valid results? An empirical test. *Psychopharmacology* 1993; **110**: 437–42.
89. Carroll KM, Rounsaville BJ, Nich C. Blind man's bluff: effectiveness and significance of psychotherapy and pharmacotherapy blinding procedures in a clinical trial. *J. Consult. Clin. Psychol.* 1994; **62**: 276–80.
90. Noseworthy JH, Ebers GC, Vandervoort MK, Farquhar RE, Yetisir E, Roberts R. The impact of blinding on the results of a randomized, placebo-controlled multiple sclerosis clinical trial. *Neurology* 1994; **44**: 16–20.
91. Poy E. Objectives of QC systems and QA function in clinical research. *Quality Assurance* 1993; **2**: 326–31.
92. Wood DJ. Quality assurance in phase II and III studies. *Quality Assurance* 1993; **2**: 353–8.
93. van Gijn J. Who is in Charge? Investigator and sponsor alliances. *Cerebrovasc. Dis.* 1995; **5**: 22–6.
94. Julian D. Trials and tribulations. *Cardiovasc. Res.* 1994; **28**: 598–603.
95. Warlow C. How to do it: organise a multicentre trial. *Br. Med. J.* 1990; **300**: 180–3.
96. Hogg RJ. Trials and tribulations of multicenter studies. Lessons learned from the experiences of the Southwest Pediatric Nephrology Study Group (SPNSG). *Pediatr. Nephrol.* 1991; **5**: 348–51.
97. McCandlish R, Renfrew M. Trial and tribulation . . . treatments for inverted nipples . . . difficulties involved in research. *Nursing Times* 1991; **87**: 40–1.
98. Bogousslavsky J. The jungle of acute stroke trials, trialists and sponsors. *Cerebrovasc. Dis.* 1995; **5**: 1–2.
99. Rockhold FW, Enas GG. Data monitoring and interim analyses in the pharmaceutical industry: ethical and logistical considerations. *Statist. Med.* 1993; **12**: 471–9.
100. Parmar MK, Machin D. Monitoring clinical trials: experience of, and proposals under consideration by, the Cancer Therapy Committee of the British Medical Research Council. *Statist. Med.* 1993; **12**: 497–504.
101. Green SJ, Fleming TR, O'Fallon JR. Policies for study monitoring and interim reporting of results. *J. Clin. Oncol.* 1987; **5**: 1477–84.
102. Rochon PA, Gurwitz JH, Simms RW, Fortin PR, Felson DT, Minaker KL, Chalmers TC. A study of manufacturer-supported trials of nonsteroidal anti-inflammatory drugs in the treatment of arthritis. *Arch. Intern. Med.* 1994; **154**: 157–63.
103. Easterbrook PJ, Berlin JA, Gopalan R, Matthews DR. Publication bias in clinical research. *Lancet* 1991; **337**: 867–72.
104. Bigby M, Gadenne AS. Understanding and evaluating clinical trials. *J. Am. Acad. Dermatol.* 1996; **34**: 555–94.
105. Peduzzi P, Detre K, Wittes J, Holford T. Intent-to-treat analysis and the problem of crossovers. An example from the Veterans Administration coronary bypass surgery study. *J. Thorac. Cardiovasc. Surg.* 1991; **101**: 481–7.
106. Lee YJ, Ellenberg JH, Hirtz G, Nelson KB. Analysis of clinical trials by treatment actually received: is it really an option? *Statist. Med.* 1991; **10**: 1595–605.
107. Nicolucci A, Grilli R, Alexanian AA, Apolone G, Torri V, Liberati A. Quality, evolution, and clinical implications of randomized, controlled

trials on the treatment of lung cancer. A lost opportunity for meta-analysis. *JAMA* 1989; **262**: 2101–7.

108. Koes BW, Bouter LM, van der Heijden GJ. Methodological quality of randomized clinical trials on treatment efficacy in low back pain. *Spine* 1995; **20**: 228–35.

109. Rabeneck L, Viscoli CM, Horwitz RI. Problems in the conduct and analysis of randomized clinical trials: are we getting the right answers to the wrong questions? *Arch. Intern. Med.* 1992; **152**: 507–12.

110. Sheiner LB, Rubin DB. Intention-to-treat analysis and the goals of clinical trials. *Clin. Pharmacol. Ther.* 1995; **57**: 6–15.

111. Olschewski M, Schumacher M, Davis KB. Analysis of randomized and nonrandomized patients in clinical trials using the comprehensive cohort follow-up study design. *Controlled Clinical Trials* 1992; **13**: 226–39.

112. Schmoor C, Olschewski M, Schumacher M. Randomized and non-randomized patients in clinical trials: experiences with comprehensive cohort studies. *Statist. Med.* 1996; **15**: 263–71.

113. Silverman WA, Altman DG. Patients' preferences and randomized. *Lancet* 1996; **347**: 171–4.

114. Pocock SJ, Hughes MD, Lee RJ. Statistical problems in the reporting of clinical trials. A survey of three medical journals. *N. Engl. J. Med.* 1985; **317**: 426–32.

115. Gøtzsche PC. Methodology and overt and hidden bias in reports of 196 double-blind trials of nonsteroidal antiinflammatory drugs in rheumatoid arthritis. *Controlled Clinical Trials* 1989; **10**: 31–56.

116. Freedman LS, Simon R, Foulkes MA, Friedman L, Geller NL, Gordon DJ, Mowery R. Inclusion of women and minorities in clinical trials and the NIH revitalization act of 1993 – the perspective of NIH clinical trialists. *Controlled Clinical Trials* 1995; **16**: 277–85.

117. Klein DF. Improvement of phase III psychotropic drug trials by intensive phase II work. *Neuropsychopharmacology* 1991; **4**: 251–8.

118. Lindgren BR, Wielinski CL, Finkelstein SM, Warwick WJ. Contrasting clinical and statistical significance within the research setting. *Pediatr. Pulmonol.* 1993; **16**: 336–40.

119. Marsoni S, Torri W, Taiana A et al. Critical review of the quality and development of randomized clinical trials (RCTs) and their influence on the treatment of advanced epithelial ovarian cancer. *Ann. Oncol.* 1990; **1**: 343–50.

120. Clarke M, Chalmers I. Discussion sections in reports of controlled trials published in five general medical journals: islands in search of continents. *JAMA* 1998; **280**: 280–2.

121. Ravnskov U. Cholesterol lowering trials in coronary heart disease: frequency of citation and outcome. *Br. Med. J.* 1992; **305**: 15–19.

122. Begg C, Cho M, Eastwood S, Horton R, Moher D, Olkin I, Pitkin RX, Rennie D, Schulz KF, Simel D, Stroup DF. Improving the quality of reporting of randomized controlled trials: the CONSORT statement. *JAMA* 1996; **276**: 637–9.

123. Altman DG. Better reporting of randomized controlled trials: the CONSORT statement. *Br. Med. J.* 1996; **313**: 570–1.

124. Chalmers TC, Frank CS, Reitman D. Minimizing the three stages of publication bias. *JAMA* 1990; **263**: 1392–5.

125. Dickersin K, Min YI. Publication bias: the problem that won't go away. *Ann. N. Y. Acad. Sci.* 1993; **703**: 135–46.

126. Davidson RA. Source of funding and outcome of clinical trials. *J. Gen. Intern. Med.* 1986; **1**: 155–8.

127. Scherer RW, Dickersin K, Langenberg P. Full publication of results initially presented in abstract: a meta-analysis. *JAMA* 1994; **272**: 158–62.

128. Hetherington J, Dickersin K, Chalmers I, Meinert CL. Retrospective and prospective identification of unpublished controlled trials: lessons from a survey of obstetricians and pediatricians. *Pediatrics* 1989; **84**: 374–80.

129. Drummond MF, Davies L. Economic analysis alongside clinical trials: revisiting the methodological issues. *Int. J. Technol. Assess. Health Care* 1991; **7**: 561–73.

130. Hansson L, Hedner T, Dahlof B. Prospective randomized open blinded end-point (PROBE) study. A novel design for intervention trials. Prospective Randomized Open Blinded End-Point. *Blood Pressure* 1992; **1**: 113–19.

131. Schwartz JS. Prostate Cancer Intervention Versus Observation Trial: economic analysis in study design and conditions of uncertainty. *Monographs – Nat. Cancer Inst.* 1995; **19**: 73–5.

132. Drummond M, O'Brien B. Clinical importance, statistical significance and the assessment of economic and quality-of-life outcomes. *Health Economics* 1993; **2**: 205–12.

133. Torgerson DJ, Ryan M, Ratcliffe J. Economics in sample size determination for clinical trials. *Q. J. Med.* 1995; **88**: 517–21.

134. Oddone E, Weinberger M, Hurder A, Henderson W, Simel D. Measuring activities in clinical trials using random work sampling: implications for cost-effectiveness analysis and measurement of the intervention. *J. Clin. Epidemiol.* 1995; **48**: 1011–18.

135. Bennett CL, Armitage JL, Buchner D, Gulati S. Economic analysis in phase III clinical cancer trials. *Cancer Invest.* 1994; **12**: 336–42.

136. Drummond M. Economic analysis alongside clinical trials: problems and potential. *J. Rheumatol.* 1995; **22**: 1403–7.

137. Bonsel GJ, Rutten FF, Uyl-de Groot CA. Economic evaluation alongside cancer trials: methodological and practical aspects. *Eur. J. Cancer* 1993; **29A**(Suppl. 7): S10–4.

138. Tannock IF. New perspectives in combined radiotherapy and chemotherapy treatment. *Lung Cancer* 1994; **10**(Suppl. 1): S29–51.

139. Drummond MF. *Economic analysis alongside clinical trials: an introduction for clinical researchers.* London: Department of Health, 1994.

140. Tilley BC, Peterson EL, Kleerekoper M, Phillips E, Nelson DA, Shorck, MA. Designing clinical trials of treatment for osteoporosis: recruitment and follow-up. *Calcified Tissue International* 1990; **47**: 327–31.

141. Welsh KA, Ballard E, Nash F, Raiford K, Harrell L. Issues affecting minority participation in research studies of Alzheimer disease. *Alzheimer Disease & Associated Disorders* 1994; **8**(Suppl. 4): 38–48.

142. Fleming ID. Barriers to clinical trials. Part I: Reimbursement problems. *Cancer* 1994; **74**(9 Suppl.): 2662–5.

143. Bigorra J, Banos JE. Weight of financial reward in the decision by medical students and experienced healthy volunteers to participate in clinical trials. *Eur. J. Clin. Pharmacol.* 1990; **38**: 443–6.

144. Silagy CA, Campion K, McNeil JJ, Worsam B, Donnan GA, Tonkin AM. Comparison of recruitment strategies for a large-scale clinical trial in the elderly. *J. Clin. Epidemiol.* 1991; **44**: 1105–14.

145. BjornsonBenson WM, Stibolt TB, Manske KA, Zavela KJ, Youtsey DJ, Buist AS. Monitoring recruitment effectiveness and cost in a clinical trial. *Controlled Clinical Trials* 1993; **14**: 52S–67S.

146. King AC, Harris RB, Haskell WL. Effect of recruitment strategy on types of subjects entered into a primary prevention clinical trial. *Ann. Epidemiol.* 1994; **4**: 312–20.

147. Research and Development Task Force. *Supporting Research and Development in the NHS.* London: HMSO, 1994.

4

Results of Clinical Trials and Systematic Reviews: To Whom Do They Apply?

DIANNE O'CONNELL, PAUL GLASZIOU,
SUZANNE HILL, JASMINKA SARUNAC,
JULIA LOWE and DAVID HENRY

SUMMARY

Background

Increasingly, clinical interventions are being evaluated by randomised controlled trials (RCTs). There have been important developments in methods for designing and conducting trials, and the quality of RCTs has improved. However, there are no acceptable methods for assessing the applicability of a clinical trial's results and for identifying individuals who will experience net treatment benefit.

Objectives

The aims were to: (1) define the methods that are currently suggested for applying clinical trial results in clinical practice; (2) assess the strengths and weaknesses of these approaches; (3) develop an appropriate method for applying clinical trial results to individual patients based on a consideration of benefit and risk; and (4) consider the implications for design and reporting of clinical trials and the development of clinical guidelines.

Methods

We conducted a systematic review of the biomedical literature using a combination of Medline searches, hand-searching of key journals, and bibliographic searches to identify reports of RCTs or systematic reviews that discussed the applicability of the findings and papers that focussed on methodological or statistical issues relating to the application of results of RCTs. Papers of potential relevance were reviewed and discussed by the multi-disciplinary research group. Annotated bibliographies of relevant papers were compiled.

Results

Of 1753 papers identified (to end of 1996), 568 were judged to be of potential relevance and, on further assessment, 419 papers formed the basis of the review and annotated bibliographies.

The main methods for assessing applicability described in the literature fall into five areas: (1) consideration of patient selection and inclusion/exclusion criteria; (2) comparison of trial subjects with those not in the trial; (3) subgroup analysis of treatment effect; (4) risk-based individualisation of benefits and harms; and (5) a mix of other approaches. The majority of papers concentrated on a consideration of the characteristics of the settings and populations in which clinical trials are conducted and to whom the estimated average treatment effect might apply. However, this approach is very limiting as, despite an overall statistically significant treatment effect, not all individuals (including some in the trial) will experience a net benefit. Also some who were not eligible for the trial may benefit from treatment. We therefore recommend an approach based on a risk–benefit model to identify in which individuals the treatment is likely to do more good than harm. This requires five questions to be addressed: (1) What are the beneficial and harmful effects of the intervention? (2) Are there variations in the relative treatment effect? (3) How does the treatment effect vary with baseline risk level? (4) What are the predicted absolute risk reductions for individuals? (5) Do the expected benefits outweigh the harms?

Conclusions

The literature on this topic is diffuse and was difficult to identify. The preoccupation with issues of patient selection, inclusion and exclusion criteria and the (un)representativeness of trial participants has inhibited the development of methods for the accurate application of trial results. The proposed method for individualising treatment decisions has implications for the design and reporting of clinical trials, for clinical practice and how groups developing clinical practice guidelines should consider the evidence when formulating treatment recommendations.

CONTEXT

Since the first randomised trial in 1948, the number of clinical interventions that have been evaluated by randomised controlled trials (RCTs) has increased dramatically. There has been considerable research into the best methods for designing and conducting trials and, as a result, the quality of the clinical trials has improved. Increasingly, clinical decisions are being made based on the results of trials and systematic reviews, rather than on opinion and clinical experience only. However, there has been relatively little research into how best to apply the results of clinical trials. The overall results of trials (or systematic reviews) represent an 'average' treatment effect. But, within the trial, some patients may have experienced a greater than 'average' improvement, and in others, the harm may have outweighed the benefit. At present, there is no generally accepted technique that allows a clinician to identify which individuals will experience net benefit from treatment.

The terms generalisability, external validity, extrapolation and applicability are often used interchangeably, but they have different meanings (Table 1). The term 'applicability' will be used throughout this chapter.

It is useful to think about the different populations involved in patient care and research, and how they do, or do not, overlap when consider-

Table 1 *Definitions of terms relating to generalisability*

- *Generalisability (or external validity)*: The extent to which a study's results provide a correct basis for generalisation beyond the setting of the study and the particular people studied, to different geographical or temporal populations.
- *Extrapolation*: The application of results to a wider population than that studied. It means to infer, predict, extend, or project beyond that which was recorded, observed or experienced. For example, can the results of a clinical trial in which patients aged 40–55 were studied be extrapolated to patients aged 55–65?
- *Applicability*: Encompasses the application of results to both individual patients and groups of patients. This is the preferred term as it includes the idea of particularising or individualising treatment, and is closest to the general aim of clinical practice. It addresses how a particular treatment, that showed an overall benefit in a study, can be expected to benefit an individual patient.

Table 2 *Definitions of populations involved in research and clinical practice. (From Collet and Boissel.[1])*

- *Sick population*: All patients suffering from the disease of interest – large and very heterogeneous and rarely precisely described.
- *Therapist's target population*: Subgroup of the sick population, corresponding to those patients who are accessible to the therapist – influenced by factors such as the technical and diagnostic facilities available.
- *Eligible population*: Patients who satisfy the inclusion criteria defined in terms of the therapist's target population – eligible patient population may differ depending on criteria used.
- *Study population*: Those patients included in the trial – depends on inclusion criteria, informed consent etc. – can differ from the eligible population.
- *Treatment target population*: Those patients to whom the study results apply should be defined after a careful, extensive, and accurate investigation of qualitative and quantitative interaction with treatment efficacy.
- *Treatment distribution population*: Those patients who will actually receive the treatment – will not include all for whom treatment is recommended and will include some for whom it is not.

ing the applicability of trial results. Collet and Boissel have defined the different populations involved in the assessment of an intervention (Table 2).[1]

Generalisability (or applicability) involves applying the results from the study population to the treatment target population, but as Collet and Boissel indicate this will be different to those who actually get the treatment.[1]

We have carried out a qualitative, but systematic review of the literature on the applicability of results of RCTs and systematic reviews of RCTs. The specific aims were to:

(a) define the methods that are currently suggested for applying clinical trial results in clinical practice;
(b) assess the strengths and weaknesses of currently suggested approaches;
(c) develop an appropriate method based on a consideration of benefit and risk to apply clinical trial results to individual patients; and
(d) consider the implications for design and reporting of clinical trials and the development of clinical guidelines.

METHODS

Our goal was to identify and review the literature about methods for generalising (or applying) the results from RCTs and systematic reviews of RCTs. We used a combination of searching electronic databases, hand-searching key medical journals and bibliographic searches of relevant papers to identify and retrieve papers that discussed methods for applying the results of clinical trials. An iterative approach was used to develop a search strategy for Medline based on keywords and MeSH headings in relevant papers, and names of authors known to have published on the topic. The search was very broad, and included papers that were reports of RCTs or systematic reviews in which the applicability of the results was considered, discussion papers, and papers focussing on methodological or statistical issues relating to the application of results of RCTs.

We hand-searched a number of key journals including: *Controlled Clinical Trials*; *Statistics in Medicine*; *Journal of the American Medical Association*; *Biometrics*; *Journal of Clinical Epidemiology*; *The Lancet*; *New England Journal of Medicine*; *Medical Decision Making*; *British Medical Journal*; *Annals of Internal Medicine*; and *International Journal of Technology Assessment in Health Care*. We also searched the Cochrane Review Methodology Database in the Cochrane Library for relevant references.

Papers identified as being of potential relevance from the title and/or abstract were downloaded from Medline into a Reference Manager database; some citations were entered manually.

Potentially relevant articles were obtained and a structured review was carried out by members of the multi-disciplinary research group, including a classification according to subject areas. Annotated bibliographies of relevant papers were compiled for each subject area.

After reviewing the methods described in the literature and a consideration of their strengths and weaknesses, we developed a 'five-step' process based on a risk–benefit model proposed by Lubsen and Tijssen for applying the results of RCTs and systematic reviews to individual patient management decisions.[2]

EVIDENCE

A total of 568 papers, published to the end of 1996, were identified as being of potential relevance, and a further 1185 papers were excluded as not relevant. After review, completion of the cover sheet and discussion, 419 papers were considered to be of direct relevance to the topic and were grouped by topic area for the annotated bibliography. The main methods for assessing generalisability described in the literature fall into five areas: (1) consideration of patient selection and inclusion/exclusion criteria; (2) comparison of trial subjects with those not in the trial; (3) subgroup analysis of treatment effect; (4) risk-based individualisation of benefits and harms; and (5) a mix of other approaches. Each of these approaches is described in more detail in the next section.

The literature on this topic is diffuse and was difficult to identify. It is our view that the predominance of papers concerned with the influences of patient eligibility, recruitment and participation in clinical trials represents an important misunderstanding of the relationships which determine the magnitude of the benefits and harms that can be expected with treatment. This preoccupation with issues of patient selection, inclusion and exclusion criteria and the (un)representativeness of trial participants has inhibited the development of methods for the accurate application of trial results.

KEY ISSUES: CURRENT METHODS

The methods described in the literature concentrated primarily on consideration of the characteristics of the settings and populations in which trials are conducted, and to whom the average treatment effect might apply.

Consideration of Subject Selection

An examination of the representativeness of the subjects who ultimately participate in randomised controlled trials and other evaluations of interventions, through consideration of the source population, the inclusion and exclusion criteria and the effects of obtaining informed consent has received most attention in the literature.[3-28] This line of reasoning is based on sampling theory and the corresponding need for a representative sample of patients.[6,12,14] Such a consideration of 'external validity' is important when the aim is to estimate the prevalence of a condition in a population, or to estimate certain characteristics such as levels of knowledge, patterns of behaviour or the range in attitudes. When this is extended to clinical trials, the conclusion that must be drawn from this approach is that the results are applicable only to subjects who resemble those included in the trial.[6,12,13,29,30]

However, the major purposes of inclusion and exclusion criteria are to improve study power (through inclusion of high-risk groups who are more likely to have the outcomes of interest, to minimise losses of subjects through death from other causes and to ensure good compliance to the intervention of interest) and to maximise safety of subjects in the trial (by minimising the occurrences of adverse effects).[31] However, there may be subjects excluded from the study who would experience an overall net benefit from the intervention, and there would certainly be subjects included who (despite a statistically significant overall treatment effect) have experienced net harm.[2,31,32]

This approach is further limited by the fact that a representative sample of eligible subjects is rarely achieved. Also, there are predictable differences between the eligible subjects and those who ultimately participate in the trial, and between those who meet the eligibility criteria and those who would be candidates for the intervention but are not eligible.[15,17-19,21,28,30,33,34]

Finally, the average treatment effect is an overall summary averaged over all subjects in the trial. The argument has been that this then applies to 'average' subjects. But, how does one define an 'average subject'? How different does a subject need to be from those in the study before one concludes that the results cannot be applied?

Comparison of Subjects Within and Outside of the Relevant Studies

Several approaches were described in the literature for comparing subjects within, and

outside of, the relevant studies and then adjusting the estimated average treatment effect for any observed differences.[35-43] Sophisticated approaches include the comprehensive cohort design and cross-design synthesis.

The *comprehensive cohort design* is a prospective cohort study with a randomised subcohort.[36-39] The idea is to compare the randomised patients with those who were eligible, but who were not randomised, on both baseline characteristics and outcomes (the non-randomised patients having been followed-up in the same way as the trial participants after receiving one of the interventions being compared). For example, a comprehensive cohort of patients with coronary heart disease was assembled to compare surgical and medical management.[36-38] The survival of patients receiving each of the treatment modalities was compared both within the randomised and the non-randomised patients. However, the analysis of the non-randomised patients is plagued by the usual sources of bias associated with observational studies, including confounding. Also, an interaction between the treatment and one or more prognostic factors (which may be distributed unevenly between the randomised and non-randomised groups) may produce an apparent difference or an apparent similarity in the results from the randomised and non-randomised components of the study.[39]

The underlying principle of *cross design synthesis* is to capture the strengths, and to minimise the weaknesses, of the randomised and non-randomised study designs.[40,41] The process, which combines the unbiased comparison of treatments from a randomised trial with the wider representativeness of a clinical database (or large cohort of patients with the condition of interest), consists of four steps:

1 Assess existing randomised studies for generalisability across the full range of relevant patients.
2 Assess databases of (non-randomised) patients for 'unbalanced comparison groups'.
3 Adjust the results of each randomised study and each database analysis, compensating for biases as needed.
4 Synthesise the studies' adjusted results within, and across, the design categories.

The main limitation of this method is the arbitrary nature of the judgements and standardisations required to make the necessary adjustments.[41] Also, the aim is to produce a single (unbiased) estimate of the average treatment effect ignoring possible variability in treatment effect and potential effect modifiers. As argued later, an exploration of the variability in estimates of treatment effect and possible sources of this variability leads to a better understanding of the underlying mechanisms through which the treatment works.

Some authors have proposed that the results of a randomised trial can be readily applied to other groups who have similar characteristics to those included in the trial(s).[35] For example, groups with a similar age range, gender mix, co-morbidities and disease severity. This represents a more formal approach to the consideration of applying the 'average' treatment effect to 'average' subjects.

Subgroup Analysis of Treatment Effects

Another common approach has been to examine the effect of the intervention in subgroups of subjects defined by characteristics such as gender, ethnicity, severity of disease, etc.[25,44–52] The idea is to compare the effect of the intervention in various subgroups, e.g. men and women, the elderly, or different ethnic groups. A common, but incorrect method is to perform a statistical test of treatment effect within each subgroup. The interpretation of the results is that the intervention should be offered only to those subgroups of patients in which a (statistically) significant treatment effect was detected. In addition, some have suggested that treatment should not be offered to those subgroups in which a significant treatment effect was not detected. Performing statistical tests for each individual subgroup can result in both false-positive (a spurious statistically significant treatment effect in some groups) and false-negative (an apparent lack of a significant treatment effect due to small numbers of subjects in some subgroups) results.[53] Such analyses have led to the interesting observation that a treatment benefit of intravenous atenolol in patients with suspected myocardial infarction only occurs in those born under the astrological birth sign Scorpio,[54] and aspirin had an effect in those patients with suspected myocardial infarction born under Capricorn, but not Gemini or Libra.[55]

The correct approach is to perform a test for treatment by subgroup interaction.[6,56–60] This results in a single statistical test, rather than multiple tests within subgroups. If a significant interaction is found, which indicates heterogeneity of treatment effect across groups, then further work can be carried out to identify which groups are different.

However, there is a difficulty in the interpretation of these analyses. Individual subjects fall into many subgroups, and the results from individual subgroup analyses may conflict. For example, how does one treat an elderly, African-American, male patient if different treatment effects are suggested in each of the subgroups defined by age, ethnicity and gender?

Risk-Based Individualisation of Benefit and Harm

A few authors have proposed methods for applying results to individual patients based on a consideration of the likely benefits and harms from treatment.[2,31,32] Based on the premise that it is inappropriate to judge the applicability of a trial's results by consideration of the subject entry criteria, and that the average treatment effect estimated in a trial is not applicable to all subjects (neither within, nor outside of the study), the idea is to identify in which individuals the treatment will do more good than harm. A model proposed by Lubsen and Tijssen suggests that patient benefit (as measured by the prevention of an adverse event such as stroke or death) increases with (untreated) risk of the outcome, but harm or rates of adverse events caused by the treatment will remain relatively fixed (Figure 1).[2] As the absolute risk reduction is related to the untreated (or baseline) risk of the event, high-risk patients are more likely to experience net benefit. Also for some low-risk patients, the likely harms may outweigh the expected benefits.

Glasziou and Irwig adapted this risk–benefit approach to identify which patients with non-rheumatic atrial fibrillation may benefit from treatment with warfarin to prevent a stroke.[31] This approach has been further developed into a

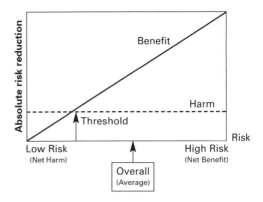

Figure 1   *Risk–benefit approach to applying the evidence to indivdiual patients (based on the model of Lubsen and Tijssen[2]).*

'five-step' process and is described in greater detail in the next section.

Other Approaches

Davis suggested that to determine the extent to which the results of a clinical trial can be generalised, several pieces of information (from various sources) are required.[61] He used the example of applying the results of the cholesterol-lowering trials in the prevention of coronary heart disease to illustrate the process. The question was whether the results could be extrapolated to women and to older men. The additional pieces of information required came from laboratory studies in which the pathogenic mechanism of the cholesterol-lowering drugs was examined to determine whether the mechanism is the same across age and genders, and from animal, genetic, observational, clinical and epidemiological studies as necessary.

Proposed Methods for Applying Results of Trials

General Issues to Consider

Firstly, applicability of the evidence to other settings and to different patient groups should be considered in its broadest context. Important issues are whether the intervention can be reproduced in the setting of interest and whether there are biological factors that may make the treatment less effective.

Can the intervention be reproduced in the setting of interest?

This needs careful consideration. Generally, if the intervention is a drug then it is readily transferable to other settings. However, the drug has to be licensed for use and it must be affordable to the patients and to the healthcare system. If the intervention is a surgical procedure, then surgeons with appropriate training and support staff are required, together with the necessary equipment.[62] The transferability of complex interventions requires a more careful consideration. For example, each component of a community health intervention programme must be taken into account and be applicable in the new setting. This includes the availability of appropriately trained personnel, the socio-cultural acceptability of the programme content, and so on.[63] Also, the availability of the required infrastructure for any type of intervention should be considered. For example, for the prescription

of warfarin to prevent stroke in patients with atrial fibrillation, the infrastructure for monitoring blood levels has to be in place and accessible to patients. This may not be the case for patients living in rural areas.

Can the results be applied in other settings and to other patients?

It is important to consider whether there are pathophysiological differences which may alter the biological mechanism through which the treatment has its effect.[64–66] For example, could the treatment effect be modified by gender, age or ethnicity, or by spectrum of the disease or timing of the intervention? A well-known example where this is true is the treatment of hypertension in blacks. The majority of trials of lipid-lowering drugs were carried out in middle-aged men, and many have debated whether the results apply to women and to older people.

Variations in the nature of the disease may also change the effect of treatment. For example, geographical patterns of antibiotic-resistant bacteria and drug-resistant malaria may alter the treatment's effectiveness. Also, the treatment may not be effective in severe disease where the patient is very sick and the disease process is now irreversible.

The timing of the intervention should be considered. Some treatments may be less effective if administration is delayed (e.g. thrombolytics after myocardial infarction), and so it may not be appropriate to prescribe the treatment beyond a certain time after the onset of symptoms or disease.

These biological effect modifiers are probably not all that common, but they may be important in a few instances.[65] However, the assumption should be made that they are unlikely, and the burden of proof really rests on demonstrating that they do modify the treatment effect, rather than assuming that they may.

A situation in which biological factors are important is the generalisation of results about a treatment for one form of disease to another variant. For example, the Diabetes Control and Complications Trial (DCCT) Research Group showed that intensive therapy and tight control in patients with insulin-dependent diabetes significantly reduced the occurrence of retinopathy, neuropathy, proteinuria and microalbuminuria.[67] However, there was also a three-fold increase in the incidence of severe hypoglycaemic reactions and an overall weight gain among those receiving intensive therapy. As patients with non-insulin-dependent diabetes mellitus (NIDDM) tend to be middle-aged or elderly, they could not tolerate this frequency of hypoglycaemic episodes and their hyperinsulinaemia may be aggravated by weight gain.[68] Therefore intensive therapy with insulin for NIDDM could aggravate, rather than ameliorate, diabetic complications.

Using evidence in primary care

A common argument against applying the results of clinical trials to clinical practice is that trials are typically carried out in tertiary care settings and so are not applicable in community hospitals, general practice and other primary care settings.[69,70] The belief is that because patients in primary care are likely to have a lower probability of the outcome being prevented (i.e. have a lower baseline risk), and milder disease, that the biological response to treatment may be different (and in particular that the treatment will be less effective). This implies that the relative risk reduction varies with baseline (or underlying) risk of the event being prevented by the treatment. That is, the relative treatment effect is lower (or it may be higher) in patients with lower baseline risk. This is an assumption that needs to be checked. However, the absolute risk reduction (which is of more relevance to the individual) is likely to be smaller for lower levels of baseline risk. Therefore an important step, which is described later in this section, is a consideration of the patient's baseline risk and a prediction of the absolute risk reduction. It may be the case that for a larger proportion of patients in primary care, the expected benefits will not justify the potential harms and costs. However, there are likely to be some patients who will benefit from treatment and therefore the treatment should not be excluded from primary care entirely.

A consideration of relative versus absolute risk reductions and their relationships with baseline risk is discussed in greater detail later in this section.

Suggested Process for Applying Evidence

As discussed in the previous section, traditional approaches for considering the applicability of results of trials and systematic reviews are very limiting, and are based on the flawed logic that if patients in the trial received an average benefit then patients like those in the trial will also, on average, benefit. However, this 'average' in the trial may include patients with greater than average benefit, some with the average benefit, and some in whom there was net harm.

The risk–benefit approach of Lubsen and Tijssen[2] was adapted to identify which patients with non-rheumatic atrial fibrillation may benefit from treatment with warfarin to prevent a stroke.[31] A modified version of this approach is recommended for use and is described in detail in this section.

Briefly, the principle underlying this approach is to apply the relative risk reduction due to the intervention (which is assumed to be constant, but this should be verified), to an individual's predicted (baseline) risk if left untreated, to obtain an estimate of their expected absolute risk reduction. This is then weighed up against the potential harms or adverse effects of the intervention to determine whether the benefits are likely to outweigh the risks.

This approach requires the consideration of five questions, each of which should be addressed when thinking about applicability (Table 3). The first three questions relate directly to the overall effect of treatment – the expected outcomes (both benefits and harms) and the robustness of the estimate of (relative) treatment effect (i.e. is it constant across a range of potential effect modifiers and levels of baseline risk?). These address the issue of transferability of the average treatment effect. The last two questions cover aspects of individualising or particularising the treatment decision through estimating the expected absolute risk reduction based on an individual's baseline risk and then taking into account patient's preferences in the weighing up of benefits and harms.

When considering each of these five issues, often there will be insufficient data to address each of them in detail. However, it is still a helpful exercise to go through these steps and to make explicit what additional information is required to be able to apply the evidence about an intervention's effectiveness in an accurate manner. With improvements in trial design, and particularly in the analysis and reporting of trials, it will become possible to use this approach in an increasing number of situations.

Transferability

What are the beneficial and harmful effects of the intervention?

The answer to the question, 'to whom should the treatment be offered so that more good than harm is achieved?' requires a careful consideration of all the potential benefits of the treatment as well as the harms (risks or side-effects) that could be attributed to the treatment. Of particular concern are patients who are at low risk of

Table 3   *Summary of suggested approach for applying the evidence*

In applying results of trials and systematic reviews in clinical practice, five questions should be addressed.

TRANSFERABILITY

What are the beneficial and harmful effects?
All patient-relevant end-points that are potentially influenced by the treatment, including, in particular, adverse effects should be considered. For example, anti-arrhythmic drugs have pro-arrhythmic effects; anticoagulants increase the risk of bleeding. Particularly for groups at low risk of the primary outcome such adverse effects may be crucial. It is helpful to begin by tabulating all that is known about possible positive and negative effects of the intervention.

Are there variations in the relative treatment effect?
Can the same (or average) treatment effect be applied to all subjects or does the effect vary according to various characteristics? For example:
a)   patient features (e.g. age, gender, biochemical markers)
b)   intervention features (e.g. the timing, compliance, or intensity of the intervention)
c)   disease features (e.g. hormone receptor status)
d)   the measure of effect used (relative risk versus risk difference)
Chance variation between subgroups is inevitable; hence without prior justification and strong evidence, we should assume there is none. The evidence should come from testing whether the factor modifies the treatment effect (i.e. interaction), and *not* by testing within each individual 'subgroup'. Ideally, this is done from individual data *within trials* (not between trials), otherwise confounding by variation in trial design may occur.

How does the treatment effect vary with baseline risk level?
Low-risk patients will usually gain less absolute benefit than high-risk patients. However, it is important to ascertain whether the relative effect varies with predicted event rate (baseline risk). If instead of the predicted rate the event rate in the control group is used, there is an intrinsic negative correlation between the relative risk and the control group rate. This has to be taken into account in any analyses performed. If there is a change across predicted event rate, then sophisticated statistical techniques are required to estimate the degree of change.

APPLICATION TO INDIVIDUALS

What are the predicted absolute risk reductions for individuals?
The relative risk is useful for assessing the biological strength of response but, to judge whether therapy is worthwhile, we need the absolute magnitude of benefit. This might be expressed as the absolute risk reduction, or as a frequency format such as the Number Needed to Treat, NNT (for both helping and harming). However it is expressed, it varies with the patient's expected event rate (PEER): for low-risk patients, absolute benefit may not outweigh the absolute harm. Thus, to apply the results, the individual's PEER or severity based on established predictors is needed. Information on prognosis, often external to the trials, should be used. Examples include the New Zealand guidelines on hypertension and predictors of stroke risk in atrial fibrillation.

Do the benefits outweigh the harms?
The absolute and net benefits of therapy, and the strength of the individual patient's preferences for these, need to be considered. If the treatment has multiple effects, e.g. adverse as well as beneficial effects, then the assessment of the absolute benefit needs to incorporate these disparate outcomes. If Step 4 is done well, the trade-offs will often be clear; however, methods developed in decision analysis may be a useful supplement, e.g. quality-adjusted life years might provide a summary measure when there are trade-offs between quality and quantity of life. The central issue is whether for the individual patient the predicted absolute benefit has greater value than the harm and cost of treatment. For example, when does the reduction in strokes outweigh the risk of bleeding from anticoagulation, or when does the benefit of surgery outweigh its risk?

Even if appropriate data are lacking, it will be helpful to think through these steps qualitatively.

the main outcome which the intervention is supposed to prevent (death, stroke, myocardial infarction, etc.). Generally, in such patients the intervention can be expected to achieve only a small absolute risk reduction, so the harms are much more important as they are likely to outweigh the benefits.

Typically, a study or systematic review evaluating the effectiveness of the intervention focuses on a single primary end-point and possibly a small number of secondary end-points. Sometimes side-effects are reported but often the number of participants with side-effects is small because the trial was not designed to detect the

Table 4   *Potential benefits and harms associated with two preventive treatments*

Benefits	Harms	
Treatment of hypertension in the elderly[71]		
Reduction in mortality due to all causes, non-cardiovascular, cardiovascular, coronary, cerebrovascular	Gout	Skin disorders
	Muscle cramps	Nausea
	Dizziness	Raynaud's phenomenon
Reduction in non-fatal stroke	Dyspnoea	Headaches
	Dry mouth	Diarrhoea
Screening high-risk individuals for colorectal cancer[72]		
Reduced risk of invasive colorectal cancer	False-positive result leading to a clinical work-	
Reduced risk of dying from colorectal cancer	up	
	Perforation of the colon	
	Discomfort	
	Inconvenience	
	Anxiety	

effects of different treatments on these outcomes (particularly long-term effects).

All patient-relevant end-points should be considered that are potentially influenced by the intervention, including, in particular, adverse effects. For example, anti-arrhythmic drugs have pro-arrhythmic effects; anticoagulants increase the risk of bleeding. Particularly for groups at low risk of the primary outcome such adverse effects may be crucial. It is helpful to begin by tabulating all that is known about possible positive and negative effects of the intervention, even if data for some outcomes are not available.

Examples of the potential benefits and harms associated with antihypertensive treatment in the elderly and screening of high-risk people for colorectal cancer are displayed in Table 4.[71,72]

Are there variations in the relative treatment effect?

To better understand how the intervention works, and how to apply the results of evaluations, it is useful to determine whether treatment effect is constant or whether it varies according to various characteristics relating to patients (e.g. age, gender, biochemical markers); the disease (e.g. hormone receptor status); the intervention (e.g. the timing, compliance, or intensity of the intervention); and the measure of effect used (relative risk versus risk difference).

In working through this, an understanding of the terms 'effect modification', 'heterogeneity' and 'interaction' is required (Table 5).

When there are several studies evaluating the intervention, the treatment effect can be

Table 5   *Definitions of heterogeneity, interaction and effect modification*

Heterogeneity: Differences in estimates of treatment effect between studies contributing to a meta-analysis. Significant heterogeneity suggests that the trials are not estimating a single common treatment effect. The variation in treatment effects may be due to differences across the trials in the patients, the setting, the mode of intervention, the way outcomes were defined and measured, and so on.

Interaction and effect modification: Refers to the relationship between a single variable (or co-variate) and the treatment effect. Significant interaction between the treatment and some variable, such as patient's age, patient's gender or ethnicity, indicates that the treatment effect varies across levels of this variable. The variable is then called an 'effect modifier' as it modifies the effect of treatment. This modification of effect may contribute to any heterogeneity detected. It may be either:

(a)   *Qualitative interaction*, where the treatment effect differs in direction across levels of the effect modifier. For example, the treatment may reduce risk of the outcome in men but increase risk in women, or

(b)   *Quantitative interaction*, which occurs when the magnitude of the treatment effect varies but is in the same direction. For example, the relative risk reduction is 50% in men and 30% in women.

It has been argued that quantitative interactions are much more likely to occur than qualitative interactions because humans are not all that different biologically. Therefore if a qualitative interaction is detected, it should be interpreted with caution.

Table 6   *Potential sources of heterogeneity in treatment effect (adapted from Guyatt et al.[73])*

Potential effect modifier	Examples
Trial design	setting, subjects, co-administered therapy, length of follow-up, outcomes measured and how, completeness of follow-up, study quality
Characteristics of:	
Patient	age, gender, race, co-morbidity, biochemical markers, genetic markers
Disease	method and accuracy of diagnosis, severity, stage, responsiveness
Intervention	form, mode of administration, dose, intensity, timing, duration, compliance

explored further by firstly conducting a test for heterogeneity. If the treatment effect appears to be heterogeneous (or non-constant) then the sources of heterogeneity (or important effect modifiers) should be examined via testing for interactions between each of the variables and treatment. In fact, since the test of heterogeneity typically has low power and sometimes heterogeneity may not be apparent even in the presence of effect modification (because the studies were homogeneous on the effect modifier), interactions should be explored regardless of the result of the test of heterogeneity.

Potential effect modifiers will vary according to the treatment and disease under investigation. For example, a number of biological/disease factors and patient features may be effect modifiers in relation to treatment of breast cancer including age/menopausal status, nodal status, receptor status, tumour size, grade, ploidy and type, vascular invasion, labelling index, S-phase fraction, body mass and family history.[57] Heterogeneity may occur by chance (but this can be checked using a statistical test) or by choosing the wrong measure of treatment effect (relative risk versus risk difference). If these causes have been dismissed, then possible sources of heterogeneity can be grouped into four areas. Some examples are shown in Table 6.

How does the treatment effect vary with baseline risk level?

A very important factor to consider when looking at whether the magnitude of benefit varies across different groups is the level of (untreated) risk. Generally, low-risk groups will have less to gain from an intervention than high-risk groups, and hence they may not gain sufficient benefit to outweigh harms from treatment (adverse effects, costs, etc.).

The benefit for an individual (as measured by the absolute risk reduction or Number Needed to Treat; NNT) is likely to depend strongly on the baseline level of risk. Table 7 shows the relationship between baseline risk and absolute risk reduction or NNT for a constant relative risk reduction.

Which patients will obtain a net benefit will depend on the harmful effects of the intervention, such as adverse drug reactions, side-effects, the burden of compliance and monitoring, etc. The greater the potential harm, the greater the benefit required to make it worthwhile. This trade-off, and how it relates to baseline risk is illustrated in Figure 1, which shows benefit increasing but harm being constant across different levels of baseline risk.

This extrapolation from the estimated relative risk to the expected absolute risk reduction for different risk groups assumes that the relative risk reduction remains constant – *an assumption that needs to be checked*. For many interventions the relative risk appears to be reasonably constant. An analysis of individual study results included in 112 meta-analyses found a statistically significant relationship between the measure of treatment effect and baseline risk in 15 (13%) meta-analyses with relative risk as the

Table 7   *Absolute reductions in risk associated with relative risk reductions of 50% and 25%*

Baseline risk	50% Relative risk reduction (RR = 0.50)		25% Relative risk reduction (RR = 0.75)	
	Risk difference	NNT	Risk difference	NNT
10%	5%	20	2.5%	40
1%	0.5%	200	0.25%	400
1 in 1000	0.05%	2000	1 in 4000	4000
1 in 10 000	1 in 20 000	20 000	1 in 40 000	40 000

measure of treatment effect, in 16 (14%) with the odds ratio, and 35 (31%) with the risk difference.[74] Thus, the relative risk was constant for 87% of the systematic reviews. However, there are clearly cases that deviate considerably from this assumption. For example, Rothwell has shown that in patients with carotid artery stenosis treated with carotid endarterectomy, the relative risk is very different for different risk groups.[32] In the high-risk groups there is a high relative risk reduction, but in the low-risk group there is no apparent benefit. By contrast, he showed that aspirin has a similar relative benefit across both groups. A second example of a non-constant relative risk reduction is the Class I anti-arrhythmic drugs. Boissel et al. found in trials of Class I anti-arrhythmics in patients after myocardial infarction, that because of different inclusion criteria, there was a large variation in the degree of risk in these trials.[75] There appeared to be a beneficial effect in the very high risk, but in lower-risk groups they appeared to do net harm. This result was confirmed by the CAST study which showed a doubling of mortality from flecainide.[76]

Since most patient groups to which trial results will be applied will not have a risk identical to the average seen in the trial, one of the crucial analyses in assessing the applicability of trial results will be a systematic study of how relative benefit varies with baseline risk. This may be done either within trials, by looking at different prognostic groups, or between trials, by making use of the variation in average baseline risk due to the different selection processes of trials.

For example, in a systematic review of 39 RCTs examining the effects of angiotensin-converting enzyme (ACE) inhibitors in the treatment of congestive heart failure, the studies were stratified according to the annual mortality rate – the low-risk group with mortality of up to 15% (28 studies) and the high-risk group with mortality greater than 15% (11 studies).[77] The relative risks for mortality in the group treated with ACE inhibitors compared with those receiving placebo were 0.88 (95% confidence interval 0.80–0.97) for the low-risk group and 0.64 (0.51–0.81) for the high-risk group. Therefore, both the absolute and relative risk reductions due to use of ACE inhibitors in patients with impaired left ventricular dysfunction and symptoms of heart failure appear to increase with mortality risk.

When examining this relationship between treatment effect and baseline risk, there are a number of methodological problems that can produce misleading results.[78–81] For example, Brand and Kragt suggested plotting the relative risk against the risk in the control group (as a

surrogate for the underlying baseline or untreated risk).[82] In their example – tocolysis for pre-term birth – there appeared to be a decreasing relative risk reduction with decreasing control group risk, i.e. a non-constant relative risk. While such an analysis is potentially very informative, a number of authors have discussed the accompanying methodological pitfalls, and alternative methods based on Bayesian and frequentist approaches have been proposed.[78–81]

The other assumption being made here is that the harms are constant across levels of baseline risk for the event being prevented. In some cases, higher-risk patients may be more susceptible to harm (e.g. surgical mortality). However, in many cases the harms may be directly associated with exposure to the intervention itself (e.g. adverse effects of drugs). However, again this assumption should be checked.

Application to Individuals

What are the predicted absolute risk reductions for individuals?

The first three steps involved the identification of all potential patient-relevant benefits and harms, identification of treatment effect modifiers and exploration of the relationship between the magnitude of the treatment effect and baseline (or untreated) risk. These all address the degree to which the estimates of treatment effect from a single study, or a systematic review of several studies, can be transferred to other settings and to other patients.

The next two issues to be considered relate directly to applying the results to an individual (or a group of similar individuals).

While the relative risk is useful for assessing the biological strength of response to the treatment, to judge whether therapy is worthwhile for an individual, the absolute magnitude of benefit should be estimated. This might be expressed as the absolute risk reduction, or as the NNT. However it is expressed, it varies with the patient's baseline risk (which is sometimes referred to as the Patient's Expected Event Rate, PEER): for low-risk patients absolute benefit may not outweigh the absolute harm. If the relative risk reduction is constant across levels of baseline risk and there is no effect modification, then the average relative risk reduction can be applied to a particular patient. If this is not the case, then the relationships need to be described so that the appropriate relative risk can be applied for a particular patient.

To estimate the absolute risk reduction for an individual, the expected relative risk reduction can be applied to the PEER. This then requires an estimate of the PEER which can be obtained from a previously developed (and preferably validated) prognostic model linking values of various (baseline/pre-randomisation) characteristics of the patient to the probability of the disease of interest.

The following example illustrates this point. In considering whether to treat two patients with aspirin to prevent a further cardiovascular event, Boissel estimated their one-year mortality risk using a previously established risk score.[83]

Patient 1: A 45-year-old man who has normal blood cholesterol and glucose levels, blood pressure and weight and who is a non-smoker. Presented with an uncomplicated inferior myocardial infarction. His one-year mortality risk is 2%.

Patient 2: A 65-year-old woman who has had hypertension for 30 years, has diabetes, had a previous myocardial infarction, smokes two packs of cigarettes a day and reports breathlessness with exercise. Presented with her second anterior myocardial infarction together with signs of heart failure. Her one-year mortality risk is 30%.

Applying a (constant) relative risk reduction of 15% in all-cause mortality, the two patients can expect absolute risk reductions of 0.3% and 4.5% respectively (NNTs of 300 and 22). These can be weighed against an excess risk of cerebral bleeding with aspirin of 0.12% for both patients.

There are many examples of prognostic models in the literature. They tend to be based on cohort (prospective) studies in which a sample of patients are recruited, various baseline characteristics are recorded, and then the patients are followed over time to see whether they develop the outcome of interest. Statistical modelling (such as logistic regression or proportional hazards models) is then used to examine which combination of variables best predict which patients experience the outcome of interest. Examples from the literature include prediction of 10-year survival after definitive surgical therapy for primary cutaneous melanoma,[84] prediction of 5-year risk of a cardiovascular event[85] and expected rates of thromboembolic stroke in patients with atrial fibrillation.[86]

Do the benefits outweigh the harms?

The final consideration in formulating recommendations about to whom the intervention should be applied is how the potential benefits and harms compare. Information on the benefits and harms by levels of baseline risk should be presented so that individuals (patients) together with their healthcare providers can, if they

choose to, make a decision about the intervention based on their preferences.

Often, there will be multiple effects associated with the intervention – both beneficial and harmful. These need to be weighed up and trade-offs made in formulating recommendations and in making individual treatment decisions.

The trade-offs between different outcomes can involve either the quality of the outcome, such as different dimensions of quality of life, or they may involve the timing of occurrence of the outcome. A particularly frequent and important trade-off between outcomes is that between quality and quantity of life. For example, many surgical procedures, such as hip replacement or cholecystectomy, involve a mortality risk that may be acceptable because of the reduction in symptoms or improvement of function. This balancing of benefits and harms requires a common scale. For example, we may need to compare having a stroke with a death from intracranial haemorrhage. This is not easy, but such a valuation is implicit in clinical decisions. If it is made explicit, discussion about individualisation of treatment will be easier. Quality of life scales, ranking outcomes on a scale between death (0) and normal good health (1) attempt to do this.[87] Where there are trade-offs between quality and quantity of life, the Quality Adjusted Life Year (QALY) attempts to combine both into a single measure.[88] Another summary measure that has been used in cancer trials is TWiST, the Time Without Symptoms and Toxicity, which deals simultaneously with survival gains and the changes in quality of life due to toxicity (loss) and delays or avoidance of relapse (gain).[89] This measure was refined to include differential weightings for quality of life while experiencing toxicity and relapse (Q-TWiST).[90,91]

Appropriate reporting and analysis of clinical trials is needed to make the trade-offs explicit, and to allow an informed decision by healthcare provider and patient. However, if the previous step of estimating an individual's potential benefits and harms is done well, and presented in a clear way, often the trade-offs will be clear. The central issue is whether, for the individual patient, the predicted absolute benefit has greater value than the harm and cost of treatment. For example, when does the reduction in strokes outweigh the risk of bleeding from anticoagulation, or when does the benefit of surgery outweigh its risk?

If no adverse events have been identified, then it may seem that only benefits need to be considered. However, serious adverse events may be rare and hence the concern is how reliably they have been excluded. This 'proof of safety' is usually more difficult, and rare adverse effects (say of drugs) may only emerge during post-marketing monitoring. Several authors have discussed the statistical difficulties of excluding such serious rare events. For example, if 300 patients have been treated in controlled trials and no serious adverse effects detected, the confidence interval for the rate of such events is from 0% to 1% – that is, we can be 95% certain that the risk of an adverse effect is less than 1%.[92]

IMPLICATIONS AND FURTHER RESEARCH

The results of this systematic review have implications for the design and reporting of clinical trials, methods for applying the results of trials and systematic reviews in clinical practice and how groups developing clinical practice guidelines should consider the evidence when formulating treatment recommendations. Each of these will be discussed in turn.

Conduct and Reporting of Clinical Trials and Systematic Reviews

The principal need in designing and reporting clinical trials is that all patient-relevant outcomes (both benefits and harms) are measured and reported. Also, effect modification and the variation in treatment effect across levels of baseline risk should be explored and discussed. The role of, and need for, inclusion and exclusion criteria should be reconsidered. There is a need for large pragmatic trials with heterogeneous patient populations to facilitate an exploration of effect modification.

People undertaking systematic reviews should examine heterogeneity, effect modification and the importance of baseline risk rather than concentrate on producing a pooled (average) estimate of treatment effect. A balance sheet of benefits and harms should be included in the report.

Clinical Practice

Practitioners, when attempting to apply the results of trials in treatment decisions, need to go beyond a consideration of the characteristics of the trial patients, settings and available clinical care and how they compare with their situation.

Rather, decision aids and clinical practice guidelines should be made available to assist in the identification of those patients in whom the treatment is more likely to do good than harm.

Development of Clinical Practice Guidelines

Guidelines-writing groups should consider broad issues regarding the applicability of the evidence including the reproducibility of the intervention in different settings and biological factors that may alter the treatment's effectiveness (although these are likely to be rare). They also need to develop more explicit processes to consider trial applicability, and the weighing of harms and benefits for individual patients. Therefore, guidelines for developing clinical practice guidelines should include methods for assessing trial applicability and should recommend more formal processes to encourage accurate application of the evidence.

Traditional methods for assessing applicability based on subject selection for the trials, inclusion/exclusion criteria, and subgroup analyses are flawed. Rather, guidelines-writing groups, using the process we have described, should identify in which individuals or homogeneous groups the treatment is more likely to do good than harm as the basis for treatment recommendations.

Guidelines should be designed to enable the clinician and patient to assess the individual's risk or prognosis and the consequent potential benefit and harm from treatment (the New Zealand guidelines on the treatment of hypertension are an excellent example[85]). Ultimately, they should not adopt a prescriptive algorithmic approach.

Areas for Further Research

Further methodological and empirical research is required to examine relationships between relative treatment effect and baseline risk, and to develop appropriate statistical methods to do this. These methods should take account of the negative correlation between a measure of treatment effect and the event rate in the control group, the error associated with the estimate of the event rate in the control group, regression–dilution bias and problems of misclassification regarding presence/absence of the outcome of interest due to limitations in the measurements.

Methods for presenting the magnitude of the treatment effect for both benefits and harms that differ in levels of severity and timing of occurrence require further development.

Further methodological development is needed to create prognostic models from studies to enable an independent estimation of predicted risk. There is a need for further investigation of the use of comprehensive cohorts for developing and testing prognostic models using both patients who entered the trial and those who did not get randomised.

Finally, research is needed into the question of whether the adoption of 'formal' approaches to the application of trial results leads to better outcomes for patients.

ACKNOWLEDGEMENTS

This work was supported by a grant from the NHS Health and Technology Assessment Research and Development Programme.

REFERENCES

1. Collet JP, Boissel JP. The sick population – treated population: the need for a better definition. The VALIDATA Group. *Eur. J. Clin. Pharmacol.* 1991; **41**: 267–71.
2. Lubsen J, Tijssen JG. Large trials with simple protocols: indications and contraindications. *Controlled Clinical Trials* 1989; **10**(Suppl.): 151S–60S.
3. Yusuf S, Held P, Teo KK, Toretsky ER. Selection of patients for randomized controlled trials: implications of wide or narrow eligibility criteria. *Statist. Med.* 1990; **9**: 73–83.
4. Sackett DL. The fourth prerequisite: the inclusion/exclusion criteria strike a balance between efficiency and generalisability. In: Shapiro SH, Louis TA (eds) *Clinical Trials: Issues and Approaches.* New York: Marcel Dekker. 1983: Vol. 46, pp. 72–4.
5. George SL. Reducing patient eligibility criteria in cancer trials. *J. Clin. Oncol.* 1996; **14**: 1364–70.
6. Simon R. Patient subset and variation in therapeutic efficacy. In: Chaput de Saintonge DM, Vere DW (eds) *Current Problems in Clinical Trials.* 1st edn. London: Blackwell Scientific Publications, 1984.
7. King AC, Harris RB, Haskell WL. Effect of recruitment strategy on types of subjects entered into a primary prevention clinical trial. *Ann. Epidemiol.* 1994; **4**: 312–20.
8. Simpson FO. Fallacies in the interpretation of the large-scale trials of treatment of mild to moderate hypertension. *J. Cardiovasc. Pharmacol.* 1990; **16**(Suppl. 7): S92–5.
9. Wittes RE. Problems in the medical interpretation of overviews. *Statist. Med.* 1987; **6**: 269–80.
10. Richmond RL, Anderson P. Research in general practice for smokers and excessive drinkers in Australia and the UK. II. Representativeness of the results. *Addiction* 1994; **89**: 41–7.
11. Feagan BG, McDonald JWD, Koval JJ. Therapeutics and inflammatory bowel disease: a guide to the interpretation of randomized controlled trials. *Gastroenterology* 1996; **110**: 275–83.
12. Schooler NR. How generalizable are the results of clinical trials? *Psychopharm. Bull.* 1980; **16**: 29–31.
13. Remington RD. Potential impact of exclusion criteria on results of hypertension trials. *Hypertension* 1989; **13**(Suppl. I): I66–8.
14. Rapaport MH, Frevert T, Babior S, Zisook S, Judd LL. A comparison of demographic variables, symptom profiles, and measurement of functioning in symptomatic volunteers and an outpatient clinical population. *Psychopharm. Bull.* 1995; **31**: 111–14.
15. Antman K, Amato D, Wood W, et al. Selection bias in clinical trials. *J. Clin. Oncol.* 1985; **3**: 1142–7.
16. Kramer MS, Shapiro SH. Scientific challenges in the application of randomized trials. *JAMA* 1984; **252**: 2739–45.
17. Juster HR, Heimberg RG, Engelberg B. Self selection and sample selection in a treatment study of social phobia. *Behav. Res. Ther.* 1995; **33**: 321–4.
18. Llewellyn-Thomas HA, McGreal MJ, Thiel EC, Fine S, Erlichmen C. Patients' willingness to enter clinical trials: measuring the association with perceived benefit and preference for decision participation. *Soc. Sci. Med.* 1991; **32**: 35–42.
19. Wilhelmsen L, Ljungberg S, Wedel H, Werko L. A comparison between participants and non-participants in a primary preventive trial. *J. Chron. Dis.* 1976; **29**: 331–9.
20. Charlson ME, Horwitz RI. Applying results of randomised trials to clinical practice: impact of losses before randomisation. *Br. Med. J. Clin. Res. Ed.* 1984; **289**: 1281–4.
21. Smith P, Arnesen H. Mortality in non-consenters in a post-myocardial infarction trial. *J. Intern. Med.* 1990; **228**: 253–6.
22. Biener L, DePue JD, Emmors KM, Linnan L, Abrams DB. Recruitment of work sites to a health promotion research trial. *J. Occup. Med.* 1994; **36**: 631–6.
23. Pincus T. Limitations to standard randomized controlled trials to evaluate combination therapies in rheumatic diseases. *Agents-Actions* 1993; **44**(Suppl.): 83–91.
24. Brundage MD, Mackillop WJ. Locally advanced non-small cell lung cancer: do we know the questions? A survey of randomized trials from 1966–1993. *J. Clin. Epidemiol.* 1996; **49**: 183–92.
25. Ziegelstein RC, Chandra NC. Selecting patients who benefit from thrombolysis. *Coronary Artery Disease* 1994; **5**: 282–6.
26. Mitchell JR. 'But will it help my patients with myocardial infarction?' The implications of

recent trials for everyday country folk. *Br. Med. J.* 1982; **285**: 1140–8.

27. Ausman JI, Diaz FG. Critique of the Extracranial–Intracranial Bypass Study. *Surg. Neurol.* 1986; **26**: 218–21.

28. Kober L, Torp-Pedersen C. On behalf of the TRACE Study Group. Clinical characteristics and mortality of patients screened for entry into the Trandolapril Cardiac Evaluation (TRACE) Study. *Am. J. Cardiol.* 1995; **76**: 1–5.

29. Pocock SJ. Organisation and planning. In: *Clinical Trials: a practical approach*. London: A Wiley Medical Publication, 1984, Chapter 3, pp. 35–8.

30. Williford WO, Krol WF, Buzby GP. Comparison of eligible randomized patients with two groups of ineligible patients: can the results of the VA total parenteral nutrition clinical trial be generalized? *J. Clin. Epidemiol.* 1993; **46**: 1025–34.

31. Glasziou PP, Irwig LM. An evidence based approach to individualising treatment. *Br. Med. J.* 1995; **311**: 1356–9.

32. Rothwell PM. Can overall results of clinical trials be applied to all patients? *Lancet* 1995; **345**: 1616–19.

33. Day AL, Rhoton AL, Little JR. The Extracranial-Intracranial Bypass Study. *Surg. Neurol.* 1986; **26**: 222–6.

34. Sundt TM. Was the international randomized trial of extracranial-intracranial arterial bypass representative of the population at risk? *N. Engl. J. Med.* 1987; **316**: 814–16.

35. Walsh JT, Gray D, Keating NA, Cowley AJ, Hampton JR. ACE for whom? Implications for clinical practice of post-infarct trials. *Br. Heart J.* 1995; **73**: 470–4.

36. Schumacher M, Davis K. Combining randomized and nonrandomized patients in the statistical analysis of clinical trials. *Rec. Results Cancer Res.* 1988; **111**: 130–7.

37. Davis K. Comprehensive cohort study: the use of registry data to confirm and extend a randomized trial. *Rec. Results Cancer Res.* 1988; **111**: 138–48.

38. Olschewski M, Schumacher M, Davis KB. Analysis of randomized and nonrandomized patients in clinical trials using comprehensive cohort follow-up study design. *Controlled Clinical Trials* 1992; **13**: 226–39.

39. Schmoor C, Olschewski M, Schumacher M. Randomized and non-randomized patients in clinical trials: experiences with comprehensive cohort studies. *Statist. Med.* 1996; **15**: 263–71.

40. Mitchell GJ, Glenn J, Pryor DB, Cohen WS. Cross design synthesis. A new strategy for medical effectiveness research. Washington DC. United States General Accounting Office, 1992, Doc. No.B-244808.

41. Droitcour J, Silberman G, Chelimsky E. A new form of meta-analysis for combining results from randomized clinical trials and medical practice databases. *Int. J. Technol. Assess. Health Care* 1993; **9**: 440–9.

42. Hlatky MA, Califf RM, Harrell FE Jr, Lee KL, Mark DB, Pryor DB. Comparison of predictions based on observational data with the results of randomized controlled clinical trials of coronary artery bypass surgery. *J. Am. Coll. Cardiol.* 1988; **11**: 237–45.

43. Hlatky MA, Califf RM, Harrell FE, et al. Clinical judgement and therapeutic decision making. *J. Am. Coll. Cardiol.* 1990; **15**: 1–14.

44. The Cardiac Arrhythmia Suppression Trial (CAST) Investigators. Preliminary report: effect of encainide and flecainide on mortality in a randomized trial of arrhythmia suppression after myocardial infarction. *N. Engl. J. Med.* 1989; **321**: 406–12.

45. Early Breast Cancer Trialists' Collaborative Group. Systemic treatment of early breast cancer by hormonal, cytotoxic, or immune therapy. Part I. *Lancet* 1992; **339**: 1–15. Part II. *Lancet* 1992; **339**: 71–85.

46. Kazempour K, Kammerman LA, Farr SS. Survival effects of ZDV, ddI and ddC in patients with $CD4 \leq 50$ cells/mm^3. *J. Acquir. Immune Defic. Syndr. Hum. Retrovirol.* 1995; **10**(Suppl. 2): S97–106.

47. Fine MJ, Smith MA, Carson CA, et al. Efficacy of pneumococcal vaccination in adults. A meta-analysis of randomized controlled trials. *Arch. Intern. Med.* 1994; **154**: 2666–77.

48. Easton JD, Wilterdink JL. Carotid endarterectomy: trials and tribulations. *Ann. Neurol.* 1994; **35**: 5–17.

49. Gruppo Italiano per lo studio della Sopavvivenza nell'Infarto Miocardico. GISSI–2: a factorial randomised trial of alteplase versus streptokinase and heparin versus no heparin among 12,490 patients with acute myocardial infarction. *Lancet* 1990; **336**: 65–71.

50. Multicentre Acute Stroke Trial-Italy (MAST-I) Group. Randomised controlled trial of streptokinase, aspirin, and combination of both in treatment of acute ischemic stroke. *Lancet* 1995; **346**: 1509–14.

51. Gheorghiade M, Schultz L, Tilley B, Kao W, Goldstein S. Effects of propranolol in non-Q-wave acute myocardial infarction in the Beta Blocker Heart Attack Trial (BHAT). *Am. J. Cardiol.* 1990; **66**: 129–33.

52. The EC/IC Bypass Study Group. Failure of extracranial-intracranial arterial bypass to reduce the risk of ischemic stroke. Results of an international randomized trial. *N. Engl. J. Med.* 1985; **313**: 1191–200.

53. Peto R. Why do we need systematic overviews of randomized trials? *Statist. Med.* 1987; **6**: 233–44.

54. Collins R, Gray R, Godwin J, Peto R. Avoidance of large biases and large random errors in the assessment of moderate treatment effects: the need for systematic overviews. *Statist. Med.* 1987; **6**: 245–54.

55. Peto R, Collins R, Gray R. Large-scale randomized evidence: large, simple trials and overviews of trials. *J. Clin. Epidemiol.* 1995; **48**: 23–40.

56. Pocock SJ, Hughes MD. Estimation issues in clinical trials and overviews. *Statist. Med.* 1990; **9**: 657–71.

57. Gelber RD, Goldhirsch A. Interpretation of results from subset analyses within overviews of randomized clinical trials. *Statist. Med.* 1987; **6**: 371–8.

58. Gail M, Simon R. Testing for qualitative interactions betweeen treatment effects and patient subsets. *Biometrics* 1985; **41**: 361–72.

59. Pocock SJ. Further aspects of data analysis. In: *Clinical trials: a practical approach*. London: A Wiley Medical Publication, 1984, Chapter 14, pp. 213–16.

60. Shuster J, van Eys J. Interaction between prognostic factors and treatment. *Controlled Clinical Trials* 1983; **4**: 209–14.

61. Davis CE. Generalizing from clinical trials. *Controlled Clinical Trials* 1994; **15**: 11–14.

62. Tannock IF. Assessment of study design in clinical trials for bladder cancer. *Urol. Clin. North. Am.* 1992; **19**: 655–62.

63. Gyorkos TW, Tannenbaum TN, Abrahamowicz M, et al. An approach to the development of practice guidelines for community health interventions. *Can. J. Public Health* (Suppl. 1) 1994; Jul–Aug: S8–13.

64. Nunnelee JD. The inclusion of women in clinical trials of antihypertensive medications: a review of twenty-four trials in one pharmacology journal. *J. Vasc. Nurs.* 1995; **13**: 41–9.

65. Piantadosi S, Wittes J. Politically correct clinical trials. *Controlled Clinical Trials* 1993; **14**: 562–7.

66. Dans AL, Dans LF, Guyatt GH, et al. Users' guides to the medical literature: XIV. How to decide on the applicability of clinical trial results to your patient. *JAMA* 1998; **279**: 545–9.

67. Diabetes Control and Complications Trial Research Group (DCCT). The effect of intensive treatment of diabetes on the development and progression of long term complications in insulin dependent diabetes mellitus. *N. Engl. J. Med.* 1993; **329**: 977–86.

68. Marshall KG. Prevention. How much harm? How much benefit? 2. Ten potential pitfalls in determining the clinical significance of benefits. *Can. Med. Assoc. J.* 1996; **154**: 1837–43.

69. Sonis J, Doukas D, Klinkman M, Reed B, Ruffin MT. Applicability of clinical trial results to primary care. *JAMA* 1998; **280**: 1746.

70. Katon W, Von Korf M, Lin E, et al. Methodologic issues in randomized trials of liaison psychiatry in primary care. *Psychosom. Med.* 1994; **56**: 97–103.

71. Thijs L, Fagard R, Lijnen P, et al. Why is antihypertensive drug therapy needed in elderly patients with systolodiastolic hypertension? *J. Hypertens. Suppl.* 1994; **12**: S25–34.

72. Eddy DM. Clinical Decision Making: from theory to practice. Comparing benefits and harms: the balance sheet. *JAMA* 1990; **263**: 2498–501.

73. Guyatt GH, Sackett DL, Sinclair JC, et al. Users' guides to the medical literature. IX. A method for grading health care recommendations. *JAMA* 1995; **274**: 1800–4.

74. Schmid CH, Lau J, McIntosh MW, Cappelleri JC. An empirical study of the effect of the control rate as a predictor of treatment efficacy in meta-analysis of clinical trials. *Statist. Med.* 1998; **17**: 1923–42.

75. Boissel JP, Collet JP, Lievre M, Girard P. An effect model for the assessment of drug benefit: example of antiarrthythmic drugs in postmyocardial infarction patients. *J. Cardiovasc. Pharmacol.* 1993; **22**: 356–63.

76. The Cardiac Arrhythmia Suppression Trial (CAST) Investigators. Preliminary report: effect of encainide and flecainide on mortality in a randomized trial of arrhythmia suppression after myocardial infarction. *N. Engl. J. Med.* 1989; **321**: 406–12.

77. North of England Evidence-based Guideline Development Project. Evidence based clinical practice guideline. ACE inhibitors in the primary care management of adults with symptomatic heart failure. Newcastle upon Tyne: Centre for Health Services Research, 1997.

78. McIntosh M. The population risk as an explanatory variable in research synthesis of clinical trials. *Statist. Med.* 1996; **15**: 1713–28.

79. Sharp S, Thompson SG, Douglas GA. The relation between treatment benefit and underlying risk in meta-analysis. *Br. Med. J.* 1996; **313**: 735–8.

80. Walter SD. Variation in baseline risk as an explanation of heterogeneity in meta-analysis. *Statist. Med.* 1997; **16**: 2883–900.

81. Thompson SG, Smith TC, Sharp SJ. Investigating underlying risk as a source of heterogeneity in meta-analysis. *Statist. Med.* 1997; **16**: 2741–58.

82. Brand R, Kragt H. Importance of trends in the interpretation of an overall odds ratio in the meta-analysis of clinical trials. *Statist. Med.* 1992; **11**: 2077–82.

83. Boissel JP. Individualizing aspirin therapy for prevention of cardiovascular events. *JAMA* 1998; **280**: 1949–50.

84. Schuchter L, Schultz DJ, Synnestvedt M, et al. A prognostic model for predicting 10-year survival in patients with primary melanoma. *Ann. Intern. Med.* 1996; **125**: 369–75.

85. Guidelines for the management of mildly raised blood pressure in New Zealand. The Core Services Committee, Wellington, New Zealand.

86. Stroke Prevention in Atrial Fibrillation Investigators. Warfarin versus aspirin for prevention of thromboembolism in atrial fibrillation: Stroke Prevention in Atrial Fibrillation II Study. *Lancet* 1994; **343**: 687–91.

87. Ware JE Jr, Sherbourne CD. The MOS 36-item short-form health survey (SF–36). I. Conceptual framework and item selection. *Med. Care* 1992; **30**: 473–83.

88. Torrance G, Feeny D. Utilities and quality-adjusted life years. *Int. J. Technol. Assess. Health Care* 1989; **5**: 559–75.

89. Price K, Gelber R, Isley M, Goldhirsch A, Coates A, Castiglione M. Time without symptoms and toxicity (TWiST): a quality-of-life-oriented endpoint to evaluate adjuvant therapy. *Adjuvant Therapy of Cancer* 1987; **V**: 455–65.

90. Goldhirsch A, Gelber RD, Simes RJ, Glasziou P, Coates AS. Costs and benefits of adjuvant therapy in breast cancer. A quality-adjusted survival analysis. *J. Clin. Oncol.* 1989; **7**: 36–44.

91. Glasziou PP, Simes RJ, Gelber RD. Quality adjusted survival analysis. *Statist. Med.* 1990; **9**: 1259–76.

92. Hanley JA, Lippman-Hand A. If nothing goes wrong is everything all right? Interpreting zero numerators. *JAMA* 1983; **249**: 1743–4.

5

The Placebo Effect: Methodological Process and Implications of a Structured Review

ROSEMARY CROW, HEATHER GAGE,
SARAH HAMPSON, JO HART, ALAN KIMBER
and HILARY THOMAS

SUMMARY

This chapter reports the processes involved in a review of the determinants of the placebo effect. In addition to the methodological considerations shared with other review subjects, the placebo effect presents particular challenges because it is such an imprecisely defined area. This chapter first considers the context of the review and three key issues of methodology designed specifically to deal with the imprecision of the topic: establishment of a conceptual framework; search, retrieval and screening in a potentially extensive literature; and the methods used in the analysis of the primary research papers. The evidence is then described, accompanied by the quality assessment, and the chapter concludes with the implications for health service delivery and directions for future research.

KEY ISSUES AND CONTROVERSIES IN DEFINING 'PLACEBO' AND 'PLACEBO EFFECT'

There is considerable debate, variability and confusion in the literature concerning the usage and interpretation of the terms 'placebo' and 'placebo effect'.[1–6] A brief overview of the main issues involved is presented here.

In its narrowest sense, a placebo is a biomedically inert substance for example, the legendary sugar pill, given by a healthcare practitioner to please a patient. Despite being inefficacious substances, placebos can produce physical effects.[7–9] The nature of these placebo effects vary with individuals, situations and medical conditions. Placebos can have diverse physical and psychological effects of a beneficial (placebo) or adverse (nocebo) nature.[10–12]

Since the advent of randomised controlled trials (RCTs), placebos have been used extensively in pharmacological research. Protected by informed consent, investigators administer placebos to a control group of patients so that the 'real' effects of an active preparation can be deduced by subtraction of the effects produced in the same clinical situation by a placebo. The use of placebos in clinical practice, however, has been subject to extensive debate since their potential therapeutic success hinges to some extent on deceiving the patient.[13–23] Whereas some commentators may argue for limited placebo use in certain well-defined clinical circumstances, there is serious concern amongst others that even the most benevolent deception will destroy the long-term trust patients place in their providers, and the general credibility of the medical profession. Significantly, these factors are thought to be important determinants of the placebo effect in its wider and more modern interpretation, which emphasises patient autonomy and involvement rather than professional paternalism and control.[24]

Probably the most widely quoted definitions of placebo and placebo effect are those of Shapiro.[25–29] Shapiro extends the definition of the placebo to 'any therapy (or component of therapy) deliberately used for non-specific psychological or psychophysiological effect . . . and without specific activity for the condition being treated'. The placebo effect, accordingly, is defined as 'the non-specific psychological or psychophysiological effect produced by placebos'. The focus on 'non-specific' in these definitions suggests that the magnitude of the placebo effect can be deduced by excluding known specific effects of the therapy on the condition in question.[30]

Grünbaum advanced on Shapiro's definition by observing that a treatment is composed of two components: characteristic factors and incidental factors.[4,5] The *characteristic* factors are those that are known or believed to affect the disease as a result of the theoretical rationale for the therapy. The *incidental* factors are those that may affect disease but cannot be derived from the theoretical rationale for the therapy. Therapies can affect the target conditions for which they are intended, and/or other aspects of patients' health. Given this framework, Grünbaum argued that the terms 'specific' and 'non-specific' to distinguish between treatment and placebo effects are not helpful. A placebo may have a highly specific effect on the target disease, for example it can make a headache go away. The specificity metaphor is borrowed from medicine, where specific therapies are developed to address specific diseases, and a general panacea is looked upon with scepticism. However, as Shepherd[31] observed, the concept of specificity in biology and medicine has always been at issue: that is, whether or not any given disease has a specific versus non-specific cause and cure.

The term 'incidental' is intended to signal that such effects are not expected on the basis of the underlying rationale behind the treatment. This point is similar to that made by Critelli and Neumann[32] when they observed that placebos may be theoretically inert, but not therapeutically inert. In other words, placebos may have beneficial effects for no apparent reason. However, that should not be taken to imply that the theoretical basis for incidental effects is inevitably mysterious.

Many commentators have noted that the placebo effect is equated to non-specific because of ignorance about its component parts. Reflecting this, it has been referred to as 'Factor X'.[33] A distinction can be made between effects that

are unspecified rather than non-specific.[34] The challenge of gaining a better understanding of the placebo effect remains, and awaits conceptual developments that isolate parameters and scientific enquiry that tests for their precise clinical significance. The end product of this process will be the transformation of the non-specific (placebo) effect into named specific therapeutic activities.[2,3,8,27,31,34–36] At that point, the term 'placebo' effect could be dispensed with since there would no longer be any mysterious, atheoretical component to therapy. Thus, there is an inherent paradox in investigating placebo effects. Once they are understood they are no longer defined as placebo effects. It was one purpose of the review to develop a framework for the study of non-specific effects, as a first step towards explicating the mechanisms by which they can enhance beneficial health outcomes.

It has been argued that eliciting the placebo effect does not require a placebo in the traditional sense of the term, and that placebos and the placebo effect should therefore be separately defined.[8,15,37,38] According to this interpretation, the placebo effect derives from the symbolic effect of treatment as determined by the total context in which healthcare is delivered. The causes of the placebo effect are located anywhere in the care delivery process, except in the inert placebo itself. Consistent with this approach is the suggestion that placebo effects are generic in applicability.[37,39] It also permits the extension of the definition of a placebo beyond that of an inert medication to encapsulate all aspects of the treatment environment. Many things, including practitioners themselves, have been described as placebos.[40] Indeed, a continuum of placebos has been suggested, ranging from tangible items such as scars, pills, injections, white coats and procedures, to intangible features of healthcare delivery such as touch, gesture, ambience and support.[41,42]

The issue of whether or not a placebo is required to produce the placebo effect reduces therefore to one of semantics, and hinges on the definitions of placebo and placebo effect that are adopted. If a placebo is narrowly defined as an inert substance it is only one aspect of the total treatment context, and one of many possible means of eliciting a broadly defined placebo effect.

For the purposes of the review, an inclusive definition of placebo was adopted. The relationship between any aspects of the healthcare delivery encounter were open to investigation for their effects on health outcomes. This included the effects of placebo medications, but extended beyond that to consider the significance of the features associated with the environment in which care is delivered and the practitioner–patient interaction. This approach acknowledges that an opportunity exists for the placebo effect to be activated in some form or another in virtually all encounters between healthcare practitioners and their patients. It suggests that with a proper understanding of the placebo effect practitioners can, through their relationships with their patients, and in conjunction with appropriate medical technologies, use a multitude of non-deceptive means to promote positive placebo responses. Ethical dilemmas associated with prescribing placebo medications are thereby avoided.[43] The advantage of this approach was that the results of the review could have potentially wide practical significance. A variety of ethically acceptable healthcare delivery improvements could subsequently be considered.

ESTABLISHING THE CONCEPTUAL FRAMEWORK

The challenge faced by the review team was a potentially large literature (searching for *placebo* as a keyword alone, produced approximately 20 000 references) and a topic that was imprecisely defined. To handle both issues, a conceptual framework was developed based on the assumption that certain indicators of the process of healthcare delivery act as placebos to produce placebo responses. This assumption enabled us to distinguish the mechanisms of the placebo effect from the placebo responses. Features of healthcare delivery were identified as 'determinants', and the placebo responses as 'outcomes'. Together with the mechanisms by which the placebo effects operate, these two related classes of factors formed the model of the placebo effect. In an initial scoping exercise, it became apparent that placebo effects had been demonstrated in numerous studies across a range of treatments for a range of disorders. To review the literature on all aspects of the model would have produced a very large literature, and would have been well beyond the scale of the project. Therefore it was decided to focus the review on the mechanisms by which the placebo effects operate, since this would increase the possibility of harnessing these effects as therapies. The background literature was used to identify the mechanisms of the placebo effect and to establish which determinants might act on them to produce the health outcomes.

Mechanisms

We turned to the psychological literature to establish which mechanisms had been associated with the placebo effect. Four were identified: expectancy, anxiety reduction, classical conditioning, and social support. The expectancy mechanism occupied the central place in the psychological literature on the placebo effect[44–47] and was therefore chosen as the focus for the review. The decision was influenced by resource considerations, and by the view held by clinicians that expectancy is the probable explanation of why treatments, once thought to be efficacious by their proponents but found more recently not to be, produce positive outcomes.[48]

Expectancy can be said to subsume anxiety reduction and classical conditioning, and so these mechanisms were not removed from the conceptual framework.[7,36,49–55] For example, anxiety reduction as a placebo mechanism, may be a consequence of positive expectancy. Similarly, in so far as past experience sets up learned expectancies, these possible classical conditioning effects may be more usefully understood in terms of expectancy mechanisms since there is some doubt as to whether humans can be classically conditioned.[56] So that, for example, positive responses to repeated association of medical care with symptom relief, even when the therapy is non-active, would be attributed to the creation of positive expectations. Similarly, negative conditioned responses ('placebo sag') to new therapies following a series of ineffective therapies[36,57] would be attributed to the creation of negative expectancies. Both mechanisms were therefore addressed in the review, but only in so far as they could be interpreted in the context of expectancy.

Social support, on the other hand, is determined by family members and outside organisations as well as healthcare practitioners. Since the review was confined to the healthcare setting, social support was addressed only in so far as the role of the patient–practitioner interactions were considered as determinants.

Determinants

Having chosen expectancy as the mechanism by which placebo effects operate, determinants could then be specified. Determinants include all aspects of the treatment environment since the causes of the placebo effect are located throughout the care delivery process.[40–42] As a large number of placebogenic variables had been advanced in the literature,[27,34,35,58–69] they were organised into four groups: patient characteristics; practitioner characteristics; patient–practitioner interaction; and the treatment and treatment setting. Within each group, factors responsible for the placebo effect were then considered in the light of their role as determinants of the expectancy mechanism.

Patient characteristics

Patient characteristics contribute to placebo effects, although placebo effects cannot be explained entirely by them. For example, the placebo effect does not remain constant even within the same individual, and no specific personality type has yet been identified that is more likely to be a placebo responder.[66,70,71] However, patient characteristics will affect the operation of the expectancy mechanism within the individual and therefore they are important determinants of the placebo effect. For example, personality traits, anxiety, age, IQ, gender, race and socio-economic status may all affect the way an individual elicits, attends to, and processes information related to the formation of expectancies. Moreover, the individual patient may possess pre-existing expectations about a particular treatment that will affect his or her response to the influences exerted by the immediate healthcare delivery process. These pre-existing beliefs will have been formed over time, and so reflect broader influences such as the macro context within which care is delivered, past healthcare experiences of the patient and the patient's family, friends and acquaintances. Patient characteristics are therefore one important class of determinants of placebo effects.

Practitioner factors

Practitioner factors have also been linked to the formation of patient expectancies.[28] They include the practitioners' personal characteristics and their own beliefs regarding the treatment they are prescribing or performing. For example, it has been observed that a practitioner who adopts a concerned, warm, supportive, caring and empathetic attitude to her/his patients may inspire trust, confidence and rapport in the relationship.[72] Conversely, a distracted, unsympathetic and abrupt practitioner may create hostility, distrust and dismay in her/his patient. There was also evidence that a confident practitioner, displaying strong beliefs in the diagnosis and the treatment can enhance positive expectancy in the patient, whilst a neutral or uncertain attitude on the part of the practitioner could have little or even a negative effect on the patient.[37,73,74] Practitioner factors were therefore included as a second class of determinants of the placebo effect.

Practitioner–patient interaction

Many commentators have emphasised the therapeutic potential of patient–practitioner interactions.[58,75–78] A practitioner's communication skills will influence the nature and extent of the interaction that takes place, but this will also be a reflection of the patient's own ability to take part in the interaction. Both parties will further be influenced by their views about the importance of communication and the appropriate balance of power in the relationship, and by the time available for consultation.[79] Patient–practitioner interactions are, therefore, opportunities when expectancies can be created and so were included as a third class of determinants of the placebo effect.

Treatment characteristics, including setting

Treatment characteristics, including the treatment setting, were the final set of factors that had been associated with the placebo effect. One example was the placebo (or nocebo) effect which the nature of the treatment may have on patients by influencing their faith or belief in the care they are receiving. Although elaborate procedures, including surgery, can be effective placebos,[80–82] routine tasks such as prescription writing have also been shown to have placebo effects.[83] The traditional placebo medication falls into this category.[84] Furthermore, the way a medication is delivered may affect its perceived action. Injections have been perceived as more effective than pills, and capsules as more effective than pills.[85,86] Even the colour of drugs can affect peoples' perceptions as to their action and their effectiveness.[86–88] Treatment and treatment setting characteristics, where they linked with expectancies, were, therefore, included as the fourth class of determinants of the placebo effect.

Outcomes

Outcomes were assessed from changes in the patient's physical and psychological condition, and changes in health service utilisation attributable to the action of the placebo. Changes in physical or psychological condition can be assessed by observations made by others, or by patient's self-report. For example, practitioners can measure reductions in swelling or judge changes in levels of discomfort, and patients can rate change in their pain, anxiety and well-being. Health service utilisation can be assessed using a number of indices including length of hospital stay, number of physicians visits and medication requirements. Accordingly, these classes of outcome measures were used to

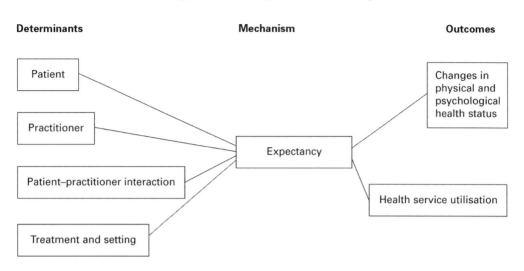

Figure 1 *Model of the placebo effect.*

categorise health outcomes, and only studies that reported one or more of these outcomes were retained for analysis. Studies that only reported intermediate behavioural outcomes (such as adherence) without any reference to health effects, were excluded.

Conceptual Framework for the Placebo Effect

The model of the determinants, expectancy mechanism and outcomes which provided the framework used to guide the review is shown in Figure 1.

By choosing expectancy as the placebo mechanism the review focused on the process by which placebos achieve their therapeutic effectiveness. It could thus test the hypothesis that changes in health status attributed to placebo effects are achieved by the manipulation of patient expectations. The theoretical exposition, although time consuming, unravelled the functional relationships of the placebo effect rendering it accessible to the review process. As the purpose of the review was to harness the placebo effect for use in the NHS, the final decision made at this stage was to confine the literature to studies concerned with healthcare delivery in the clinical sector.

Excluded Literature

In the process of developing the model of the placebo effect, four literatures were removed from the search frame.

The first literature that was removed was a set of studies that had investigated placebo effects without reference to expectancy. Therefore, mere demonstrations of placebo effects were excluded, such as all randomised trials of new treatments and drugs that are intended to demonstrate the superiority of the new therapy above and beyond placebo effects. In addition, the neurophysiological mechanisms by which expectancy affects biological processes were considered beyond the scope of the review because they are controversial (for example, the role of endogenous opiates in placebo analgesia has been debated[50,89–92]).

The second literature removed from the frame was the psychological research using laboratory based experiments to deliberately manipulate subject expectancies[93] or to manipulate the effect of instruction or expectancy on patients.[94,95] It was felt that findings from the laboratory would not generalise to clinical settings, particularly since crucial psychological variables present in patients undergoing treatment, such as distress, were not likely to be found in non-patient volunteers.[66]

The third literature that was excluded was studies concerned with measuring the effectiveness of psychotherapy over placebo treatment. This literature presents serious challenges to researchers, particularly because of the uncertainties that it raises. It has been argued that the placebo effect works like psychotherapy through transference,[96] and that since psychotherapy affects patients' expectancies by providing support, compassion, reassurance, advice, and sharing knowledge, it is in fact analogous to a placebo. Whilst some commentators argue that the specific and non-specific (or expectancy or placebo) effects of psychotherapy cannot be separated because of the problem of finding a credible placebo,[8,97–102] others argue that credible placebos are possible[32] and that a treatment effect can be discerned.[103,104] There is, however, significant debate about this conclusion, and many investigations have found no evidence of a treatment effect from psychotherapy above the placebo effect.[105–109]

There is a similar controversial debate about the alternative, or complementary medical sector, which is frequently discussed as an entity, although in reality it includes a range of varied therapeutic modalities. Some commentators suggest that the therapeutic value of these alternative approaches may be largely, if not entirely, accounted for by the placebo effect, rather than by specific physiological effects of the treatments themselves.[59,75,84,110–112] There is

little empirical evidence to assist the debate, and what exists is subject to methodological difficulties, not least the problem of finding appropriate placebo controls.[113–118] In view of the diversity of the complementary sector and the methodological difficulties associated with identifying the placebo effect in it, this fourth literature was also excluded from the review.

SEARCH, RETRIEVAL AND SCREENING OF LITERATURE

Search and Retrieval

The search and retrieval procedure that was used is illustrated in Figure 2. The initial scoping

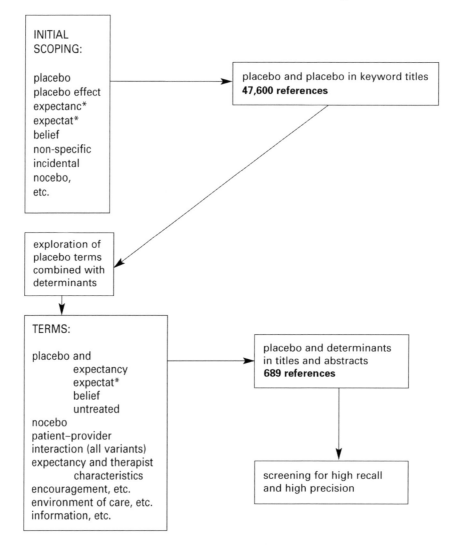

Figure 2   *Search and retrieval procedure.*

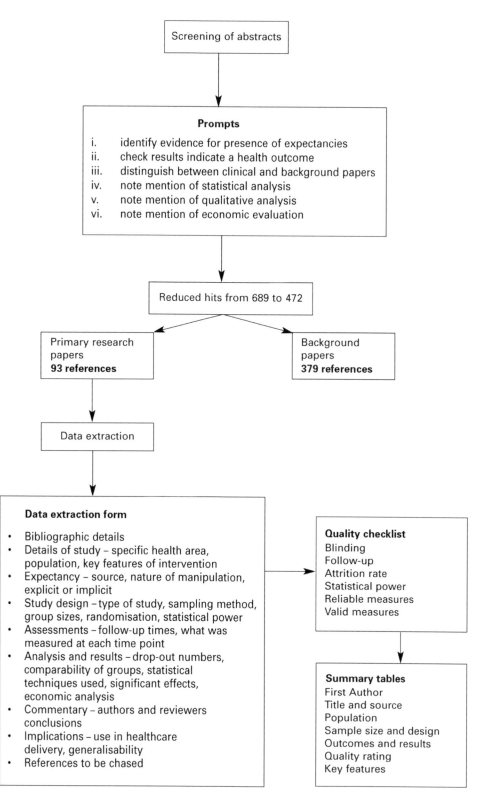

Figure 3 *Development of summary tables for data analysis.*

exercise used terms which included placebo, synonyms of placebo, expectancy, and synonyms of expectancy and identified 47 600 abstracts. The terms were subsequently restricted to placebo combined with synonyms of expectancy, and to determinants of the placebo mechanism and their synonyms. After testing these restricted terms for recall (sensitivity) and precision (specificity) the retrieval process was repeated. This reduced the references that were located to 689.

Sources used in the search

The search included journal articles, books, chapters of books, letters and editorials. The major source was the electronic databases chosen to span a broad range of disciplines and including both European and American material. Although electronic sources were not searched before 1980, pre-1980 studies were included if they had been identified by other means. Moreover, a comprehensive bibliography of placebo studies prior to 1980 was already available.[119] The same search terms were used for each database, although there were slight differences in the strategy that was used because of differences in the databases.

Other literature sources included reference lists of identified papers (known as exploding references), personal contacts with known experts in the field and conferences. The latter sources provided information about ongoing work.

Screening and Data Extraction Process

The second flow diagram (Figure 3) illustrates the screening and data extraction process. Using a set of prompts, each abstract was screened by at least two members of the team. This process reduced the numbers of papers to be retrieved from 689 to 472, 93 of which were primary research papers and 379 background papers. Using a set of guidelines developed from pilot work, data from the primary research papers were extracted and entered onto a proforma. Information concerning the quality of the research was extracted with the help of a checklist. The information entered onto the proforma was then used to develop a summary table for each primary research paper. The table included information of first author, title and source, study population, sample size, study design and quality rating, key features of the intervention, the health outcomes that had been measured, and the results.

The primary research papers (93) identified in the search strategy described studies in which a number of research approaches had been used to test a range of different clinical hypotheses. In order that the review could test the hypothesis that changes in health status were achieved by the manipulation of patient expectations, a method of extracting data appertaining to the expectancies created by the investigations was needed. To this end, a working definition of expectancy was developed, together with criteria that verified expectancy as a key target of the investigation.

Working Definition of Expectancy

Definitions of expectancy as the mechanism of the placebo effect, were developed from Bandura's theorising about expectancy. Bandura[120,121] distinguished two types of expectancies: outcome expectations and self-efficacy expectations. For the purposes of this review, his concept of outcome expectancy[120–122] was interpreted as a treatment-related expectancy and his concept of self-efficacy expectation[120,122] was interpreted as a patient-related self-efficacy. These two interpretations of expectancy were further developed as follows.

Treatment-related expectancy

Treatment-related expectancy was developed into three separate categories.

1 *Process expectancy* was used to refer to expectations about medical interventions created for patients either with no knowledge of an unfamiliar medical procedure, or with inaccurate expectations about the actual processes involved.
2 *Positive outcome expectancy* was used to refer to expectancies created by practitioners when they convey their own faith and enthusiasm in the treatment. This particular concept of outcome expectancy went further than simply providing accurate information about what experiences the patient can expect.
3 *Negative outcome expectancy* was used to refer to expectancies created either when the practitioner conveys uncertainty or even lack of faith in the procedure or when the practitioner informs the patient of the negative consequences of treatment such as possible side effects.

Patient-related self-efficacy expectations

Self-efficacy expectations are beliefs that one can successfully execute the actions required to achieve valued outcomes. Self-efficacy is derived from four sources: previous performance accomplishments; vicarious experiences such as seeing others succeeding; verbal persuasion; and the individual's psychological state. Self-efficacy has been demonstrated to affect behaviour in a range of health and non-health areas,[120,121] and formed the basis for the concept of patient-related self-efficacy expectations. Building up a patient's confidence and self-worth all contribute to self-efficacy and are part of good practitioner skills. Changing self-efficacy is, therefore, considered to be one of the most important components of any behavioural healthcare intervention.[123] It is promoted whenever an intervention is designed to provide the patient with confidence that he/she can cope or behave in such a way that he/she can manage the disease or its treatment. Based on these assumptions, patient-related self-efficacy was developed into two separate categories

1 *Interaction self-efficacy* was said to be promoted when interventions are designed to increase the patient's involvement in decision-making regarding their care, and is achieved by empowering or activating the patient so enabling him/her to participate more effectively in the medical consultation.
2 *Management self-efficacy* was said to be promoted by teaching the patient specific skills for coping with, or managing, the effects of treatment or the disease itself to augment the patient's self-efficacy beliefs for these particular skills, so increasing the likelihood of the patient putting these skills into action.

Criteria for Verifying the Presence of Expectancy

The criteria developed to verify that an expectancy had been created by the investigation were the presence in the study methods section of one or all of the following:

(a) An explicit statement/description of the content of any practitioner information given to patients which formed a key feature of the intervention and created an expectancy which met the definition developed for the purpose of the analysis.
(b) An explicit statement/description of the information given to the patient, either orally, during audio or videotaped messages or during group teaching sessions which formed a key feature of the intervention and created an expectancy which met the definition developed for the purpose of the analysis.
(c) An explicit statement/description of the skills provided in the training given to the patient which formed a key feature of the intervention and created an expectancy which met the definition developed for the purpose of the analysis.

Application of the above criteria screened out a further eight papers. This final set of 85 papers provided the information used in the review to assess the determinants of the placebo effect.

Preparation of Tables which Specified Type of Expectancy

Using the summary table for each study, a second table was prepared which covered type of expectancy, clinical area, health outcomes, type and quality of data. Using the working definition of expectancy, information about the expectancies was extracted from the descriptions given to patients of the procedures they were to experience, the training programmes they were being invited to undergo, or the likely effectiveness of the treatment they were to be prescribed. This information was reported in the methods section of each paper. To establish the reliability of the extraction procedure, each paper was read, independently, by two members of the research team, obtaining an agreement of 98%. To illustrate the extraction process, three examples are provided to show how the instructions/descriptions described in the methods section of the paper were interpreted as expectancies.

In the first example (Table 1), information about expectancies was available in the instructions used to prepare patients for cardiac catheterisation.[124] The instructions included details about the procedures patients would experience and training in how to cope with a stressful event. The information concerning the procedures was considered *process expectancy*, and that concerning the training programme was considered *management self-efficacy*.

In the second example (Table 2), information about expectancies was available in the training used to help patients participate in their medical care.[125] The instructions involved coaching in how to seek information from the practitioner during the consultation and were said to represent *interaction self-efficacy*.

In the third example (Table 3), information about expectancies was available in the information given to patients about the effectiveness of the drugs they were to receive.[71] Patients were

Table 1   *Process and management self-efficacy during preparation of a patient for cardiac catheterisation*

Description of the intervention	Expectancy
Individual education about the heart and the impending cardiac catheterisation and individual training in how to cope using a cognitive-behavioural intervention	*Process expectancy* created by procedural information *Management self-efficacy* created by training patients in cognitive-restructuring

Table 2   *Interaction self-efficacy to help patients become involved in decision making*

Description of the intervention	Expectancy
Diabetic algorithm used in conjunction with medical records to teach patients how to focus on treatment issues so that they could improve their information seeking skills and negotiate treatment with the doctor	*Interaction self-efficacy* created by encouraging patients to be involved in decision making

Table 3   *Positive and negative outcome expectancies when prescribing treatment*

Description of the patient instructions	Expectancy
Patients were either instructed that the pill was very effective at reducing tension, anxiety and pain (oversell condition) or they were instructed that it may be effective (undersell condition)	*Positive outcome expectancy* created by dentist's belief in the success of treatment (oversell condition) *Negative outcome expectancy* created by the dentist's belief that treatment was not very effective (undersell condition)

either told that the drug was very effective or that it *may be* effective. Instructions which said the drug was very effective were said to be *positive outcome expectancies*, and those which only told patients that the drugs may be effective were said to be *negative outcome expectancies*.

Grouping the Studies for Analysis

Because of the heterogeneity of the studies used in the review, the papers needed to be grouped so that the benefits of the placebo effect could be evaluated across subgroups of similar studies. A number of strategies were employed includ-

ing the classification of types of expectancy by clinical area, clinical setting, and class of determinants. Some 60% of papers were located in three cells when types of expectancy were classified by class of determinants. Three main relationships were identified: management self-efficacy and the treatment and treatment setting (30); process expectancy and the treatment and treatment setting (24); and positive outcome expectancy and practitioner factors (15) (Table 4).

Three clinical categories classified all the studies: preparation for medical procedures; management of illness; and medical treatment. Studies in which patient expectancies were

Table 4   *Frequency with which type of expectancy[a] was associated with class of determinant*

	Patient expectation	Practitioner factors	Practitioner–patient interaction	Treatment and treatment setting	Total
Process expectancy	–	2	1	24	27
Positive outcome expectancy	5	15	5	9	34
Negative outcome expectancy	2	5	3	4	14
Interaction self-efficacy	–		6	1	7
Management self-efficacy	3	1	–	30	34
Total	10	23	15	68	116

[a] Some investigations included more than one type of expectancy.

created by the treatment and treatment setting either concerned the preparation for medical procedures or the management of illness. Studies in which patient expectancies were created by practitioner factors mostly concerned the effectiveness of medical treatments (usually drug therapy).

EVIDENCE

Eighty-five studies were used to assess the role of expectancies in the placebo effect. Of these studies, 25 concerned the preparation for medical procedures, 20 of which were clinical trials and five observational studies. Using the criteria for verifying expectancy (see earlier), there was evidence that process expectancy and management self-efficacy had either been created alone or in combination. The results are summarised in Table 5a.

Taken together, the results suggest that process expectancy, when combined with management self-efficacy, produces the greatest benefits by enhancing the quality of the patients' hospital experience. Management self-efficacy when created alone, on the other hand, was most likely to reduce patient anxiety. There was also a suggestion in a few of the studies that the effect of expectancy may be counteracted by personality. For the NHS, there are potential cost savings in reduced use of analgesics and reductions in the length of stay, although only one of the studies calculated the financial ramifications of the education and training programme.

Forty studies were concerned with the management of illness, 23 of which examined patient-centred management of chronic illness. Eighteen were clinical trials and five were observational studies. The effects of manipulating management self-efficacy either alone or in combination with positive outcome expectancy or process expectancy are summarised in Table 5b.

Fifteen studies examined aspects of the patient–provider consultation. Ten of the studies were observational, and five were clinical trials. The effects of expectancies for these studies are summarised in Table 5c.

The remaining two of the 40 studies concerned with chronic illness examined patients' levels of positive outcome expectations for treatment, but were poor in quality and so no conclusions could be drawn.

Taken together, the results reported in the studies concerned with the management of illness also show positive health outcomes. From the 23 studies which examined patient-centred

Table 5a *Summary of expectancy effects in studies[a] of preparation for medical procedures: Percentage of studies reporting significant improvements in outcome for each type of expectancy manipulation*

Outcomes	Process ($n = 13$)	Process + Management ($n = 11$)	Management ($n = 5$)
Anxiety	38%	72%	80%
Analgesics	8%	64%	40%
Recovery	8%	55%	–
Pain	–	36%	–
Hospital stay	15%	27%	40%

[a] The same study may appear in more than one column.

Table 5b *Summary of expectancy effects in studies of patient-centred management of illness: Percentage of studies reporting significant improvements in outcomes for each type of expectancy manipulation*

Outcomes	Management ($n = 16$)	Management + Positive ($n = 2$)	Management + Positive[a] ($n = 3$) Management only	Positive only	Management + Process ($n = 2$)
Physical symptoms	44%	50%	33%	33%	100%
Psychological status	19%	–	33%	–	–
Disease state	25%	–	66%	33%	–
Service use	25%	–	–	–	–

[a] Studies in which the effects of management expectancy and positive outcome expectancy were separated.

Table 5c *Summary of expectancy effects in studies of patient–provider interaction: Percentage of studies reporting significant improvements in outcomes for each type of expectancy manipulation*

Outcomes	Interaction (Provider) (n = 11)	Interaction (Patient) (n = 4)
Physical symptoms	45%	–
Disease status	18%	50%
Functional ability	–	100%

Table 5d *Summary of expectancy effects in studies[a] of medical treatment: Percentage reporting significant improvements in outcomes for each type of expectancy manipulations*

Outcomes	Positive practitioner (n = 11)	Negative practitioner (n = 3)	Positive other (n = 5)	Positive patient (n = 2)	Negative patient (n = 2)
Anxiety	100%	–	100%	–	–
Weight	100%	–	–	–	–
Pain-decrease	100%	–	100%	100%	–
Pain-increase	–	–	–	–	100%
Swelling	100%	–	–	–	–
Headache-decrease	–	–	100%	–	–
Headache-increase	–	67%	–	–	–
Minor gastro-intestinal increase	–	67%	–	–	–

[a] The same study may appear in more than one column.

management there is the suggestion that it is the creation of management self-efficacy that leads to beneficial health outcomes. Positive outcome expectancy alone was not as successful. For the NHS, the potential cost benefits are a reduction in the use of health services. From the 15 studies which investigated the effects of creating interaction self-efficacy there is also the suggestion of health benefits for the patients. However, the mechanism through which these positive health outcomes effects are achieved needs further investigation.

Twenty studies concerned the outcomes of medical treatment in which the effects of various factors on the patients' responses, including their own beliefs, were reported. Eighteen were clinical trials and one was an observational study, with one study providing insufficient information. The results are summarised in Table 5d.

Taken together, the results from the studies concerned with the outcomes of medical treatment show the power of positive outcome expectancy to enhance the effects of medical treatment. The effects of negative outcome expectancy are ambiguous.

Given the evidence of the subjective and objective benefits of creating expectancy, the studies reviewed provide support for the hypothesis that expectancies are the mechanism by which placebos have their effects. However, because of the heterogeneity of outcomes assessed and the uneven distribution of the expectancies across the three clinical areas, it was not possible to use meta-analysis to combine effect sizes across studies.

Quality Assessment

These conclusions must be tempered by a lack of methodological excellence characterising both the clinical trials (62) and observational studies (23) that were reported. Weaknesses of the clinical trials was their lack of methodological detail, making it difficult to judge the validity of the findings. For instance, in some cases there was no information on whether groups were comparable at baseline, so confounding the results. Other weaknesses included a failure to ensure that the control group had not been given information similar to the treatment group and a failure to use all cross-over orderings in a cross-over trial. As well as their lack of methodological detail, the shortcomings of the observational studies was their weak research designs, high dropout rates, the lack of adequate controls, multiple testing of hypotheses leading to statistically significant correlations that were small in magnitude, a heavy reliance on retrospective reporting, and the use of patient groups that were not comparable in terms of the medical procedures they were to undergo. The quality of the studies tended to show an improvement over time, with ones published more recently demonstrating greater rigour. It is not surprising that studies drawn from such diverse literatures would be of mixed quality. Our conclusions must, therefore, be limited by the methodological shortcomings, and the scarcity of studies conducted in the UK since a large proportion of the studies (66%) were conducted in the USA.

Implications for Health Service Staff and Practitioners

The principal implication of the results of the review for both health service staff and practitioners is the importance of the psychological components of healthcare delivery. The most important message coming out of the review is the influence on health outcomes of: (a) the information/training provided (or not provided) for patients; (b) the patient's ability to manage their own care; and (c) the attitudes and interpersonal skills of practitioners during the delivery of care. All three aspects need to be seen as health technologies in their own right, not as incidental, non-specific aspects of the medical/nursing care. As such, when evidence is being sought, whether it be to inform health policy or medical decision making, the effectiveness of these psychological interventions should be included in cost–benefit analyses.

Suggestions for Further Research

Two particular areas for further research follow from the review.

Firstly, there is a need for reviews of health technologies which focus on the psychological as well as the physical therapies. The health technologies identified from the review are the various self-management interventions used to help patients cope with stress in acute clinical studies, particularly as preparation for medical procedures, and those which help patients manage their illness. Insights into the benefits of these psychological health technologies were drawn from studies reporting health effects from a range of clinical areas which included illness associated with cardiac rehabilitation, diabetes, asthma, chronic headache, chronic pain, rheumatoid arthritis and Parkinson's disease. Reviews of the literature which focus only on single clinical groups may not, therefore, show the beneficial effects which psychological health technologies can have on health outcomes. Reviews of other psychological health technologies which are also drawn from different clinical groups could contribute further understanding that could also be usefully harnessed by the NHS. We identified gaps in the clinical literature; for example, we located no studies concerned with the management of chronic illness resulting from some of the major degenerative diseases. Further research is also needed in these and possibly other clinical areas as well.

The second area concerns the development of statistical methods for handling studies that are heterogeneous with respect to outcome variables. For example, the studies we identified on preparation for medical procedures typically used a measure of post-procedure recovery such as number of pain-killing medications requested over a certain period of time period, days in hospital, or self-ratings of physical discomfort. Rarely did two studies use exactly the same outcome measure. Therefore, our analysis was limited to a narrative review and we were not able to perform any quantitative meta-analysis. Methods for combining diverse outcomes that are essentially measuring the same effects (in this case patient recovery) are currently being considered by our group so that statistical methods of meta-analysis can be used to quantify findings from reviews that encompass such diversity as we found for the placebo effect. One such statistical method has developed a technique for combining multiple outcomes involving, in particular, a mixture of discrete and continuous responses.[126] In the simplest case these outcomes can be bivariate, comprising a binary and continuous response as, for example, the patient's health status reported as improved/stable or deteriorated (binary response) and their level of anxiety (continuous response). Another difficulty which our review pinpointed was the complex two-level structure (determinants and mechanisms) of factors affecting outcomes of the placebo effect. Statistical methods that handle one level of dependence and require that the determinants be specified in advance as covariates are readily available.[127,128] However, more research is needed to develop statistical methods to handle routinely the type of data encountered here.

ACKNOWLEDGEMENTS

The review of the determinants of the placebo effect and its use in the delivery of health care was supported by a grant from the Health Technology Assessment Programme, part of the NHS R and D Executive. The Surrey review team would also like to acknowledge Dr I.G. Vlachonikolis, Reader in Medical Statistics, EIHMS contribution concerning the new developments in meta-analytical techniques. Our thanks are also due to Mrs J. King for her help in the preparation of this manuscript.

REFERENCES

1. Beecher HK. The powerful placebo. *JAMA* 1955; **159**: 1602–6.
2. Borkovec TD. Chapter 4, Placebo: redefining the unknown. In: White L, Tursky B, Schwartz GE (eds). *Placebo: Theory, Research and Mechanisms.* New York: The Guilford Press; 1985; pp. 59–66.
3. Gotzsche PC. Is there logic in the placebo? *Lancet* 1994; **344**: 925–6.
4. Grünbaum A. The placebo concept. *Behav. Res. Ther.* 1981; **19**: 157–67.
5. Grünbaum A. Chapter 2, Explication and implications of the placebo concept. In: White L, Tursky B, Schwartz GE (eds). *Placebo: Theory, Research and Mechanisms.* New York: The Guilford Press; 1985; pp. 9–36.
6. Kienle GS, Kiene H. Placebo effect and placebo concept: a critical methodological and conceptual analysis of reports on the magnitude of the placebo effect. *Alternative Therapies in Health and Medicine* 1996; **2**: 39–54.
7. Byerly H. Explaining and exploiting placebo effects. *Perspect. Biol. Med.* 1976; **19**: 423–36.
8. Wilkins W. Chapter 6, Placebo controls and concepts in chemotherapy and psychotherapy research. In: White L, Tursky B, Schwartz GE (eds). *Placebo: Theory, Research and Mechanisms.* New York: The Guilford Press; 1985; pp. 83–109.
9. Wolf S. The pharmacology of placebos. *Pharmacol. Rev.* 1959; **22**: 689–704.
10. Pogge RC. The toxic placebo. *Medical Times* 1963; **91**: 773–8.
11. Rosenzweig P, Brohier S, Zipfel A. Pharmaco-epidemiology and drug utilization. *Clin. Pharmacol. Ther.* 1993; **54**: 578–83.
12. Wolf S, Pinsky RH. Effects of placebo administration and occurrence of toxic reactions. *JAMA* 1954; **155**: 339–41.
13. Barham Carter A. The placebo: its use and abuse. *Lancet* 1953; **1**: 823.
14. Bok S. The ethics of giving placebos. *Scientific American* 1974; **231**: 17–23.
15. Brody H. The lie that heals: The ethics of giving placebos. *Ann. Intern. Med.* 1982; **97**: 112–18.
16. Elander G. Ethical conflicts in placebo treatment. *J. Advanced Nursing* 1991; **16**: 947–51.
17. Handfield-Jones, M. A bottle of medicine from the doctor. *Lancet* 1953; **2**: 823–5.
18. Kluge EH. Placebos: Some ethical considerations. *Can. Med. Assoc. J.* 1990; **142**: 293–5.
19. Krouse JH, Krouse HJ. Placebo debate. *Am. J. Nursing* 1981; **81**: 2146–8.
20. Lynoe N, Mattsson B, Sandlund M. The attitudes of patients and physicians toward placebo treatment – A comparative study. *Soc. Sci. Med.* 1993; **36**: 767–74.
21. Oh VMS. The placebo effect: Can we use it better? *Br. Med. J.* 1994; **309**: 69–70.
22. Rawlinson MC. Chapter 22, Truth-telling and paternalism in the clinic: Philosophical reflections on the use of placebos in medical practice. In: White L, Tursky B, Schwartz GE (eds). *Placebo: Theory, Research and Mechanisms.* New York: The Guilford Press; 1985; pp. 403–18.
23. Simmons B. Problems in deceptive medical procedures: An ethical and legal analysis of the administration of placebos. *J. Med. Ethics* 1978; **4**: 172–81.
24. Bakan D. Chapter 11, The apprehension of the placebo phenomenon. In: White L, Tursky B, Schwartz GE (eds). *Placebo: Theory, Research and Mechanisms.* New York: The Guilford Press; 1985; pp. 211–14.
25. Shapiro AK. Attitudes toward the use of placebos in treatment. *J. Nerv. Mental Disord.* 1960; **130**: 200–11.
26. Shapiro AK. Factors contributing to the placebo effect. *Am. J. Psychother.* 1961; **18**: 73–88.
27. Shapiro AK. Chapter 22, The placebo response. In: Howells JG (ed.). *Modern Perspectives in World Psychiatry.* London: Oliver and Boyd; 1968, pp. 596–619.
28. Shapiro AK. Iatroplacebogenics. *Int. Pharmacopsychiatry* 1969; **2**: 215–48.
29. Shapiro A, Morris L. Chapter 10, The placebo effect in medical and psychological therapies. In: Garfield S, Bergin A (eds). *Handbook of Psychotherapy and Behavioural Change.* New York: Wiley; 1978, pp. 369–410.
30. Levine J, Gordon N. Chapter 21, Growing pains in psychobiological research. In: White L, Tursky B, Schwartz GE (eds). *Placebo: Theory, Research and Mechanisms.* New York: The Guilford Press; 1985; pp. 395–402.
31. Shepherd M. The placebo: from specificity to the non-specific and back. *Psychol. Med.* 1993; **23**: 569–78.
32. Critelli JW, Neumann KF. The placebo: Conceptual analysis of a construct in transition. *Am. Psychol.* 1984; **39**: 32–9.
33. White KL. Factor X. In: *Epidemiology, Medicine and the Public's Health.* New York: 1991; pp. 150–66.

34. White L, Tursky B, Schwartz GE. Chapter 1, Placebo in perspective. In: White L, Tursky B, Schwartz GE (eds). *Placebo: Theory, Research and Mechanisms*. New York: The Guilford Press; 1985; pp. 3–7.

35. Shapiro AK, Shapiro E. Chapter 25, Patient-provider relationships and the placebo effect. In: Matarazzo JD, Weiss SM, Herd JA, Miller NE (eds). *Behavioural Health – A Handbook of Health Enhancement and Disease Prevention.* 1984; pp. 371–83.

36. Wickramasekera I. Chapter 15, A conditioned response model of the placebo effect: Predictions from the model. In: White L, Tursky B, Schwartz GE (eds). *Placebo: Theory, Research and Mechanisms*. New York: The Guilford Press; 1985; pp. 255–87.

37. Brody H, Waters DB. Diagnosis is treatment. *J. Family Practice* 1980; **10**: 445–9.

38. Brody H. Chapter 3, Placebo effect: An examination of Grunbaum's definition. In: White L, Tursky B, Schwartz GE (eds). *Placebo: Theory, Research and Mechanisms*. New York: The Guilford Press; 1985; pp. 37–58.

39. Moerman DE. Perspectives on the placebo phenomenon. *Medical Anthropology Q.* 1983; **14**: 3–19.

40. Gelbman F. The physician, the placebo and the placebo effect. *Ohio State Med. J.* 1967; **63**: 1459–61.

41. Chaput de Saintonge M, Herxheimer A. Harnessing placebo effects in healthcare. *Lancet* 1994; **344**: 995–8.

42. Ernst E, Herxheimer A. The power of placebo. *Br. Med. J.* 1996; **313**: 1569–70.

43. Vogel AV, Goodwin JS, Goodwin JM. The therapeutics of placebo. *Am. Family Physician* 1980; **22**: 105–9.

44. Ross M, Olson JM. An expectancy-attribution model of the effect of placebos. *Psychol. Rev.* 1981; **88**: 408–37.

45. Evans F. Chapter 12, Expectancy, Therapeutic Instructions and the Placebo Response. In: White L, Tursky B, Schwartz GE (eds). *Placebo: Theory, Research and Mechanisms*. New York: The Guilford Press; 1985; pp. 215–28.

46. Kleijnen J, de Craen AJM, Van Everdingen J, Krol L. Placebo effect in double-blind clinical trials: A review of interactions with medications. *Lancet* 1994; **344**: 1348–9.

47. Kleijnen J, de Craen AJM. Chapter 3, The importance of the placebo effect: A proposal for further research. In Ernst E (ed.). *Complementary Medicine: An Objective Appraisal*. Oxford: Butterworth Heinemann; 1996; pp. 30–41.

48. Roberts AH, Kewman DG, Mercier L, Hovell M. The power of nonspecific effects in healing: Implications for psychosocial and biological treatments. *Clin. Psychol. Rev.* 1993; **13**: 375–91.

49. Ernst E. Make believe medicine: The amazing powers of placebos. *Eur. J. Phys. Med. Rehab.* 1996; **6**: 124–5.

50. Peck C, Coleman G. Implications of placebo theory for clinical research and practice in pain management. *Theor. Med.* 1991; **12**: 247–70.

51. Richardson PH. Placebo effects in pain management. *Pain Rev.* 1994; **1**: 15–32.

52. Wall PD. The placebo effect: an unpopular topic. *Pain* 1992; **51**: 1–3.

53. Wall PD. Pain and the placebo response. In: Bock GR, Marsh J (eds). *Experimental and Theoretical Studies of Consciousness*. 174th edn. Chichester: John Wiley; 1993; pp. 187–216.

54. Voudouris NJ, Peck CL, Coleman G. Conditioned response models of placebo phenomena: further support. *Pain* 1989; **38**: 109–16.

55. Voudouris NJ, Peck CL, Coleman G. The role of conditioning and verbal expectancy in the placebo response. *Pain* 1990; **43**: 121–8.

56. Brewer WF. There is no convincing evidence for operant or classical conditioning in adult humans. In: Weimer WB, Palermo DS (eds). *Cognition and the symbolic processes*. New Jersey: Lawrence Erlbaum; 1974; pp. 1–42.

57. Turkkan JS, Brady JV. Chapter 18, Mediational theory of the placebo effect. In: White L, Tursky B, Schwartz GE (eds). *Placebo: Theory, Research and Mechanisms*. New York: The Guilford Press; 1985; pp. 324–31.

58. Benson H, Epstein MD. The placebo effect – a neglected asset in the care of patients. *JAMA* 1975; **232**: 1225–7.

59. Benson H, Friedman R. Harnessing the power of the placebo effect and renaming it 'remembered wellness'. *Annu. Rev. Med.* 1996; **47**: 193–9.

60. Berg AO. Placebos: a brief review for family physicians. *J. Family Practice* 1977; **5**: 97–100.

61. Cousins N. Belief becomes biology. *California School of Medicine* 1989; **6**: 20–9.

62. Ernst E. Placebos in medicine. *Lancet* 1994; **345**: 65–6.

63. Ernst E, Resch KL. The science and art of the placebo effect. *Curr. Therap.* 1994; **10**: 19–22.

64. Honigfeld G. Nonspecific factors in treatment: I. Review of placebo reactions and placebo reactors. *Dis. Nervous System* 1964a; **25**: 145–56.

65. Honigfeld G. Non-specific factors in treatment: II. Review of social-psychological factors. *Dis. Nervous System* 1964b; **25**: 225–39.

66. Jospe M. *The placebo effect in healing*. Toronto: Lexington Books; 1978.

67. Liberman R. An analysis of the placebo phenomenon. *J. Chron. Dis.* 1962; **15**: 761–83.

68. Miller NE. Placebo factors in treatment: Views of a psychologist. In: Shepherd M, Sartorius N (eds). *Non-specific aspects of treatment*. Hans Huber Publishers; 1989; pp. 39–56.

69. Turner JA, Deyo RA, Loeser JD, Von Korff M, Fordyce WE. The importance of placebo effects

in pain treatment and research. *JAMA* 1994; **271**: 1609–14.

70. Buckalew LW, Ross S, Starr BJ. Nonspecific factors in drug effects: Placebo personality. *Psychological Reports* 1981; **48**: 3–8.

71. Gryll SL, Katahn M. Situational factors contributing to the placebo effect. *Psychopharmacology* 1978; **57**: 253–61.

72. Letvak R. Putting the placebo effect into practice. *Patient Care* 1995; **29**: 93–102.

73. Finkler K, Correa M. Factors influencing patient perceived recovery in Mexico. *Soc. Sci. Med.* 1996; **42**: 199–207.

74. Thomas KB. The placebo in general practice. *Lancet* 1994; **344**: 1066–7.

75. Benson H. Commentary: placebo effect and remembered wellness. *Mind/Body Medicine* 1995; **1**: 44–5.

76. Di Matteo MR. The physician-patient relationship: Effects on the quality of health care. *Clin. Obstet. Gynecol.* 1994; **37**: 149–61.

77. Friedman HS, Dimatteo MR. Chapter 4, Patient-physician interactions. In: Shumaker SA, Schron EB, Ockene JK (eds). *The Handbook of Health Behavior Change*. New York: Springer Publishing Company; 1990; pp. 84–101.

78. Rogers S. Facilitative affiliation: Nurse-client interactions that enhance healing. *Issues in Mental Health Nursing* 1996; **17**: 171–84.

79. Ong LML, de Haes JCJM, Hoos AM, Lammes FB. Doctor-patient communication: A review of the literature. *Soc. Sci. Med.* 1995; **40**: 903–18.

80. Beecher HK. Surgery as placebo: A quantitative study of bias. *JAMA* 1961; **176**: 1102–7.

81. Cobb LA, Thomas GI, Dillard DH, Merendino KA, Bruce RA. An evaluation of internal-mammary-artery ligation by a double-blind technic. *N. Engl. J. Med.* 1959; **260**: 1115–18.

82. Johnson AG. Surgery as a placebo. *Lancet* 1994; **344**: 1140–2.

83. Fessel WJ. Strategic aspects of prescription writing. *Postgrad. Med.* 1981; **70**: 30–7.

84. Brown WA. The placebo effect. *Scientific American* 1998; **278**: 68–73.

85. Buckalew LW, Ross S. Relationship of perceptual characteristics to efficacy of placebos. *Psychological Rep.* 1981; **49**: 955–61.

86. Buckalew LW, Coffield KE. An investigation of drug expectancy as a function of capsule color and size and preparation form. *J. Clin. Psychopharmacol.* 1982; **2**: 245–8.

87. de Craen AJM, Roos PJ, de Vries AL, Kleijnen J. Effect of colour of drugs: Systematic review of perceived effect of drugs and of their effectiveness. *Br. Med. J.* 1996; **313**: 1624–6.

88. Jacobs KW, Nordan FM. Classification of placebo drugs: Effect of color. *Perceptual and Motor Skills* 1979; **49**: 367–72.

89. Graceley RH, Dubner R, Deeter WR, Wolskee PJ. Clinicians expectations influence placebo analgesia. *Nature* 1985; **305**: 43.

90. Grevart P, Goldstein A. Chapter 19, Placebo analgesia, naloxone, and the role of endogenous opioids. In: White L, Tursky B, Schwartz GE (eds). *Placebo: Theory, Research and Mechanisms*. New York: The Guilford Press; 1985; pp. 332–50.

91. Levine JD, Gordon NC, Fields HL. The mechanism of placebo analgesia. *Lancet* 1978; **2**: 654–7.

92. Straus JL, Von Ammon Cavanaugh S. Placebo effects: Issues for clinical practice in psychiatry and medicine. *Psychosomatics* 1996; **37**: 315–26.

93. Ross S, Buckalew LW. The placebo as an agent in behavioral manipulation: A review of problems, issues, and affected measures. *Clin. Psychol. Rev.* 1983; **3**: 457–71.

94. Butler C, Steptoe A. Placebo responses: An experimental study of psychophysiological processes in asthmatic volunteers. *Br. J. Clin. Psychol.* 1986; **25**: 173–83.

95. Luparello T, Leist N, Lourie CH, Sweet P. The interaction of psychologic stimuli and pharmacologic agents on airway reactivity in asthmatic subjects. *Psychosom. Med.* 1970; **32**: 509–13.

96. Gordon EE. The placebo: an insight into mind-body interaction. *Headache Q.* 1996; **7**: 117–25.

97. Kazdin AE. Therapy outcome questions requiring control of credibility and treatment-generated expectancies. *Behavior Therapy* 1979; **10**: 81–93.

98. Kirsch, I. Unsuccessful redefinitions of the term placebo. *Am. Psychol.* 1986; **4**: 844–5.

99. Kirsch, I. The placebo effect as a conditioned response: Failures of the 'Litmus Test'. *Behav. Brain Sci.* 1991; **14**: 200–4.

100. Laporte JR, Figueras A. Placebo effects in psychiatry. *Lancet* 1994; **344**: 1206–9.

101. O'Leary KD, Borkovec TD. Conceptual, methodological, and ethical problems of placebo groups in psychotherapy research. *Am. Psychol.* 1978; **33**: 821–30.

102. Wilkins W. Placebo problems in psychotherapy research: Social psychological alternatives to chemotherapy concepts. *Am. Psychol.* 1986; **41**: 551–6.

103. Bowers TG, Clum GA. Relative contribution of specific and non specific treatment effects: Meta-analysis of placebo-controlled behavior therapy research. *Psychol. Bull.* 1988; **103**: 315–23.

104. Smith ML, Glass GV, Miller TL. *The Benefits of Psychotherapy*. Johns Hopkins University Press, 1980.

105. Bootzin RR. Chapter 10, The Role of Expectancy in Behavior Change. In: White L, Tursky B, Schwartz GE (eds). *Placebo: Theory,*

Research and Mechanisms. New York: The Guilford Press; 1985; pp. 196–210.

106. Brody N. Is psychotherapy better than a placebo? *Behav. Brain Sci.* 1984; **7**: 758–63.

107. Brown WA. Placebo as a treatment for depression. *Neuropsychopharmacology* 1994; **10**: 265–9.

108. Dago PL, Quitkin FM. Role of the placebo response in the treatment of depressive disorders. *CNS Drugs* 1995; **4**: 335–40.

109. Prioleau L, Murdock M, Brody N. An analysis of psychotherapy versus placebo studies. *Behav. Brain Sci.* 1983; **7**: 756–7.

110. Frank JD. Biofeedback and the placebo effect. *Biofeedback and Self-Regulation* 1982; **7**: 449–60.

111. Kaptchuk TJ, Edwards RA, Eisenberg DM. Chapter 4, Complementary medicine: Efficacy beyond the placebo effect. In Ernst E (ed.). *Complementary Medicine. An Objective Appraisal.* Oxford: Butterworth Heinemann; 1996; pp. 42–70.

112. Lynoe N. Is the effect of alternative medical treatment only a placebo effect? *Scand. J. Soc. Med.* 1990; **18**: 149–53.

113. Buckman R, Lewith G. What does homeopathy do and how? *Br. Med. J.* 1994; **309**: 103–6.

114. Joyce CRB. Placebo and complementary medicine. *Lancet* 1994; **344**: 1279–81.

115. Kleijnen J, Knipschild P, Ter Riet G. Clinical trials of homeopathy. *Br. Med. J.* 1991; **302**: 316–23.

116. Reilly TD, Taylor MA, McSharry C, Aitchison T. Is homoeopathy a placebo response? Controlled trial of homoeopathic potency, with pollen in hayfever as model. *Lancet* 1986; **2**: 881–6.

117. Smith, I. Commissioning complementary medicine. *Br. Med. J.* 1995; **310**: 1151–2.

118. ter Riet G, Kleijnen J, Knipschild P. Acupuncture and chronic pain: A criteria-based meta-analysis. *J. Clin. Epidemiol.* 1990; **43**: 1191–9.

119. Turner JL, Gallimore R, Fox-Henning C. An annotated bibliography of placebo research. *J. Supplement Abstract Service Am. Psychol. Assoc.* 1980; **10**: 22.

120. Bandura A. Self-efficacy: Toward a unifying theory of behavioral change. *Psychol. Rev.* 1977; **84**: 191–215.

121. Bandura, A. *Social Foundations of Thought and Action: A Social Cognitive Theory.* Englewood Cliffs, NJ: Prentice Hall, 1986.

122. Bandura, A. *Self-efficacy: The exercise of control.* New York: Freeman, 1997.

123. Lorig KR, Mazonson PD, Holman HR. Evidence suggesting that health education for self-management in patients with chronic arthritis has sustained health benefits while reducing health care costs. *Arthritis Rheum.* 1993; **36**: 439–46.

124. Kendall PC, Williams L, Pechacek TF, Graham LE, Shisslak C, Herzoff N. Cognitive-behavioral and patient education interventions in cardiac catheterization procedures: The Palo Alto medical psychology. *J. Consult. Clin. Psychol.* 1979; **47**: 49–58.

125. Greenfield S, Kaplan SH, Ware JE, Yano EM, Frank HJL. Patient participation in medical care: Effects on blood sugar control and quality of life in diabetes. *J. Gen. Intern. Med.* 1988; **3**: 448–57.

126. Berkey CS, Anderson JJ, Hoaglin DC. Multiple-outcome meta-analysis of clinical trials. *Statist. Med.* 1996; **15**: 537–57.

127. Berkey, CS, Hoaglin, DC, Mostellar, F., Corditz, CA. A random-effects regression model for meta-analysis. *Statist. Med.* 1995; **14**: 395–411.

128. Thompson, SG (1994) Why sources of heterogeneity should be investigated. *Br. Med. J.* 1994; **309**: 1351–5.

Part II
OBSERVATIONAL AND QUALITATIVE METHODS

INTRODUCTION by RAY FITZPATRICK

As the previous section of this volume has demonstrated, the randomised controlled trial (RCT) can in principle be considered the optimal study design in order to evaluate the benefits of an intervention. A well-designed and conducted RCT comparing outcomes in two or more groups of patients receiving different interventions is most likely to be able to minimise the biases that may arise because groups differ in other respects such as disease severity, co-morbidity or other factors that may influence outcomes in addition to study interventions. However, there are circumstances where an RCT may be unethical because potential participants do not have equipoise to permit random allocation or may not be feasible because adverse outcomes are so rare or so distant in time from the intervention that the study costs become prohibitive.[1] Given that the scope for RCTs to be poorly designed is potentially enormous, it is essential to re-examine the advantages, disadvantages and future potential of observational (i.e. non-randomised) evidence in health technology assessment.

This section considers the distinctive role and merits of three broadly distinguished types of observational evidence. Firstly, the section considers quantitative data derived from dedicated observational studies set up especially to address particular research questions. Usually this in-volves data-gathering in the context of a research study established to address specific questions. Such data form a continuum with a second type of quantitative data, that in summary terms may be termed routine. In the healthcare systems of most advanced societies, there is a wide array of quantitative data gathered routinely and regularly for administrative, financial, surveillance or other purposes rather than to address specific research questions. Because they have largely not been set up specifically to address evaluative questions, the role of routine data in health technology assessment needs to be examined very carefully. The third kind of data considered in this section is quite distinctive in that it is qualitative; in other words, data which may relate to or be capable of being rendered into quantitative form but are primarily of significance as non-numerical narrative or verbal evidence. Generally qualitative data most resemble our first type of quantitative data since they are invariably collected in the context of dedicated research rather than as a by-product of health service routines.

The first two chapters of this section provide important and complementary analyses of the relative advantages and disadvantages of randomised compared with observational evidence to evaluate healthcare interventions. Sanderson and colleagues report a number of reviews addressing aspects of this comparison. Firstly, they examine studies on four specific and contrasting healthcare interventions: surgery in the form of coronary artery bypass grafting and coronary angioplasty, calcium antagonists, stroke units, and malaria vaccines. They conclude that differences in results between randomised and observational evidence in these four fields are smaller than might be expected and show no consistent tendency for RCTs to report smaller effects, as claimed by some earlier reviews.[2] From other evidence, Sanderson and colleagues conclude that many differences in results between the two types of studies may arise from differences in samples recruited into studies rather than study design. Where appropriate adjustments are made in non-randomised studies, results may more closely resemble those of randomised designs. The overall message of this chapter is to caution the reader against the instinctive assumption that observational evidence of effectiveness of interventions is inherently more biased and flawed.

Reeves and colleagues address similar questions about inferences that may be drawn from randomised compared with observational designs, using data from research on effectiveness in other fields, for example, mammographic screening and folic acid supplementation. When observational studies rated by the team as of high methodological quality were compared with results obtained from RCTs, evidence of effectiveness was found to be rather similar in the two types of study. Only when observational studies of poorer quality were included did evidence of effectiveness of interventions begin to diverge more significantly. Whilst they are cautious in generalising beyond the areas of healthcare captured in their literature review, their conclusions are strikingly similar to those of Sanderson and colleagues. With appropriate use of conventional methods of adjustment for possible confounding factors, well-designed observational quantitative studies can prove as valid estimates of effectiveness of interventions as do RCTs.

Routine data of the kind collected by healthcare systems for administrative or quality assurance purposes normally attract the most negative comments in terms of potential value in health technology assessment.[3] Raftery and colleagues use the diverse array of routine data available in the UK national health service as a test case to reassess the value of such data. Their review demonstrates what is likely to be the case for many other healthcare systems, which is that routine data vary very considerably in their potential relevance to health technology assessment. In the best instances it is possible to make linkages between interventions and health outcomes; commonly however, data on health outcomes do not exist or cannot be linked informatively. Raftery and colleagues point out that the evaluation of healthcare interventions is not solely concerned with effectiveness. We are often concerned with other issues such as how successfully effective treatments diffuse and how fairly and equitably between social groups they are provided. Routine data sets may be a unique resource to address such broader evaluative questions.

Lewsey and colleagues also address the central question of the value of routinely collected data in evaluative research. They examine the role of linked Scottish healthcare and health status data in two case studies, one to address questions regarding surgery for subarachnoid haemorrhage, the other comparing coronary artery bypass grafting with percutaneous coronary angioplasty. They conclude that limitations in the quality of routinely collected data (for example in terms of diagnostic imprecision) make it difficult to perform appropriate adjustments to produce unbiased estimates of treatment benefits. However, they also make a case for the benefits that would flow from strengthening the quality of routine data.

Finally, the role of qualitative evidence in health technology assessment is addressed by Murphy and Dingwall. Qualitative research is a relatively recent arrival to the field of health technology assessment and, as they acknowledge, its role is more contested. In an authoritative overview, they consider why this should be the case. They consider and challenge views that qualitative research is inherently less generalisable and its inferences less well validated. They argue that qualitative research has a vital role to play in the evaluation of healthcare, in for example, identifying mechanisms underlying the effects of services and, more generally, providing policy-makers and other audiences with deeper understanding of the nature of healthcare organisations that deliver interventions. As the authors put it, qualitative methods address the 'how' rather than 'how many' questions that modern healthcare constantly raises. Currently the quality of qualitative contributions to healthcare research is more variable, but the potential role is considerable.[4]

There have been long-standing debates about the most informative and most creative study designs to examine causal relationships both in the wider field of human behaviour, and more narrowly in the evaluation of the impact of health services.[5,6] The lesson of this section is that evidence must replace dogma in choice of study design to optimise the value and impact of data to inform decisions about health services.

REFERENCES

1. Black N. Why we need observational studies to evaluate the effectiveness of health care. *Br. Med. J.* 1996; **312**: 1215–18.
2. Colditz G, Miller J, Mosteller F. How study design affects outcomes in comparisons of therapy: I Medical. *Statist. Med.* 1989; **8**: 441–54.
3. Sheldon TA. Please bypass the PORT. *Br. Med. J.* 1994; **309**: 142–3.
4. Boulton M, Fitzpatrick R, Swinburn C. Qualitative research in health care. II A structured review and evaluation of studies. *J. Eval. Clin. Pract.* 1996; **2**: 171–9.
5. Cook T, Campbell D. *Quasi-experimentation Design and Analysis Issues for Field Settings.* Boston: Houghton Mifflin, 1979.
6. Cochrane A. *Effectiveness and Efficiency.* London: Nuffield Provincial Hospitals Trust, 1972.

6

Randomised and Non-Randomised Studies: Threats to Internal and External Validity

COLIN SANDERSON, MARTIN McKEE,
ANNIE BRITTON, NICK BLACK, KLIM McPHERSON
and CHRIS BAIN

SUMMARY

Potential threats to the validity of evaluative studies have been extensively reviewed. In terms of *internal* validity (of inference for the kinds of patient recruited), the preferred approach has been to eliminate bias through study design and execution (randomisation; blinding; complete follow-up, etc.) rather than to try to allow for it in the analysis. Threats to *external* validity (of inference for a wider population) have generally had less attention.

Difficulties arise when the measures taken to eliminate one potential source of bias exacerbate another. Orthodox randomisation should eliminate bias due to baseline differences, but may create other problems for internal validity if there are differential effects on outcome associated with patients being involved in choice of therapy. More generally, there may be conflict between the pursuit of internal and external validity. Randomisation and blinding may affect willingness to participate, which may in turn result in unrepresentative recruitment – as may restricting eligibility to the patients most likely to be compliant and to provide follow-up data. This raises questions about how far and in what circumstances: (1) non-randomised studies *are* misleadingly biased; and (2) randomised trials *are* misleadingly unrepresentative – questions which must be addressed empirically.

A series of reviews was undertaken, based largely on searches of Medline and EMBASE, with follow-up of cited references. The first reviewed comparisons of results from randomised and non-randomised studies, with case studies of four different types of intervention. Differences in the results obtained by the different types of design were:

(a) often within the margins of statistical error, and frequently smaller than those between different randomised controlled trials (RCTs) or between different non-randomised studies; and

(b) generally in the magnitude rather than the direction of estimated treatment effect, with no evidence of consistent bias towards smaller reported effects in RCTs.

The second review addressed the issues of exclusion as a matter of study design, and recruitment bias resulting from decisions about participation by centres, doctors and patients. On the very limited direct evidence, differences in measured outcome between RCTs and non-randomised studies could be reduced by restricting the analysis of non-randomised studies to subjects who met RCT eligibility criteria. On the indirect evidence:

1 Trials of similar interventions vary widely in the proportions of potential candidates excluded by design, with eligibility criteria often the main barrier to recruitment.

2 The limited data supported the widely perceived tendency for RCTs to be mainly undertaken in single university or teaching hospitals, with non-randomised studies more likely to be multi-centre and include non-teaching centres.

3 Comparing participants in RCTs with eligible non-participants, there was evidence, mainly from studies of heart disease, that participants in some *treatment* trials were poorer, less educated and more ill, whereas in some *prevention* trials they were better off, better educated and healthier in lifestyle. The impact on external validity was unclear.

The third review addressed the question of whether differences in results between RCTs and non-randomised studies could be attributed to baseline differences between intervention groups, and could be adjusted for. It was found that the effect of adjustment on treatment effect size was often of the same order as the margins of statistical error; but that the impact of adjustment was hard to assess because of between-study differences in selection criteria.

In the fourth review, of the effect of patient preference on outcome in RCTs, it was found that in spite of proposed new designs, assessment of preference effects remains problematic; only four actual studies were found, and these were small or had yet to report full results.

Clinical and policy decision-makers should look for pragmatic studies with clearly defined reference populations and data on indicators of recruitment bias.

There were a number of implications for researchers:

1 There are gaps in our empirical knowledge of the biases that can arise during different kinds of study which make it difficult to strike the best balance between competing design considerations. Major studies, both randomised and non-randomised, should involve collecting data on potential sources of bias, including selective participation.

2 Restrictive studies may have advantages in terms of internal validity, but these may be offset by costly or slow recruitment, and uncertainty about extrapolation of results.

3 Meta-analyses, and comparisons of results from different study designs, should include analyses in which the same set of eligibility criteria are applied to as many studies as possible. Prospectively, eligibility criteria for different trials in the same field should be harmonised, unless this leads to material conflict with other design objectives.

CONTEXT

Recognition of the need to base healthcare decisions on sound evidence, whether in commissioning services for populations or in clinical practice, has heightened awareness of methodological issues in evaluative studies. Random allocation to treatment groups has been widely accepted on theoretical grounds as the methodological gold standard, but many RCTs are weak in other ways, and the coverage of RCT-based evidence is patchy at best. Meanwhile attitudes to non-randomised studies vary from selective enthusiasm, through 'better than nothing', to 'worse than nothing'. (In this review the primary concern is with non-randomised studies using high-quality data collected prospectively for research purposes, rather than data from routine information sources.) The starting point for this review is that choice of design by researcher, and interpretation of results by practitioner, should be informed by empirical information on the practical impact of the various theoretical threats to validity; and that these should include threats to *external* validity (generalisation from the trial subjects to the wider population of interest) such as selective recruitment as well as threats to *internal* validity (relevance of the results for the subjects studied and patients similar to them) such as baseline differences, losses to follow-up, and inadequate blinding.

These are controversial matters, and it is important to identify at the outset the main areas of common ground. Firstly, it is clear that given properly conducted randomisation, double blinding where appropriate, and comprehensive follow-up, RCTs provide good estimates of the relative effectiveness of interventions in the types of subject recruited to the study. It is also accepted that without randomisation, even with satisfactory blinding and follow-up, observed differences in outcomes may be due to differences in the initial composition of the groups rather than in the effects of the interventions. In terms of internal validity, the properly conducted RCT is incontestably the design of choice.

However, this has led to the suggestion that evidence from randomised trials is the only kind that should be taken seriously. The dissenters (Black,[1] for example) argue that randomisation is unnecessary when the effect of an intervention is so dramatic that the contribution of unknown confounding factors can plausibly be ignored, as with the example of defibrillation for ventricular fibrillation; that the cost of an RCT may be unjustifiable if long-term or rare events are involved (particularly if the intervention or product at issue is expected to have a limited 'life'); and that ethical recruitment is impossible when individual clinicians and/or patients do not accept that there is sufficient uncertainty about the effectiveness of alternative treatments. Even where randomisation is practical, there can be problems with internal validity if the process of randomisation affects outcome in different ways for different treatment groups, or when subjects have preferences and cannot be effectively blinded to the intervention;[2] and there can be problems with external validity if the process through which patients become involved in randomised studies is highly selective.[3] Also in practice, randomised trials may have been less free from bias than many have supposed, with systematic differences arising from faulty randomisation and incomplete blinding.[4,5]

Thus, it is contended, there can be an important complementary role for non-randomised studies, provided that the same attention is paid to data collection processes as in good randomised studies, and that adequate steps can be taken to avoid or allow for material baseline differences. Such studies have the potential, at least, for less selective recruitment and more rapid accumulation of subjects at lower administrative cost – or greater sample size. The randomisers' riposte is that external validity is pointless without internal validity, that one can never be sure that adequate steps have been taken to deal with baseline differences, that selective recruitment does not seriously bias measures of relative effect, and that pragmatic randomised designs give as much external validity as is necessary.

This debate has been characterised by strongly held views based on limited empirical evidence. In this review we seek to define some of the unresolved questions; to examine the evidence in support of the differing positions; and to suggest priorities for further research. The material presented here is a summary of a report that addresses these issues in more detail.[6]

DEFINING THE QUESTIONS

Systematic Differences in Measured Treatment Effectiveness

When the same intervention is assessed in different RCTs, the results can differ for a number of reasons. This truism also applies to non-randomised studies. However, it has been claimed that non-randomised studies have a consistent tendency to report larger treatment effects than RCTs.[7,8] The concern is that in the absence of rigorous randomisation, a bias –

conscious or otherwise – may creep into the allocation process, with those receiving the new treatment tending to have greater underlying potential to benefit. The first question is, what evidence is there for this?

Selection of Subjects and External Validity

Evaluation studies vary widely in the extent to which the range of potential future recipients of treatment is represented. Some groups of subjects may be excluded as part of the design for *medical* reasons (a high risk of adverse effects in relation to expected benefits; a belief that benefit will be relatively small or absent – or has already been established for the group in question). Exclusions of this kind can be problematic if there is a tendency towards, say, a more cautious attitude to risk of adverse effects in trials than in regular clinical practice.

Subjects may also be excluded for *scientific* reasons (increased precision in estimates of effect by studying relatively homogeneous groups; reduced vulnerability to bias by excluding subjects who may be at high risk of failure to comply with treatment, or loss to follow-up[9]). The pursuit of homogeneity can lead to exclusion of large groups of people who are quite plausible candidates for treatment.

A further threat to the external validity of both randomised and non-randomised studies comes from selective participation, the cumulative effect of decisions by centres, practitioners and eligible patients about whether to take part.

This suggests a second set of questions: what evidence is there on the contribution of eligibility criteria and selective participation to differences between randomised and non-randomised studies in measured relative effect? And if the evidence is sparse – which it turns out to be – what is known about differences between these study designs in terms of: (i) the extent and nature of the selection involved; and (ii) subjects at baseline?

Accounting for Baseline Differences

The assumption has been that if randomised and non-randomised studies produce different results, then decision-making should be based on the results of the randomised study because of its superior internal validity. However, if non-randomised studies have (potentially at least) greater external validity, the question arises of how far, and in what circumstances, allocation bias can be allowed for at the analysis stage.

One test of this is whether, given similar eligibility criteria, adjustment for confounding brings the results of non-randomised studies closer to those from RCTs; and if the answer is 'sometimes', then under what circumstances?

Patient Preferences

The idea that randomisation itself can give rise to biased results about outcome may seem surprising. However, when treatments are allocated randomly, practitioners and patients are deprived of expressing a preference and, if choice and control are of therapeutic benefit, then a blinded randomised comparison might provide a misleading estimate of the relative effect of treatment in 'regular' practice.[10] The difficulty is that if such preference effects exist, attempts to detect them are compromised by potential confounding by selection:[11] people who tend to prefer something may well tend to be different in other ways, plausibly related to prognosis.[12,13] There are several possible mechanisms for patient preferences having an effect. These have been examined in research on the psychology of the placebo[14] as well as in studies showing that the extent of a person's social or professional control over their lives has a role in the aetiology of coronary heart disease.[15] Where people have strong preferences, randomising is difficult.[16] Thus, an important and neglected part of the research agenda is to disentangle the main physiological effect of a treatment from any possible preference-dependent effect.

In summary, the questions that will be addressed in this review are first, 'do non-randomised studies differ from RCTs in measured magnitude of treatment effect?', and if they do, 'to what extent can these differences be explained by:

(a) selective recruitment;
(b) baseline differences between groups in non-randomised studies (and can these be allowed for); and
(c) the differential impact, in a randomised study, of any therapeutic effect arising from patient participation in treatment decisions?'

METHODS

The search strategy used to address the four questions identified above has been described in detail elsewhere[6] but, in brief, it involved searches of Medline (1966–1996) and EMBASE (1980–1996) using, among others, variants on the words participation, inclusion, exclusion, recruitment and preference. Cited references

were followed-up. As published evidence was lacking, data from two recently completed systematic reviews that included both RCTs and non-randomised studies[17,18] were reanalysed to assess the effect of differential participation by teaching and non-teaching facilities.

In addition, four case studies were undertaken, examining the results of RCTs and non-randomised studies of interventions representing four different modes of therapeutic action: coronary artery bypass grafting (CABG) and percutaneous transluminal coronary angioplasty (PTCA) (surgical); calcium antagonists (pharmacological); stroke units (organisational); and malaria vaccines (preventive). Of necessity, the overview provided here is a brief summary of the evidence examined, and a full review provides more details.[6]

Our thinking about external validity has been informed by a simple conceptual model (Figure 1). The horizontal axis represents an indicator or predictor of potential benefit from treatment A relative to treatment B, such as blood pressure or symptom score. The vertical axis represents numbers of people. The population is represented by an outer triangular 'envelope', of which only the right-hand part is shown; most of the population are to the left of the broken line. This represents schematically the common situation in which there are relatively few people with the highest levels of potential benefit and increasing numbers with lower levels. In reality the envelope will take a variety of shapes depending on the intervention being studied.

For a substantial proportion of the population there will be little doubt that the expected potential advantage of treatment A over treatment B is outweighed by risks or other 'costs'. These, indicated as *me* (medical exclusions), should be excluded by design – from randomised studies as ineligible, and from non-randomised studies as inappropriate. (The diagram also shows an 'upper' threshold, above which there is little doubt that benefits outweigh risks.) That leaves the grey band in the diagram, indicating the reference population for which results are needed.

However, as we have seen, some subjects (*se:* scientific exclusions) may be 'designed out' to improve precision or reduce bias. Then, eligible patients may not participate for a variety of reasons: non-participation in study by treatment centre or doctor (*d*); patient not invited to participate (*i*); patient choice not to participate (*p*). The study population becomes a progressively smaller subset of the reference population, with opportunities for recruitment bias arising at each stage. There may also be some deliberate sampling process, but as random sampling, at least, should be 'neutral', this is not shown. In the diagram the distributions of (and hence

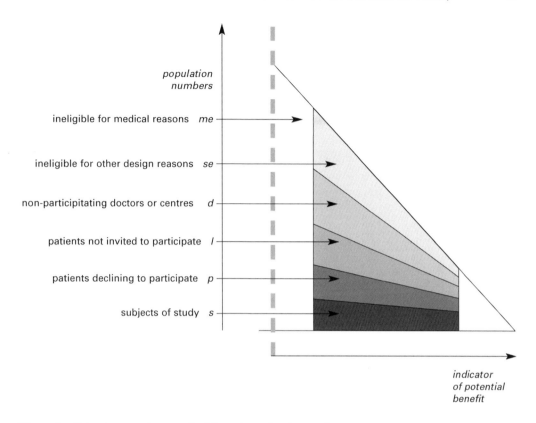

Figure 1   *Selective recruitment of subjects in evaluative studies.*

mean values of) potential benefit in the study and reference populations are different, signalling the question of whether it is valid to generalise from one to the other.

THE EVIDENCE

Do Non-Randomised Studies and RCTs Produce Systematically Different Results?

The proposition that non-randomised studies 'produce' greater treatment effects than randomised studies appears to be based on two kinds of evidence. The first consists of a few frequently quoted comparisons of the two methods. The second comes from studies of RCTs with varying quality of randomisation, which have shown that inadequate or unclear methods are associated with exaggerated intervention effects.

In this review, 18 papers were identified that directly compared the results of RCTs and non-randomised studies of the same intervention.[12,19–35] The results are summarised in Table 1. The table is difficult to summarise further because different papers involved different types of comparison; but in a very crude analysis of differences in effect, seven papers reported larger effect sizes in non-randomised studies, but in only three of these was the difference significant (or test-based conclusions from the two types of study different) at the 5% level; in three, differences were not significant, and in one, significance was not reported. Eleven papers reported larger effect sizes for RCTs, but only four of these were significant; six were not significant, and one did not report significance.

- For CABG versus PTCA, the RCTs tended to favour CABG although confidence intervals were wide; unadjusted results of the non-randomised studies favoured PTCA.
- For calcium antagonists, effects for randomised studies (overall risk ratio for nine RCTs: 1.10 [0.95 to 1.27]) and non-randomised (unadjusted RR for one study: 1.18 [1.04 to 1.34]) were similar.
- For stroke units versus conventional care, the Cochrane meta-analysis for RCTs gave OR = 0.81 (0.68 to 0.96) for survival to final follow-up (median 12 months) as against 0.6

Table 1 Comparison of effects from RCTs and non-randomised studies

Authors	Ref.	Topic	Same eligibility criteria	Adjustment used?	Treatment groups	Outcome indicator	Randomised studies				Non-randomised studies				Different effect size
							n	risk	relative risk	p	n	risk	relative risk	p	p
McKay et al. (1995)	12	Alcohol rehab	yes	yes	day care inpatients	% days > 3 drinks at 1 yr	24 / 24	20.0% / 55.0%	0.36	?	65 / 31	35.1% / 39.1%	0.90	?	<0.05
					day care inpatients	% treated again in rehab at 1 yr	24 / 24	15.0% / 10.0%	0.50	?	65 / 31	12.3% / 30.4%	0.40	?	(ns)
CASS (1984)	19	CHD	yes	no	Surgery Medical	5-yr survival	390 / 390	95.0% / 92.0%	1.03	ns	570 / 745	94.0% / 92.0%	1.02	?	ns
Hlatky et al. (1988)	20	CHD	yes	yes	Surgical Medical	5-yr survival	686	83.0% / 78.0%	1.064	?	719	85.5% / 80.9%	1.057	?	ns
		CHD	yes	yes	Surgical Medical	5-yr survival	767	92.0% / 84.0%	1.10	?	512	91.9% / 86.3%	1.06	?	
Horwitz et al. (1990)	21	Myocardial infarction	yes	no	Beta-blockers no BB	Mortality at 24 m	1916 / 1912	7.3% / 9.2%	0.79	?	417 / 205	7.2% / 10.7%	0.67	?	ns
			yes	yes	Beta-blockers no BB	Mortality at 24 m	1916 / 1912	7.3% / 9.2%	0.79	?	417 / 205	7.6% / 9.7%	0.78	?	
Paradise et al. (1984)	22	Throat infection	yes	no	Tonsillectomy Control	Infections/pers in yr 1	38 / 35	1.24 / 3.09	na	0.001	44 / 34	1.77 / 3.09	na	0.04	?
Paradise et al. (1990)	23	Otitis media	yes	no	Adenoidectomy Control	% of days with otitis media in y1	52 / 47	15.0% / 28.5%	0.53	0.04	47 / 67	17.8% / 23.3%	0.76	0.55	sdtr
Schmoor et al. (1996)	24	Breast cancer	yes	yes	chemotherapy control	treatment effect	289	? / ?	0.90	0.45	176	? / ?	0.90	?	0.99
					hormone therapy control	treatment effect	184	? / ?	0.75	0.085	71	? / ?	0.53	?	0.20
			yes	yes	radiotherapy control	treatment effect	199	? / ?	0.79	0.32	129	? / ?	0.76	?	0.94
Yamamoto et al. (1992)	25	Peptic strictures	yes	no	Eder-Puestow Balloon	recurrence of dysphagia	16 / 15	69.0% / 80.0%	0.86	<0.05	58 / 34	88.0% / 94.0%	0.94	>0.05	nsdtr
			yes	no	Eder-Puestow Balloon	% needing redilation	16 / 15	38.0% / 27.0%	1.41	<0.05	58 / 34	43.0% / 50.0%	0.86	>0.05	

Study	No.	Condition			Treatment / Comparison	Outcome	n	value	ratio	p	n	value	ratio	p	final
Nicolaides et al. (1994)	26	Pregnancy	yes	no	cvs / amino	spontaneous loss	250 / 238	1.2% / 5.9%	0.20	<0.05	320 / 493	3.1% / 5.1%	0.61	ns	sdtr
Emanuel (1996)	27	Terminal cancer	no	no	hospice / conventional	cost/patient	247	$16,000 / $15,493	na	?	5853	$7,719 / $11,729	na	?	?
Garenne et al. (1993)	28	Measles	no	no	vaccine / none	measles absent	740 / 348	? / ?	0.97	?	1224 / 4403	? / ?	0.93	?	ns
Antman et al. (1985)	29	Sarcoma	yes	no	chemotherapy / control	disease-free at follow-up	20 / 22	75.0% / 72.7%	1.03	0.81	21 / 27	61.9% / 44.4%	1.39	0.001	sdtr
			yes		chemotherapy / control	disease-free at follow-up	20 / 22	? / ?	?	0.26	21 / 27	? / ?	?	0.03	
Shapiro et al. (1994)	30	Breast cancer	no	no	chemotherapy surgery / radiation	% with acute non-lymphocytic leukaemia	? / ? / ?	? / ? / ?	24.0 / 2.6 / 10.3	<0.01 / ns / <0.01	? / ? / ?	? / ? / ?	8.10 / 1.40 / 3.70	<0.01 / ns / <0.01	nsdtr
Jha et al. (1995)	31	Cardio-vascular	no	yes	vitamin E / no vitamin suppl	% CVD mortality per 10000 yrs fu	14564 / 14569	5.0% / 6.0%	0.98	ns	11342 / 75903	5.2% / 8.5%	0.61	<0.05	sdtr
Pyorala et al. (1995)	32	Crypto-orchism	no	no	LHRG / hCG	descent of testes	872	21.0% / 19.0%	1.11	ns	2410	47.0% / 33.0%	1.42	<0.05	sdtr
RMTIG (1994)	33	Spontaneous abortion	no	no	immuno / control	live birth rates	240 / 209	61.7% / 51.7%	1.19	0.024	877 / 256	59.0% / 55.1%	1.07	0.216	sdtr
Watson et al. (1994)	34	Infertility	no	no	hysterosalpin / control	pregnancy rate	287 / 513	30.3% / 18.7%	1.62	?	1072 / 734	41.8% / 25.9%	1.61	?	ns
Reimold (1992)	35	Atrial fibrillation	yes	no	quinidine / control	sinus rhythm at 3 m	372 / 354	69.4% / 45.1%	1.54	<0.00	471 / 290	44.3% / 35.1%	1.26	<0.05	ns
					quinidine / control	sinus rhythm at 12 m	372 / 354	50.2% / 24.7%	2.03	<0.00	471 / 290	13.7% / 10.9%	1.26	0.29	ns

Key: in body of table   ?:   not stated in reference
      in final column   na: not applicable
      ns: effect sizes not significantly different at 5% level
      sdtr: test results significant at 5% level for one type of study and not the other
      nsdtr: test results significant at 5% level in both types of study, or neither

(0.4 to 0.9) and 0.59 (0.42 to 0.84) for the two unadjusted non-randomised studies.

- For malaria episodes within 12 months of vaccination, a meta-analysis of five RCTs gave an odds ratio of 0.62 (0.53 to 0.71) as against 0.78 (0.52 to 1.17) for a non-randomised study.

In summary, contrary to the proposition, we found no evidence for a consistent pattern or bias when the results of RCTs and non-randomised studies were compared. Some will find this result surprising, but there are a number of possible explanations:

1   The biases that the RCT is designed to guard against are in practice too small to have been detected in this analysis, and have been swamped by 'random' variation or heterogeneity.
2   Most of the RCTs in this study were of such poor quality that in practice the differences in study design became blurred.
3   There *are* various biases involved in non-randomised studies, but they tend to cancel out.

All of these explanations may have a part to play. If the last is a significant one, the implication is that although non-randomised designs may be unbiased, their results may be subject to larger mean absolute error.

To What Extent can Differences between the Results of Randomised and Non-Randomised Studies be Explained by Differences in Eligibility Criteria?

The key question here is the possible impact of eligibility criteria specifically (as opposed to the whole recruitment process) on measured effects. The direct evidence is very limited. We found only one paper, by Horwitz et al.[21] in which the relative effectiveness of two treatments found in a randomised trial was compared with results from non-randomised cohorts subject to first some, and then all, of the same eligibility criteria. Their findings are summarised in Table 2. It shows that the effect estimate for the trial was closer to that for a 'restricted' observational cohort (who satisfied all the trial's eligibility criteria) than that for an 'expanded' observational cohort (with the trial's age and diagnostic criteria, but without its contra-indications and factors designed to enhance follow-up).

Results from the study by Ward et al.[36] may throw some light on this because although they did not address relative effectiveness, their trial of adjuvant chemotherapy for stomach cancer found no significant effect. They compared 960 cancer registry patients with 493 trial-eligible patients and 249 trial patients, and found median survivals of 9, 11 and 13, months respectively.

Some indirect light is thrown on this issue by the growing interest in heterogeneity of trials that has accompanied meta-analyses. Thompson for example has shown a relationship between measured risk reduction and average age at coronary event for subjects in different trials.[37] However, heterogeneity is a product of the whole process of trial design and recruitment, not just of variations in eligibility criteria.

In terms of *extent* of selection, very little is known about non-randomised studies, even though they are (at least potentially) less vulnerable to selective recruitment than RCTs. This may be at least partly because they have been widely seen as so flawed as to be of little interest to methodologists. For RCTs, the impact of

Table 2   *Candidates for treatment with beta-blockers (BB): comparison of baseline characteristics and outcomes for subjects in a trial, in a restricted database with the same eligibility criteria as the trial, and an expanded database*

| | | Database | | | | | |
| | | BHAT trial | | Restricted cohort | | Expanded cohort | |
		BB	no BB	BB	no BB	BB	no BB
Baseline	Number	1916	1921	417	205	626	433
	Mean age	55	55	57	60	58	60
	males (%)	84	85	75	73	73	68
	mild (%)	58	61	72	68	64	51
Outcome: Crude	24 m mortality	7.3	9.2	7.2	10.7	9.3	16.4
	reduction (%)	21		33		43	
Outcome: Adjusted for age and severity	24 m mortality	7.3	9.2	7.6	9.7	10.2	14.4
	reduction (%)	21		22		29	

Source: Horwitz et al.[21]

Table 3 *Percentage of eligible patients/subjects included in RCTs of selected interventions*

Malaria vaccines		Calcium antagonists		CABG/PTCA		Hypertension	
Alonso[80]	98.20%	TRENT[81]	48.20%	CABRI[82]	4.60%	SHEP[83]	1.06%
D'Alessandro[84]	97.30%	SPRINT II[85]	66.60%	EAST[86]	16.40%	MRC '92[97]	3.49%
Sempertegui[87]	91.80%	SPRINT I[88]	49.70%	GABI[89]	4.00%	MRC '85[98]	3.37%
Valero '93[90]	84.80%	Branigan[91]	12.40%	LAUSANNE[92]	7.90%		
Valero '96[93]	77.60%	Sirnes[94]	c.30.0%	ERACHI[95]	40.20%		
				BARI[96]	16.30%		

eligibility criteria on numbers recruited appears to vary widely. For example, one of the early studies of losses prior to randomisation[38] was based on 16 trials in the 1979 inventory of the National Institute of Health. Overall, 73% of those screened were deemed ineligible, the rate ranging from 10% to 99% for different studies. In a more recent overview of eight trials of intravenous thrombolysis by Muller and Topol,[39] the percentage of patients screened that was deemed eligible ranged from 9% to 51%.

These results are difficult to interpret because much of this variation may be attributable to differences in use of the word 'screening'. It may, for example, mean surveillance of all hospital admissions to provide possible *candidates* for proper diagnostic screening rather than diagnostic screening itself. This is illustrated by Table 3, which draws largely on material from our case studies. The generally low proportions excluded from vaccine trials in which there was no sickness- or risk-related selection prior to screening, and very high proportions for primary prevention of hypertension in which those screened were again whole populations, are unsurprising. More striking are the fairly high proportions excluded from a set of secondary prevention trials in which screening was typically based on chest pain on hospital admission, and for cardiac surgery, in which those screened were patients with multiple-vessel disease.

The relative importance of exclusions for scientific reasons (to improve precision and/or reduce vulnerability to bias) rather than medical ones (to focus on groups without contraindications and for whom outcome is uncertain) is unclear, partly because of lack of data, but partly because for many common exclusion criteria both medical and scientific factors are involved. For example, people with serious co-morbidities may be excluded not only because the expected balance of benefit and risk is adverse, but also because they may not survive to the trial endpoint, and they may add to the heterogeneity of likely treatment effect.

Those with severe disease[40] or strong preferences are also commonly excluded,[41] and many RCTs have 'blanket' exclusions, such as women,[42] the elderly[43] and ethnic minorities, for reasons that are often unspecified. For example, Gurwitz et al. reviewed 214 RCTs of specific pharmacotherapies for treatment of acute myocardial infarction between 1960 and 1991, and found that over 60% formally excluded people aged 75 or more. However, explicit exclusion from trials on the basis of age seems to be less common in cancer trials.[44]

In summary, high levels of exclusions can bring some benefits for the researcher in terms of precision and risk of bias, as well as the medical benefits of avoiding potential harm, but there are also important disadvantages:

(a) uncertainty about extrapolation of results to other populations;

(b) denial of potentially effective treatment to those who might benefit; and

(c) delay in obtaining definitive results and/or the likelihood of added research costs because of reduced recruitment rate.

To What Extent can Differences between the Results of Randomised and Non-Randomised Studies be Explained by Selective Participation?

Again, there are very few data on the impact of selective participation on measured effect in randomised and non-randomised trials. There have, however, been some studies of the extent and nature of the selection involved.

In the 1979 National Institutes of Health study, in addition to the 73% deemed ineligible, 15% were not randomised (4% withdrawn by the doctor, 4% patient refusals, and 7% withdrawn by the investigators),[38] leaving 12% of those screened participating in studies.

A few reports of individual studies have given the proportions of patients under treatment not recruited for different reasons: Lee and Breuax: 34% excluded, 29% clinician refusal, 5% patient refusal;[45] Begg et al.: 70% excluded, 8% clinician refusal, 3% patient refusal;[46] Martin et al.: 69% excluded, 15% clinician or patient refusal;[47] EORTC: 60% ineligible, 4% patient refusal.[48] If at all representative, these figures suggest that doctor or patient preferences are less of a barrier to recruitment than eligibility criteria.

Of course studies of participation which take patients under treatment in participating treatment centres or hospitals as their denominator reveal nothing about selective participation by centres. In a reanalysis of two recently completed systematic reviews[17,18] it was found that non-randomised studies were more likely to be multicentre than RCTs, with some weaker support for the proposition that non-randomised studies were more likely to extend beyond teaching or specialist centres.[6]

There is some evidence for socio-demographic differences between those who participate in trials and those who do not. Earlier reviews found that subjects of RCTs that evaluated treatments tended to be less affluent and less educated than those who declined to participate, whilst those in RCTs evaluating preventive interventions tended to be more affluent, and better educated.[49] Rochon et al. have shown that although 64 out of 83 RCTs of non-steroidal anti-inflammatory drugs had no specified upper age limit, only 10% of the 9664 subjects were reported as being aged 50 or more.[50]

In our own review of 16 RCTs of treatments, we also found studies in which patients were younger (significantly so in four studies out of the 11 in which age was examined), more likely to be male (five studies out of 12), non-white (three out of seven) and of lower socio-economic status (three out of four). The three studies that were biased in favour of younger males all involved post-infarction anticoagulants or anti-arrhythmics. By contrast, in one RCT of diabetic care[51] the trial subjects tended to be older than the trial-eligible patients in a primary care database.

In our review the four prevention trials all addressed the issue of age. Subjects were relatively young in one. Of the three that considered gender selection, the excess of males was significant in one and borderline in another.

There have also been studies of whether baseline severity or prognostic indicators were similar for subjects in RCTs and non-randomised studies. In our review, 14 treatment trials examined this in one way or another. In seven trials the participants tended to have the poorer prognoses, but in one (non-Hodgkin's lymphoma) prognoses were better. The prevention trials were more mixed in this respect.

In our case-study of CABG versus PTCA, patients in the non-randomised Medicare study[52] had markedly higher baseline risks of mortality than those in the Duke non-randomised study and the nine RCTs .

Overall, the amount of direct evidence on the effects of selective participation was very limited. However, it does seem that where there are differences between the results of randomised and non-randomised studies, explanations should be sought in differences in the populations participating, as well as in the method of allocating subjects.

To What Extent can Differences in Results be Attributed to Baseline Differences Between Intervention Groups, and be Allowed for?

There are a number of theoretical objections to relying on adjustment to deal with baseline differences. Particular problems arise where large numbers of factors contribute to the risk of an adverse outcome.[53] Many of these factors may be unknown, stratified analysis may fail because of small numbers in each stratum, and adjustment models may be vulnerable to high levels of correlation between treatment and prognostic factors.

The papers reviewed again gave mixed results. Horwitz et al., in the Beta-Blocker Heart Attack Trial,[21] found that adjustment of non-randomised findings for age and severity, when combined with exclusion of subjects that did not meet the corresponding trial eligibility criteria, gave similar results to their randomised trial (see Table 2). However, the authors of a paper evaluating treatment for sarcoma were unable to reconcile the results of the different approaches.[30]

In our four case studies:

1   For CABG versus PTCA, there were marked baseline differences between treatment groups in the non-randomised studies. Adjustment improved the consistency of the 'dose–response' relationship between baseline severity and relative mortality in the non-randomised studies (low-risk: PTCS better, high-risk: CABG better), but did nothing to improve agreement with RCTs. This is an area in which results may well be sensitive to selective recruitment.

2   For the calcium antagonist non-randomised study, the patients were generally similar at baseline, apart from there being more hypertensives in the treatment group and more patients on beta-blockers and digoxin among the controls. The effect on the crude result (1.18; 1.04 to 1.34) of adjustment for baseline differences was progressive as more

factors were added, first closing the gap with the RCT meta-analysis result of 1.10 (0.95 to 1.27) and then overshooting to 0.94 (0.82 to 1.08).

3 For stroke units, in the Copenhagen non-randomised study there were no significant differences at baseline in terms of age, sex and a range of cardiovascular and neurological parameters; but stroke unit patients were more likely to have a history of hypertension. In the Edinburgh study the effect of adjustment for baseline differences was again progressive as more factors were added, closing the gap with the RCT and then overshooting.

4 For malaria vaccine the two groups in the non-randomised study were similar in age, sex and occupation at baseline, but those receiving vaccination tended to come from areas with high risks of transmission. An attempt to adjust for this brought the odds ratio down from 0.78 (0.52 to 1.17) to 0.45 (0.25 to 0.79), again overshooting the RCT meta-analysis value of 0.62 (0.53 to 0.71).

To summarise, for the CABG/PTCA studies there were differences in results for the two study designs, but also differences in the populations studied, which confuses assessment of adjustments aimed at remedying within-study baseline differences. For calcium antagonists, stroke units and malaria vaccine, the evidence that RCTs and non-randomised studies produce different results was weak in the first place. Adjustment affected the results, but the studies involved were too small for firm conclusions.

The Impact of Patient Preference

In theory, patient preference could have an important impact on results of RCTs, especially where the difference between treatments being compared is small, and could account for some of the observed differences between results of RCTs and non-randomised studies. Methods have been proposed to detect preference effects reliably, but while these approaches may contribute to our understanding of this phenomenon, none provide a complete answer.[11] This is mainly because, as preference is a characteristic of the subject, randomisation between preferring a treatment and not is impossible and confounding may bias any observed comparison.

There has been relatively little empirical research in this field. Only four studies have sought to measure preference effects,[54] and they were either small or have yet to report full results.

CONCLUSIONS

The results of randomised and non-randomised studies do differ, but in most of the studies we reviewed, differences in effect-size were within the margins of statistical error, and we found no evidence that they were consistent in direction.

Where there are differences, they can be attributed to bias arising from differences in eligibility criteria, participation, allocation to treatment groups, preference effects, compliance with regimens, blinding and completeness of follow-up. A wholly satisfactory study of the reasons for inter-study differences would address all these potential sources of bias at the same time, and apart from unresolved difficulties over the assessment of preference effects, there is no reason in principle why such studies should not be carried out. However, none of the studies reviewed here achieved this. The nearest was the study by Horwitz et al.,[21] in which both eligibility criteria and differences in composition of the treatment groups were shown to contribute. Allowing for each of these in turn led to convergence of results for the two designs. Allowing for both at once made the results very similar, suggesting that for this beta-blocker study at least, other possible sources of bias had minor roles – or cancelled each other out.

With regard to selective recruitment, both randomised and non-randomised studies are vulnerable. There are a priori reasons for supposing that non-randomised studies may generally be less vulnerable, but RCTs are better documented in this respect. There is abundant evidence to show that the extent of selection varies very widely between trials. It would seem that eligibility criteria may be more of a barrier than doctor or patient participation, but little is known about the impact of selective recruitment on the validity of extrapolation from study to reference populations.

Non-randomised studies may be subject to allocation bias. A number of studies have compared the results of RCTs with adjusted and unadjusted results from non-randomised studies. However, in most cases the subjects of the two kinds of study had different baseline characteristics overall, and this undermines any assessment of how successful adjustment has been in dealing with baseline differences between treatment groups in non-randomised studies.

Recognition of the potential significance of patient preference effects is becoming widespread, but measurement of preference effects is problematic. New designs have been proposed, but evidence is only beginning to come through.

This review provides little support for the proposition that non-randomised studies are inherently biased, but the power of the analysis was limited. Some biases lead to greater treatment effects in non-randomised studies, and some to smaller effects, the resultant or net bias reflecting the relative importance of each component in a particular case (see Table 4).

At the same time, in the absence of good empirical data on the circumstances in which non-randomised studies can be expected to be (i) internally valid and (ii) superior to RCTs in terms of selective recruitment, there is nothing in this review to challenge the proposition that a well-conducted RCT is likely to be the most reliable source of evidence of clinical effectiveness.

The key question for the clinical practitioner is how to use the results of evaluative studies to inform the treatment of an individual patient. This embraces a number of issues. For example, what does a group-level measurement such as an odds ratio imply for:

(a) a patient who is a member of a heterogeneous group that was studied in the trial?
(b) a patient who is a member of a group that was excluded from the trial for scientific, but not medical, reasons?
(c) a patient who is a member of a group that was excluded from the trial for medical reasons that were more conservative than might obtain in regular practice?
(d) a patient who is going to be treated in a non-teaching, non-specialist hospital, when the evaluative study was conducted in a different context?

A number of researchers have sought to link differences in effect size with variation in baseline risk among participants in RCTs.[55–57] If such links can be established, it may become possible to estimate a patient's expected benefit from baseline prognostic features.[41] For example, Glasziou and Irwig[58] have suggested that, with increasing baseline risk, the per cent *reduction* in risk attributable to treatment may remain constant, so that the expected absolute benefit from treatment increases, but that the risk of harm from treatment may remain relatively constant. They propose meta-analysis of RCTs to check the consistency of, and provide estimates of, relative risk reduction and risk of harm, and multivariate risk equations from cohort studies to provide individualised estimates of baseline risk.

Miettinen has described 'confounding by indication' in which those whom practitioners think are most likely to benefit from a particular treatment are most likely to receive it.[59] This, he contends, provides a strong argument against non-randomised studies of intended effects, as the combination of often subtle clues that practitioners use to identify those whom they expect to benefit most from an intervention often cannot be captured by the researcher. He suggests, however, that when seeking as yet unknown adverse effects of treatment, this is not a problem.

Cowan and Wittes have argued that the closer an intervention is to a purely biological process, the lesser the dangers of extrapolation,[60] but this begs the question of what is a purely biological process. Strategies to determine how far study results may be generalised have been developed,[61] but problems remain,[62] and it is not possible at this stage to make clear recommendations.

Table 4 *Contributions to differences between estimates of effects from different types of study*

A greater treatment effect may be seen with a RCT if:

- quality of care influences relative effectiveness and RCT subjects receive higher-quality care;
- RCT subjects are selected in such a way as to have a greater relative capacity to benefit than those in non-randomised studies.

On the other hand, a greater treatment effect may be seen in a non-randomised study if:

- patients are typically allocated to treatments considered most appropriate for their individual circumstances, such as the presence of co-existing disease;
- RCT subjects are selected in such a way as to have a lower relative capacity to benefit than those in non-randomised studies, as for example in some prevention trials;
- those with strong preferences for a particular treatment show an enhanced response, whether as a result of active participation in decision-making or because the intervention itself requires the patient to take on an active role;
- negative results are less likely to be published from non-randomised studies than from RCTs.

The implications for external validity of selective participation by treatment centre are unclear. Strategies have been developed to evaluate the effect of individual institutions in multi-centre trials,[63,64] and these could be instructive if used more widely.

Meanwhile, this review confirms the proposition that participants in RCTs can be highly selected groups that have had to pass through a series of hurdles of eligibility, invitation and decision to participate. Thus clinical decision-makers, and also policy-makers, need to:

(a) pay particular attention to eligibility criteria, and any analyses of the characteristics of those in the trial as compared to those who were eligible and to any more broadly defined reference population; and

(b) be aware of the distinction between *efficacy* studies (of effectiveness under ideal circumstances) and *pragmatic* studies (of effectiveness in 'normal' practice); and base their decisions on pragmatic studies where possible.

Exclusive versus Inclusive Trials

The pros and cons of restrictive eligibility criteria for trials need to be more widely debated and understood. Commentators such as Chalmers have long been arguing for less restrictive trials.[65] Unless subgroups are pre-specified, less restrictive trials provide less precise information on a wider range of patient groups rather than more precise information on one group and none at all on others. The irony seems to be that if heterogeneity is a real problem, extrapolation from one subgroup to a wider population may be particularly hazardous, and restrictive trials are of limited relevance. Meanwhile, Yusuf et al. among others have argued that worthwhile gains in homogeneity require good predictors of treatment effect, and that since these are seldom available, in practice restricting eligibility does little to improve precision.[66]

Assessment of External Validity

One immediate priority is to improve the quality of reporting evaluative research. Information on eligibility and selective participation is often lacking in spite of the evidence that recruitment rates vary widely. As a minimum, authors should be required to state:

(a) the reference population to whom their results may be applied;

(b) the steps they have taken to ensure that the study population is representative of this wider population in relevant respects; and

(c) information on how study and reference populations differ.

Further, until these issues are better understood it would be desirable for authors to describe:

(a) the characteristics of those centres participating, and any that declined; and

(b) the numbers and characteristics of those eligible to be included, those who were not invited, and those invited who declined.

There will be advantage doing this for both RCTs and non-randomised studies.

Effective implementation of the CONSORT statement,[67] which requires authors to report the number in the eligible population and the number not randomised for each reason, will partly address this issue. The statement does not, however, require information on the proportion of the treated population screened, and the characteristics of those included and excluded.

One obstacle to explicit assessment of representativeness will be the lack of information on the spectrum of potential candidates for treatment. Involving more 'normal' treatment settings in trials would help, although extraneous factors, such as competition between professionals or hospitals can work against this; in the USA, research is increasingly concentrated in the less competitive parts of the healthcare market as pressures from healthcare funders squeeze out research.[68]

Improving External Validity

The evidence concerning behaviour change, either lay or professional, suggests that it may be difficult to overcome the failure (whether deliberate or unintended) to invite certain centres or subjects to participate, or to obtain consent. Any strategy must address not only the lack of recognition among both practitioners and the public that patients often benefit simply from being in RCTs and that a new treatment may be harmful instead of beneficial,[69] but also attitudes and practices. It should take into account the emerging body of research on patients' expectations of researchers and how recruitment might be improved.[70–72] In particular, where there is opposition to randomisation from practitioners, methods such as that advocated by Zelen (Figure 2), in which subjects are randomised before being asked to give consent, should be considered.[73] This has been shown to increase participation by practitioners in certain circumstances, although it is difficult to predict how many subjects will be recruited to each category

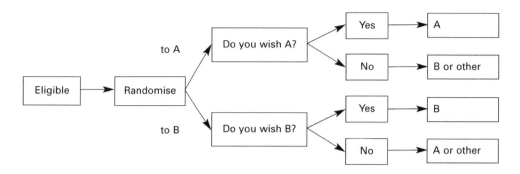

Figure 2   *Double consent randomised design (Source: Zelen[73]).*

and thus to estimate how long it will take to accumulate a given sample size. The approach may also be cause for ethical concern.[74]

Dealing with Baseline Differences in Non-Randomised Studies

The proposition that in the past, imperfections in the randomisation process[75] have resulted in baseline differences in RCTs is increasingly accepted by researchers and, in major trials at least, such imperfections are being rectified. Thus, the focus here is on non-randomised studies.

The theoretical superiority of RCTs in dealing with unknown confounders is clear, but how effective can adjustment be in dealing with unbalanced treatment groups? The evidence reviewed is not sufficient to provide an answer. One test would be progressive convergence with the results of RCTs, but this requires the subjects recruited to non-randomised studies to be similar at baseline to those in RCTs, and in most of the studies reviewed they were not. Some papers have shown how results can be affected by increasing the number of variables adjusted for, but often sample sizes were too small for confidence in the findings.

Evidently, adjustment methods should be developed in a rigorous fashion, based primarily on an understanding of the biological, clinical and social, as well as the statistical issues involved. A range of precautionary measures is suggested by Concato[76] (see Table 5).

Certain key messages emerge:

1   heterogeneity among studies, both in terms of the populations and the interventions studied, should be addressed explicitly.
2   Where there is a difference in effect size between randomised and non-randomised studies, differences in the study population or lack of power should be considered as well as differences in treatment allocation procedures.

Any differences in the measurement of effect size by the two methods are likely to reflect the interaction of several different factors. The more obvious threats to validity, and some of the accepted counter-measures have been set out in Table 6.

Table 5   *Issues in developing multivariate models of risk*

Problem	Potential remedy
Under- or over-fitting	Ensure > 10 outcome events per independent variable
Non-conformity with linear gradient	Check for linearity throughout range, and stratify if necessary
Violation of proportional hazards	Check for proportionality throughout range, and stratify or use time-dependent variables if necessary
Interactions	Include interaction terms, but be cautious about over-fitting
Variation in coding of variables	Specify how variables coded and use them consistently
Selection of variables	Specify how variables selected
Co-linearity	Select only one of several clinically similar variables or select using principal components analysis
Influential outliers	Be aware
Inadequate validation	Use independent sample/split sample/bootstrap sample

Adapted from Concato et al.[76]

Table 6   *Threats to validity and possible solutions*

	Threatening factors	Proposed solution
Internal validity	Allocation bias (risk of confounding)	Randomisation Risk adjustment and subgroup analysis (analysis)
	Patient preference	Preference arms or adjustment for preference (design)
External validity	Exclusions (eligibility criteria)	Expand inclusion criteria
	Non-participation (centres/practitioners)	Multicentre, pragmatic design
	Not-invited (practitioner preference or administrative oversight)	Encourage practitioners to invite all eligible patients
	Non-participation (patients)	Less rigorous consent procedures

Studying the Effect of Patient Preferences

Preferences can change while physiological effects may be less volatile. To be able to interpret results from unblind RCTs properly, it is necessary to know when estimates of treatment effects are likely to be free from important preference components, and when they are not. For example, it seems plausible that interventions designed to affect behaviour might be relatively susceptible to strong patient preferences.

Preference trials[77] can answer pragmatic questions about which treatment works best, incorporating both individual choice and their preference effects, but double-blind trials are more likely to control for any psychological effects and hence detect the physiological effects only. Physiological effects cannot be reliably observed from unblind trials.

Rucker has postulated a two-stage design (Figure 3) where randomisation between two groups is described.[11] However, even if it were possible for people with strong preferences to be recruited into such a trial (Torgerson et al.,[13] for example, demonstrate that it is possible in one instance at least), the estimation of any preference effect would remain complex. The problem is one of interpretation since, in this case, subtracting the means from the two randomised groups provides an estimate of a complex combined algebraic function of the main physiological effects and any preference effect. As has been emphasised, measuring the existence of main physiological effects is, in the known absence of preference effects, relatively straightforward, but estimating interactions is difficult. Complicated models could be imagined in which the effects of preference were multiplicative, graded, different for each treatment

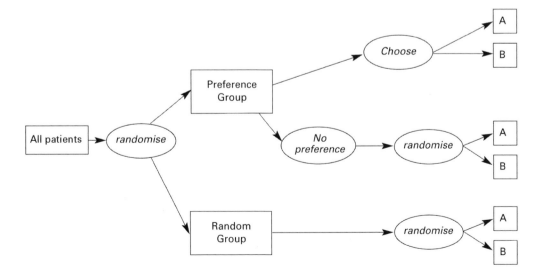

Figure 3   *Possible means of incorporating preference (Source: Rucker[11]).*

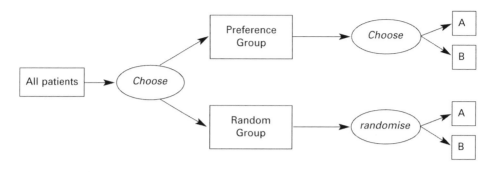

Figure 4   *Possible means of incorporating preference (Source: Brewin and Bradley[79]).*

and/or asymmetric, but these effects are poorly understood.

The physiological effect can be estimated from the randomised arm, but with an unknown preference component. A preference effect might thus be estimated from comparison of the results from the two arms, but the error structures are formidable.[78]

It may be easier to put into practice the trial design described by Brewin and Bradley[79] (Figure 4), but this will produce results for which a preference effect cannot be disentangled from the possible confounding arising from differences between patients with strong treatment preferences. Alternative methods[13] involve recording preferences before randomisation as a co-variate and estimating a preference effect by including a term in a regression equation estimating the main effects. Unless the trial is extremely large, such estimates will probably be too imprecise to distinguish them reliably from the main physiological effects.

Does Selective Participation in Evaluative Studies affect Generalisability?

There is good evidence that participants in RCTs are different from the wider population, but little on when and how far this selection has a material impact on the generalisability of measured effects. There is less evidence for non-randomised studies.

If selective participation is indeed an issue for RCTs, there are two implications:

1   An understanding of the effects involved is necessary for interpretation of trial results.

2   If non-randomised studies are less vulnerable in this respect, this would suggest a potential complimentary role for such studies, even where RCTs are ethical, feasible and affordable.

To clarify this issue, the first step for researchers would be to define reference populations more explicitly. Studies could then be carried out for different conditions (heart disease, cancer, etc.), different types of intervention (primary and secondary prevention, pharmaceutical, surgical, organisational, etc.) and different types of study (RCT, non-randomised) to establish the impact on measured effect of selection at each 'stage' in Figure 1. Ideally, all the categories of patient would be followed and their outcomes compared.

Those commissioning research could have an important role in encouraging organisers of evaluative studies to gather and report such information.

Understanding Heterogeneity in Study Findings

Differences in results can be attributed to bias arising from differences in eligibility criteria, participation, method of allocation to treatment groups, preference effects, compliance with regimens, blinding and completeness of follow-up, as well as chance variation. Collecting the data suggested above would also provide the basis for analyses in which the contributions of the various factors could be assessed for a variety of circumstances.

Increasing numbers of meta-analyses involve re-analysis of data from contributing studies. One such re-analysis could involve a consistent set of eligibility criteria. This would be of limited value for estimating effect sizes, as the analysis would have to be based, for each criterion, on the most restrictive range used in any of the studies involved, and large numbers of cases would be excluded. However, it would provide some impression of the contribution of differences in eligibility criteria to differences in measured effect.

The Role of Non-Randomised Studies

There will continue to be situations in which RCTs cannot be carried out, in particular where the ethical concerns are beyond remedy. It is in these situations that a good understanding of when, why and how non-randomised studies can be misleading would be invaluable.

It has been suggested earlier that non-randomised studies could also have an important role to play if they turn out to be less vulnerable than RCTs to problematic selective recruitment. Another requirement for this is that problems of allocation bias can be resolved or managed.

The literature reviewed here does not support the contention that RCTs tend to produce smaller effects than non-randomised studies, but margins of statistical error were large and the evidence not very discriminating. Even if they are not biased overall, non-randomised studies may be subject to larger absolute errors than RCTs, but these should be reduced if the same standards of data collection, blinding and follow-up are applied. This, of course, may create barriers to recruitment, and such studies would begin to lose their advantage unless it is randomisation *per se* that is the prime cause of problematic recruitment in RCTs.

The effectiveness of adjustment in dealing with allocation bias was difficult to judge from studies comparing RCTs with adjusted results from non-randomised studies because of differences in subject selection. There is a need for more studies like that of Horwitz et al.,[21] in which adjustment was made after applying consistent selection criteria. It should be possible to do this retrospectively on existing datasets.

Where there are likely to be difficulties with an RCT due to selective or slow recruitment, one approach that has been adopted in the past is to nest the RCT within a prospective cohort study, ideally using the same participating centres and methods of data collection, ensuring compliance, blinding, follow-up, etc. If the results for the subset of the cohort that match the RCT subjects are found to be similar to those of the RCT, possibly after adjustment for known confounders, confidence in the results of the wider cohort (and to a lesser extent for other subsets within it) may be increased.

What, If Any, is the Effect of Patient Preference?

The case for patient preferences affecting therapeutic efficacy is theoretically plausible. However, even if such effects exist, finding the empirical evidence will require a major effort, and interested researchers are in the common bind of there being insufficient evidence for their importance to convince funders of the need for the complex trials needed to *establish* their importance.

There is, however, some scope for greater use of preference trials. With this design, patients are carefully and fully informed about the relevant scientific uncertainties and encouraged to actively choose their treatment. Those with no clear preference for treatment are encouraged to accept randomisation. The systematic follow-up of such cohorts would offer the opportunity to establish through randomisation the physiological effects of treatment among those with no preference, and to learn whether patients with apparently similar prognostic characteristics who actively choose their treatments have different outcomes than those predicted by randomisation.

ACKNOWLEDGEMENTS

We are grateful to Simon Thompson, Tom Jefferson and Diana Elbourne for helpful advice during the project.

REFERENCES

1. Black N. Why we need observational studies to evaluate the effectiveness of health care. *Br. Med. J.* 1996; **312**: 1215–18.
2. Black NA. The relationship between evaluative research and audit. *J. Publ. Health Med.* 1992; **14**: 361–6.
3. Tools for effectiveness research. In: *Identifying health technologies that work*. Office of Technology Assessment, Washington DC, 1994.
4. Schulz KF, Chalmers I, Hayes RJ, Altman DG. Empirical evidence of bias: dimensions of methodological quality associated with estimates of treatment effects in controlled trials. *JAMA* 1995; **273**: 408–12.
5. Majeed AW, Troy G, Nicholl JP, Smythe A, Reed MW, Stoddard CJ, Peacock J, Johnson AG. Randomised, prospective, single-blind comparison of laparoscopic versus small-incision cholecystectomy. *Lancet* 1996; **347**: 989–94.

6. Britton A, McKee M, Black N, McPherson K, Sanderson C, Bain C. Choosing between randomised and non-randomised studies: a systematic review. *Health Technol. Assessment* 1998; **2**(13).

7. Colditz GA, Miller JN, Mosteller F. How study design affects outcomes in comparisons of therapy. I: Medical. *Stat. Med.* 1989; **8**: 441–54.

8. Miller JN, Colditz GA, Mosteller F. How study design affects outcomes in comparisons of therapy. II: Surgical. *Stat. Med.* 1989; **8**: 455–66.

9. Lumley J, Bastian H. Competing or complimentary? Ethical considerations and the quality of randomised trials. *Int. J. Tech. Assess. Health Care* 1996; **12**: 247–63.

10. McPherson K. The best and the enemy of the good: randomised controlled trials, uncertainty, and assessing the role of patient preference in medical decision making. The Cochrane Lecture. *J. Epidemiol. Community Health* 1994; **48**: 6–15.

11. Rucker G. A two-stage trial design for testing treatment, self-selection and treatment preference effects. *Stat. Med.* 1989; **8**: 477–85.

12. McKay JR, Alterman AI, McLellan T, Snider EC, O'Brien CP. Effect of random versus nonrandom assignment in a comparison of inpatient and day hospital rehabilitation for male alcoholics. *J. Consult. Clin. Psychol.* 1995; **63**: 70–8.

13. Torgerson DJ, Klaber-Moffett J, Russell IT. Patient preferences in randomised trials: threat or opportunity. *J. Health Serv. Res. Policy* 1996: **1**: 194–7.

14. Redd WH, Anderson BL, Bovbjerg DH, Carpenter PJ, Dolgin M, Mitnick L, Schover LR, Stevens J. Physiologic and psychobehavioural research in oncology. *Cancer* 1991; **67**: 813–22.

15. Marmot MG, Bosma H, Hemingway H, Brunner E, Stansfield S. Contribution of job control and other risk factors to social variations in coronary heart disease incidence. *Lancet* 1997; **350**: 235–9.

16. Lilford RJ, Jackson G. Equipoise and the ethics of randomisation. *J. Roy. Soc. Med.* 1995; **88**: 552–9.

17. Downs SH, Black NA, Devlin HB, Royston CMS, Russell RCG. Systematic review of the effectiveness and safety of laparoscopic cholecystectomy. *Ann. R. Coll. Surg. (Engl.)* 1996; **78**: 241–323.

18. Black NA, Downs SH. The effectiveness of surgery for stress incontinence in women. A systematic review. *Br. J. Urol.* 1996; **78**: 497–510.

19. CASS Principal Investigators and their Associates. Coronary artery surgery study (CASS): A randomised trial of coronary artery bypass surgery. Comparability of entry characteristics and survival in randomised patients and nonrandomised patients meeting randomisation criteria. *J. Am. Coll. Cardiol.* 1984; **3**: 114–28.

20. Hlatky MA, Califf RM, Harrell FE, et al. Comparison of predictions based on observational data with the results of randomised controlled clinical trials of coronary artery bypass surgery. *J. Am. Coll. Cardiol.* 1988; **11**: 237–45.

21. Horwitz RI, Viscoli CM, Clemens JD, Sadock RT. Developing improved observational methods for evaluating therapeutic effectiveness. *Am. J. Med.* 1990; **89**: 630–8.

22. Paradise JL, Bluestone CD, Bachman RZ, et al. Efficacy of tonsillectomy for recurrent throat infection in severely affected children. Results of parallel randomised and nonrandomised clinical trials. *N. Engl. J. Med.* 1984; **310**: 674–83.

23. Paradise JL, Bluestone CD, Rogers KD, et al. Efficacy of adenoidectomy for recurrent otitis media in children previously treated with tympanostomy-tube replacement. Results of parallel randomised and nonrandomised trials. *JAMA* 1990; **263**: 2066–73.

24. Schmoor C, Olschewski M, Schumacher M. Randomised and non-randomised patients in clinical trials: experiences with comprehensive cohort studies. *Stat. Med.* 1996; **15**: 236–71.

25. Yamamoto H, Hughes RW, Schroeder KW, et al. Treatment of esophageal stricture by Eder-Puestow or balloon dilators. A comparison between randomized and prospective nonrandomized trials. *Mayo Clin. Proc.* 1992; **67**: 228–36.

26. Nicolaides K, de Lourdes Brizot M, Patel F, Snijders R. Comparison of chorionic villus sampling and amniocentesis for fetal karyotyping at 10–13 weeks' gestation. *Lancet* 1994; **344**: 435–9.

27. Emanuel, EJ. Cost savings at the end of life. What do the data show? *JAMA* 1996; **275**: 1907–14.

28. Garenne M, Leroy O, Beau JP, Sene I. Efficacy of measles vaccines after controlling for exposure. *Am. J. Epidemiol.* 1993; **138**: 182–95.

29. Antman K, Amoto D, Wood W, et al. Selection bias in clinical trials. *J. Clin. Oncol.* 1985; **3**: 1142–7.

30. Shapiro CL, Recht A. Late effects of adjuvant therapy for breast cancer. *J. Natl Cancer Inst. Monographs* 1994; **16**: 101–12.

31. Jha P, Flather M, Lonn E, et al. The antioxidant vitamins and cardiovascular disease – a critical review of epidemiological and clinical trial data. *Ann. Intern. Med.* 1995; **123**: 860–72.

32. Pyorala S, Huttunen NP, Uhari M. A review and meta-analysis of hormonal treatment of cryptorchidism. *J. Clin. Endocrinol. Metab.* 1995; **80**: 2795–9.

33. The Recurrent Miscarriage Immunotherapy Trialists Group. Worldwide collaborative observational study and meta-analysis on allogenic leukocyte immunotherapy for recurrent spontaneous abortion. *Am. J. Repro. Immunol.* 1994; **32**: 55–72.

34. Watson A, Vail A, Vandekerckhove P, et al. A meta-analysis of the therapeutic role of oil soluble contrast media at hysterosalpingography: a surprising result? *Fertil. Steril.* 1994; **61**: 470–7.

35. Reimold SC, Chalmers TC, Berlin JA, Antman EM. Assessment of the efficacy and safety of antiarrhythmic therapy for chronic atrial fibrillation: Observations on the role of trial design and implications of drug-related mortality. *Am. Heart J.* 1992; **124**: 924–32.

36. Ward LC, Fielding JWL, Dunn JA, Kelly KA for the British Stomach Cancer Group. The selection of cases for randomised trials: a registry survey of concurrent trial and non-trial patients. *Br. J. Cancer* 1992; **66**: 943–50.

37. Thompson SG. What sources of heterogeneity in meta-analyses should be investigated? *Br. Med. J.* 1994; **309**: 1351–5.

38. Charlson ME, Horwitz RI. Applying results of randomised trials to clinical practice: impact of losses before randomisation. *Br. Med. J.* 1984; **289**: 1281–4.

39. Muller DWM, Topol EJ. Selection of patients with acute myocardial infarction for thrombolytic therapy. *Ann. Intern. Med.* 1990; **113**: 949–60.

40. Col NF, Gurwitz JH, Alpert JS, Goldberg RJ. Frequency of inclusion of patients with cardiogenic shock in trials of clinical therapy. *Am. J. Cardiol.* 1994; **73**: 149–57.

41. Bailey KR. Generalizing the results of randomised clinical trials. *Controlled Clinical Trials* 1994; **15**: 15–23.

42. Stephenson P, McKee M. Look twice. *Eur. J. Publ. Health* 1993; **3**: 151–2.

43. Institute of Medicine. Effectiveness and outcomes in health care: Proceedings of an invitational conference by the Institute of Medicine Division of Health Care Services. Heithoff KA, Lohr KN (eds). National Academy Press, Washington DC, 1990.

44. Begg CB, Engstrom PF. Eligibility and extrapolation in cancer clinical trials. *J. Clin. Oncol.* 1987; **5**: 962–8

45. Lee JY, Breaux SR. Accrual of radiotherapy patients to clinical trials. *Cancer* 1983; **52**: 1014–16.

46. Begg CB, Zelen M, Carbonne PP, et al. Cooperative groups and community hospitals: measurement of impact on community hospitals. *Cancer* 1983; **52**: 1760–7.

47. Martin JF, Henderson WG, Zacharaski LR et al. Accrual of patients into a multi hospital cancer clinical trial and its implications. *Am. J. Clin. Oncol.* 1984; **7**: 173–82.

48. Fentiman IS, Julien JP, Van DJ, et al. Reasons for non-entry of patients with DCIS of the breast into a randomised trial (EORTC 10853). *Eur. J. Cancer* 1991; **27**: 450–2.

49. Hunninghake DB, Darby CA, Probstfield JL. Recruitment experience in clinical trials: literature summary and annotated bibliography. *Controlled Clinical Trials* 1987; **8**: 6S–30S.

50. Rochon PA, Fortin PR, Dear KBG, Minaker KL, Chalmers TC. Reporting age data in clinical trials of arthritis. *Arch. Intern. Med.* 1993; **153**: 243–8.

51. The Diabetes Control and Complications Trial Research Group; Klein R, Moss S. A comparison of the study populations in the diabetes control and complications trial and the Wisconsin epidemiologic study of diabetic retinopathy. *Arch. Intern. Med.* 1995; **155**: 745–54.

52. Hartz AJ, Kuhn EM, Pryor DB et al. Mortality after coronary angioplasty and coronary artery bypass surgery (the National Medicare Experience). *Am. J. Cardiol.* 1992; **70**: 179–85.

53. Iezzoni LI (ed.). Dimensions of risk. In: *Risk adjustment for measuring health outcomes.* AHSR, Ann Arbor, 1994.

54. Fallowfield LJ, Hall A, Maguire GP, Baum M. Psychological outcomes of different treatment policies in women with early breast cancer outside a clinical trial. *Br. Med. J.* 1990; **301**: 575–80.

55. Davey Smith G, Song F, Sheldon T. Cholesterol lowering and mortality: the importance of considering initial risk. *Br. Med. J.* 1993; **206**: 1367–73.

56. Brand R, Kragt H. Importance of trends in the interpretation of an overall odds ratio in the meta-analysis of clinical trials. *Stat. Med.* 1992; **11**: 2077–82.

57. Antman EM, Lau J, Kupelnick B, Mosteller F, Chalmers TC. A comparison of results of meta-analyses of randomized controlled trials and recommendations of clinical experts: Treatments for myocardial infarction. *JAMA* 1992; **268**: 240–8.

58. Glasziou PP, Irwig LM. An evidence based approach to individualising treatment. *Br. Med. J.* 1995; **311**: 1356–9.

59. Miettinen OS. The need for randomization in the study of intended effects. *Stat. Med.* 1983; **2**: 267–71.

60. Cowan CD, Wittes J. Intercept studies, clinical trials, and cluster experiments: to whom can we extrapolate? *Controlled Clinical Trials* 1994; **15**: 24–9.

61. Davis CE. Generalizing from clinical trials. *Controlled Clinical Trials* 1994; **15**: 11–14.

62. Sharp SJ, Thompson SG, Altman DG. The relationship between treatment benefit and underlying risk in meta-analysis. *Br. Med. J.* 1996; **313**: 735–8.

63. Gray RJ. A Bayesian analysis of institutional effects in a multi-centre clinical trial. *Biometrics* 1994; **50**: 244–53.

64. Pacala JT, Judge JO, Boult C. Factors affecting sample selection in a randomised trial of balance enhancement: the FISCIT study. *J. Am. Geriatr. Soc.* 1996; **44**: 377–82.

65. Chalmers TC. Ethical implications of rejecting patients for clinical trials (editorial). *JAMA* 1990; **263**: 865.

66. Yusuf S, Held P, Teo KK. Selection of patients for randomized controlled trials: implications of wide or narrow eligibility criteria. *Stat. Med.* 1990; **9**: 73–86.

67. Begg C, Cho M, Eastwood S, Horton R, Moher D, Olkin I, et al. Improving the quality of reporting of randomized controlled trials: the CONSORT Statement. *JAMA* 1996; **276**: 637–9.

68. McKee M, Mossialos E. The impact of managed care on clinical research. *Pharmacoeconomics* 1998; **14**: 19–25.

69. Chalmers I. Assembling comparison groups to assess the effects of health care. *J. Roy. Soc. Med.* 1997; **90**: 379–86.

70. Corbett F, Oldham J, Lilford R. Offering patients entry in clinical trials: preliminary study of the views of prospective participants. *J. Med. Ethics* 1996; **22**: 227–31.

71. Snowden C, Garcia J, Elbourne D. Reactions of participants to the results of a randomised controlled trial: exploratory study. *Br. Med. J.* 1998; **337**: 21–6.

72. Snowden C, Garcia J, Elbourne D. Making sense of randomisation: responses of parents of critically ill babies to random allocation of treatment in a clinical trial. *Soc. Sci. Med.* 1998; **45**: 1337–55.

73. Zelen M. Randomized consent designs for clinical trials: an update. *Stat. Med.* 1990; **9**: 645–56.

74. Snowden C, Elbourne D, Garcia J. Zelen randomisation: attitudes of parents participating in a neonatal clinical trial. *Controlled Clinical Trials* 1999; **20**: 149–71.

75. Schulz KF, Chalmers I, Grimes DA, Altman DG. Assessing the quality of randomization from reports of controlled trials published in obstetrics and gynecology journals, *JAMA* 1994; **272**: 125–8.

76. Concato J, Feinstein AR, Holford TR. The risk of determining risk with multivariate models. *Ann. Intern. Med.* 1993; **118**: 201–10.

77. Wennberg JE. What is outcomes research? In: Gelijns AC (ed.) *Medical innovations at the crossroads. Vol. 1. Modern methods of clinical investigation.* Washington DC: National Academy Press, 1990, pp. 33–46.

78. McPherson K, Britton AR, Wennberg J. Are randomised controlled trials controlled? Patient preferences and unblind trials. *J. Roy. Soc. Med.* 1997; **90**: 652–6.

79. Brewin CR, Bradley C. Patient preferences and randomised clinical trials. *Br. Med. J.* 1989; **299**: 313–15.

80. Alonso PL, Smith T, Schellenberg JRM et al. Randomised trial of efficacy of SPf66 vaccine against *Plasmodium falciparum* malaria in children in southern Tanzania. *Lancet* 1994; **344**: 1175–81.

81. Wilcox RG, Hampton JR, Banks DC, et al. Trial of early nifedipine in acute myocardial infarction. The TRENT study. *Br. Med. J.* 1986; **293**: 1204–8.

82. CABRI Trial Participants. First year results of CABRI (Coronary Angioplasty vs Bypass Revascularisation Investigation). *Lancet* 1995; **346**: 1179–84.

83. SHEP Cooperative Research Group. Prevention of stroke by antihypertensive drug treatment in older persons with isolated systolic hypertension. *JAMA* 1991; **265**: 3255–64.

84. D'Alessandro U, Leach A, Drakeley CJ, et al. Efficacy trial of malaria vaccine SPf66 in Gambian infants. *Lancet* 1995; **346**: 462–7.

85. Goldbourt U, Behar S, Reicher-Reiss H, et al. Early administration of nifedipine in suspected acute myocardial infarction: the SPRINT 2 study. *Arch. Intern. Med.* 1993; **153**: 345–53.

86. King SB, Lembo NJ, Kosinski AS et al. A randomised study of coronary angioplasty compared with bypass surgery in patients with symptomatic multi-vessel coronary disease. *N. Eng. J. Med.* 1994; **331**: 1044–50.

87. Sempertegui F, Estrella B, Moscoso J, et al. Safety, immunogenicity and protective effect of the SPf66 malaria synthetic vaccine against *Plasmodium falciparum* infection in a randomized double-blind placebo-controlled field trial in an endemic area of Ecuador. *Vaccine* 1994; **12**: 337–42.

88. The Israeli SPRINT Study Group. Secondary Prevention Reinfarction Israeli Nifedipine Trial (SPRINT). A randomised intervention trial of nifedipine in patients with acute myocardial infarction. *Eur. Heart J.* 1988; **9**: 354–64.

89. Hamm CW, Reimers J, Ischinger T, et al. A randomised study of coronary angioplasty compared with bypass surgery in patients with symptomatic multi-vessel disease. *N. Eng. J. Med.* 1994; **331**: 1037–43.

90. Valero MV, Amador LR, Galindo C, et al. Vaccination with SPf66, a chemically synthesised vaccine, against *Plasmodium falciparum* in Columbia. *Lancet* 1993; **341**: 705–10.

91. Branigan JP, Walsh K, Collins WC, et al. Effect of early treatment with nifedipine in suspected acute myocardial infarction. *Eur. Heart J.* 1986; **7**: 859–65.

92. Goy JJ, Eeckhout E, Burnand B, et al. Coronary angioplasty versus left main internal mammary grafting for isolated proximal left anterior descending artery stenosis. *Lancet* 1994; **343**: 1449–53.

93. Valero MV, Amador R, Aponte JJ, et al. Evaluation of SPf66 malaria vaccine during a 22-month follow-up field trial in the Pacific coast of Columbia. *Vaccine* 1996; **14**: 1466–70.

94. Sirnes PA, Overskeid K, Pedersen TR, et al. Evaluation of infarct size during the early use of

Nifedipine in patients with acute myocardial infarction: The Norwegian Nifedipine Multicentre Trial. *Circulation* 1984; **70**: 638–44.

95. Rodriguez A, Boullon F, Perez-Balino N, et al. Argentine randomised trial of percutaneous transluminal coronary angioplasty versus coronary artery bypass surgery in multi-vessel disease (ERACHI): in-hospital results and 1-year follow up. *J. Am. Coll. Cardiol.* 1993; **22**: 1060–7.

96. BARI Investigators. Comparison of coronary bypass surgery with angioplasty in patients with multi-vessel disease. *N. Eng. J. Med.* 1996; **335**: 217–25.

97. MRC Working Party. Medical Research Council trial of treatment of hypertension in older patients: principal results. *Br. Med. J.* 1992; **304**: 405–12.

98. MRC Working Party. Medical Research Council trial of treatment of mild hypertension: principal results. *Br. Med. J.* 1985; **291**: 97–104.

7

A Review of Observational, Quasi-Experimental and Randomised Study Designs for the Evaluation of the Effectiveness of Healthcare Interventions

BARNABY C. REEVES, RACHEL R. MACLEHOSE,
IAN M. HARVEY, TREVOR A. SHELDON,
IAN T. RUSSELL and ANDREW M.S. BLACK

SUMMARY

Objective

The review investigated the internal validity of quasi-experimental and observational (QEO) estimates of effectiveness. The size and direction of discrepancies between randomised controlled trials (RCTs) and QEO estimates of effectiveness were compared systematically for specific interventions and the extent to which the discrepancies were associated with variations in methodological quality, study design and other attributes of studies were investigated. Two strategies were used to minimise the influence of differences in external validity between studies: RCT and QEO estimates were compared: (i) for any intervention where both estimates were reported in a single paper; and (ii) for mammographic screening and folic acid supplementation, interventions for which external validity was anticipated to be homogeneous across studies, where respective estimates were reported in different papers.

Methods

Relevant studies were identified by searches of electronic databases, reference lists of papers already identified, experts, and 'hand searches' of databases of abstracts, and were not limited to the English language. Assessment of the methodological quality of papers focused on the comparability of study populations, bias, confounding and quality of reporting.

Results

Strategy one identified 14 papers which yielded 38 comparisons between RCT and QEO estimates. Using a variety of measures of discrepancy, QEO estimates derived from high-quality studies were found not to differ from estimates from RCTs, whereas QEO estimates from low-quality studies often differed considerably. Strategy two identified 34 papers, 17 for each of the interventions reviewed. Pooled estimates of effectiveness for RCTs and cohort studies did not differ significantly for either intervention ($P > 0.80$), but the pooled estimates for case control studies indicated more benefit for mammographic screening ($P = 0.06$) and less benefit for folic acid supplementation ($P = 0.05$).

Conclusions

These findings suggest that QEO estimates of effectiveness from high-quality studies can be valid. Although the majority of the QEO evidence reviewed was of poor quality, we recommend that QEO designs should not be rejected for evaluations of effectiveness just because most past studies have had serious flaws in their designs or analyses.

INTRODUCTION

The debate about the respective advantages and disadvantages of different research designs for evaluating the effectiveness of healthcare interventions is one of the most controversial in the field of health services research, with strong advocates for randomised controlled trials (RCTs) on the one hand[1-7] and observational or quasi-experimental (QEO) research designs on the other.[8-10]

High-quality RCTs are widely perceived as the gold standard research design for evaluating effectiveness[5,11-14] because they increase the comparability of the groups being compared and so minimise confounding of the intervention of interest by differences in known and unknown prognostic factors between groups. This property is particularly important for evaluations of interventions for two reasons. Firstly, small effects of comparable size to those arising from bias and confounding are often clinically important.[2,13] Secondly, quantifying the effect of an intervention, rather than merely whether or not it is statistically significantly different from an alternative, is very important; interventions have financial costs, and often side-effects or complications, as well as benefits and the decision to adopt an intervention therefore depends on weighing up the relative magnitudes of the benefits and the costs. These considerations have led some proponents of RCTs to adopt an extreme position about the value of non-randomised study designs, stating for example that '. . . observational methods provide no useful means of assessing the value of a therapy',[14] or that '. . . they [observational studies] cannot discriminate reliably between moderate differences and negligible differences in outcome, and the mistaken clinical conclusions that they engender could well result in the under-treatment, over-treatment or other mistreatment of millions of future patients'.[13]

QEO research designs[15] have nevertheless been advocated for evaluating effectiveness, because there are perceived to be many circumstances in which RCTs may be unnecessary, inappropriate, impracticable or inadequate.[9] Black and others[9,10,16,17] contend that the polarity of the debate about the value of QEO methods for evaluating effectiveness arises because

non-randomised designs are seen as alternatives to experimentation, rather than as a set of complementary approaches. QEO studies can provide estimates of the effectiveness of interventions when RCTs are not possible, and can help to interpret the findings of RCTs and their applicability in circumstances that do not exactly match those of the RCTs (external validity). A recent editorial attempted to reconcile the two points of view, arguing that the complementary nature of different study designs reflects the different types of research questions that they are best suited to address.[18]

The internal validity of these non-randomised approaches must always be suspect, since it is impossible to be certain that all important confounding factors have been identified and adequately controlled for.[4,5] QEO studies also offer less opportunity to control for biases since, although outcome assessment can often be blinded, healthcare providers and study participants are usually aware of treatment allocations. The extent of the distrust of evidence derived from these non-experimental approaches is illustrated by the above quotations, although Black[10] comments that 'it is unclear how serious and how insurmountable a methodological problem *the threat to internal validity* is in practice'.

Previous comparisons of estimates of effectiveness derived from RCTs and QEO studies have suggested that the latter tend to report larger estimates of the benefit of the treatment being evaluated.[19-21] The perception that QEO estimates consistently favour new treatments has led to the assumption that discrepancies arise from bias. However, comparisons from the literature are often cited selectively. They may not have been carried out systematically and may have failed to consider alternative explanations for the discrepancies observed, for example differences in the populations, interventions, or outcomes studied, a greater susceptibility of QEO studies than RCTs to publication bias, or a tendency for RCTs to underestimate effectiveness.[10]

A 'sister' review[22] (see Chapter 6) focused on ways in which possible differences in external validity between RCT and QEO studies can give rise to discrepant estimates of effect size. Our review[23] is complementary, and focuses on the internal validity of QEO estimates of effect size. The objective was to compare systematically estimates of effectiveness for specific interventions derived from RCTs and QEO studies, and we adopted two strategies to minimise the influence of differences in external validity:

1. Compare RCT and QEO estimates of effectiveness for an intervention where both estimates were reported in a *single paper*, on the assumption that such papers were more

likely to compare 'like with like' than comparisons across papers; evaluations of any intervention were eligible.

2. Compare RCT and QEO estimates of effectiveness for an intervention where the respective estimates were reported in *different* papers and where the intervention, population and outcome investigated were anticipated to be homogeneous across studies.

Our primary interest was in the size and direction of discrepancies between RCT and QEO estimates, and the extent to which the discrepancies were associated with variations in methodological quality, study design and other attributes of studies. We reasoned that being able to quantify such associations would be valuable to healthcare decision makers in guiding the weight that they should attach to observational evidence about the effectiveness of interventions.

METHODS

Eligibility

Two types of evidence were eligible for the first strategy:

1. Primary studies, which reported both RCT *and* QEO estimates of effect size for the *same* intervention.
2. Secondary studies, which compared pooled RCT and QEO estimates of effect size for the *same* intervention by synthesising evidence from primary studies which reported either an RCT *or* QEO estimate of effect size for the intervention. (The second strategy carried out this type of study for two interventions.)

Secondary studies, which compared pooled RCT and QEO estimates of effect size for many interventions by aggregating evidence from primary studies which reported either an RCT *or* QEO estimate of effect size,[20,21] were not eligible. These studies were excluded because of the possibility of 'confounding' of any association between study design and discrepancy in effect size by intervention. We also excluded studies which reviewed RCT and QEO studies for the same intervention in a comparative way, but which did not attempt to calculate an estimate of effect size for different study designs.

For the second strategy, our choice of interventions to review was made through a multistage selection process. An initial list of 31 interventions was drawn up by the project steering group on the basis of their personal expertise, focusing on the availability of a substantial number of both RCTs and QEO studies. This number was reduced to seven by preliminary

Medline searches to estimate the amount of literature available for each of the interventions. Our final choice of interventions required three aspects of evaluations to be uniform across studies: (i) the intervention under consideration; (ii) the outcome used to measure effectiveness; and (iii) the population in which the intervention was investigated. The two interventions which best satisfied these criteria were selected for review:

1. Mammographic screening (MS; intervention) for women aged 50–64 years (population) to reduce mortality from breast cancer (outcome);
2. Periconceptional folic acid supplementation (FAS; intervention) for women trying to conceive (population) to prevent neural tube defects (outcome).

Papers were eligible if they evaluated either of the interventions being reviewed, and matched the definitions for the intervention, population and outcome described above. We considered this latter point to be very important, since only by ensuring that all studies were evaluating the same intervention on the same population could we be confident of minimising any confounding of the association between study quality and effect size by differences in these attributes.

Searching for Evidence

A range of methods were used to identify relevant literature, including (i) searches of electronic databases (Medline 1966–June 1996; EMBASE 1980–June 1996; Cochrane Library); (ii) reference lists of relevant papers already identified; (iii) experts; and (iv) 'hand searches' of databases of abstracts (Cochrane Library, Database of Abstracts of Reviews of Effectiveness, and a database of 1535 abstracts created by another review team[24]) which we anticipated might contain a higher proportion of relevant material than specific journals. Searches were not limited to the English language.

Our efforts to design electronic search strategies for the first strategy were frustrated by the inadequacy of the indexing of methodological aspects of studies. Terms typically used to identify RCTs, such as 'comparative studies' and 'prospective studies',[25] are ambiguous and can also describe observational studies. The term 'randomised controlled trial' is available as a publication type, but this classification was only introduced in 1992. Because of these limitations, search strategies designed to identify papers that included *both* RCT *and* QEO study design elements in fact detected studies that used a single study design. Traditional hand-searching methods were rejected for this strategy because it was not obvious which journals should be searched, and because eligible papers were exceedingly rare. Most references were therefore identified from expert knowledge and from the reference lists of papers already obtained for the review.

For the second strategy, papers were identified primarily by electronic searches of Medline and EMBASE, and the databases of abstracts. EMBASE searches were always carried out last and were designed to be less restrictive. They were intended to represent a final 'trawl' for papers which may have been missed by other searches.

Quality Assessment

Papers reviewed for the first strategy often reported more than one comparison between RCT and QEO effect sizes, for example for different outcomes, populations or interventions. The 'quality' of each *comparison* was assessed by three reviewers using a checklist of six items to identify the comparability of the populations studied (1–2 below) and the susceptibility of the comparison to bias (3–6 below):

1. Were the same eligibility criteria used for RCT and non-randomised study populations?
2. Were RCT and non-randomised populations studied contemporaneously?
3. Was the assessment of outcome 'blinded' (both RCT and non-randomised studies)?
4. Did the non-randomised estimates take account of the effects of confounding by disease severity?
5. Did the non-randomised estimates take account of the effects of confounding by comorbidity?
6. Did the non-randomised estimates take account of the effects of confounding by other prognostic factors?

For each comparison, a reviewer indicated whether the items were satisfied or not, and an overall score was calculated by averaging the scores allocated by the three reviewers. Scores greater than 3/6 were classified as high quality, and scores less than or equal to 3/6 as low quality.

The first three items were considered to be matters of fact, and the few discrepancies between assessors were resolved by discussion and reference to the papers. The extent to which QEO estimates of effect size were adjusted for confounding was considered to be a judgement, and disagreements between assessors were respected. Disagreements mainly concerned adjustment for co-morbidity and other prognostic factors, and probably arose because assessors were asked to assign a dichotomous

(yes/no) score. For example, in some papers authors may have adjusted for some, but not all, prognostic factors. No attempt was made to mask the authorship or other details of these papers because many were already familiar to the reviewers, having been identified through their expertise. We did not use a more complex method of measuring quality because none of the available checklists were suitable for assessing the RCT *versus* QEO *comparison* (as opposed to the individual design elements).

For the second strategy, that is comparison of RCT and QEO estimates of effectiveness for the same intervention but published in different papers, three reviewers used a detailed instrument to evaluate all eligible papers. Details of journal, author, year of publication, and all references were removed before the papers were distributed for evaluation. If the methods of the study were reported in detail in a separate paper, relevant sections of the additional paper were also distributed with the paper under evaluation.

The instrument used for measuring methodological quality was based on an existing instrument,[26] which had been developed to provide a measure of external as well as internal validity for both randomised and observational study designs. The instrument was modified to try to satisfy our aim of quantifying the relationship between study quality and effect size; additional questions were included to measure the extent to which factors likely to influence effect size (for example adjustment for confounders) were addressed, and the original questions about external validity were also modified. Questions were classified as pertaining to one of four dimensions of quality on the basis of face validity: (i) quality of the reporting of the study; (ii) external validity; (iii) features of the study designed to reduce bias; and (iv) features of the study designed to reduce confounding. A score for each question for each paper was calculated by averaging the scores allocated by the three reviewers.

For both strategies, additional information about the interventions, populations studied, sample sizes and estimates of effectiveness were extracted from the papers by one reviewer and checked by another.

Data Analyses and Synthesis

For the first strategy, measures of the size of discrepancies between RCT and QEO estimates of effect size and outcome frequency for intervention and control groups were calculated, where possible, for each comparison. There are

Table 1   *Indices used to compare the findings of RCT and QEO study design elements using strategy one*

1	$\dfrac{RR(RCT)}{RR(QEO)}$	RR effect size for the RCT element divided by the RR effect size for the QEO element
2	RD(RCT) − RD(QEO)	Difference between RD effect sizes (risk or rate difference), i.e. RD for the QEO element subtracted from RD for the RCT element
3	IOF(RCT) − IOF(QEO)	Difference between OFs for intervention groups, i.e. the OF for the QEO intervention group subtracted from the OF for the RCT intervention group
4	COF(RCT) − COF(QEO)	Difference between OFs for control groups, i.e. the OF for the QEO control group subtracted from the OF for the RCT control group

RR – relative risk (risk, odds or rate ratio); RD – risk difference; IOF – outcome frequency (risk, rate) for intervention group; COF – outcome frequency (risk, rate) for control group.

no established indices for comparing the findings from two studies. We therefore constructed four indices, described in Table 1, to reflect different ways of quantifying discrepancies in measures of effect size and outcome frequency.

The rationale for considering discrepancies in outcome frequencies, as well as discrepancies in measures of effect size, arose from our primary objective of evaluating the internal validity of the QEO estimates. The quality criteria required the RCT and QEO elements to compare the same populations, as well as to control for confounding. Under these circumstances, the outcome frequencies as well as the effect estimates should be the same for RCT and QEO elements. If we had considered only effect size estimates, these might have disguised substantial differences in outcome frequencies.

It was not possible to calculate all indices for all comparisons considered, because some of the data required were not reported either in the papers which were reviewed, or in previous papers by the same research teams describing the same investigations. At least one index was calculated for each comparison.

Distributions showing the size and direction of discrepancies were compared for high- and low-quality comparisons. No analytical statistics were calculated because several papers included multiple comparisons, and it was considered unlikely that comparisons within papers were statistically independent.

For the second strategy, we described the performance of the instrument as well as the relationship between effect size estimates and study design, quality and other attributes. Inter-rater reliabilities for each question (pooled across all papers for the two interventions) were determined by two methods: (i) unweighted Kappa (calculated using the statistical package STATA Version 4.0; the use of three assessors precluded the calculation of weighted Kappas for ordinal responses); (ii) percent agreement

(three points were awarded where the three reviewers agreed, and one point where two of the three reviewers agreed; points were summed across papers and expressed as a percentage). The internal consistency of the different quality dimensions was investigated using Cronbach's alpha.

Simple multiple regression was used to investigate predictors of different dimensions of quality and the sum of the scores for different dimensions of quality, in order to try to validate the instrument. Independent variables that were investigated included the intervention (MS or FAS), study design (RCT, cohort or case control study; other designs were omitted from the analysis) and the interaction of intervention and study design.

Meta-regression was used to investigate factors associated with the magnitude of the effect size estimates, taken as the natural logarithm of the relative risk estimate (ln(RR)), weighting each estimate by the inverse of its variance. Dummy variables were created for cohort studies and case control studies, using RCTs as the baseline comparison. Associations between other independent variables, characterising the quality of studies and their heterogeneity with respect to population and intervention, and effect size were also investigated.

RESULTS

Strategy One

Fourteen papers were identified from a variety of sources and a wide range of journals. Three papers were reviews,[19,27,28] four were comprehensive cohort studies,[29–32] and seven compared primary data for RCT and QEO populations indirectly.[33–39]

The comprehensive cohort studies consisted of a cohort study of all subjects who were eligible for a RCT, with the subjects who participated in the RCT nested in the cohort.[40] Schmoor and colleagues[32] used this study design to compare mastectomy and breast preservation treatments, and other adjuvant treatments for breast cancer.

The study by Hlatky and colleagues,[34] which compared coronary artery bypass surgery *versus* medical treatment for coronary artery disease, provides an example of other studies which compared RCT and QEO primary data indirectly. Their QEO data were obtained from a prospective database, which included information about important clinical and prognostic factors; data from the database were compared with data from three independent RCTs. Outcomes for medical and surgical patients in the prospective database who would have been eligible for one of the RCTs were analysed to provide a treatment effect which was then compared with the treatment effect found by the RCT. The three RCTs used different eligibility criteria, allowing the researchers to make three independent comparisons.

The papers reported 38 comparisons between RCT and QEO findings. The numbers of comparisons based on different study designs and their average quality are shown in Table 2. Some comparisons were indirect, when the QEO element of a study consisted of a single group; this usually occurred when the RCT found no difference between intervention and control groups. For these comparisons, we compared one or both groups in an RCT with the single non-trial group; the QEO population could either be the same (randomisable patients who received a single treatment) or different from the RCT population. Three of the 14 papers focused on a comparison between trial and non-trial patients,[32,37,39] but did not include all of the details which were considered relevant to the review. In these cases, relevant data were extracted from earlier papers[41–43] reporting the findings of the study by the same research groups.

The inclusion of studies which compared one or both groups in an RCT with a single non-trial group might be considered controversial, since they cannot provide a QEO estimate of effect size directly. QEO estimates for these studies were calculated by comparing the single QEO outcome frequency with the outcome frequency

Table 2 *Quality scores for different types of study reviewed using strategy one. The percentage for each cell is calculated from the number of quality items scored as present by three assessors for all comparisons of each study type*

Quality criterion	Reviews ($n = 13$)	CCH ($n = 8$)	IC:IC ($n = 8$)	IC:I ($n = 6$)	IC:C ($n = 3$)
Contemporaneity	0%	100%	38%[‡]	0%	75%
Eligibility	0%	100%	75%	33%	100%
Blinding of outcome assessment[†]	23%[§]	13%	100%	33%[#]	100%
Confounding by severity	0%	50%	85%	100%	75%
Confounding by co-morbidity	0%	0%	0%	33%[$]	75%[$]
Confounding by other prognostic factors	0%	29%	100%	100%	75%
Overall quality score	4%	49%	67%	50%	83%

CCH – comprehensive cohort; IC:IC – indirect comparison where the QEO study design element comprised both intervention and control groups; IC:I – indirect comparison where the QEO study design element comprised an intervention group only; IC:C – indirect comparison where the QEO study design element comprised a control group only.

[†] Only two papers mentioned blinding of outcome assessment;[32,37] this criterion was scored as 'yes' for other papers only where the outcome was unequivocal, i.e. survival/all-cause mortality.

[‡] Three IC:IC comparisons[33] were given credit for contemporaneity because the analyses took account of the date of entry of each subject.

[§] One review paper[18] considered a number of outcomes; credit for blinding of outcome assessment was only given for all-cause mortality.

[$] Credit for adjustment of co-morbidity (and other confounders) was given to two IC:I[37] and two IC:C comparisons.[36] Because the QEO and RCT samples were drawn from the same population and the QEO population received only one treatment, the QEO sample should have balanced on all factors with both intervention and control RCT samples.

[#] Credit was given for blinding of outcome for only one of the outcomes considered in each of the two IC:I studies, i.e. for endometrial cancer but not any disease event[37] and for all-cause mortality but not intra-breast recurrence, distant metastasis or contralateral breast cancer.[38]

for the 'missing' group from the RCT element of the study. We believe that this approach is justified because the criteria for eligibility for this strategy meant that RCT and QEO elements had to investigate the same intervention and outcome and similar populations (except, perhaps, in the case of reviews).

The distributions of discrepancies in relative risk (RR), risk difference (RD) and outcome frequencies for high- and low-quality comparisons are shown in Figure 1. Discrepancies for all indices were much smaller for high- than low-quality comparisons. The distribution of the

direction of discrepancies in RR and RD cannot be inferred from the figure, because some outcomes were adverse and some favourable. Discrepancies are therefore shown in Table 3, according to whether the RCT or the QEO effect size estimate was more extreme. For high-quality comparisons, there was no evidence at all that QEO effect size estimates were more extreme, although there was some evidence of this tendency for low-quality comparisons.

The same *caveat* applies to the distributions of discrepancies in intervention and control outcome frequencies, which were clearly skewed,

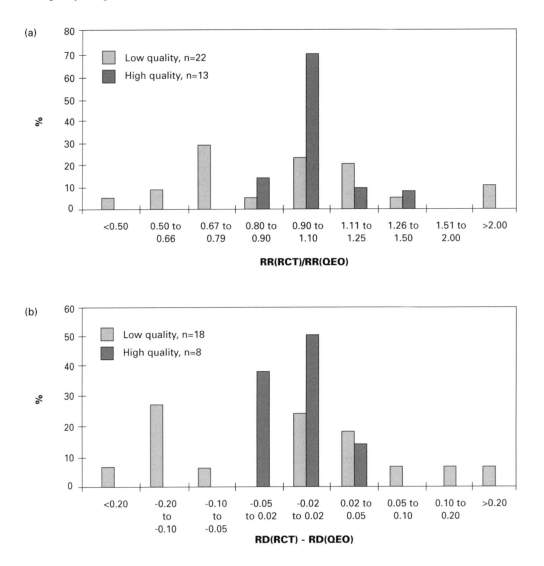

Figure 1   *Distributions of the discrepancies between the effect size estimates of RCTs and QEO study design elements for low- and high-quality comparisons reviewed for strategy 1; (a) ratios of RCT and QEO relative risks (RR); (b) differences between RCT and QEO risk differences (RD);*

indicating that QEO outcome frequencies tended to be larger than RCT outcome frequencies. Because of the prevailing view that eligibility criteria for RCTs tend to exclude patients who have a higher risk of an adverse outcome, discrepancies in outcome frequency are shown in Table 4 according to whether or not the RCT or QEO outcome frequency was greater for an adverse outcome or smaller for a favourable outcome. Discrepancies in outcome frequency for high-quality comparisons were equally distributed, but those for low-quality comparisons were more likely to indicate a higher adverse,

or lower favourable, QEO outcome frequency. The latter finding, is consistent with the above view.

It is interesting to consider the extent to which differences in internal validity and differences in the populations contributed to discrepancies. In two papers,[35,36] the authors reported how the effect size estimate changed for the QEO element as differences between the RCT and QEO populations and confounding factors were taken into account. In both these cases, restricting the QEO population to subjects who would have been eligible for the RCT brought about the

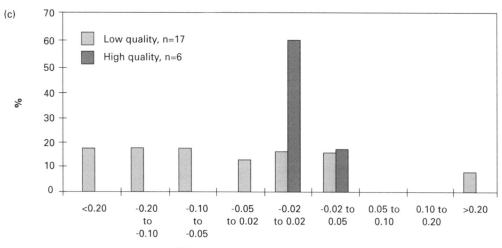

RCT intervention OF - QEO intervention OF

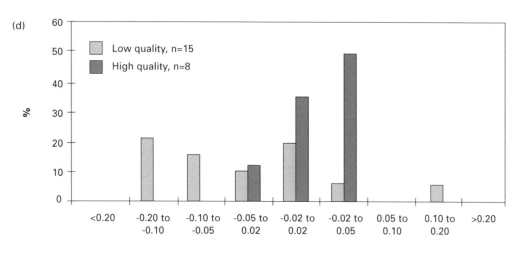

RCT control OF - QEO control OF

(c) differences between RCT and QEO intervention group outcome frequencies (OF); and (d) differences between RCT and QEO control group outcome frequencies (OF).

Table 3 *Direction of discrepancies between RCT and QEO estimates of effect size. The number of comparisons in which the RCT and QEO elements gave the more extreme estimate of effect size are tabulated separately (a) for measures of relative risk and (b) risk or rate difference*

(a)

	RCT more extreme	=	QEO more extreme	Total[†]
Low quality	9	0	13	22
High quality	6	1	6	13

[†] Relative risk estimates were not available for three comparisons.

(b)

	RCT	=	QEO	Total[†]
Low quality	9	0	12	21
High quality	7	0	3	10

[†] Risk or rate difference estimates were not available for seven comparisons.

Table 4 *Direction of discrepancies between RCT and QEO estimates of (a) intervention and (b) control outcome frequencies. The number of comparisons for which the RCT and QEO outcome frequencies of an adverse event was higher, or a favourable event lower, are shown*

(a)

	RCT	=	QEO	Total[†]
Low quality	5	0	16	21
High quality	3	0	5	8

[†] RCT or QEO intervention outcome frequencies were not available for nine comparisons.

(b)

	RCT	=	QEO	Total[†]
Low quality	4	1	13	18
High quality	4	1	3	8

[†] Risk or rate difference estimates were not available for twelve comparisons.

largest step in the convergence between RCT and QEO estimates, with adjustment for confounding producing relatively little subsequent change.

The comparison of studies of high and low quality with respect to the size and direction of

discrepancies between RCT and QEO elements may itself be 'confounded' by other factors; that is, other attributes of comparisons may be associated both with size and direction of discrepancy and with study quality. It was not possible to investigate confounding formally, because of the likely non-independence of the discrepancies between RCT and QEO design elements across comparisons within papers. Instead, we described either the relationship between quality and size and direction of discrepancies within strata of a possible confounding factor (see I and III below), or the relationship between possible confounding factors and the size and direction of discrepancies (see II below). The former approach allows inspection of the relationship in the absence of the confounding factor; using the latter approach, if no relationship between the confounding factor and size or direction of discrepancy is apparent, confounding is extremely unlikely. Three confounding factors were considered.

I. Confounding due to the inclusion of reviews

By their nature, reviews were scored as being of low quality. If comparisons in review papers tend to give rise to larger discrepancies than comparisons made on the basis of primary data, the inclusion of reviews may be a confounding factor. It should also be pointed out that, because reviews included data from several primary studies, discrepancies for review comparisons were more likely to arise from differences in the characteristics of the populations studied. Because all of the review comparisons were of low quality, the findings for the high-quality comparisons were unaltered. The distributions of the discrepancies for the low-quality comparisons based on primary data still showed a greater spread and a slight tendency to produce more extreme effect size estimates.

II. Confounding by whether or not the intervention is effective

When an intervention is ineffective, the RCT versus QEO comparison becomes harder to interpret. If prognostic factors are reasonably balanced, the outcome frequencies should be very similar for intervention and control groups in both RCT and QEO populations and the discrepancies between RCT and QEO effect size estimates should be small. The observation that high-quality comparisons show smaller discrepancies might therefore arise because they tend, on average, to have evaluated less effective interventions. If confounding by the effectiveness of an intervention were having an important effect, we would expect discrepancies to be larger, on average, for comparisons involving effective interventions. On the basis of the prevailing view that QEO studies are more likely to yield exaggerated effect sizes, we might also expect the discrepancies involving effective interventions to be more extreme for QEO study design elements.

Confounding by the effectiveness of the intervention was explored by tabulating size and direction of discrepancies for comparisons by a proxy marker of the effectiveness of an intervention, namely whether or not the RCT study design element yielded a statistically significant result. The distributions of the discrepancies for 'effective' and 'ineffective' comparisons showed no marked difference in either their dispersion or symmetry, suggesting that confounding by the effectiveness of an intervention was unlikely to explain the difference in the size of discrepancies for high- and low-quality comparisons.

III. Confounding by sample size

One would expect a direct relationship between the size of discrepancies and sample size, because sample size (in conjunction with outcome frequency) determines the precision of an effect size estimate; that is, discrepancies for comparisons based on small sample sizes would be expected on average to be larger than those based on large samples. If high-quality comparisons tend on average to be based on larger sample sizes, the relationship between quality and size of discrepancy might be substantially reduced by taking account of sample size. (It could be argued that sample size is itself a factor that should be considered in assessing quality, but it was not included in the quality assessment which was carried out for this strategy.) With respect to the direction of discrepancies, one would expect any general tendency for QEO estimates to produce more extreme estimates of effect size to be more evident when the effect size estimates are more precise, that is for larger sample sizes.

Confounding by sample size was explored by examining size and direction of discrepancies for comparisons by low and high quality separately for 'small' and 'large' sample size strata. Classification was based on the total RCT sample size only, because QEO sample size was affected for some comparisons by the absence of either an intervention or control group; a cut-off of 750 subjects was chosen since this created two groups with approximately equal numbers of comparisons in each.

Stratifying by sample size reduced the number of comparisons in each stratum and makes it more difficult to interpret the distributions of the discrepancies. Overall, however, the distributions of the size of discrepancies appeared to be similar across strata, and showed the same pattern as without stratification, that is larger discrepancies for low-quality comparisons. With respect to the direction of discrepancies, the tendency for QEO estimates to be more extreme was most apparent for low-quality comparisons based on large sample sizes, as predicted and shown in Table 5. There was no evidence from high-quality comparisons, whether based on small or large sample sizes, to support the view

Table 5 *Direction of discrepancies between RCT and QEO results classified by quality and stratified by the sample size of the RCT study design element, (a) for measures of relative risk and (b) risk or rate difference*

(a)

RCT sample size ≤750 (n = 21)	RCT more extreme	=	QEO more extreme	Total[†]
Low quality	8	0	4	12
High quality	2	1	3	6

[†] Relative risk estimates were not available for three comparisons.

RCT sample size >750 (n = 16)	RCT more extreme	=	QEO more extreme	Total
Low quality	1	0	8	9
High quality	4	0	3	7

(b)

RCT sample size ≤750 (n = 21)	RCT more extreme	=	QEO more extreme	Total[†]
Low quality	7	0	4	11
High quality	3	0	0	3

[†] Risk or rate difference estimates were not available for seven comparisons.

RCT sample size >750 (n = 16)	RCT more extreme	=	QEO more extreme	Total
Low quality	2	0	7	9
High quality	4	0	3	7

that QEO effect size estimates tend to be more extreme than RCT estimates.

Strategy Two

Thirty-four eligible papers were identified, 17 evaluating MS[44–60] and 17 evaluating FAS.[61–77] For MS and FAS respectively, eight[44,45,48,51,54,56,60] and four papers[61,70,72,73] were RCTs, five[49,52,55,58,59] and six[62,63,64,67,68,69] were non-randomised trials or cohort studies, and three[46,47,50,52] and six[65,66,71,74,75,77] were matched or unmatched case control studies; one study of MS[57] and one of FAS[76] used some other design.

Inter-assessor agreement was similar for MS and FAS, and is reported here for all papers combined. The majority of Kappa statistics indicated only slight (0–0.2) or fair (>0.2–0.4) agreement, yet percent agreement exceeded 60% for all but two questions. One explanation for this apparent contradiction is that the majority of papers were given the same rating on many items (see Note a). The moderate overall level of agreement can be attributed to problems experienced by reviewers in using the instrument; despite piloting, some questions remained ambiguous and difficult to apply to all study designs.[23]

Cronbach alpha values for different quality dimensions were low, suggesting that the items were not assessing a homogeneous aspect of quality. Surprisingly, the highest alpha value was obtained for the sum of the four dimensions, although the increase in the value of alpha for the total quality score is due in part to the larger number of items. There were modest correlations between the quality of reporting and measures taken to avoid bias (0.28) and confounding (0.56), but no correlation between bias and confounding (−0.03). We had expected a strong inverse correlation between external validity and confounding (since RCTs, which are often considered to have poor external validity, were automatically given credit for controlling for confounding) but found none (−0.07).

Average scores for different aspects of quality for each type of study design are shown in Table 6. Both cohort and case control studies had significantly poorer total quality than RCTs (mean quality differences −4.9, 95% CI −6.5 to −3.3, $P < 0.0001$, and −1.8, 95% CI −3.5 to −0.1, $P = 0.03$, respectively). The difference in total quality between cohort and case control studies was also statistically significant (mean difference 3.1, CI 1.2 to 5.0, $P = 0.003$). There was no independent effect of intervention, nor interaction of intervention and study design, i.e. the findings were the same for both interventions.

Considering the individual dimensions of quality, cohort studies but not case control studies had worse reporting scores than RCTs (mean difference −2.3, CI −3.2 to −1.4, $P < 0.0001$). Cohort studies also had poorer reporting scores than case control studies (mean difference −2.0, CI −3.4 to −0.9, $P < 0.001$). For confounding, both cohort and case control studies had poorer scores than RCTs (mean quality differences −2.8, 95% CI −3.4 to −2.3, $P < 0.001$, and −2.4, 95% CI −3.0 to −1.8, $P = 0.001$, respectively); cohort and case control studies did not differ significantly. There were no differences in external validity or bias between study designs or interventions.

The fact that RCTs were given significantly higher scores than both cohort and case control studies provides some evidence of the content validity of the instrument. However, the finding that case control studies scored higher than cohort studies ran counter to the widely accepted view that cohort studies provide higher quality evidence than case control studies. The explanation for this finding may lie in the fact that cohort studies were a mix of quasi-experiments and observational studies, whereas all case control studies were observational. Some reviewers commented that observational studies seemed to be of higher quality than quasi-experiments, and this perception is supported by the difference in reporting scores for different study designs, which followed the same pattern. The observation may, therefore, having nothing to do with study design *per se*, that is cohort versus case control study, but

Table 6 *Scores for different quality dimensions and total quality scores (and standard deviations) for different types of study reviewed for strategy two*

	RCTs	Cohort studies	Case control studies	Other study designs
Reporting	10.6 (0.9)	8.2 (1.3)	10.2 (0.9)	6.9 (1.6)
External validity	0.7 (0.2)	0.8 (0.2)	0.9 (0.1)	0.5 (0.2)
Internal validity – bias	4.8 (0.7)	5.0 (0.9)	5.6 (1.0)	4.3 (0.0)
Internal validity – confounding	4.9 (0.8)	2.0 (0.7)	2.5 (0.5)	1.7 (0.4)
Total quality	21.0 (1.6)	16.1 (2.3)	19.2 (1.6)	13.5 (2.2)

result from the fact that the quasi-experiments tended to be of low quality.

The number of papers was limited by the strict criteria which we laid down in order to achieve homogeneity of the intervention, population and outcome investigated. There were some difficulties in applying these criteria, and they were relaxed in some instances; we also found that studies differed in ways which we had not anticipated at the outset.

For MS, we originally defined the population of interest to be women aged 50–64 years. However, several of the studies which were identified did not limit their study populations to this age group, and did not report findings for this age range separately. If the original population criterion had been applied strictly, several studies would have had to have been excluded. The population criterion was therefore relaxed to include women aged between 35 and 74 years, the range of ages investigated in the studies which we identified.

Variation in the intervention/exposure was also a major source of heterogeneity across studies. Some studies used 1-view mammography, some used 2-view mammography, and others used both (on different screening visits, or when the screening protocol changed during the course of the study); in some studies, mammography was combined with breast examination by a physician or with the teaching of breast self-examination. The interval between screens varied across studies from once each year to once every four years, and some studies used a variable screening interval. The duration of the intervention varied across studies from four to 17 years. Provision for the control group varied across studies; in some cases control participants received nothing, but in others they were taught breast self-examination. Case control studies were carried out in the context of an entire population being offered screening, and the only exposure that could be compared across studies was 'ever screened' (compared to never screened). Screening provision for participants at the end of the studies varied; in some studies, both intervention and control groups were offered screening, while in others both intervention and control groups received no screening.

A key factor that limited the number of MS studies reviewed for this strategy was the choice of breast cancer mortality as the outcome measure. Breast cancer mortality was chosen to minimise the problems of lag and lead time biases that affect survival studies of the effectiveness of screening interventions. Despite choosing this outcome, there was some variation across studies in the precise outcome measured. The duration of follow-up varied considerably

across studies, although we tried to minimise this source of heterogeneity by choosing the duration of follow-up which was closest to 10 years when findings for a particular study were reported for different follow-up durations. Alexander and colleagues[56] also highlighted the possibility that the definition of a breast cancer death might have varied across studies.

For FAS, eight studies investigated women without a previous history of a neural tube defect, that is the effect of FAS on the *occurrence* of neural tube defects, and nine studied women with a previous history of a neural tube defect, that is the effect of FAS on the *recurrence* of neural tube defects. Since our eligibility criteria did not specify whether FAS should be intended to prevent occurrence or recurrence, and because excluding either would have halved the number of studies available, both types of study were included. Researchers defined a neural tube defect in different ways so that there may have been further heterogeneity within populations of women with a previous history of a neural tube defect. The definition of a control subject in case control studies also varied; some studies recruited a control group of healthy babies, some recruited malformed control babies without a neural tube defect, and others recruited both types of control groups.

As was found in studies of MS, several sources of heterogeneity in the FAS interventions were observed. Some studies used folic acid alone and others used multivitamins which contained folic acid; one study used a factorial design to investigate the effect of both folic acid and multivitamins simultaneously. The dose of folic acid that was used varied from 0.3 mg/day to 5 mg/day. The time period during which women had to have taken FAS in order to be considered 'fully supplemented' varied, particularly with respect to supplementation prior to conception. (If FAS was used prior to conception, most researchers generally assumed that supplementation continued during the critical first three weeks after conception.) In some studies the control group received multivitamins or a trace supplement, and in others the control group received nothing; this variation was confounded by study design, since RCTs or quasi-experiments were more likely to give some intervention to the control group than observational studies.

For MS, the pooled RR estimate for case control studies (0.51) was about 0.6 times less (indicating greater benefit) than for RCTs (RR = 0.85; mean difference ln(RR) = −0.50, 95% CI = −1.04 to 0.03, $P = 0.06$). In contrast, the pooled RR estimate for cohort studies was the same as for RCTs (RR = 0.82; mean difference ln(RR) = −0.03, 95% CI = −0.34 to 0.28,

$P = 0.82$). Neither total quality, nor any component of the quality score, were significantly associated with effect size. Including any of these variables resulted in lower values of r^2(adj), without affecting the mean differences in effect size between different study designs. The lack of relationship between study quality and effect size for different study designs can be seen in Figure 2. None of the other independent variables, singly or in combination, were sig-

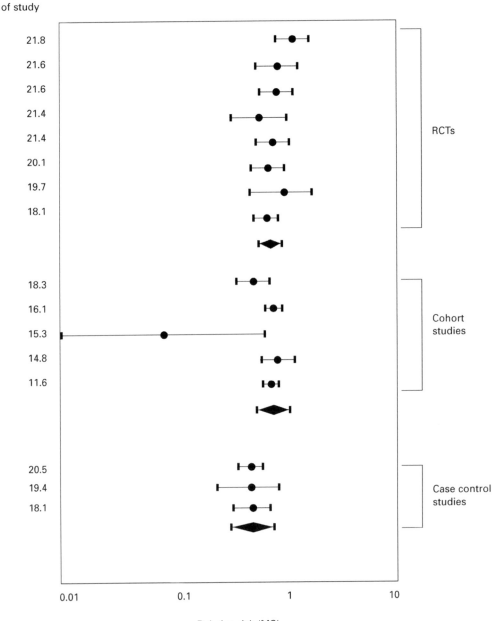

Quality
of study

Relative risk (MS)

Figure 2   *Blobbogram showing the effect size point estimates and confidence intervals for MS studies reviewed for strategy two. Pooled estimates are shown separately for RCTs, cohort studies and case control studies. Within each type of design, studies are ranked in order of quality.*

nificantly associated with effect size. Nor did they affect the mean differences in effect size between different study designs. Coefficients for case control and cohort studies in different models varied little (−0.47 to −0.61 and −0.12 to 0.13 respectively) compared to their standard errors.

For FAS, the pooled RR estimate for case control studies (0.72) was about 2.6 times higher (indicating less benefit) than for RCTs (RR =

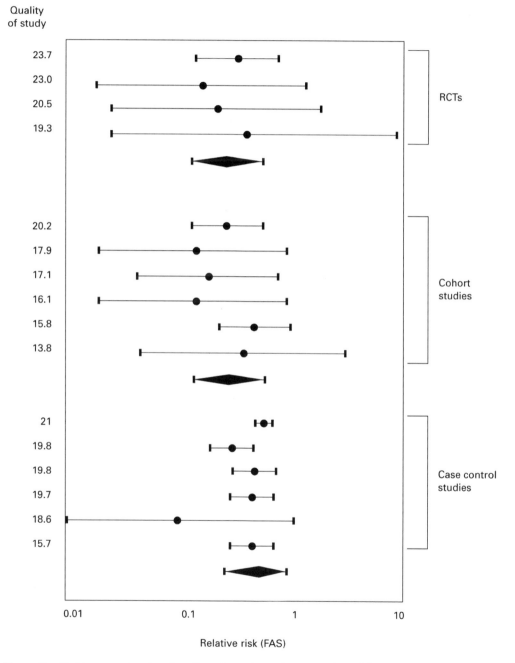

Figure 3   *Blobbogram showing the effect size point estimates and confidence intervals for FAS studies reviewed for strategy two. Pooled estimates are shown separately for RCTs, cohort studies and case control studies. Within each type of design, studies are ranked in order of quality.*

0.28; mean difference ln(RR) = 0.96, 95% CI = 0.02 to 1.89, $P = 0.05$). As in the analysis of MS studies, the pooled RR estimate for cohort studies was the same as for RCTs (RR = 0.27; mean difference ln(RR) = −0.03, 95% CI = −1.13 to 1.08, $P = 0.96$), and neither total quality, nor any component of the quality score, were significantly associated with effect size. The lack of relationship between study quality and effect size for different study designs can be seen in Figure 3.

Time of starting and stopping supplementation, but none of the other independent variables, were marginally associated with effect size; however, including these variables had no impact on the coefficients for cohort and case control studies. The RR was increased (that is less benefit) by a factor of 1.04 for each unsupplemented week prior to conception (coefficient = 0.04, 95% CI −0.001 to 0.08, $P = 0.05$), and the RR was reduced (that is greater benefit) by a factor of 0.95 for each additional week supplemented after conception (coefficient = −0.05, 95% CI −0.10 to 0.01, $P = 0.10$). These associations are not entirely consistent with the critical period for closure of the neural tube, but may simply reflect that women who were supplemented for longer were more fully supplemented.

CONCLUSIONS

The results of the first strategy suggest that QEO estimates of effectiveness may be valid (as measured by agreement with the results of RCTs), providing that important confounding factors are measured and controlled for using standard epidemiological methods of analysis, that is stratification or regression modelling. The small size of the discrepancies for high-quality comparisons between RCT and QEO estimates also suggests that psychological factors, for example treatment preferences or willingness to be randomised, had a negligible effect on outcome. Previous comparisons reported in the literature may have overemphasised the differences between RCT and QEO estimates of effectiveness because of the poor quality of most non-randomised, and especially quasi-experimental, evidence.

We do not recommend generalising the results found using the first strategy to other contexts, for three main reasons. Firstly, few papers were reviewed, and our findings may depend on the specific interventions evaluated in these papers. For example, evaluations of

interventions for cardiovascular disease predominated amongst the comparisons which were reviewed.

Secondly, most high-quality comparisons studied RCT and QEO populations with the same eligibility criteria; this may have had the effect of creating relatively uniform risk strata, reducing the possibility of confounding. In contrast, QEO studies typically use more relaxed selection criteria than RCTs, recruiting populations which are more heterogeneous with respect to prognostic factors.

Thirdly, the papers that were reviewed may have been subject to some form of publication bias. Authors did not appear to be disinterested about the comparison between RCT and QEO estimates, and findings appeared to support authors' viewpoints. Therefore the papers may not be a representative sample of all instances in which researchers have set out to compare RCT and QEO effect size estimates, and researchers may have chosen to report examples that supported their points of view.

The second strategy found no difference in effect size between RCTs and cohort studies, suggesting that evidence from cohort studies can be valid when this evidence is considered collectively. However, for both interventions that were reviewed, significantly different RR effect size estimates were obtained for case control studies compared with either RCTs or cohort studies. Interestingly, the direction of the discrepancy was not consistent across interventions, with RR estimates from case control studies indicating on average more benefit than those from RCTs and cohort studies for MS, but less benefit for FAS. No association was found between study quality and effect size for either MS or FAS interventions, after taking account of different study designs.

The lack of association between quality and effect size is difficult to interpret because this result could have arisen for a variety of reasons. The first, and most relevant to the review, is that study quality is truly not associated with RR in a predictable way. Second, the two reviews may have had inadequate power to detect an important association. Third, the instrument may have been an insensitive measure of quality, and may have failed to characterise relevant study attributes adequately. Fourth, using a quality score that was the sum of many items may have disguised the opposing influences of particular subgroups of items on effect size.

We believe that the second and fourth explanations are unlikely, since there was no evidence of any trend in effect with study quality, nor of associations between components of study quality and effect size. The fact that the quality scores for papers reviewed varied considerably from 11.6 to 23.7, and that RCTs were given significantly higher quality scores on average than both the cohort and case control studies, provides some evidence of the construct validity of the instrument and goes some way to refute the third explanation. However, the difficulty we experienced using the instrument for measuring methodological quality means that we are not confident in concluding that the first explanation is correct.

There are similar difficulties in interpreting the failure to show associations between aspects of heterogeneity, considered likely to be associated with outcome for a priori reasons, and effect size. The analyses may have had inadequate power, or the independent variables included in the analysis may have been unreliable measures of the relevant attributes. Information about other variables of interest, for example dose of folic acid, was not always available or was inadequately specified. Therefore, despite being unable to demonstrate significant associations between sources of heterogeneity and effect size, we are wary of interpreting the pooled results for different study designs. Investigating reasons for discrepancies, rather than providing a pooled estimate, was the primary objective of the review.

There are several possible reasons for the different direction of the discrepancy for the two interventions, although it should be recognised that any such explanations are *post hoc*. Case control studies of MS provide estimates of screening with 100% coverage, albeit ever versus never screened; both RCTs and cohort studies included substantial proportions of unscreened women in their intervention groups for intention-to-treat analyses, with coverage for MS varying considerably between studies that reported this information. Case control studies of FAS also provide estimates of supplementation with 100% coverage. However, coverage amongst women assigned to supplementation in RCTs and cohort studies is likely to have been much higher than for MS.

Almost all case control studies also required women to recall their 'exposure'. Recalling supplementation, which often required remembering the particular supplement taken in order to confirm the folic acid content, is likely to have been much less reliable than asking women to recall whether they had ever had a mammogram. Unreliable recall could easily lead to bias, with women whose pregnancy was affected by a neural tube defect being more likely to report they had taken supplementation when they had not than women who did not have an affected pregnancy.

We therefore conclude, in common with standard methodological texts,[78] that case control studies designed to estimate effectiveness should be interpreted with caution, and that the direction of any discrepancy between RR estimates for case control studies and other study designs is likely to depend on the intervention being evaluated. There was no evidence that discrepant estimates for case control studies could be attributed to confounding by quality or sources of heterogeneity.

RECOMMENDATIONS

Our aim was to establish 'safety limits' for QEO studies of different levels of quality, that is the size of effect which would be unlikely to be explained by bias, in order to guide interpretation of QEO evidence. This aim was thwarted for both strategies, for different reasons. For strategy one, we felt unable to draw strong conclusions because of the paucity of evidence, and the potentially unrepresentative nature of the evidence we reviewed. For strategy two, the aim was thwarted by our inability to distinguish, and measure, the influences of variations in internal and external validity between studies. Our recommendations relate directly to these obstacles.

Our first recommendation is a general one. We strongly recommend that the use of quasi-experimental designs to evaluate healthcare interventions should not be rejected on the basis of past QEO evidence because, for both strategies, most quasi-experiments that were reviewed were of poor quality.

This leads to our second recommendation, namely that there is a need for more direct evidence about the comparability of findings from RCTs and QEO studies. We believe that the comprehensive cohort study is the best study design to use to obtain such evidence with the addition that *ineligible* patients who receive one or other of the treatments being investigated, not usually included in comprehensive cohorts, should also be followed-up. Studies need to be carried out in areas where RCTs are the preferred design, as well as areas where RCTs are problematic, in order to assess the generalisability of evidence about the validity of QEO evidence. Analyses of comprehensive cohort studies should focus on using the RCT estimate of effectiveness, and estimates of the effect of other prognostic factors from the entire cohort, to predict outcome frequencies for different groups of patients who were not randomised;

close agreement between predicted and observed results would be strong evidence of the validity of QEO studies. However, this approach cannot take account of interactions between an intervention and prognostic factors.

Comprehensive cohort studies are expensive, since they need at least double the sample size of a conventional RCT. It would therefore be attractive to nest RCTs in established high-quality prospective databases, where relevant prognostic factors and outcomes are routinely recorded and where large numbers of patients can be studied at reasonable cost. Consideration also needs to be given to the optimal way of obtaining consent and offering randomisation or treatment choices to patients.

Our third recommendation arises from the considerable problems we experienced in measuring study quality and other aspects of study design which may influence effect size. The instrument that we used was not entirely successful, largely because of the compromises and ambiguities that arose from using the same instrument for all study designs. Developing an instrument to assess the quality of different studies is an urgent priority. We believe that it is not worthwhile comparing the results of evaluations using different designs observed in different studies for other interventions (i.e. strategy two) until a more suitable instrument has been developed to assess different attributes of studies. The instrument must be able to assess all aspects of study design that may influence effect size and should make explicit the aspect which each item is intended to assess and the anticipated direction of its influence on effect size. Separate instruments are likely to be required for different study designs, necessitating some method of standardising quality scores when comparisons are made across study designs.

NOTE

a. Kappa is a 'chance corrected' measure of agreement, and is therefore usually preferred over simpler measures such as % agreement. However, the interpretation of Kappa becomes difficult when the scores for the examples being rated are distributed across the available response categories in a grossly unequal manner; the marginal totals become severely constrained, and a high degree of agreement is expected by chance. In these circumstances, a high value of Kappa is almost impossible to attain, and a low value may not necessarily imply poor agreement.

REFERENCES

1. Cochrane AL. *Effectiveness and efficiency.* London, Nuffield Provincial Hospitals Trust, 1972.
2. Chalmers I. Evaluating the effects of care during pregnancy and childbirth. In: Chalmers I (ed.) *Effective care in pregnancy and childbirth.* Oxford, Oxford University Press, 1989; pp. 3–79.
3. Jaeschke R, Sackett DL. Research methods for obtaining primary evidence. *Int. J. Technol. Assess. Health Care* 1989; **5**: 503–19.
4. Byar DP. Problems with using observational databases to compare treatments. *Stat. Med.* 1991; **10**: 663–6.
5. Davey Smith G. Cross design synthesis: a new strategy for studying medical outcomes? *Lancet* 1992; **340**: 944–6.
6. Peto R, Collins R, Gray R. Large-scale randomized evidence: large, simple trials and overviews of trials. *Ann. N. Y. Acad. Sci.* 1993; **703**: 314–40.
7. Sheldon T. Please bypass the PORT. *Br. Med. J.* 1994; **309**: 142–3.
8. Hlatky MA. Using databases to evaluate therapy. *Stat. Med.* 1991; **10**: 647–52.
9. Black N. Experimental and observational methods of evaluation. *Br. Med. J.* 1994; **309**: 540.
10. Black N. Why we need observational studies to evaluate the effectiveness of health care. *Br. Med. J.* 1996; **312**: 1215–18.
11. Sackett DL, Haynes RB, Guyatt GH, Tugwell P. *Clinical Epidemiology. A Basic Science for Clinical Medicine.* 2nd edn. Toronto, Little Brown and Company, 1991.
12. Guyatt GH, Sackett DL, Cook DJ. Users' guides to the medical literature. II. How to use an article about therapy or prevention. A. Are the results of the study valid? *JAMA* 1993; **270**: 2598–601.
13. Peto R, Collins R, Gray R. Large-scale randomized evidence: large, simple trials and overviews of trials. *J. Clin. Epidemiol.* 1995; **48**: 23–40.
14. Doll R. Doing more good than harm: the evaluation of health care interventions. *Ann. N. Y. Acad. Sci.* 1993; **703**: 313.
15. Cook TD, Campbell DT. *Quasi-experimentation: Design and Analysis Issues for Field Settings.* Boston, Houghton Mifflin, 1979.
16. Eddy DM. Should we change the rules for evaluating medical technologies? In: Gelijns AC (ed.) *Medical Innovation at the Crossroads, Volume 1, Modern Methods of Clinical Investigation.* Washington: National Academy Press 1990; pp. 117–34.
17. Hennekens C, Buring JE. Observational evidence. *Ann. N. Y. Acad. Sci.* 1993; **703**: 18–24.
18. Sackett DL, Wennberg JE. Choosing the best research design for each question. *Br. Med. J.* 1997; **315**: 1636.

19. Chalmers TC, Matta RJ, Smith H, Kunzler AM. Evidence favouring the use of anticoagulants in the hospital phase of acute myocardial infarction. *N. Engl. J. Med.* 1977; **297**: 1091–6.

20. Colditz GA, Miller JN, Mosteller F. How study design affects outcomes in comparisons of therapy. I: Medical. *Stat. Med.* 1989; **8**: 441–54.

21. Miller JN, Colditz GA, Mosteller F. How study design affects outcomes in comparisons of therapy. II: Surgical. *Stat. Med.* 1989; **8**: 455–66.

22. Britton A, McKee M, Black N, McPherson K, Sanderson C, Bain C. Choosing between randomised and non-randomised studies: a systematic review. *Health Technol. Assessment* 1998; **2**: 1–115.

23. MacLehose RR, Reeves BC, Harvey IM, Black AM, Sheldon TA, Russell IT. A review of randomized controlled trials, quasi-experimental and observational study designs for evaluating the effectiveness of health care. *Health Technol. Assessment*; in press.

24. Prescott R, Counsell CE, Gillespie WJ, et al. Factors that limit the quality, number and progress of randomized controlled trials. *Health Technol Assessment* 1999; **3**(20).

25. Dickersin K, Scherer R, Lefebvre C. Identifying relevant studies for systematic reviews. *Br. Med. J.* 1994; **309**: 1286–91.

26. Downs SH, Black N. The feasibility of creating a checklist for the assessment of the methodological quality both of randomized and non-randomized studies of health care interventions. *J. Epidemiol. Community Health* 1998; **52**: 344–52.

27. Wortman PM, Yeaton WH. Synthesis of results in controlled trials of coronary artery bypass graft surgery. In: Light R (ed.) *Evaluation Studies Review Annual.* Sage Publications, 1983; **8**: 536–57.

28. Reimold SC, Chalmers TC, Berlin JA, Antman EM. Assessment of the efficacy and safety of antiarrhythmic therapy for chronic atrial fibrillation: observations on the role of trial design and implications of drug-related mortality. *Am. Heart J.* 1992; **124**: 924–32.

29. CASS principal investigators and their associates. Coronary artery surgery study (CASS): A randomized trial of coronary artery bypass surgery. Comparability of entry characteristics and survival in randomized and non-randomized patients meeting randomization criteria. *J. Am. Coll. Cardiol.* 1984; **3**: 114–28.

30. Paradise JL, Bluestone CD, Bachman RZ, et al. Efficacy of tonsillectomy for recurrent throat infection in severely affected children: results of parallel randomized and non randomized clinical trials. *N. Engl. J. Med.* 1984; **310**: 674–83.

31. Blichert-Toft M, Brincker H, Andersen JA, et al. A Danish randomized trial comparing breast preserving therapy with mastectomy in mammary

carcinoma. Preliminary results. *Acta Oncol.* 1988; **27**: 671–7.

32. Schmoor C, Olschewski M, Schumacher M. Randomized and non-randomized patients in clinical trials: experiences with comprehensive cohort studies. *Stat. Med.* 1996; **15**: 263–71.

33. Gray-Donald K, Kramer MS. Causality inference in observational vs. experimental studies. *Am. J. Epidemiol.* 1988; **127**: 885–92.

34. Hlatky MA, Facc MD, Califf RM, et al. Comparison of predictions based on observational data with the results of RCT of coronary artery bypass surgery. *J. Am. Coll. Cardiol.* 1988; **11**: 237–45.

35. Horwitz RI, Viscoli CM, Clemens JD, Sadock RT. Developing improved observational methods for evaluating therapeutic effectiveness. *Am. J. Med.* 1990; **89**: 630–8.

36. Kirke PN, Daly LE, Elwood JH, for the Irish Vitamin Study Group. A randomized trial of low dose folic acid to prevent NTD. *Arch. Dis. Child.* 1992; **67**: 1442–6.

37. Ward L, Fielding JWL, Dunn JA, Kelly KA, for the British Stomach Cancer Group. The selection of cases for randomized trials: a registry of concurrent trial and non-trial participants. *Br. J. Cancer* 1992; **66**: 943–50.

38. Fisher B, Costantino JP, Redmond CK, et al. Endometrial cancer in tamoxifen-treated breast cancer patients: findings from the National Surgical Adjuvant Breast and Bowel Project (NSABP) B-14. *J. Natl Cancer Inst.* 1994; **86**: 527–37.

39. Marubini E, Mariani L, Salvadori B, et al. Results of a breast cancer-surgery trial compared with observational data from routine practice. *Lancet* 1996; **347**: 1000–3.

40. Olschewski M, Scheurlen H. Comprehensive cohort study: an alternative to randomized consent design in a breast preservation trial. *Methods Inf. Med.* 1985; **24**: 131–4.

41. Veronesi U, Banfi A, Salvadori B, et al. Breast conservation is the treatment of choice in small breast cancer: long-term results of a randomized trial. *Eur. J. Cancer* 1990; **26**: 668–70.

42. Schumacher M, Bastert G, Bojar H, et al. A randomized 2 × 2 trial evaluating hormonal treatment and the duration of chemotherapy in node-positive breast cancer patients. *J. Clin. Oncol.* 1994; **12**: 2086–93.

43. Allum WH, Hallissey MT, Kelly KA, for the British Stomach Cancer Group. Adjuvant chemotherapy in operable gastric cancer. 5 year follow-up of first British stomach cancer group trial. *Lancet* 1989; **i**: 571–4.

44. Dales LG, Friedman GD, Collen MF. Evaluating periodic multiphasic health check ups: a controlled trial. *J. Chron. Dis.* 1979; **32**: 385–404.

45. Shapiro S, Vent W, Strax P, Venet L, Roeser R. Ten- to fourteen-year effect of screening on breast

cancer mortality. *J. Natl Cancer Inst.* 1982; **69**: 349–55.

46. Collette HJA, Rombach JJ, Day NE, de Waard F. Evaluation of screening for breast cancer in a non-randomized study (The DOM Project) by means of a case-control study. *Lancet* 1984; **i**: 1224–6.

47. Verbeek ALM, Holland R, Sturmans F, et al. Reduction of breast cancer mortality through mass screening with modern mammography. First results of the Nijmegen Project, 1975–1981. *Lancet* 1984; **i**: 1222–4.

48. Andersson I, Aspergren K, Janzon L, et al. Mammographic screening and mortality from breast cancer: the Malmo mammographic screening trial. *Br. Med. J.* 1988; **297**: 943–8.

49. Morrison AS, Brisson J, Khalid N. Breast cancer incidence and mortality in the Breast Cancer Detection Demonstration Project. *J. Natl Cancer Inst.* 1988; **80**: 1540–7.

50. Palli D, Rosselli Del Turco M, Buiatti E, et al. Time interval since last test in a breast cancer screening programme: a case-control study in Italy. *J. Epidemiol. Community Health* 1989; **43**: 241–8.

51. Frisell J, Eklund G, Hellstrom L, et al. Randomized study of mammography screening – preliminary report on mortality in the Stockholm trial. *Breast Cancer Res. Treat.* 1991; **18**: 49–56.

52. Collette HJA, de Waard F, Rombach JJ, Collette C, Day NE. Further evidence of benefits of a (non-randomized) breast cancer screening programme: the DOM project. *J. Epidemiol. Community Health* 1992; **46**: 382–6.

53. Miller AB, Baines CJ, To T, Wall C. Canadian National Breast Screening Study: 2. Breast cancer detection and death rates among women aged 50 to 59 years. *Can. Med. Assoc. J.* 1992; **147**: 1477–88.

54. Miller AB, Baines CJ, To T, Wall C. Canadian National Breast Screening Study: 1. Breast cancer detection and death rates among women aged 40 to 49 years. *Can. Med. Assoc. J.* 1992; **147**: 1459–76.

55. UK Trial of Early Detection of Breast Cancer Group. Breast cancer mortality after 10 years in the UK trial of early detection of breast cancer. *The Breast* 1993; **2**: 13–20.

56. Alexander FE, Anderson TJ, Brown HK, et al. The Edinburgh randomized trial of breast cancer screening: results after 10 years of follow-up. *Br. J. Cancer* 1994; **70**: 542–8.

57. Thompson RS, Barlow WE, Taplin SH, et al. A population-based case-cohort evaluation of the efficacy of mammographic screening for breast cancer. *Am. J. Epidemiol.* 1994; **140**: 889–901.

58. Hakama M, Pukkala E, Kallio M, Godenhjelm K, Svinhufvud U. Effectiveness of screening for breast cancer in women under 50 years at entry: the Kotka pilot project in Finland. *Int. J. Cancer* 1995; **63**: 55–7.

59. Peer PGM, Werre JM, Mravunac M, et al. Effect on breast cancer mortality of biennial mammographic screening of women under age 50. *Int. J. Cancer* 1995; **60**: 808–11.

60. Tabar L, Fagerberg G, Chen HH, et al. Efficacy of breast cancer screening by age. New results from the Swedish two-county trial. *Cancer* 1995; **75**: 2507–17.

61. Laurence KM, James N, Miller MH, Tennant GB, Campbell H. Double-blind randomized controlled trial of folate treatment before conception to prevent recurrence of neural-tube defects. *Br. Med. J.* 1981; **282**: 1509–11.

62. Smithells R, Sheppard S, Schorah CJ, et al. Apparent prevention of neural tube defects by periconceptional vitamin supplementation. *Arch. Dis. Child.* 1981; **56**: 911–18.

63. Smithells R, Seller MJ, Harris R, et al. Further experience of vitamin supplementation for prevention of neural tube defect recurrences. *Lancet* 1983; **i**: 1027–31.

64. Seller MJ, Nevin NC. Periconceptional vitamin supplementation and the prevention of neural tube defects in south-east England and Northern Ireland. *J. Med. Genet.* 1984; **21**: 325–30.

65. Mulinare J, Cordero JF, Erickson JD, Berry RJ. Periconceptional use of multivitamins and the occurrence of neural tube defects. *JAMA* 1988; **260**: 3141–5.

66. Mills JL, Rhoads GG, Simpson JL, et al. The absence of a relation between the periconceptional use of vitamins and neural-tube defects. *N. Engl. J. Med.* 1989; **321**: 430–5.

67. Milunsky A, Jick H, Jick SS, et al. Multivitamin/folic acid supplementation in early pregnancy reduces the prevalence of neural tube defects. *JAMA* 1989; **262**: 2847–52.

68. Smithells R, Sheppard S, Wild J, Schorah CJ. Prevention of neural tube defect recurrences in Yorkshire: final report. *Lancet* 1989; **ii**: 498–9.

69. Vergel RG, Sanchez LR, Heredero BL, Rodriguez PL, Martinez AJ. Primary prevention of neural tube defects with folic acid supplementation: Cuban experience. *Prenat. Diag.* 1990; **10**: 149–52.

70. MRC Vitamin Study Research Group. Prevention of neural tube defects: results of the Medical Research Council vitamin study. *Lancet* 1991; **338**: 131–7.

71. Bower C, Stanley FJ. Periconceptional vitamin supplementation and neural tube defects; evidence from a case-control study in Western Australia and a review of recent publications. *J. Epidemiol. Community Health* 1992; **46**: 157–61.

72. Cziezel AE, Dudas I. Prevention of the first occurrence of neural-tube defects by periconceptional vitamin supplementation. *N. Engl. J. Med.* 1992; **327**: 1832–5.

73. Kirke PN, Daly LE, Elwood JH, for the Irish Vitamin Study Group. A randomized trial of low dose folic acid to prevent neural tube defects. *Arch. Dis. Child.* 1992; **67**: 1442–6.

74. Martinez-Frias ML, Rodriguez-Pinilla E. Folic acid supplementation and neural tube defects. *Lancet* 1992; **340**: 620.

75. Werler MM, Shapiro S, Mitchell AA. Periconceptional folic acid exposure and risk of occurrent neural tube defects. *JAMA* 1993; **269**: 1257–61.

76. Chatkupt S, Skurnick JH, Jaggi M, et al. Study of genetics, epidemiology, and vitamin usage in familial spina bifida in the United States in the 1990s. *Neurology* 1994; **44**: 65–70.

77. Shaw G, Schaffer D, Velie EM, Morland K, Harris JA. Periconceptional vitamin use, dietary folate, and the occurrence of neural tube defects. *Epidemiology* 1995; **6**: 219–26.

78. Elwood M. *Critical Appraisal of Epidemiological Studies and Clinical Trials*. 2nd edn. Oxford, Oxford University Press, 1998.

8

The Potential Use of Routine Datasets in Health Technology Assessment

JAMES RAFTERY, ANDREW STEVENS
and PAUL RODERICK

SUMMARY

The international growth of Health Technology Assessment (HTA) calls out for increasing levels of research and information beyond randomised controlled trials. In theory, routine data offer a considerable contribution, but they have been underused to date. There is a vicious circle of poor data and lack of use.

Routine data are identified by characteristics of regular and continuous collection, using standard definitions, with comprehensive coverage of the target group, service or technology, with some, usually considerable, degree of obligation to collect the data completely and regularly, and with collection at national or regional level.

HTA is considered in this chapter to include not only the measurement of efficacy and effectiveness, but also equity and diffusion and the cost impact of health technologies.

If routine datasets are to help assess the effectiveness of new technologies, they need to possess certain key characteristics which are available to the other methods of HTA. These include:

1   A clear identification of the health technology and the relevant comparator health technology.
2   Measurement of patients' health state at patient or population level, before and after the intervention.
3   Relevant patient characteristics such as severity, co-morbidity and socio-demographics and any other likely confounders.

From this it follows that one can classify datasets as follows:

1   Those datasets which have health technology plus patient and/or health status information including Registries, administrative datasets, and aggregated datasets. Only Registries are likely to even approach passing the criteria required for measurement of effectiveness. Administrative databases often do not distinguish important healthcare technologies, and are slow at capturing new technologies when they do. Aggregated datasets do not identify individuals, but population level data can be used to assess the effectiveness of specific populative or population-oriented inventions such as national immunisation and vaccination programmes.
2   Health-technology-only datasets contain data on the use of the health technology by time and place, but without any linkage to patients or to their conditions. They can occasionally be used to assess diffusion by geographical area and hence also equity. The prescription pricing authority data in the UK is an example. Other uses are very limited, however.
3   Health-status-only datasets specify outcomes or health states, but without reporting either the health technology or the patients. These include adverse event notification schemes,

disease-specific databases and health surveys. While adverse event datasets can be useful for assessing the performance of organisations, they have little else to offer HTA except where linkage can be established.

4   Census-based datasets are important because they provide the population denominator for other analyses.

In assessing the cost of health technologies, four different types of cost-related datasets can be distinguished: health technology plus unit cost (prices) directly linked to specific health technologies; grouped health technology plus unit costs; linkable unit costs, i.e. unit costs based on combining two datasets, at least one of which is routine; and survey unit costs, i.e. unit costs based on special surveys.

In interpreting the scope of HTA widely, much evidence already exists of the use of routine data at least in some aspects of HTA. However, for mainstream evaluation of effectiveness and efficiency, the scope is restricted by data limitations and quality problems. There is, however, some potential widening of that scope given the growth of high-quality, technology-specific clinical datasets, developments in information technology and healthcare coding schemes. But if routine datasets are to fulfil their potential, a strategic overview is required plus support for potentially promising databases, greater linkage, assessment of gaps in current datasets, and greater use of routine data in the clinical (and therefore also potentially health technology assessment) setting need to explored.

INTRODUCTION

Routine data have arguably been under-used in health technology assessment (HTA). A vicious circle applies; 'the data are poor, so they cannot be used, so they remain limited and of poor quality'. One of the purposes of this report is to help instil a virtuous circle; 'good quality data which, because used, must be improved'.

The international 'effectiveness revolution' in healthcare cries out for much more research and information. Better information is required on both the effectiveness and the costs of the multiple and varied health technologies that make up healthcare. Healthcare exhibits the familiar data-information gap in an extreme way. While masses of detail on patients' health states and their use of health technologies are collected in most healthcare systems, they generally fail to become 'data' in the sense of being available for analysis; and only through analysis can data become information.

Conventional wisdom suggests ever more and larger randomised controlled trials (RCTs) measuring differences in efficacy using 'customised' data. The relative merits of trials have been pitted against other approaches (modelling, observational studies) which rely on non-customised or routinely collected data. The limitations of RCTs in providing generalisable information, particularly on effectiveness (as opposed to efficacy), plus the cost of trials, and the large number of technologies to be assessed, mean that alternative approaches will continue to be explored.

The information deficit is greater if HTA is recognised to include not only the measurement of efficacy and effectiveness, but – as argued here – also assessment of the diffusion, equity and cost of health technologies. Diffusion of health technologies can be seen as closely related to assessment of equity in access or use, in that both issues require data on the use of technologies by time and place or group. Assessments of diffusion/equity and cost of health technologies, by contrast with those focused on efficacy, rely heavily on routine data.

Routine data (see full definition below) include not only administrative data, but also registry data, adverse event reporting and regular health-related surveys. The quantity and quality of routine datasets vary widely. They depend partly on how particular healthcare systems are organised, with more administrative data in more market-oriented systems. Registers of diseases, long established in clinical practice, are partly an attempt to improve routine data. Computerisation and automated data collection are dramatically increasing the scope for registers.

Improvement of routine datasets requires a knowledge of their flaws. These include problems around data collection (coverage, accuracy, frequency, delays in publication), plus limited scope (imperfect capture of health technologies, their outcomes, and likely confounding factors). Routine datasets are often poor at picking up fine but clinically relevant distinctions between technologies, and at identifying new technologies (often constrained by the standard classification systems). For example, coronary stenting would not be picked up as a distinct technology in routine hospital statistics despite its high cost and questions over its effectiveness. Concerns over confidentiality of data, coupled historically with inability to link different datasets, have prevented technologies and treatments being connected to patients, and hence to health status.

Nonetheless, routine data are being used more widely in HTA. An analysis of the effectiveness of in-vitro fertilisation (IVF) based on data collected routinely by the UK Human Fertility and Embryology Authority identified factors associated with successful conception, including age, number of previous children if any, and duration of infertility[1] and in turn formed the basis of evidence based guidelines on managing the infertile couple.[2]

In the UK, Hospital Episode Statistics (HES) data have been used to explore variations in clinical health status and diffusion patterns. The National Health Service (NHS) clinical indicators published in 1999, covering specific types of hospital mortality, readmission and discharge, are entirely based on HES.[3] The impact of GP Fundholding (arguably a health technology) on waiting times,[4] prescribing[5] and day case rates,[6] has been assessed using NHS routine data.

In the US, the PORT studies[7] used administrative claims data to assess the effectiveness of a range of common treatments, but were criticised[8] for potential bias. Many other studies have explored equity and diffusion issues in the US context.

This chapter proposes a more optimistic-than-usual view of the potential use of routine data in HTA, based partly on a wider definition of health technology assessment, because of encouraging evidence of several specific registries, discussed below.

AIMS AND METHODS

The aim of the project reported here was to explore how routine data can be relevant to health technology assessment, taking into account its planned development, rules of access, previous use in HTA, and potential for future use. Methods used in this review to assess the role of routine data included:

(a) a review of the literature on the potential use of routine data;

(b) a structured compilation of sources of routine data in the UK, both NHS[9] and more generally;[10]

(c) information from key informants on characteristics of each dataset planned development, and the rules for access; and

(d) annotation of each source according to the aims outlined above.

While the main focus is on the UK, the proposed classifications of HTA and the typology of routine datasets will apply to most modern healthcare systems.

KEY TERMS AND CONCEPTS

Each of the key terms – routine data, health technology and health technology assessment – requires clarification.

Routine[a] Data

In the absence of an unequivocal definition in the literature[b], this chapter identifies the following important characteristics in routine datasets[c]:

(a) regular and continuous collection;

(b) using standard definitions;

(c) with comprehensive coverage of the target group, service or technology;

(d) with some (usually considerable) degree of obligation to collect the data completely and regularly; and

(e) with collection at national or regional level (depending partly on the degree of compulsion involved).

This definition excludes single site (hospital or health authority) datasets, of which there have been many a often short-lived datasets of limited generalisability. Some deliberate 'fuzziness' remains around the level of compulsion and about the role of 'regional' datasets.

Routine datasets cover not only administrative data (such as hospital episode statistics), but go beyond these to include disease or technology-specific databases established for epidemiological research, and evaluation purposes, provided they meet the above criteria. It thus includes disease registers such as those for cancer, and technology-specific registers such as those for renal replacement therapy, which have developed in many countries. This wider definition breaks with the (largely US) literature which discusses mainly administrative data.

Some indication of the scope of routine data in relation to health and healthcare can be gleaned by briefly reviewing the history of UK routine data.

The decennial *Census* of Population since 1801 has provided the most basic data on population size and composition. *Mortality* data have long been collected, largely for probate reasons. Mortality statistics collected at national level in England since the Births and Deaths Registration Act 1836, became compulsory in 1874. Natural and unnatural causes of death have been distinguished and classified, partly for legal reasons, partly for epidemiological reasons. Stillbirths were added to notifiable causes of death in 1927, and amended in 1992 in line with the changed legal definition of stillbirth. Limited *morbidity* data, particularly in relation to infectious diseases, have also been required by law to be collected.

Some disease-specific registries have long been established, notably for cancer. Registries have been defined as 'data concerning all cases of a particular disease or other health relevant condition in a defined population such that the cases can be related to a population base'.[11] Cancer registries were developed on a voluntary basis from 1962[12] in the UK after follow-up studies of patients treated with radium in the 1930s. Registries for particular diseases (also known as case registers) have come in and out of existence in the different countries of the UK.[13] Clinicians have often kept designated lists of patients, identifying their illnesses, severity, health service contact and health status. Psychiatric case registers were developed in the 1960s but fell out of use in the 1980s.[14] More recently there has been interest in registers of diabetes and stroke.[15]

Some data on the *use of healthcare* have also long been routinely collected. Mental hospital admissions data date from the 1845 Lunacy Act. Compulsory detention required such data for legal reasons, and covered patients in both public and privately funded hospitals.[16] Data on admissions to other hospitals came later. NHS acute hospital data have been collected and published from 1948; these include demographic, administrative and some clinical headings (surgical interventions and ICD coding of conditions, but generally not medical interventions or technologies). Although these are not subject to legal statute, they have the force of administrative law.

The establishment of the NHS in 1948, by covering the entire population increased the scope for use of comprehensive data. Of particular note is the NHS Central Register, which has been used since 1948 to pay GPs in relation to the number of patients registered. This register, based on a special 1939 Census of Population and subsequently used for rationing food in the Second World War, was computerised in 1991. The Central Health Register Inquiry System (CHRIS) contains 'flags' relating to both cancer registration and membership of some 240 ongoing medical research studies, in which around 2 million people or some 4% of the UK population, are included.[17]

Data on *privately provided services* have often been lacking in the UK except for services whose legal regulation required such data (compulsory psychiatric admissions, terminations, IVF). In the 1990s, both US and France imposed a legal obligation on private providers of acute hospital services to provide minimum datasets to the state. In England, only occasional survey data are available, even though as much as 20% of all elective surgery is carried out in the private sector.[18] Although nursing home and residential care are increasingly provided privately (if often publicly funded), few routine data are required. Routine data on personal social services are also largely absent in the UK.

The potential usefulness of routine data has increased due to information technology, improved record linkage, and coding.

Information Technology

This has dramatically increased the scope of routine data in healthcare, as in other sectors of the economy. Although much patient-specific information is recorded in the course of healthcare delivery (such as patient characteristics, disease severity, co-morbidity, diagnostic and treatment data plus some information on outcomes), it is usually stored in inaccessible casenotes. A useful distinction can be made between 'data' (given) and 'capta' (captured or taken). Health services capture enormous amounts of detail, often in casenotes, but these are seldom translated into data. Casenotes in England still tend to be handwritten,[19] specific to the site of treatment, and difficult to interpret. Problems include lack of standard formats, variation between doctors in completeness and accuracy of data recording (such as the difficulty in defining cancer stage from medical notes), poor integration with other professions' entries (nurses, physiotherapists), or with other settings of care. A high proportion of casenotes have been untraceable in various studies. Computerisation of casenotes offers great scope for their 'routinisation'. Electronic patient records have already become a reality in some hospitals and their widespread use is an objective of the NHS Information and Communications Technology strategy.[20]

Linking of Data

Linking of data between routine datasets provides a powerful way of greatly extending their use as well as validating data items. Besides the NHS Central Register, more detailed linkage including hospital records has been pioneered in the Oxford Region and in Scotland.[21,22] Historically, the lack of a single computable NHS patient number has limited health record linkage, but the change to a single NHS number from 1997 greatly increased the scope for such linkage.

If healthcare 'capta' are to be turned into useful data, *standardised coding systems* of diseases and health technologies are essential. The International Classification of Diseases (ICD) was originally developed for classifying causes of death but from 1948 was extended to cover morbidity.[23] ICD has been regularly updated to keep up with new diseases (currently on ICD10), and has the major advantage of being international.

Standard definitions of treatments have been slower to develop. Surgical interventions are captured in different ways in different countries. The UK uses the OPCS codes (Office of Population Census and Surveys – since changed to Office of National Statistics), and the US the Classification of Procedures and Treatments (CPT). Standard definitions apply to drugs via the British National Formulary (which can be linked to both World Health Organization and European Union classifications, but which do not readily map to International Classification of Disease headings).

Several systems,[24] including Read, offer means of translating all terms used by doctors to describe diseases, conditions and treatments into standard codes by way of an electronic thesaurus. Despite the NHS adoption of Read codes, their development has been slow.

Even when codes exist, their usefulness is limited by the lack of detail in most standard coding definitions. For example, ICD does not cover disease severity and in practice, many conditions are coded as 'unspecified'. Whilst procedure coding systems (such as OPCS and CPT) capture detail of the surgical interventions, detail is lacking on the specific surgical technologies used. All standard coding systems inevitably lag new diseases and procedures. Health status is seldom recorded, partly due to problems of the coding systems (no severity), but also due to limitations with ICD (no quality of life measurement, or disease-specific symptom profiles). These difficulties are exacerbated by variations in medical diagnosis. To remedy these limitations, clinical trials usually go beyond standard classifications by using more detailed terms. As argued below, clinical trials provide criteria against which to gauge the potential usefulness of routine data in assessing efficacy and effectiveness.

HEALTH TECHNOLOGIES

'Health technology' tends to be defined broadly. In the UK health technologies are defined as:

'all methods used by health professionals to promote health, prevent and treat disease,

and to improve rehabilitation and long term care'.[25]

And in the US:

'the set of techniques, drugs, equipment and procedures used by health care professionals in delivering medical care to individuals and the systems within which such care is delivered'.[26]

The ability of routine data to capture health technologies thus depends on how well defined the health technologies are, and the purposes of the dataset. Those technologies that are regulated by law tend to have fuller, more precise definitions. Pharmaceuticals make up a specific class of health technologies, due to having long been subject to licensing in most countries both to ensure quality and to prevent harm. Most pharmaceuticals are manufactured and marketed by private enterprises. The regulation of pharmaceuticals reflects a history of harm and subsequent litigation. The most notorious episode was probably the thalidomide scandal in the 1960s, which led to tighter controls in many industrialised countries. Within pharmaceuticals, different regulations apply depending on whether drugs are available only on prescription, over-the-counter in pharmacies only, or in all shops.

Medical and surgical devices tend to be less regulated, but since they are often privately provided, they are also subject to litigation (the extent of which varies internationally). Litigation has led to the establishment of registers of patients who have had certain devices implanted, for example cardiac pacemakers or silicone breast implants. The main regulation of diagnostic testing has to do with quality control, such as the national external quality scheme for pathology laboratories.

Other health technologies are subject to less regulation and tend to be less well defined. Surgical procedures are recorded in routine datasets for in-patient and day cases (but not for outpatients or when carried out in GP surgeries), but are not regulated other than by clinical audit of outcomes (both in general and of adverse events), and voluntary means such as the UK's Safety and Efficacy Register of New Interventional Procedures (SERNIP).

Changes in the setting or organisation of healthcare are less regulated, but the recent history of community care for the mentally ill may indicate a move towards auditing of adverse events (spurred in part by media reports). The move in many countries to increased reliance on primary care may have the effect of reducing the extent to which routine data systems capture treatment data (such as minor surgery). Against that, primary care organisations may over time come to collect more detailed relevant data than at present.

HEALTH TECHNOLOGY ASSESSMENT

Health technology assessment is widely used to include assessment of efficacy, effectiveness and cost effectiveness. This section suggests broadening the definition explicitly to include equity, diffusion and cost. For the purposes of understanding the scope of routine data, assessments can be classified as measuring:

(a) efficacy and/or effectiveness;
(b) equity and/or diffusion; and
(c) the cost impact of health technologies, whether alone or in conjunction with their efficacy/effectiveness.

Assessment of Efficacy and/or Effectiveness

Efficacy measures patient benefit and short-term harm in scientific, usually experimental, studies. Effectiveness, by contrast, is concerned with patient benefit and harm in everyday practice.

Health technology assessments concerned with efficacy place particular emphasis on RCTs and systematic reviews of trials. The conventional wisdom is that only trials can provide the requisite data on efficacy/effectiveness, and perhaps on cost effectiveness. However, effectiveness can only be measured in costly large pragmatic trials with wide entry criteria. The degree to which efficacy as established in trials translates into everyday practice depends on many factors, including the transferability of the technology and its application to groups not included in trials.

The advantages of trials in measuring efficacy have been well rehearsed.[27] The random allocation of patients to intervention and control arms prevents differences in patients (including selection bias and confounders unknown to the experimenter) affecting the results. The blinding of outcome assessment minimises the possibility of information bias. However, the limitations of trials in relation to efficacy have also been outlined.[28] Assessment of effectiveness requires both large simple trials and detailed registers of particular diseases and their treatments.[29]

If routine datasets are to help assess effectiveness, *they should possess the key characteristics of data generated by trials*, including information on patients' health before and after treatment, together with data on relevant confounders. Specifically this implies:

(a) clear identification of the health technology along with relevant comparator health technology;
(b) measurement of patients' health state at patient or population level, before and after intervention; plus
(c) relevant patient characteristics such as severity, co-morbidity and socio-demographics, and any other likely confounders.

Assessment of Diffusion and Equity of Health Technologies

Equity can be defined in terms of which groups use particular health technologies. Assessment of equity *requires that datasets show which particular groups receive the relevant technology*. Groups can be defined in many ways (age, sex, ethnicity, socio-economic group, geography). Diffusion is concerned with the factors influencing the uptake of health technologies by place and time, and requires broadly the same information as equity. Both require data on the use of technologies by time, place and relevant group.

Health technology assessments concerned with equity or diffusion need less information than those concerned with efficacy or effectiveness. It remains necessary to have the health technology specifically identified at one or more points in time and place. Some NHS routine datasets have been extended in recent years to include group identifiers (ethnic group). Postcoding of patients' records in the UK has enabled service use to be linked to the Census of Population enumeration districts allowing ecological analysis of socio-economic factors.[30]

Assessment of the Costs of Technologies

To be useful for costing, datasets must identify the relevant health technology and its cost. Cost-related assessments include the range of economic evaluations: cost efficacy, cost effectiveness, 'cost of illness', cost consequences and cost impact studies. Costing is complicated by several factors, including the wide definition of cost used by economists and the lack of prices or unit costs (used equivalently here) for many health technologies. Economics defines costs in terms of societal opportunity costs, which requires data on the range of knock-on effects of particular health technologies (both in terms of the full range personal costs and benefits, and over the entire life of the patient). Difficulties around the assessment of such knock-on cost effects are most extreme in trials (which tend to be short term and focused on outcomes), but is shared by all approaches.

Only some datasets that identify a health technology have a price linked to the technology. Pharmaceuticals and some packages of healthcare tend to be priced, depending on the healthcare system, but few other health technologies are priced. Costing then involves estimating unit costs for those technologies. Prices (and unit costs) vary, depending on patent, industrial processes, and competition.

For costing purposes, the key criteria are that the health technology is identified in the dataset and linked to either a price/unit cost or to a pattern of resource use which can be priced/costed. Ideally, the knock-on effects of use of one technology on use of others would be identified, but as the requisite long-term follow-up data are rarely available, this usually involves modelling.

ROUTINE DATASETS FOR EFFICACY/EFFECTIVENESS AND EQUITY/DIFFUSION

The above discussion suggests four broad types of datasets relevant to assessing issues around efficacy/effectiveness or equity/diffusion:

I   Health technology, plus patient and/or health status;
II   Health technology only;
III Health status only;
IV   Census based datasets.

A similar but less refined classification has been suggested by WHO researchers.[31] This classification is applicable widely and not just to the UK.

For assessing effectiveness, only datasets in type I are potentially useful, due to their inclusion of both health technology and health status. Health status can be measured directly (as in registers and to some extent in enhanced administrative datasets) or indirectly (through linkage based on the individual patient records or at aggregate population level). Type I datasets can also be used to assess equity/diffusion, as they usually include data on groups and place, by time.

The other types fail to include both health technology and health status. Type II contain health technologies only and so can potentially be used for equity/diffusion analysis. Type III contain health status only and can only exceptionally be linked back to a particular health technology. Type IV refer to Census of Population datasets which provide the denominator data for rates and which can sometimes be linked to other datasets. Systems enabling linkage to mortality or to Census of Population data are discussed separately below.

Type I: Health Technology + Patient and/or Health Status Datasets

These databases specify a particular health technology plus patient characteristics (such as age, sex, condition, severity, co-morbidity, and socio-demographics). Although generally patients are identified directly, for some population-oriented programmes only aggregate population characteristics are needed. Within this premier group of databases, three subtypes can be distinguished: registries; enhanced administrative datasets; and population-based datasets.

Registry-type databases

New disease-specific or health technology-specific databases have been developing, partly due to the limitations of traditional routine administrative datasets. Some are statutory and many are led by clinicians. These are routine in the sense of being regularly collected, but are registries in reporting additional clinically relevant data and following-up patients.

Only registry-type datasets are likely to even approach the criteria required for measurement of effectiveness. The criteria require measurement of patients' health state, before and after intervention, plus relevant patient characteristics such as severity, co-morbidity and socio-demographics, and any other likely confounders. While good quality registry-type datasets include relevant patient health states, the possibility of bias due to uncontrolled circumstances is difficult to overcome.

The ability of registries to contain the data required for assessing effectiveness depends on the condition or disease and the relevant health technologies. Some outcomes can be more readily linked to well-defined effective interventions or patient characteristics. For example, in the Human Fertility and Embryology Authority database, successful conceptions are the outcome of IVF, with relevant details of patient groups and the interventions. In some datasets, extension of life is the main target outcome. Examples include the Renal Registries in England & Wales and in Scotland, and the UK Transplant Support Services Authority (TSSA). The Renal Registry collects data on the characteristics of all new patients starting renal replacement therapy, types and details of treatment, and a range of health statuses including death, modality switches and intermediate biochemical and haematological markers. As planned, this database will eventually give long-term health statuses – including those rare outcomes which are beyond trials. Some registries provide proxies for health status. The National Prospective Monitoring Scheme for HIV provides not only data on drugs prescribed but also on CD4 blood count (which defines the transition from HIV to AIDS).

Cancer registries provide data on the incidence, stage and progression of disease. Although they contain some treatment data, their lack of precise data on specific forms of chemotherapy and radiotherapy, and on subsequent healthcare use, limits their usefulness in health technology assessment. The effectiveness of interventions varies both by cancer site and stage and specific intervention. Nonetheless, differences in survival rates internationally for particular cancers have spurred action in the reorganisation of cancer services. Cancer registries arguably need to develop their ability to capture the diffusion and equity of use of major evidence based interventions such as adjuvant chemotherapy for particular stages of cancers.

Enhanced administrative datasets

The main UK dataset under this heading is the Hospital Episode Statistics (HES) and its Welsh and Scottish equivalents (PEDW and COPPISH). These large databases (10 million records annually in England alone) contain demographic, administrative and clinical data of cases treated as in-patients or daycases in NHS hospitals. By including surgical interventions, as captured by OPCS4 surgical codes, a range of important health technologies is identified. Diseases are noted using ICD codes, but medical treatments and diagnostic tests, which are itemised in casenotes, are not included.

Within HES, important health technologies, such as stroke unit and ICU beds are not distinguished. Health status data in HES are limited to ICD coding of events plus deaths while in hospital, as in the 1999 NHS Clinical Indicators which focus on in hospital mortality post surgery or admission with a fractured hip or a myocardial infarction.[3] Mortality rates post discharge require linking to the NHS Central Register. 'Destination on discharge' to normal home provides a crude proxy outcome for certain conditions – for stroke and fractured hip in the NHS Clinical Indicators. More specific outcome measures are being developed for the NHS, including mortality and complications after discharge, which require additional linked data. The use of the single NHS number in this dataset will enable records to be linked from year to year and to other datasets. Lack of data on out-patients and on diagnostic data remain major barriers. HES has been criticised, not least for its definition of finished consultant episodes,[32] but it has also performed well when validated against one disease register.[33] Its use in the Clinical Indicators, which has been

accompanied by quality checks, may over time lead to quality improvement.

Although in-patients in NHS hospitals are recorded in HES, only limited data are collected on out-patients (ambulatory care), GP and community health services. The Minimum Data Set for outpatients, introduced in 1996 (yet to report) is limited due partly to the nature of ambulatory care – much of the service is either diagnostic or monitoring with many repeat visits. The large number of contacts with GPs means that no routine patient-based data are collected centrally, other than that for the payment of prescriptions, so that analysis of trends relies on surveys such as the periodic GP Morbidity survey or various ongoing data collections from samples of practices, such as the General Practice Research Database (GPRD) and the Doctors Independent Network (DIN). The scale and complexity of diagnostic imaging means that only rudimentary data are collected.

Aggregated datasets useful for population effectiveness

Although patients are not identified at an individual level in these datasets, population level data can be used to assess the effectiveness of specific population-oriented interventions. The national immunisation and vaccination programmes are examples. Since the effectiveness of these interventions is well established, data on the coverage of these programmes enables their overall effectiveness to be assessed. Screening programmes, such as national breast and cervical programmes, where again coverage, incidence and mortality are the critical target variables, also fall under this heading.

While such datasets can be used for selective analyses of effectiveness/efficacy, they can also be used for equity/diffusion and costing. Those discussed in the next section can only be used for diffusion/equity and costing.

Type II: Health-Technology-Only Datasets

Datasets in this group contain data on use of a health technology by time and place, but without any linkage to patients or their conditions. Such datasets can be used to assess the diffusion by geographical area, and hence in assessment of equity. A prime example is the Prescription Pricing Authority data which specifies the amount of each drug dispensed by GPs in each UK country each year. These data are fed back to GPs and play a role in monitoring and controlling prescribing. Other databases in this heading include the National Breast Implant Register (which records who has had silicone implants) and the family planning returns (NHS Return KT31).

Type III: Health-Status-Only Datasets

Databases in this group specify health status or health states, but without necessarily reporting either the health technology or the patient. Three subtypes can be identified: adverse events/confidential enquiries, disease-specific databases, and health surveys. While adverse event-type datasets can be useful for assessing the performance of organisations, the other two types have little to offer HTA except where event linkage, such as to mortality, can be established.

Adverse events/confidential enquiries

The Adverse Drug Reaction notification system identifies adverse events associated with particular drugs, with doctors reporting on a voluntary basis by filling in a widely available yellow card. Individual pharmaceutical companies carry out similar monitoring via 'post-marketing surveillance'. The Medical Devices Agency has recently developed a voluntary reporting scheme for adverse events associated with use of particular devices.

The four Confidential Inquiries run by the English Department of Health which audit selected causes of death (stillbirths, perioperative deaths, maternal deaths, suicides) also fit under this heading. These provide an assessment of the relevant system and can indicate the need for more detailed inquiry. While adverse event reporting clearly has an important role to play, it also has severe limitations. First, the process means that only extreme events are likely to be detected. Second, reporting is usually voluntary. Third, lack of data on the totality of events means that rates cannot be estimated. Fourth, limited control population data prevents estimation of the relative magnitude of any effects. Finally, the necessary standardised definitions required for comparisons over time and place, are not always available.

Limited disease registers

This group includes long-standing disease registers, such as for the blind, deaf or physically handicapped. These differ from the registers classified in group Ia above by lacking data on health technologies. Such registers of the number of people who are blind or deaf are of no use for assessing current health technologies.

Health surveys

Health surveys provide data on health status, but without identifying either patients or health technologies. Without linkage to health technologies these datasets have little to offer health technology assessment. Some surveys such as the Health Survey for England collect data on patient health states and on prescribed drug use.

Type IV: Census-Related Datasets

The decennial Census of Population which contains several questions on long-standing illness must be included in any inventory of datasets, not least because it provides the population denominator for all epidemiological analyses. Beyond this, a number of long-standing studies based on record linkage to the Census have developed, most notably the Longitudinal Study, which links an anonymised 1% of the 1971 Census to subsequent censuses, and to vital events (deaths, births) using the NHS Central Register. Only by linkage to datasets which identify a health technology can such datasets be used to assess health technologies, and then mainly for assessment of equity/diffusion and for effectiveness as captured by mortality.

Linkage-Enabling Systems

The two main UK linkage-enabling systems are Central Health Register Inquiry Service (CHRIS) and postcodes. Linkage by CHRIS by means of the NHS number enables records with that number to be linked. The most immediate scope applies to Hospital Episode Statistics, along the lines of the Oxford Record Linkage Study. As the use of the NHS number gradually extends to cover other health services, more integrated records can be built up. The new NHS number, which became mandatory in 1997, will in time, assuming full coverage and accuracy, enable greatly improved linkage.

Assessing the Cost of Health Technologies

Assessing the costs of health technologies requires a similar set of distinctions between datasets as discussed above. Cost-related datasets can be classified by the extent to which they can identify a health technology and attribute a price or unit cost to it.

Four different types of cost-related routine datasets can be distinguished:

(a) *Health technology* plus *unit cost*, that is unit costs (or prices) which are directly linked to specific health technologies, with subclassifications linked to levels of patient treatment.

(b) *Grouped health technology plus unit cost.* These are the unit costs of groups of different, related health technologies or treatments.

(c) *Linkable unit costs*, that is unit costs based on combining of two datasets, at least one of which is routine.

(d) *Survey unit costs*, that is unit costs based on special surveys, whether one-off or repeated or updated annually.

Remarkably few cost-related datasets specify health technologies. Of the 127 NHS Financial Returns for England only eight could be linked to health technologies. Two main exceptions exist – the costs of drugs dispensed by GPs (as published by the Prescription Pricing Authority) and the English NHS acute hospital reference costs.

Health Technology plus Unit Costs

The most readily available unit costs are prices, which apply when the NHS purchases a technology from some other organisation. Prices for products purchased from the pharmaceutical industry provide the obvious example.

Routine data on unit costs of non-drug health technologies has historically been much less common. The National Schedule of Reference Costs[34] provides data on cost per surgical health-related group (HRG) in each acute NHS hospital trust in England. Since HRGs are based on the HES data, their level of specificity is limited by the coding systems used there. The aim is to roll out this approach to costing the medical specialities and to reconcile the data with Trust annual accounts[35] – which should improve the accuracy of HRG costs. HRGs can be divided into those which identify a single technology, such as total hip replacement, and those which comprise a group of technologies. The former fit group (a) in being health technology plus unit cost, while the latter make up group (b) grouped health technology plus unit cost.

Grouped Health Technology Unit Costs

HRG unit costs that refer to a group of health technologies, typically surgical interventions, in a particular specialty are similar to the average cost per FCE per specialty which has long been available via the Trust Financial Return 2 (TFR2). Health technology assessments have tended to use these in both cost per finished consultant episode and per in-patient day. Many but not all of the non-surgical costed HRGs provide unit costs for similar groups of cases (casemix), which necessitates further estimation to obtain the unit costs of particular interventions.

Linked Health Technology Unit Costs

Many cost evaluations of health technologies (other than drugs and hospital stays) have had to improvise, either by combining customised data with routine data or by special surveys. Examples of the former include those evaluations which have combined data on number and duration of contacts with healthcare personnel and valued these using national pay scales. The most usual source for pay scales has been the Annual Pay Review Body Reports[d].[36,37] Any moves to local pay levels would pose problems for this approach. The reported 14 ways of costing a GP consultation[38] result from the lack of agreed routines in use of such data. However, standardised estimates are now produced annually for these and a range of other personnel such as district nurses and health visitors.[39]

Survey Health Technology Unit Costs

The annual report from the Personal Social Services Research Unit 'Unit costs of community care',[39] provides an example of the use of surveys to establish unit costs. This important source contains unit costs not only for consultations but also for packages of care such as for mental health services. Estimated on a standardised basis, these rely heavily on surveys carried out for research projects. A major advantage is its use of consistent and transparent methods for deriving unit costs.

This group of datasets might also include individual examples of bottom-up costing to the extent that such costing is achieved without use of any routine data. Although such an approach is recommended in recent guidelines,[40] few UK studies have attempted this.

CONCLUSIONS

This chapter has suggested that the potential use of routine data varies by type of HTA. While there is scope for the use of routine data in each of the three types of HTA we have distinguished, i.e. the measurement of efficacy and effectiveness, of equity and diffusion and of costs, that scope is greater the less the focus of the HTA is on efficacy. Where possible, efficacy should be assessed in trials, partly because of requirements in relation to measurement of health status but particularly in relation to controlling for confounding and bias. Routine data-sets have an essential role in monitoring effectiveness, especially where large and long-term pragmatic trials are not possible. To play this role however, they need development. For assessment of equity and diffusion and for costing, routine data are widely used, but may also need development.

A major encouraging theme emerging from the review of routine datasets was the growth of high-quality technology-specific clinical datasets in the UK. These offer scope for assessing the effectiveness of key technologies, as well as assessing diffusion and equity. Few of these databases include costs, however.

Information technology is rapidly increasing the scope for use of routine data in health technology assessment. The increasing data capture of details (capta) of healthcare using computers is transforming the meaning of routine data. Although healthcare spending on computerisation has lagged other sectors,[41] there are already signs of how healthcare is being transformed. Electronic patient records, computerised work stations, bar-coding, use of smart cards, and telemedicine are only some of the key developments. Improved methods of coding (Read) and grouping (Healthcare Resource Groups), again relying on information technology, may facilitate extraction and collation of real-time data which may for the first time contain clinical health state data. The sensitivity and specificity of these data will depend on the underlying coding systems used, which will always be partly out of date and hence of less relevance for new health technologies. The challenge may be around how best to absorb and interpret the enormous amount of routine data that will shortly be available within healthcare. Health technology assessment has the opportunity to become routinised to the extent that it rises to this challenge.

For the above reasons, the common equations 'routine = rubbish' and 'customised = good' is much too simple. The scope for reliable, validated routine data is increasing rapidly, and there are examples of excellent datasets which have already been used for assessing health technologies such as IVF. That said, it must be noted that the bulk of routine administrative datasets collected by the NHS (and other health systems) are of no use to health technology assessment. Ideally to be useful for health technology assessment, a dataset should identify a health technology, the patient, the health status and its unit cost. One UK dataset which has long identified unit cost – that from the Prescription Pricing Authority – lacks any data on patients, thus precluding any information on health status or equity. Some of the more recent developments with registry-type datasets could include unit cost, but none does so at present.

For assessment of equity and diffusion, routine datasets provide clear indications of differential patterns of service use. Ingenuity in linking these to other datasets, notably to the Census of Population, has indicated problems and led to policy changes (e.g. capitation formula based on linking census to hospital use data).

Finally, a number of issues require attention if routine datasets are to fulfil the potential outlined above. Those databases collecting data on health technology, patients and health status need to be supported, perhaps initially by means of a strategic overview. The scope for greater linkage of datasets requires active exploration, including facilitation and monitoring of the use of the unique patient identifiers. The gaps in existing datasets must be addressed. These, we have suggested are largely around diagnostic activity, medical procedures in hospital and outpatient and ambulatory activity. Regular surveys of organisation and delivery of care, such as stroke units, should be seen as part of routine intelligence. The lack of data in the UK from the private sector needs to be remedied. More systematic surveillance of adverse events needs to be encouraged, including use of standardised definitions and fuller coverage. Improved training should be provided in the use of routine datasets and their potential use in the different kinds of health technology assessment.

NOTES

a. The *Shorter Oxford English Dictionary* defines 'routine' as follows:

'1.a. Routine- a regular course of procedure, a more or less mechanical or unvarying performance of certain acts or duties.
1.b. A set form of speech, a regular set or series (of phrases etc)
2. regular, unvarying or mechanical procedure or discharge of duties'.

b. Literature searches provided very few references under 'routine data' but very many under 'administrative data', particularly from countries whose healthcare systems generate masses of administrative data (notably the US).

c. The term 'Datasets' is used to refer to excerpts from databases. In the past, datasets were often published one-off analyses of paper based datasets. The computerisation of databases means that what matters in assessing their usefulness is the extent to which the relevant fields are included, such as use of a health technology, patient identification, and outcomes.

d. Both the Review Body for Nursing Staff, Midwives, Health Visitors and Professions Allied to Medicine and the Review Body for Doctors and Dentists Remuneration publish annual reports which include data on pay scales.

References

1. Templeton A, Morris J K, Parslow W. Factors that affect outcome of in vitro fertilisation treatment. *Lancet* 1996; **348**: 1402–6.
2. Royal College of Obstetrics and Gynaecology. How to treat the infertile couple. London: RCOG, 1998. (available at http://www.rcog.org.uk/guidelines/secondary.html)
3. National Health Service Executive Leeds. Quality and Performance in the NHS: Clinical Indicators. Leeds: NHSE, 1999. (available at http://www.doh.gov.uk/dhhome.htm)
4. Dowling B. Effect of fundholding on waiting times: database study. *Br. Med. J.* 1997; **315**: 290–2.
5. Baines D, Tolley K, Whynes DK. *Prescribing, budgets and fundholding in general practice.* London: Office of Health Economics, 1997.
6. Raftery J, Stevens A. Day case surgery trends in England: the influences of target setting and of general practitioner fundholding. *Journal of Health Service Research and Policy* 1998; **3**: 149–52.
7. Warren KS, Mosteller F (eds). Doing more harm than good: the evaluation of health care interventions. *Ann. N. Y. Acad. Sci.* 1993; **703**: 1–341.
8. Sheldon T. Please bypass the PORT. *Br. Med. J.* 1994; **309**: 142–3.
9. NHSE Leeds. Central Data Collections from the NHS. HSC 1999; 070. (www.open.gov.uk/doh/outlook/htm)
10. Central Statistics Office. *Guide to Official Statistics.* London: CSO, 1997.
11. Last JM. *A Dictionary of Epidemiology.* Oxford: Oxford University Press, 1988.
12. Knox EG. Information needs in public health. In: Holland WW, Detels R, Knox G (eds). *Oxford Textbook of Public Health*, 2nd edn. Oxford: Oxford University Press, 1991.
13. Ashley JSA, Cole SK, Kilbane MP. Health information resources in the United Kingdom. In: Detels R, Holland W, McEwan J. Omenn G (eds). *Oxford Textbook of Public Health*, 3rd edn. Oxford: Oxford University Press, 1997.
14. Wing J. *Health Services Planning and Research – contributions from psychiatric case registers.* London: Gaskell, 1989.
15. Wolfe CDA, Taub NA, Woodrow J, Richardson E, Warburton FG, Burney PGJ. Patterns of acute stroke care in three districts in southern England. *J. Epidemiol. Community Health* 1993; **47**: 144–8.
16. Raftery J. Economics of psychiatric services in counties of the UK 1845–1985. Unpublished PhD Thesis, University of London, 1993.
17. Botting B, Reilly H, Harris D. The OPCS records in medical research and clinical audit. *Health Trends* 1995; **27**: 4–7.
18. Williams B, Nicholl J. Patient characteristics and clinical workload of short stay independent hospitals in England & Wales 1992/3. *Br. Med. J.* 1994; **308**: 1699–701.
19. Audit Commission. *Setting the record straight. A study of hospital medical records.* London: Audit Commission, 1995.
20. Information for Health: an information strategy for the Modern NHS 1998–2005. Leeds: NHS Executive, 1998. (http://www.doh.gov.uk/dhhome.htm)
21. Goldacre M. Cause specific mortality. *J. Epidemiol. Community Health* 1993; **47**: 491–6.
22. Newcombe HB. *Handbook of Record Linkage.* Oxford: Oxford University Press, 1988.
23. Israel RA. The history of the International Classification of Diseases. *Health Trends* 1990; **22**: 43–4.
24. Campbell JR, Carpenter P, Sneiderman C, Cohn S, Chute CG, Warren J. Phase II evaluation of clinical coding schemes: completeness, taxonomy, mapping, definitions, and clarity. CPRI Work Group on Codes and Structures. *J. Am. Med. Informatics Assoc.* 1997; **4**: 238–51.
25. Department of Health. *Assessing the Effects of Health Technologies: Principles, Practice, Proposals.* London: Department of Health, 1992.
26. Office of Technology Assessment, U.S. Congress. *Development of medical technology: Opportunities for assessment.* Washington DC: U.S. Government Printing Office, 1976. Quoted in Klawansky S, Antczak-Bouckoms A, Burdick E, Roberts MS, Wyshak G, Mosteller F. Using Medical Registries and data sets for Technology Assessment: an overview of seven case studies. *International Journal of Technology Assessment in Health Care* 1991; **7**: 194–9.
27. Sheldon TA. Problems of using modelling in economic evaluation of health care. *Health Economics* 1996; **5**: 1–11.
28. Black N. Why we need observational studies to evaluate the effectiveness of health care. *Br. Med. J.* 1996; **312**: 1215–18.
29. Stochart DH, Long, AJ, Porter, ML. Joint responsibility: the need for a national arthroplasty register. *Br. Med. J.* 1996; **313**: 66–7.
30. Carr-Hill R, Hardman G, Martin S, et al. A formula for distributing NHS revenues based on small area use of hospital beds. York: Centre for Health Economics, Univ. of York, 1994.
31. Hansluwka H, Chrzanowski RS, Gutzwiller F, Paccaud F. Importance of databases for technology assessment. *Health Policy* 1988; **9**: 277–84.
32. Clarke A, McKee M, Appleby J, Sheldon T. Efficient purchasing [editorial]. *Br. Med. J.* 1993; **307**: 1436–7.
33. Mant J, Mant F, Winner S. How good is routine information? Validation of coding of acute stroke

in Oxford hospitals. *Health Trends* 1997; **29**: 96–9.

34. NHS Executive. The National Schedule of Reference Costs (NSRC) and National Reference Cost Index (NRCI). Leeds: NHSE 1999. (available on http://www.doh.gov.uk/dhhome.htm)

35. Raftery J. Benchmarking costs in the NHS. *Journal of Health Service Research and Policy* 1999; **4**: 63–4.

36. Review Body for Nursing Staff, Midwives, Health Visitors and Professions Allied to Medicine. London: Department of Health, annually.

37. Review Body for Doctors and Dentists. London: Department of Health, annually.

38. Graham B, McGregor K. What does a GP consultation cost? *Br. J. Gen. Pract.* 1997; **47**: 170–2.

39. Netten A, Dennett J. Unit costs of community care PSSRU. Univ. of Kent, annual 1998.

40. Gold M, Siegel J, Russell L, Weinstein M. *Cost effectiveness in health and medicine*. Oxford University Press, 1996.

41. Anonymous. Healthcare lags in spending on information technology. *Financial Times*, 23 November, 1998.

9

Using Routine Data to Complement and Enhance the Results of Randomised Controlled Trials

JAMES D. LEWSEY, GORDON D. MURRAY,
ALASTAIR H. LEYLAND and F. ANDREW BODDY

SUMMARY

This chapter considers ways of using routinely collected data as a means of enhancing information from clinical trials. This may be done through the sharpening of treatment comparisons – either by using the routine data as the entire basis of analysis in situations in which ethical or other constraints mean that trials are not feasible, or as a supplement to trial data, for example during subsequent meta-analysis. Alternatively, such data may be used as a means of exploring the impact of randomised controlled trials (RCTs) on clinical practice and patient outcomes through an examination of the uptake of new technologies, or through the monitoring of outcomes in subpopulations, where routine data are particularly beneficial for rare conditions or when rare or long-term outcomes are being considered.

Two case studies were selected to illustrate the potential of routine data for these purposes. The first of these was a study of the timing of surgery following aneurysmal subarachnoid haemorrhage as a way of informing the design of a trial of early versus late surgery. The second was a study comparing percutaneous transluminal coronary angioplasty with coronary artery bypass grafting as approaches to coronary revascularisation, with the routine data being used to augment information available from a meta-analysis of randomised clinical trials and also to explore the uptake and impact of the two procedures.

The routine data present problems regarding their adequacy and precision for the two studies, but can still be used to complement trials in the intended manner. However, they also provide valuable information concerning the context of trials: in terms of the epidemiology of subarachnoid haemorrhage and, in the case of coronary revascularisation, providing detail as to the treatment and subsequent outcomes of those patients who would not meet eligibility criteria for trials.

INTRODUCTION

It is widely acknowledged that the randomised controlled trial (RCT) is the best available tool for evaluating the risks and benefits of medical interventions. There are, however, many situations where for ethical or other more pragmatic reasons it is not feasible to conduct an RCT. For example, a randomised trial of delivery by caesarean section would be considered unethical, despite the existence of large unexplained differences in rates between consultants or obstetric units.[1] Similarly, a trial investigating a rare outcome or side-effect (such as common bile duct injury in laparoscopic cholecystectomy, or deep vein thrombosis in low-risk surgical groups) may require so many patients to detect a clinically relevant difference that the costs of a study would be difficult to justify in terms of its potential benefits.

When a trial is feasible, its design is generally based on specifying the desired power and significance levels. Routine data may allow reliable estimates of the treatment effect likely to be observed in a clinical trial, with the consequence that power calculations will be more accurate or realistic. Estimating the 'patient horizon' (the number of present and future patients, including those taking part in the trial) can only be done realistically by using routine data; this has implications not only for the estimation of sample size but also for the method of treatment assignment.[2]

Even when trials have been completed, important questions are often left unanswered. For example, the use of angiotensin-converting enzyme (ACE) inhibitors following an acute myocardial infarction is arguably one of the most comprehensively researched questions in clinical medicine, and yet it is still unclear whether the use of such drugs should be restricted to 'high-risk' patients. Equally, it is not clear how soon the treatment should be initiated after the myocardial infarction, or for how long it should be continued.[3,4] Data also exist which show that in spite of overwhelming evidence of the efficacy of these drugs, their uptake is very low.[5,6]

There is thus a need to augment information from clinical trials: this project explores the uses of routine NHS data in this context. We examine the use of routine data, firstly, as a way of 'sharpening' the treatment comparisons derived from RCTs, either by informing the trial design, or – more directly – by using routine data to estimate treatment effects and, secondly, as a means of exploring the impact of RCTs on clinical practice and patient outcomes.

Sharpening Treatment Comparisons

Although RCTs may be the only unambiguous method of equalising risk among groups of patients receiving different treatments,[7] there may be ethical or financial constraints which mean that RCTs are not feasible; in these situations, forming pseudo-trials from routine data is an alternative. There are limitations and problems associated with this approach: routine data sets tend to include limited information on potential confounding variables (such as educational status or smoking), and the allocation of patients to treatments will tend to reflect clinical factors whose effects cannot be fully captured in a covariate adjustment.[8]

Routine data may also be used as a supplement to clinical trials for subsequent Bayesian analysis. This may be for a specific trial, when the data provide prior information regarding the expected outcomes of one or more of the treatment groups, or during subsequent meta-analysis, when the routine data may be regarded as comprising a large single or multi-centre trial. Such analyses take the form of a weighted average of the information provided by the routine data set and that provided by the trial, with the weighting depending on both the numbers involved (favouring routine data) and the likelihood of bias (favouring RCT data).[9]

Routine data may be used before a trial begins by providing estimates of likely event rates or even treatment effects. They can thus be of value when performing power calculations, estimating sample sizes or deciding when to stop a trial. The decision to stop or continue a trial is made by weighing the consequences of the possible actions, averaging over the distribution of future observations.[10] Observational data can then be used in conjunction with trial data to improve estimates of the probability that an apparent difference occurred by chance, leading to the trial being either stopped early or continued until decisive evidence has been accumulated.

The Impact and Uptake of New Technologies

After the initial introduction of new technology, there is a period before it becomes a recommended treatment during which its use may be refined and clinicians gain experience with it. Little is known about the rate of uptake of new technologies and the factors which influence this process. As an example, fewer than 10% of hospitals in Pennsylvania were using laparoscopic cholecystectomy one year after the introduction of the technique; after a further year, this proportion had increased to 80%.[11]

When an RCT recommends the uptake of a new technology, it anticipates an expected improvement in outcomes. Routine data make it possible to examine observed outcomes and to evaluate whether the expected benefits have been realised. This may be in terms of the difference between alternative treatments (current and historical) or differences between centres and subgroups of patients. If a treatment is recommended for a particular subpopulation, then it is possible to assess the extent to which appropriate patients have been targeted, whether the benefits are also seen in other subpopulations and whether there has been a change in trends in outcomes (such as survival rates).

Large routine data sets also permit assessments of the importance of an RCT result, particularly for rare conditions or when rare outcomes are being considered.

Case Studies

The two key areas in which routinely assembled data have uses in the field of clinical trials are for improving treatment comparisons and for assessing the generalisability and impact of the results of RCTs. The two case studies presented below illustrate their potential for:

(a) sharpening treatment comparisons: as an aid to power calculations; as the entire basis of an analysis; or as a supplement to a meta-analysis; and

(b) putting trial results into context in terms of: the representativeness of their populations; the uptake of new technologies; and the impact of new technologies on outcomes.

LINKED SCOTTISH MORBIDITY RECORDS

General Description

The data for the two case studies were taken from the linked hospital discharge and mortality data set created by the Information and Statistics Division of the NHS in Scotland.[12] Summaries of hospital in-patient episodes are completed on Scottish Morbidity Record Form 1 (SMR1) for 100% of non-psychiatric and non-obstetric in-patient and day cases in Scotland, and provide some information about the background of the patient as well as detailing case management, diagnoses and surgical procedures. The data are linked by individuals and are also linked to statutory death records from the Registrar General for Scotland and registrations in the Scottish Cancer Register. They provide information about hospital care and mortality for individuals in the whole Scottish population for the period 1981–1995, and are unique in Britain. Because the SMR1 records and the death records both include the individual's postcode sector of residence, they can be related to population denominators and socio-demographic area descriptions derived from the 1991 census. The content of these records is listed in Table 1.

Selection of Case Studies

The scope of the data meant that we were restricted to considering surgical interventions; other interventions are not recorded. Although desirable in the light of current debate, it would

Table 1   *Data recorded on SMR1*

Data item	Comment
Patient 'identifier'	Not permitting the identification of individual patients, but a unique number which permits linkage of hospital discharge, death and cancer registry records
Continuous in-patient stay marker	SMR1 forms are completed for each episode of care; a patient may have several episodes within a period of hospital stay
Hospital code	The identifier for the hospital attended
Area of residence	Health Board, Local Government District, postcode sector and census enumeration district
Age	The patient's age in months
Sex	
Marital status	
Admitted from	Home, other NHS hospital, other unit in this hospital, other
Type of admission	Deferred, waiting list/diary/booked, repeat admission, transfer, emergency
Wait	Days on the waiting list
Discharge code	Irregular (e.g. self discharge), home, convalescent hospital or home, other hospital, local authority care, transfer to other specialty in same hospital, died
Date of admission	
Date of discharge	
Date of operation	
Length of stay	
Specialty	
Diagnoses	Up to six diagnoses, coded using ICD9 (WHO, 1997)[38]
Operation	Up to four procedures, coded using OPCS4 (OPCS, 1987)[22]

not have been possible, for example, to use the linked SMR1 database to investigate the uptake of thrombolysis for the treatment of acute myocardial infarction.

Given this restriction, we chose first to study the timing of surgery following aneurysmal subarachnoid haemorrhage (SAH) as a way of informing the design of a trial of early versus late surgery. The second study compares percutaneous coronary angioplasty (PTCA) with coronary artery bypass grafting (CABG) as approaches to coronary revascularisation. This latter study illustrates the use of routine data to augment a meta-analysis of RCT data, and to explore the uptake and impact of the two procedures.

CASE STUDY 1: THE TIMING OF SURGERY AFTER SUBARACHNOID HAEMORRHAGE

Introduction

Spontaneous aneurysmal subarachnoid haemorrhage is a common and often devastating event: there are approximately 6000 cases each year in the United Kingdom. The case fatality rate is of the order of 40%, and there is significant residual morbidity in about 50% of survivors.[13–16] In about two-thirds of cases the haemorrhage results from the rupture of an aneurysm on a major cerebral blood vessel but, even after complete angiography, no source can be identified in about 25% of cases.[14] This risk is greatest in the few days following the initial haemorrhage but operative intervention can be technically more difficult in this period, and the patient may be less able to withstand the added trauma of surgery. For these reasons, there is controversy about the optimal timing of surgical interventions.

Epidemiology

Epidemiological reports suggest that the incidence of SAH is of the order of 10 to 15 cases per 100 000 population per year, although more recent reports yield estimates in the range of six to eight cases per 100 000 per year. A recent meta-analysis[15] reviews this literature and shows that the apparent fall in incidence can be explained by more precise diagnosis, following the wider availability of computed tomography (CT) scanning. SAH is more common in women (unselected series are typically 60% female). There is strong evidence that genetic factors predispose individuals to the risk of SAH, and some populations have much higher incidence rates: Finland, for example, has an incidence

rate that is almost three times greater than those of other parts of the world.[15]

Clinical Presentation

With a major haemorrhage, consciousness is lost rapidly, and death can occur very quickly. Smaller leaks lead to a severe headache, with a characteristic rapid onset. Despite its characteristic presentation, SAH is commonly misdiagnosed[17–19] – more severe cases with headache, vomiting and neck stiffness can be diagnosed as meningitis, resulting in admission to an infectious diseases unit – but misdiagnosis can have serious outcomes because a minor 'warning leak' may precede a potentially devastating rupture, which could have been prevented by early intervention.[14]

Diagnosis

CT scanning is the key initial investigation: if the scan is performed within 24 hours of the onset of symptoms, then a high-density clot in the subarachnoid space will be identified in over 90% of cases,[14] but diagnostic sensitivity declines progressively after the first day. A negative CT scan should be followed by a diagnostic lumbar puncture; if this is also negative then the diagnosis of a warning leak is effectively excluded and the prognosis is excellent. If a positive diagnosis of SAH is reached, then cerebral angiography is the next standard investigation to identify the source of the haemorrhage.

Timing of Surgery

The only published randomised trial of the timing of surgery[20] randomised a total of 216 patients to: acute surgery (days 0–3); intermediate surgery (days 4–7); or late surgery (day 8 or later). Only good grade patients (Grades I to III according to the Hunt and Hess classification[21]) were recruited, but in this selected subgroup – and in what was an under-powered trial – there was some evidence to support acute surgery. This conclusion appears to reflect current practice, where there has been a drift towards early surgery, especially for patients in a good clinical condition.[14]

Endovascular techniques as an alternative to clipping intracranial aneurysms have evolved over the last 10–15 years. The aneurysm is occluded either by inflating a detachable balloon, or by releasing coils of platinum wire to induce thrombosis. The 'state of the art' is arguably the Guglielmi Detachable Coil device

(GDC) which has been available in North America since 1991 and in Europe since 1992. Uncontrolled series have provided encouraging results, especially with patients in poor clinical condition or with difficult surgical aneurysms. Formal evaluation of the GDC device continues, most notably in a MRC-funded trial of coiling versus conventional surgery (ISAT – International Subarachnoid Aneurysm Trial).

SMR1 Data in the Study of SAH

Against this background, there was a sequence of questions that it seemed possible to explore using the linked SMR1 data. These were, first, whether it was possible to describe the epidemiology of the condition in the whole population and thus establish a context for its management in specialist centres and the outcomes they achieved. Second, given the problem of misdiagnosis and the sequence of events needed to establish a definitive diagnosis prior to surgical intervention, was it possible to describe the patterns of care on which the practice of specialised centres was actually based? Third, acknowledging the difficulties in conducting formal trials of one form of intervention or another, could the SMR1 data be used to describe patients treated by the open clipping of aneurysms with those treated by embolisation? What had been the pattern of uptake of the newer embolisation treatment? Finally, providing that satisfactory answers could be found for these questions, was it possible to devise a pseudo-trial of early or late interventions?

It quickly became evident that the SMR1 data presented a number of difficulties in addressing these questions. One was that of identifying 'true' cases of SAH amongst multiple patient transfers either between hospitals or between specialities within a hospital. It was not uncommon, for example, to have an initial diagnosis of meningitis which changed to SAH in a subsequent episode record, or an initial diagnosis of SAH meriting transfer to a neurosurgical unit where the diagnosis of SAH is subsequently refuted. What were the criteria for accepting a diagnosis of SAH, and at what stage in a patient's history should they be applied? This question was complicated further by the lack of a record of the onset of symptoms or of the patient's condition on admission to hospital or later deterioration. This meant that it was not possible to discern what had been the *intended* management of the patient: was early surgery planned or would this be the consequence of a further haemorrhage? Although death was available as an outcome measure, there was no other information about the patient's condition on discharge from hospital or subsequently.

There were other technical problems. In the SMR1 data, surgical interventions are coded according to the OPCS codes with a change from OPCS3 to OPCS4 between 1988 to 1989;[22] codes for embolisation are only included in OPCS4 so that it was not possible to analyse the data for earlier periods. The form of the record makes it difficult to reconstruct sequences of operative events and so it was not always possible to distinguish between a definitive procedure to repair a ruptured aneurysm and the surgical treatment of a later complication.

With these qualifications, the potential of the SMR1 data for studying subarachnoid haemorrhage appeared to be:

(a) Epidemiology: the linked data and death records provide an opportunity for estimating the incidence of SAH, and the case fatality rate; the inclusion of place of residence allows the use of Census-derived population denominators.

(b) Admissions to neurosurgical units: the linkage of 'episode' data allows an account of the sequences of patient care – for example, the numbers of patients who died before being admitted to hospital, the numbers admitted to a neurosurgical unit, and their prior in-patient care. Doing so can provide a useful account of admission policies, although the absence of data on the patients' clinical state limits this capability.

(c) Timing of surgery: the data report the numbers of patients undergoing clipping of an aneurysm, and the timing of surgery can be related to the date of first hospital admission. Linking this information to the date of death allows the construction of best- and worst-case scenarios for early surgery versus late surgery.

(d) Other treatments: the potential of SMR1 data to investigate other treatments is limited because, for example, information about drugs is not included. The data could have uses, for example, for exploring changes in case fatality rates following the publication (in the late 1980s) of evidence about the value of nimodipine in reducing cerebral infarction.

The case study we describe focussed on the uses of these data as a means of assessing the optimal timing of surgical interventions.

Methods

For the reasons we describe above, subgroups reflecting different degrees of confidence in the diagnosis of SAH were extracted from the complete SMR1 data set. The main analysis was restricted to records from 1989–95, when surgical interventions were coded according to OPCS4. The data were for the whole of Scotland, with no attempt to compare the different neurosurgical units involved.

The first sample (Sample I) comprised all cases of *suspected SAH*, defined as all cases with a primary diagnosis of SAH not otherwise specified (ICD9 430.9) in an SMR1 record or as the principal cause in a death record. A total of 4903 cases were identified, comprising 1796 males (37%) and 3107 females (63%); this total provides an incidence rate of 13.7 per 100 000 population per year.

Sample I consisted of three disjoint subsamples: (i) individuals with a death record but no record of hospital admission for SAH; (ii) individuals admitted to hospital but not to a neurosurgical unit during the relevant continuous in-patient stay (CIS); and (iii) patients who were admitted to a neurosurgical unit during the relevant CIS. We then excluded two subgroups of patients where it might be argued that the diagnosis of SAH had not been established, to obtain Sample II which can be considered as cases of *presumed SAH*. For patients who were hospitalised but not admitted to a neurosurgical unit, we excluded cases where the final SMR1 record did not mention SAH as any of the recorded diagnoses. When patients had been admitted to a neurosurgical unit, we excluded cases where there was no primary diagnosis of SAH for the records relating to the period of neurosurgical care. These two rules excluded 51 male and 478 female cases, leaving Sample II with 4374 cases of presumed SAH. This total provides an annual incidence of 12.3 cases per 100 000 population.

Sample III comprised all individuals in Sample I who were admitted to a neurosurgical unit – that is, *patients with suspected SAH admitted to neurosurgery*. This sample was further reduced to 3091 individuals comprising 1163 males (38%) and 1928 females (62%). This sample provided a means of exploring the admission policies of the different neurosurgical units.

The final Sample IV included individuals from Sample II who were admitted to a neurosurgical unit – that is, *patients with a presumed SAH who were treated in a neurosurgical unit*. This sample comprised 2613 individuals (949 males and 1664 females) and is the relevant sample for exploring the potential for trials of the timing of surgery or of embolisation. (One might, however, take a wider view and regard the admission policies of neurosurgical units as

needing review if trial populations are to be optimised.)

The Timing of Surgery

Patients who were treated within a neurosurgical unit for presumed SAH (Sample IV) comprised 2613 individuals, of whom 1628 (62.3%) underwent surgery (when this was defined as clipping of the aneurysm). Figure 1 shows the distribution of the timing of surgery, in days from first hospital admission, and is virtually the same as the corresponding results from the International Co-operative Study on the Timing of Aneurysm Surgery,[23] although in the latter study the timing was from onset of symptoms of SAH rather than from admission to hospital.

Table 2 reports the numbers of patients undergoing clipping in each of three age groups (<45 years, 45–64 years, and ≥65 years): about half of those patients aged 64 or less underwent definitive procedures, but this proportion was only 32% for those at older ages. Figure 2 shows the timing of surgery for these three groups. It is clear that the tendency towards earlier surgical intervention decreases with increasing age; Figure 2c indicates that 15% of those aged 65 and over who underwent surgery were not operated on within two weeks of admission.

One-fifth of this sample died from any cause within 90 days of their first admission. Table 3 details 90-day survival for the three age groups, when again mortality was higher (32%) in the oldest group. There were only 61 deaths (5%) in the 1252 operated cases compared with 441 deaths (32%) amongst the 1361 patients who did not receive clipping. Table 4 shows the survival time following hospital admission for the two groups when 33% of cases with no operation compared to only 11% of those who did have operations died within three days of admission; 30% of deaths in the operated cases and 28% in the group who did not have operations occurred between 15 and 90 days after the first admission to a neurosurgical unit.

Table 5 shows the timing of the 61 operated deaths broken down according to the timing of surgery. Collectively, the tables allow one to perform various 'what if . . .?' calculations. Taking a very pessimistic view of early surgery, we could assume that all deaths following surgery performed within three days of admission could have been prevented if surgery had been delayed. This would have prevented 45 deaths (28 following surgery performed on days 0–1 and a further 17 following surgery performed on days 2–3), reducing the overall mortality rate for the whole sample of 2613 patients from 19.2%

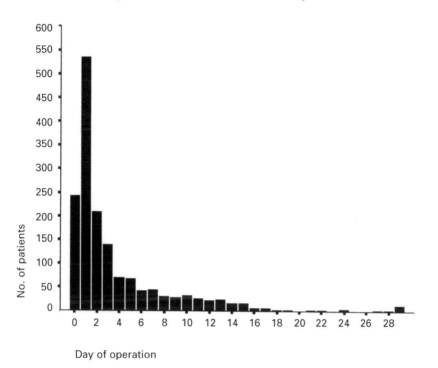

Figure 1 *Distribution of timing of surgery, in days from first hospital admission to clipping of the aneurism.*

to 17.5%. In contrast, by taking a very optimistic view of early surgery, we could assume that all deaths in unoperated patients occurring from day 2 to day 10 could have been prevented by early surgery, and that deaths in patients operated on after day 3 could have been prevented by early surgery. This would have prevented 190 deaths – 174 unoperated (Table 4) and 16 deaths among patients operated upon after day 3 (Table 5) – reducing the overall mortality rate from 19.2% to 11.9%.

These are extreme scenarios; in practical terms, they mean that a comparison between early and late surgery in an unselected neurosurgical population would require a trial with sufficient power to detect a reduction in mortality of the order of 1.7%. This implies a trial in which an unfeasibly large total sample size of about 21 800 would be needed in order to

achieve 90% power to detect a reduction in mortality from 19.2% to 17.5% at the 5% significance level. The SMR1 data could be used to refine these calculations – for example, by imposing an upper age limit on the trial population – but they would not permit more precise inclusion/exclusion criteria based on the patient's clinical state. These would be important considerations in the design of an actual trial.

CASE STUDY 2: CORONARY REVASCULARISATION

Introduction

Coronary artery bypass grafting (CABG) was first reported in 1968[24] as a technique for coronary revascularisation in patients with symptomatic coronary artery disease. There is strong evidence that the technique results in prolonged survival and improved quality of life in specific patient subgroups when the procedure is compared to medical therapies.[25] The rate of coronary artery surgery in the United Kingdom has risen steadily from 212 per million in 1986 to 341 per million in 1993–94.[26]

Percutaneous transluminal coronary angioplasty (PTCA) was described in 1979[27] as an

Table 2 *Number and proportion of patients undergoing surgery, according to age group*

Age group (years)	Number of patients	Number (proportion) undergoing surgery
<45	902	493 (54.7%)
45–64	1273	619 (48.6%)
≥65	438	140 (32.0%)

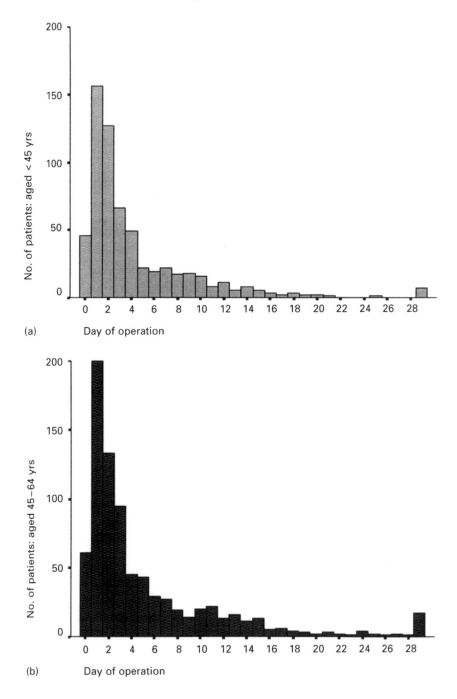

(a)   Day of operation

(b)   Day of operation

Table 3   *Number and proportion of patients dying within 90 days of their first admission to hospital, according to age group*

Age group (years)	Number of patients	Number (proportion) dying within 90 days of first admission
<45	902	123 (13.6%)
45–64	1273	241 (18.9%)
≥65	438	138 (31.5%)

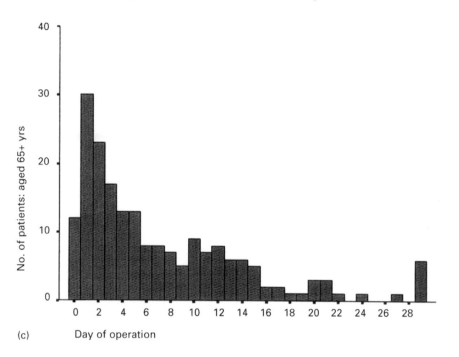

(c) Day of operation

Figure 2 *Distribution of timing of surgery, in days from first hospital admission to clipping of the aneurism, for (a) patients aged < 45 years, (b) patients aged 45–64 years and (c) patients aged 65+ years.*

Table 4 *Timing of deaths within the first 90 days following first admission to hospital, according to operational status*

Days to death	0–1	2–3	4–7	8–10	11–14	15–28	29–90	Total
Operated cases	2 (3%)	5 (8%)	13 (21%)	15 (25%)	8 (13%)	4 (7%)	14 (23%)	61 (100%)
Unoperated cases	100 (23%)	47 (11%)	62 (14%)	65 (15%)	44 (10%)	66 (15%)	57 (13%)	441 (100%)

Table 5 *Timing of deaths within the first 90 days following admission to first hospital for operated cases, according to timing of surgery*

Timing of surgery (days from first admission)	Days to death (days from first admission)							
	0–1	2–3	4–7	8–10	11–14	15–28	29–90	Total
0–1	2	5	7	5	4	1	4	28
2–3	–	0	5	6	2	2	2	17
4–7	–	–	1	4	1	0	2	8
8–10	–	–	–	0	0	0	3	3
11–14	–	–	–	–	1	0	2	3
15+	–	–	–	–	–	1	1	2
All operated cases	2 (3%)	5 (8%)	13 (21%)	15 (25%)	8 (13%)	4 (7%)	14 (23%)	61 (100%)

alternative revascularisation technique. It was used initially in patients with single vessel disease, but as the technology advanced the procedure has also been employed for patients with multi-vessel disease. A more recent development has been that of placing coronary stents as part of the PTCA procedure: it is estimated that more than 500 000 such procedures will take place worldwide in 1998. These will comprise between 60% and 90% of all PTCA procedures.[28]

Clearly, there are fundamental differences between the two techniques. With PTCA there is a risk of further stenosis as a result of elastic recoil, or from the progression of atherosclerosis. PTCA does, however, retain future options for revascularisation. CABG places venous conduits which are largely immune from advancing disease,[29] although they do tend to deteriorate over time. Repeating the bypass surgery can be compromised if the 'prime' veins have been used in an initial procedure.

The Evidence from Trials

There are several well-defined subgroups of patients where one or other procedure is clearly indicated, but there is a large 'grey area' where either procedure might be thought appropriate. Several clinical trials comparing CABG and PTCA as the first intervention in patients with symptomatic coronary artery disease have been conducted or are on-going. In 1995, a meta-analysis summarised the results of eight trials in which a total of 3371 patients (1661 CABG and 1710 PTCA) had been followed for a mean of 2.7 years.[30] The number of deaths was 73 in the CABG group and 79 in the PTCA group, resulting in a relative risk (RR) of 1.08 with a 95% confidence interval (CI) of 0.79 to 1.50. This number of deaths is too small for this result to establish the equivalence of the two mortality rates: a more sensitive comparison of the two procedures employed the composite end-point of cardiac death or non-fatal myocardial infarction (MI). The results of the eight trials were relatively consistent, with a total of 127 end-points in the CABG group during the first year compared to 135 end-points in the PTCA group (RR 1.03, 95% CI 0.84–1.27). Over the entire follow-up period there were 154 end-points in the CABG group and 169 in the PTCA group (RR 1.10, 95% CI 0.89–1.37). In contrast to these findings, there was evidence that CABG – relative to PTCA – gave better control of angina and required less frequent subsequent intervention. A subgroup analysis based on three of the eight trials suggested that CABG was to be preferred to PTCA in patients with single-vessel disease in terms of the end-point of cardiac death or non-fatal MI. This is, perhaps, a counter-intuitive finding to be interpreted with caution given the very small number of events on which the subgroup analysis was based.

These findings are limited by the short follow-up period, and so it is helpful to consider the results of the BARI trial which had an average follow-up of 5.4 years.[31] The 5-year survival rate was 89.3% for the CABG group and 86.3% for the PTCA group ($P = 0.19$, 95% CI for difference -0.2% to 6.0%). Again, there is no strong evidence of a difference in outcomes, although the limited number of deaths is reflected in a wide confidence interval which does not exclude the possibility of a clinically relevant difference. A *post hoc* subgroup analysis suggested that CABG is to be preferred to PTCA in patients with treated diabetes.

Limitations of the Trial Data

In a commentary accompanying the Pocock meta-analysis, White pointed out that the trials of CABG versus PTCA leave many questions unanswered.[32] There is, firstly, the problem of generalising these findings: the trials have only randomised a minority of the patients who were eligible for revascularisation. Secondly, even when taken together in a meta-analysis, trials up to the present have been under-powered, and their results do not exclude what may be clinically relevant differences in mortality and or later myocardial infarction. Thirdly, there is the question of the most appropriate outcome measures: one could, for example, consider PTCA as a 'package' or a holding procedure, accepting as a 'cost' the possibility of further intervention in return for the perceived benefit of delaying a CABG procedure that it might not be possible to repeat. For this argument, follow-up periods of the trials have been too short, because CABG procedures would not be expected to fail for about six years. Fourth, there is the question of subgroup effects. Various trials have suggested that there are such effects, but none has had sufficient power to investigate this issue. This is a crucial difficulty because the clinical question is not so much a simple comparison of CABG with PTCA, but rather one of narrowing the indeterminate area between them by improving the identification of patients where one or other procedure is indicated. Finally, the trials report outcomes that may have been overtaken by major advances in the procedures themselves. Anaesthetic and surgical techniques have improved, and the use of stents in conjunction with PTCA is becoming widespread.[28] How relevant are comparisons of yesterday's technology for today's practice?

Some of these problems are inherent in any approach to health technology assessment. By definition, evaluation must lag behind the development of new technologies – in particular, and for questions of this kind, it takes time to accumulate adequate long-term follow-up data. Routine data do, however, have the potential to address some of these problems. They provide a powerful means of assessing the relationship of trial populations to the 'real world' from which they are drawn, and they have the potential for assembling much larger numbers of cases than can be achieved in trials. Routine data could be used to augment a meta-analysis of trial data, and could be used to explore subgroup effects.

SMR1 Data in the Study of Coronary Revascularisation: Limitations

In practice, several problems limited the usefulness of the linked SMR1 data for analysing the outcomes of coronary artery revascularisation. The first of these was that there was no definitive way to identify patients who were undergoing their first coronary revascularisation outwith the data themselves. The linked data had to be used to identify records of previous procedures; doing so was further complicated by the fact that an operative code for PTCA was not included in the OPCS3 codes (used before 1989) so that patients who had this procedure before this date could not be confidently identified. The records did not include a description of the patients' clinical state (specifically, the severity of angina). This information would have been invaluable as a way of stratifying case-mix, and in interpreting outcome measures. There was no record of the extent of the underlying pathology – particularly, whether patients had single or multiple-vessel disease, used in many trials as an entry criterion or as a stratifying factor. It was possible to approximate to this pathological classification by using procedure codes which permitted a distinction between single- or multiple-vessel interventions, whether for CABG or PTCA. Doing so introduced a degree of confounding because it was possible for patients with multi-vessel disease to have a first procedure performed on only one of the affected vessels.

SMR1 Data in the Study of Coronary Revascularisation: Their Potential

The two main limitations with trial data in this area are, first, that – even with meta-analysis – patient numbers are insufficient for detecting modest but relevant differences in mortality between the two procedures, and are inadequate for exploring subgroup effects. The length of follow-up is unlikely to detect late failures of CABG. A further problem is that trial subjects are highly selected and likely to be unrepresentative of the vast majority of patients who undergo coronary revascularisation. Hundreds of thousands of these operations are conducted

around the world each year, and so the poverty of trial data is an interesting commentary on the perceived importance of trials as a support for major invasive procedures when compared to those expected for pharmaceutical innovations. It is, of course, a reflection of differing regulatory standards and requirements.

Routine data do provide the potential to study very large numbers of patients, with prolonged follow-up. Unlike trial data, they also provide the opportunity to study epidemiological trends in the uptake of different procedures, and to characterise their use in the entire patient population. In this case study we describe these epidemiological aspects of their use briefly, but chiefly focus on trying to combine information from the routine data with the trial data in order to make formal comparisons of outcome following the two procedures.

Methods

The initial sample comprised all patients with an SMR1 record of CABG or PTCA between 1989 and 1995. These records were then divided between patients who had procedures for single- or multi-vessel disease on the basis of the OPCS4 operative codes. A subset of this sample was then generated to reflect as closely as possible the entry criteria for the major trials. Specifically, patients were excluded if there was a record of an earlier CABG (1981 onwards) or PTCA (1989 onwards), or if any of the following diagnoses were recorded as being present at the time of surgery: diseases of mitral valve (ICD9 394); diseases of aortic valve (ICD9 395); diseases of mitral and aortic valves (ICD9 396); acute myocardial infarction (ICD9 410); other diseases of endocardium (ICD9 424); cardiac dysrhythmias (ICD9 427); heart failure (ICD9 428); ill-defined descriptions and complications of heart disease (ICD9 429). Within the limits of the SMR1 data, these were patients undergoing their first coronary revascularisation. This subset became the 'Pseudo-RCT Sample' below. It included 12 238 individuals, of whom 8524 (70%) underwent CABG. Those failing to meet these criteria are described as the 'Excluded Sample' and comprised 2359 individuals, of whom 1825 (77%) underwent CABG.

Epidemiology: Coronary Revascularisation in Scotland between 1989 and 1995

Figure 3 plots the number of CABG and PTCA procedures undertaken in Scotland from 1989 to 1995 for patients in the 'Pseudo-RCT' sample. At 33 per 100 000, the rate of CABG operations

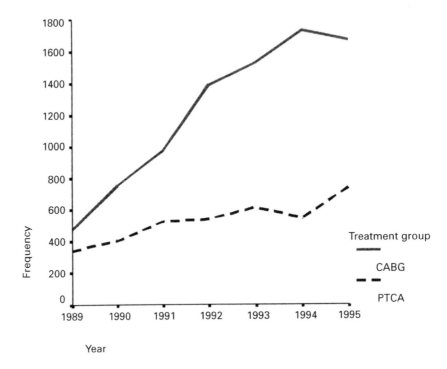

Figure 3   *Frequency of undertaking CABG and PTCA in Scotland, 1989 to 1995.*

was considerably greater in 1995 than the 9 per 100 000 in 1989; the rate for PTCA was 14 per 100 000 in 1995 – an increase from 7 per 100 000 in 1989. In absolute numbers, CABG was substantially greater than PTCA, and until 1994 the rate of increase was also greater for CABG. This increase was mostly attributable to the largest of the three main Scottish centres performing these operations.

An initial analysis, based on logistic regression, investigated case-mix differences between patients undergoing the two procedures. As expected, there was strong evidence of selection bias: female patients, patients with multi-vessel disease and patients with hypertension were more likely to receive CABG. Patients with a record of MI in the previous four weeks and patients with angina as a recorded co-morbidity were more likely to receive PTCA. This pattern was clearly evident in the 'Pseudo-RCT' sample, and even more apparent in the 'Excluded' sample.

Comparing RCT Subjects with 'Routine' CABG/PTCA Patients

Table 6 compares the baseline characteristics of the two samples derived from the SMR1 data with a major trial published after the Pocock meta-analysis,[31] and the three largest trials from the meta-analysis.[33–35] The 'Pseudo-RCT'

Table 6   *A comparison of the baseline characteristics between the routine data patients and four published trials*

	'Pseudo-RCT'	'Excluded'	BARI	CABRI	RITA	EAST
Number of patients	12 238	2359	1829	1054	1011	393
Mean age (years)	58	62	61	60	57	62
Female (%)	24	33	27	22	19	26
Diabetes mellitus (%)	7*	7*	25	12	6	23
Previous myocardial infarction (%)	40*	41*	55	43	43	41
Single-vessel disease (%)	43†	48†	2	1	45	0

* Determined from previous hospital admission.
† Determined from operation not diagnosis code.

Table 7   *Event rates for death and/or myocardial infarction within one year*

	Pseudo-RCT	Excluded	CABRI	RITA	EAST	GABI	Toulouse	MASS	Lausanne	ERACI
Total number of events	377	288	72	65	57	28	12	6	8	15
Event rates (%):										
CABG	3.7	13.6	5.7	6.2	18.4	10.2	7.9	1.4	3.0	10.9
PTCA	4.1	27.6	7.9	6.7	13.7	5.5	7.9	6.9	8.8	12.7

patients are broadly similar to the trial populations, although a major difference between the trials is whether or not they focussed on multivessel disease. The 'Excluded' sample had a higher proportion of females, but was otherwise broadly similar to the other populations.

Cardiac Death and/or Myocardial Infarction following CABG/PTCA

The primary end-point for the Pocock meta-analysis was cardiac death and/or MI within one year. Table 7 shows the relevant event rates in each of the trials from the meta-analysis, together with those from the two routine data samples. In general, the 'Pseudo-RCT sample had event rates for the two procedures that were lower than those for most individual trials. One might note, however, that the range of these rates across the eight trials was between 1.4% and 18.4% for CABG, and between 5.5% and 13.7% for PTCA, with only very small numbers of events in some studies. As expected, the event rates for the 'Excluded' sample were considerably higher.

The meta-analysis combining the results from these eight trials reported a relative risk for PTCA compared to CABG of 1.03 (95% confidence interval 0.84 to 1.27). A logistic regression was used to estimate this same relative risk, controlling for case-mix, for the 'Pseudo-RCT' sample. The point estimate was 1.15, with a 95% confidence interval of 0.90 to 1.48. A more detailed analysis, which modelled potential interactions between covariates and the treatment effect, provided evidence supporting an interaction with patients who had had a MI within four weeks prior to their intervention. This approach thus has the potential for exploring subgroups effects, which in this context are plausible a priori.[32]

Revascularisation following CABG/PTCA

Figure 4, derived from the Cox regression model, shows survival free from revascularisation in the CABG and PTCA groups, for the

'Pseudo-RCT' and 'Excluded' samples. It is clear that PTCA patients are far more likely to require reintervention than CABG patients. The BARI and EAST trials reported similar analyses, and the similarity in the shape of the survival curves from the two sources is striking. For the PTCA patients, the rate of reintervention was higher for the 'Pseudo-RCT' sample than for the 'Excluded' sample.

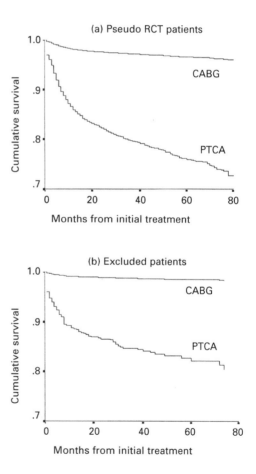

Figure 4   *Survival free from revascularisation in CABG and PTCA groups for (a) the 'Pseudo RCT' sample and (b) the 'Excluded' sample.*

Table 8   *Mortality rates at one year*

	Mortality rate		Relative risk (RR) PTCA:CABG	95% CI	Adjusted RR PTCA:CABG	95% CI
	CABG	PTCA				
'Pseudo-RCT' patients	3.2%	1.7%	0.54	0.40–0.73	0.68	0.49–0.93
'Excluded' patients	13.5%	7.1%	0.53	0.36–0.78	0.41	0.25–0.68

Table 9   *Mortality rates at five years*

	Mortality rate		Relative risk (RR) PTCA:CABG	95% CI	Adjusted RR PTCA:CABG	95% CI
	CABG	PTCA				
'Pseudo-RCT' patients	8.9%	7.2%	0.81	0.59–1.11	1.00	0.70–1.43
'Excluded' patients	27.0%	3.3%	0.12	0.03–0.48	0.12	0.03–0.59

Mortality following CABG/PTCA

Table 8 summarises mortality at one year for the 'Pseudo-RCT' and 'Excluded' groups, and Table 9 gives the corresponding results for deaths within 5 years. The 5-year results are based on relatively small numbers of cases from early in the study period. For the 'Pseudo-RCT' patients, both unadjusted and adjusted one-year outcomes show that the deaths among the CABG patients were significantly more frequent than those in the PTCA patients. This finding contrasts with the results from the randomised trials where, on the basis of substantially smaller numbers, no significant difference in mortality has been reported. The 1-year mortality rate of 3.2% for CABG patients is comparable to the rate of 2.7% reported in the CABRI trial. This trial reported a rate of 3.9% for the PTCA patients, however, and this is more than twice the rate observed for the 'Pseudo-RCT' patients.

In the 'Pseudo-RCT' sample, neither the unadjusted nor the adjusted results provide evidence of a difference in mortality at 5 years between the CABG and PTCA groups. This is consistent with the results from the randomised trials, but there is a similar pattern to that observed at 1 year: the 'Pseudo-RCT' mortality rate for CABG was similar to that observed in the randomised trials, but the rate for PTCA (at 7.2%) was lower than that reported for the BARI and EAST trials.

The results for the 'Excluded' patients show the expected high mortality rates in the CABG group. The low 5-year mortality rate for the 'Excluded' PTCA patients possibly reflects very careful selection of patients with complicated coronary disease in the early years of developing this procedure.

Synthesising Evidence

Continuing research on this topic is concerned with ways of combining the evidence on treatment differences from the routine data set with the evidence provided by the meta-analysis. Two Bayesian approaches are being developed.

1   To derive a posterior predictive distribution for the treatment difference based on the meta-analysis data. Compare this with the posterior (using a vague prior) distribution for the treatment difference based on the routine data in order to examine possible discrepancies.
2   To derive a posterior distribution from the routine data and use this as a prior for the meta-analysis. Doing so will allow investigation of the extent to which beliefs based solely on the routine data change in the light of evidence from the RCTs.

CONCLUSIONS AND RECOMMENDATIONS

The Uses of Routine Data

The case studies on which this chapter is based were undertaken to test the proposition that routinely assembled NHS data can either substitute for RCTs in situations where they are not feasible or can supplement the information that RCTs provide in assessing the benefits ensuing from new technologies or interventions. There are three main ways in which routine data can provide this supplementary function:

1   In situations where formal RCT designs are inappropriate – as in the SAH study.
2   For evaluating outcomes over longer periods or in a wider context than is practical even with meta-analyses – as in the CABG assessment.

3 By providing a link between the methodologically constrained conclusions of RCTs and their later adoption in health services practice.

The investigation of surgical interventions for SAH illustrates both the strengths and weaknesses of routine data as an alternative to RCTs: the major problem of the analysis we describe was simply the adequacy and precision of the data for the purposes of the enquiry. This is not a very surprising conclusion given that routine data are, at best, summaries of case records assembled for other (usually administrative) purposes. As we are able to demonstrate, however, the data do have value as a means of describing the epidemiological features of the condition, the patterns of surgical intervention relating to it, and rates of survival. The lack of additional data made it difficult to go beyond this stage (for example, in assessing outcomes other than death). In other ways, the data did not permit treatment comparisons that might have made it possible to address the question of the benefits of early or late surgery. This is not to say, however, that the study was without value in understanding the context of the original question. The need to develop case-definitions through different stages is illustrative of the ways in which RCT populations may not be typical of the complete diagnostic entity, and thus of the extent to which RCT findings can be generalised to expectations for the healthcare system as a whole. Whilst it may appear at first sight that there were 4903 instances of SAH, based upon the principal cause of death or the recorded primary diagnosis in hospital, further evidence available from routine data suggests that this may be an over-count. In 11% of such cases the diagnosis was altered in neurosurgery or prior to discharge from hospital if the patient was never admitted to neurosurgery, so only 89% of all the 'suspected' cases of SAH could be considered 'presumed' SAH. If the interest is in surgery, as in this case, the numbers are further limited since only 63% of all 'suspected' cases of SAH are admitted to neurosurgery, and just 53% of all 'suspected' cases may be considered 'presumed' SAH and are admitted to neurosurgery. Such a comment has a bearing on other possible uses of RCT findings – for example, as baseline standards for audit studies or as anticipated measures of hospital performance. Other uses of routine data are illustrated by the 'what if . . .' speculation we include as an indication of the trial conditions necessary to answer certain kinds of question. In this example, an almost impossibly large trial would be necessary in order to answer the question we first posed, given the gain in death rates suggested by the analysis of the routine data.

Two different kinds of question were posed for the second case study: firstly, were the outcomes promised by earlier trials achieved when these interventions were adopted in more routine practice; and secondly – against this background – was it possible to evaluate the relative uses and benefits of CABG and PTCA as complementary, rather than alternative, interventions? Both questions depended on earlier RCT findings, but both required longer follow-up and larger numbers than RCTs (even as meta-analyses) were likely to provide. As with SAH, initial analyses of the SMR1 records identified the lack of diagnostic precision necessary for formal RCT designs as a problem, but the study also illustrates the diffusion of procedure to other patients: 77% of the patients excluded from the 'Pseudo-RCT' we devised also underwent CABG.

This said, and with the exception of data about multi-vessel disease, it was possible to devise a sample of patients who were broadly similar to trial patients and to compare their outcomes with the results of RCTs – notably the meta-analysis of Pocock et al. Its importance is not (or not only) that it provides information that can be set alongside earlier RCT findings when these procedures are undertaken in the less precisely defined context of surgical practice. It is also an answer to the question of whether the potential for 'health gain' implicit in RCT results finds realisation in the wider healthcare system.

The Limitations of Routine Data

The link between the benefits to clinical practice that accrue from RCTs and the gain to the health of the population that might then be expected is important for considering the future content and uses of routinely assembled data. It forms part of the rationale for evidence based practice because routine data will continue to provide the basis for the epidemiological monitoring of morbidity and its outcomes. Present data have a number of deficiencies for these purposes. The most significant is the lack of diagnostic precision in regard to both their content (considered as diagnostic-mix) and the slow response of ICD The difficulty of sequencing of events and the lack of information about medication and non-surgical interventions are other constraints as is the limited reporting of a patient's condition at the end of an episode of care. Case-severity and case-complexity are perhaps the most significant deficiency, even though scoring systems such as POSSUM[36] and APACHE III[37] are increasingly well-established and, perhaps with modification, could be included in routine information systems.

Data gathered for routine purposes will always fall short of those needed to answer clinical questions: if only for this reason, routine data will never replace the RCT as a way of evaluating new treatments or interventions. The main conclusion of the case studies we report, however, is that routine data could – with relatively straightforward development – provide a stronger framework for more focussed enquiries. Routine data can contribute to understanding the context and applicability of RCT results, partly by contributing to their design, partly through longer-term assessments of the effectiveness of new technologies, and partly as a means of evaluating the process of translating evidence into practice.

ACKNOWLEDGEMENTS

We are grateful to the Information and Statistics Division of the National Health Service in Scotland for the provision of the linked hospital discharge records and mortality data. This project was funded by the UK National Health Service as part of its Health Technology Assessment programme. The Public Health Research Unit is supported financially by the Chief Scientist Office of the Scottish Office Department of Health. Opinions and conclusions contained in this report are not necessarily those of the Scottish Office Department of Health.

REFERENCES

1. Joffe M, Chapple J, Paterson C, Beard RW. What is the optimal caesarean section rate? An outcome based study of existing variation. *J. Epidemiol. Community Health* 1994; **48**: 406–11.
2. Berry DA, Eick SG. Adaptive assignment versus balanced randomization in clinical trials: a decision analysis. *Stat. Med.* 1995; **14**: 231–46.
3. Ball SG. ACE inhibition in acute myocardial infarction. In: Ball SG (ed.). *Myocardial Infarction: From Trials to Practice*. Wrightson Biomedical Publishing, Petersfield, 1995, pp. 157–66.
4. Hall AS, Murray GD, Ball SG. ACE inhibitors in and after myocardial infarction. In: Pitt B, Julian D, Pocock S (eds). *Clinical Trials in Cardiology*. Saunders, London, 1997, pp. 261–70.
5. The ASPIRE Steering Group. A British Cardiac Society survey of the potential for the secondary prevention of coronary disease: ASPIRE (Action on Secondary Prevention through Intervention to Reduce Events). *Heart* 1996; **75**: 334–42.
6. Sapsford RJ, Hall AS, Robinson MB. Evaluation of angiotensin-converting enzyme inhibitor dosage and prescription rates in post-myocardial infarction patients. *Eur. Heart J.* 1996; **17**: 62 (Abstract).
7. Cochrane AL. *Effectiveness and Efficiency: Random Reflections on Health Services*. Nuffield Provincial Hospitals Trust, London, 1972.
8. Byar DP. Why data bases should not replace randomised clinical trials. *Biometrics* 1980; **36**: 337–42.
9. Spiegelhalter DJ, Freedman LS, Parmar MKB. Bayesian approaches to randomized trials (with Discussion). *J. Roy. Statist. Soc., Ser. A* 1994; **157**: 357–416.
10. Berry DA. A case for Bayesianism in clinical trials. *Statistics in Medicine* 1993; **12**: 1377–93.
11. Fendrick AM, Escarce JJ, McLane C, Shea JA, Schwarz JS. Hospital adoption of laparoscopic cholecystectomy. *Medical Care* 1994; **32**: 1058–63.
12. Kendrick S, Clarke J. The Scottish record linkage system. *Health Bull.* 1993; **51**: 72–9.
13. Hop JW, Rinkel GJE, Algra A, van Gijn J. Case-fatality rates and functional outcome after subarachnoid haemorrhage. A systematic review. *Stroke* 1997; **28**: 660–4.
14. Jennett B, Lindsay KW. *An Introduction to Neurosurgery*, 5th edn. Butterworth Heinemann, Oxford, 1994.
15. Linn FHH, Rinkel GJE, Algra A, van Gijn J. Incidence of subarachnoid haemorrhage. Role of region, year, and rate of computed tomography: a meta-analysis. *Stroke* 1996; **27**: 625–9.
16. Mayberg MR, Batjer H, Dacey R, et al. Guidelines for the management of aneurysmal subarachnoid hemorrhage. A statement for healthcare professionals from a special writing group of the Stroke Council, American Heart Association. *Circulation* 1994; **90**: 2592–605.
17. Craig JJ, Patterson VH, Cooke RS, Rocke LG, McKinstry CS. Diagnosis of subarachnoid haemorrhage (letter). *Lancet* 1997; **350**: 216–17.
18. van Gijn J. Slip-ups in diagnosis of subarachnoid haemorrhage. *Lancet* 1997; **349**: 1492.
19. Mayer PL, Awad IA, Todor R, et al. Misdiagnosis of symptomatic cerebral aneurysm. Prevalence and correlation with outcome at four institutions. *Stroke* 1996; **27**: 1558–63.
20. Ohman J, Heiskanen O. Timing of operation for ruptured supratentorial aneurysms: a prospective randomized study. *J. Neurosurg.* 1989; **70**: 55–60.
21. Hunt WE, Hess RM. Surgical risk as related to time of intervention in the repair of intracranial aneurysms. *J. Neurosurg.* 1968; **28**: 14–20.

22. Office of Population Censuses and Surveys. *Classification of surgical operations and procedures.* Fourth revision. London: OPCS, 1987.

23. Kassell NF, Torner JC, Haley EC, et al. The international co-operative study on the timing of aneurysm surgery. Part 1: Overall management results. *J. Neurosurg.* 1990; **73**: 18–36.

24. Favaloro RG. Saphenous vein autograft replacement of severe segmental coronary artery occlusion. Operative technique. *Ann. Thorac. Surg.* 1968; **5**: 334–9.

25. Killip T, Ravi K. Coronary Bypass Surgery. In: Pitt B, Julian D, Pocock S (eds). *Clinical Trials in Cardiology.* Saunders, London, 1997, pp. 173–84.

26. Black N, Langham S, Coshall C, Parker J. Impact of the 1991 NHS reforms on the availability and use of coronary revascularisation in the UK (1987–1995). *Heart* 1996; **76**(Suppl. 4): 1–30.

27. Grüntzig AR, Senning A, Siegenhaler WE. Non-operative dilatation of coronary-artery stenosis. *N. Eng. J. Med.* 1979; **301**: 61–8.

28. EPISTENT Investigators. Randomised placebo-controlled and balloon-angioplasty-controlled trial to assess safety of coronary stenting with use of platelet glycoprotein-IIb/IIIa blockade. *Lancet* 1998; **352**: 87–92.

29. Knudtson ML. Commentary. *Evidence-Based Medicine* 1996; **1**: 83–4.

30. Pocock SJ, Henderson RA, Rickards AF, Hampton JR, King SB III, Hamm CW, Puel J, Hueb W, Goy J, Rodriguez A. Meta-analysis of randomised trials comparing coronary angioplasty with bypass surgery. *Lancet* 1995; **346**: 1184–9.

31. BARI Investigators. Comparison of coronary bypass surgery with angioplasty in patients with multivessel disease. *N. Eng. J. Med.* 1996; **335**: 217–25.

32. White HD. Angioplasty versus bypass surgery. *Lancet* 1995; **346**: 1174–5.

33. CABRI Trial Participants. First year results of CABRI (Coronary Angioplasty versus Bypass Revascularization Investigation). *Lancet* 1995; **346**: 1179–83.

34. RITA Trial Participants. Coronary angioplasty versus coronary artery bypass surgery: the Randomised Intervention of Angina (RITA) trial. *Lancet* 1993; **341**: 573–80.

35. King SB III, Lembo NJ, Weintraub WS, et al. A randomised trial comparison of coronary angioplasty with coronary bypass surgery. *N. Eng. J. Med.* 1994; **331**: 1050–5.

36. Copeland GP, Jones D, Walters M. POSSUM: a scoring system for surgical audit. *Br. J. Surg.* 1991; **78**: 355–60.

37. Knaus WA, Wagner DP, Draper EA, et al. The APACHE III prognostic system: risk prediction of hospital mortality for critically ill hospitalized adults. *Chest* 1991; **100**: 1619–36.

38. World Health Organization. *Manual of the international statistical classification of diseases, injuries and causes of death.* Ninth revision. Geneva: WHO, 1977.

10

Qualitative Methods in Health Technology Assessment

ELIZABETH MURPHY and ROBERT DINGWALL

SUMMARY

There are some problems in Health Technology Assessment (HTA) that cannot be resolved using quantitative methods alone, and there are some circumstances in which qualitative methods represent a technically superior option. However, qualitative research is a highly contested field in which there are extensive disagreements about the nature, purpose, status and practice of its methods. Some versions are more compatible with the goals of HTA than others, which means that both those who wish to commission research and those who intend to use qualitative methods need to be clear about which particular version is being proposed. In this chapter we review some key dimensions of the debates among qualitative researchers and identify those positions that we see as most promising in relation to HTA. We then consider the claim that the relevance of qualitative research to policy-makers and practitioners is limited by the impracticability of probability sampling in most such work. We suggest that qualitative researchers need not, and should not, abandon the pursuit of empirical and/or theoretical generalisability in their research. Finally, we turn to the evaluation of qualitative research. Recently there have been a number of attempts to develop check-lists that can be used to judge the quality of qualitative research. We argue that the evaluation of qualitative research is always a matter of informed judgement and that it is impossible to side-step this by means of check-list criteria, which may, all too easily, come to be treated as an end in themselves rather than enhancing the validity of a study. We discuss some of the central issues around which such informed judgement about the quality of a study may be made. Finally, we make some observations about the circumstances in which qualitative work is likely to be the preferred option for an HTA research commissioner.

INTRODUCTION

This chapter reviews the appropriate application of qualitative methods to Health Technology Assessment (HTA). The use of qualitative methods – observation, informal interviewing, interactional analysis, documentary analysis, focus groups and the like – has been a controversial development in HTA research in recent years. The controversy has two dimensions. On the one hand, there is a debate over whether qualitative methods are usable at all in HTA. Some people would argue that only quantitative methods can deliver a sufficient degree of precision and objectivity to allow planners, policy-makers and practitioners to make rational decisions about the adoption or rejection of new technologies. Against this, others would contend that the exclusion of qualitative methods is like playing a round of golf with one club. There is a range of questions in HTA that cannot be addressed by quantitative methods, but have considerable practical importance. If qualitative work is not commissioned, then either the decision-maker is proceeding on a basis of ignorance or, perhaps more dangerously, on the basis of misinformation arising from an inappropriate use of a quantitative method. This applies particularly when examining the delivery and organisational contexts of new technologies – how can a national roll-out achieve the same results as the demonstration projects? – or some of the inter-personal dimensions of the technology. New drugs depend for their effectiveness on patient concordance with specific regimens which, in turn, seems to be affected by the interactional environment within which prescription and dispensing occur and the ways in which information and advice about appropriate use are delivered. Some new technologies, of course, are non-material – the rise of counselling in primary care would be a good example. Even a material technology may have some dimensions that imply qualitative research. How can consistent reading of DNA maps be achieved? It seems to be difficult enough with the established technology of cervical smears!

However, there is also considerable disagreement amongst users of qualitative methods about their nature, status and employment. This chapter attempts to demonstrate this diversity of view, while indicating which positions can make particular contributions to HTA. For this reason it is not based on a conventional systematic review, which was both materially and intellectually impracticable in this context. The literature to be searched was too large, and the search engines inadequate for the task. Moreover, in the absence of an agreement about how to resolve disagreements about the methodological foundations of qualitative research, it is impossible to produce an incontestable 'Best Buy'. The most that one can achieve is to review the range of options and to assess their fitness for the purposes of HTA. The test of this chapter is the representativeness of the range of positions reviewed rather than the exhaustiveness of the reading on which it is based. Nevertheless, if the objectives of HTA are taken as given, it is possible to make some fairly firm assessments of the value of particular positions for this programme.

This chapter does not provide a 'how to do it' guide. There are numerous excellent textbooks and courses available for that.[a] However, it does attempt to explain why qualitative research has a place in the HTA armamentarium, how to identify when it is appropriate, how to evaluate it and how to think sensibly about it.

Key Issues and Controversies

Debates in HTA, as in other fields, about the use of qualitative research often homogenise this intellectual tradition as if it were to be adopted or dismissed en bloc. This obscures the contested nature of qualitative research, and the extent to which different versions exist which may be more or less appropriate to the goals of HTA. There is little agreement among practitioners of qualitative research about what it is, what it is for, how it should be done or how it should be evaluated. Given this dissensus, it is meaningless to argue for or against qualitative research in general. Whether for the prosecution or the defence, the case needs to be made in relation to particular versions in particular contexts for particular purposes.

At the most fundamental level, the methodological literature on qualitative research reflects two conflicting sets of basic philosophical assumptions. Some writers[1,2,3] argue that qualitative and quantitative research methodologies derive from radically incompatible paradigms or world-views.[4] The proponents of this 'two paradigms' approach hold that the differences are so pervasive and ineluctable[5,6] that it is impossible to 'mix and match' between them.

The separatist position is consistently argued by Smith, for example.[1,2,7–10] The fundamental philosophical divide between qualitative and quantitative research reflects the former's grounding in Idealism and the latter's in Scientific Realism. (The opposition between these two positions has a long history in philosophy, which will not be reviewed here.) Smith[8] sums up Realism, which he sees as antithetical to qualitative research, as 'the idea that reality exists independent of us. Independent means that this reality exists whether or not we are aware of it or take any interest in it.' (p. 8). Idealism, on the other hand, is the view that what we take to be the external world is merely a creation of our minds.[11] Idealists do not necessarily deny the possibility that a material world exists, they hold that it is impossible to 'know' such a world. While Realists pursue what Smith[9] has called a 'God's eye point of view' (p. 381), or one single 'true' reality, Idealists hold that there are multiple realities or 'as many realities as there are persons'[9] (p. 386).

The Constructivism of some qualitative methodologists leads to similar conclusions. Guba and Lincoln,[12] for example, argue that 'there exist multiple, socially constructed realities, ungoverned by laws, natural or otherwise . . . these constructions are devised by individuals as they attempt to make sense of their experiences . . . constructions can be and usually are shared . . . this does not make them more *real* but simply more *commonly* assented to' (p. 86, original emphasis). The quotation highlights the problem of this position for HTA research. HTA is committed to pursuing truth as a secure basis for action. Idealists and Radical Constructivists hold that multiple, even contradictory, true versions of reality can exist simultaneously. There is no ultimate basis on which we can choose between them. If this is the case, and researchers simply produce yet another version that has no better claim to truth, then one wonders about the justification for spending public money on their work.[13] Radical relativism has deeply negative consequences for the value of research findings in practice and/or policy making.[14] It leads either to a 'debilitating nihilism'[15] (p. 252) or the chaos of 'anything goes'.

In rejecting Idealism and Radical Constructivism as a basis for HTA research, it should not be thought that the pursuit of 'truth' in any research (qualitative or quantitative) is unproblematic. There are profound difficulties with the conception of truth in conventional (or as Hammersley[13] terms it 'naïve') Realism. Researchers cannot escape the social world to make their observations.[16] A researcher's observation is always and inevitably shaped by the 'biological-cultural lenses through which it is seen'[17] (p. 157). As a result we can never know, in an absolute sense, that our research findings are true. Likewise, any given reality can be represented from a range of different perspectives and it is futile to search for 'a body of data uncontaminated by the researcher'[16] (p. 16). It is possible to have multiple descriptions or explanations of the same behaviour or event that are all valid, as long as they are compatible with each other. What is not possible is to have multiple *contradictory* versions that are all true. As Phillips[18] suggests, we can combine an acceptance that multiple perspectives are possible without abandoning truth as a 'regulatory ideal'.

This position (sometimes known as 'Subtle Realism') is equally appropriate for qualitative and quantitative research. It is an alternative to the polarising rhetoric of some qualitative researchers which is neither an accurate analysis of the current state of qualitative and quantitative research, nor a necessary or helpful distinction between these two traditions. It also allows that qualitative and quantitative research methods may be used in combination.

A second controversy within qualitative research, which is of fundamental importance in relation to HTA, concerns the frequent assertion that a defining characteristic of qualitative research is its commitment to uncovering the meanings that underpin human action. Health technologies are applied by people (be they doctors, nurses or technicians) to people (usually patients). One of the distinctive features of *human* action is that it is endowed with meaning.[19] This has the very practical consequence that what people *think* each other's actions mean (their interpretation) may be more important

than so-called 'objective reality' in determining how they respond.[20] People act on the basis of what they *believe* to be true[21] rather than what might be 'objectively true'. This has important implications for the successful implementation of technologies in health, as in other fields, in that advocates for change will need to engage the beliefs of intended users and beneficiaries rather than relying purely on rationalist justifications.

A number of methodologists have moved from this uncontroversial assertion of the importance of interpretation in human action and interaction to argue that the *central* role of qualitative research should be to uncover the meanings behind such action.[22–31] This is sometimes presented as a defining difference between qualitative and quantitative research. Henwood and Pidgeon[29] argue, for example, that qualitative researchers seek to avoid quantitative research's tendency to 'fix meanings' without reference to the meanings employed by the participants in the context being studied. The understanding of participants' meanings is associated with a preference for methods that allow the researcher to 'get close' to those being studied. These include prolonged periods of observation,[32] which allow researchers to put themselves 'in the shoes' of their subjects, and/or in-depth interview techniques, which are thought to encourage people to express their understandings and perspectives in their own words according to their own priorities.

The identification of qualitative research with uncovering participants' meanings is flawed in a number of respects. First, it is inaccurate to suggest that a focus on participant meanings defines qualitative research.[33–35] Much of this type of work has been less concerned with participants' perspectives than with their practices.[35] It focuses not on what people think, but upon what they do. These researchers are more concerned with studying the *function* rather than the *meaning* of such practices.[35] For example, Silverman et al. studied the organisation and reception of advice giving in HIV counselling sessions in ten medical centres. The analysis was based on audio-tapes of sessions.[36] Silverman et al. found that such advice giving was typically truncated and non-personalised – features which may be expected to be related to low patient uptake of advice. They considered the functions that such demonstrably ineffective practices might serve within the context in which they were performed. They showed how such truncated and non-personalised advice giving can be effective in handling the delicate issues which arise in relation to sexual practices. Generalised advice allowed counsellors to avoid singling out particular patients' sexual activities for discussion. It also meant that patients were not required to discuss their own behaviour. Such practices also avoided the embarrassment that might have arisen if the counsellors appeared to be telling comparative strangers what they should be doing in their intimate lives. Finally, these practices minimised the likelihood of any overt conflict within the consultation. Overall, Silverman et al. concluded that such truncated and non-personalised advice-giving was functional, not least because it enabled counsellors to limit the amount of time such counselling sessions require.

The second problem raised by the identification of qualitative research with the search for participants' meanings is that there are serious questions about the feasibility of 'uncovering' such meanings.[33] How are we to access these meanings? *Homo sapiens* is not known to be a telepathic species. Participants can be asked to explain the meanings that underlie their actions; indeed, this is the justification for much qualitative interviewing. However, this immediately presents two problems. Firstly, there is the possibility that participants have knowledge and experience which are relevant, but which they are unable to articulate, leading to distortion and over-simplification. Secondly, even more problematically, asking participants to explain why they behave in certain ways leads them to produce 'accounts'.[37–39] Their answers are not straightforward reproductions of the mental states which lay behind the actions they are intended to explain. They are versions of the respondent's experience specifically designed to make their behaviour seem meaningful and contextually appropriate to their interlocutor. As such they have, as Gould and his co-workers[24] have observed, an indeterminate relationship to the original decision to act in one way rather than another.

QUALITATIVE RESEARCH IN HTA

A frequently expressed reservation about qualitative research is its alleged failure to meet the criterion of generalisability, often held to be the hallmark of science.[40,41] Quantitative research usually pursues generalisability by sample to population inference, using probabilistic sampling methods. Much qualitative research is carried out in a single setting or with a small sample of informants, and does not meet the requirements for statistical inference.[42] The relative absence of probability sampling generates concerns that qualitative work is merely anecdotal and therefore of no practical use to policy-makers or practitioners.

Qualitative researchers are again divided on this issue. Some appear to reject generalisability as an appropriate goal[43,44] as being 'unimportant, unachievable or both'[45] (p. 201). In HTA research, of course, generalisability is extremely important, since research commissioners are normally less interested in particular settings for their own sake than in the extent to which findings from one can be extrapolated to others. If qualitative research is to be acceptable to practitioners and policy-makers, then its approaches to sample selection, representativeness and generalisability must be understood.[46]

Some qualitative methodologists, such as Stake,[44] argue that concern with representativeness may have a distorting effect. He suggests that the researcher's object should be to understand the uniqueness of individual cases and to offer the reader a vicarious experience of each. Readers are invited to engage in 'naturalistic generalization' as they relate these case studies to their existing knowledge of other settings. If the primary function of qualitative research is to provide 'vicarious experience' and 'experiential understanding' in order to allow readers to make 'naturalistic generalizations' then probability sampling does appear to be both inappropriate and impractical. However, this position places qualitative research closer to an exercise in communication than to a public science. As Kennedy[41] has wryly remarked, if this is the case then the researcher would need 'the talent of Tolstoi to be able to describe . . . events in the way that allow the reader to draw the appropriate inference' (p. 664).

There are, in fact, no fundamental reasons why probabilistic sampling methods could not be adopted in qualitative research.[43,47–51] Practical and resource constraints, however, mean that they are normally unlikely to be efficient or cost-effective. Because of the intensive and time-consuming nature of qualitative research, the ratio of settings studied to the number in the population of interest can rarely be raised to a sufficient level to allow statistical inference.[52,53] In qualitative research the general use of non-probability sampling methods is best understood as a trade-off between depth and breadth.

However, the impracticality of probability sampling need not, and should not, lead qualitative researchers to abandon concerns for generalisability. The basis for sampling decisions in qualitative research has too often been pure opportunism. Pragmatic considerations such as ease of access (both geographical and organisational) are, of course, important in sampling decisions for both qualitative and quantitative research. In some cases, particularly where the research topic is highly sensitive or the population of interest is mobile or inaccessible, opportunistic sampling may, of course, be the only option. If, though, the role of research in HTA is to provide cumulative knowledge about technologies and their implementation, then opportunistic sampling will be the method of last resort in anything but the most exploratory research. In all other qualitative research, samples should be drawn in a systematic and principled way.[45]

The research objective will determine which of two such systematic approaches is appropriate in a particular study. Where researchers are primarily concerned with the representativeness or typicality of their findings, they will adopt purposive sampling strategies that maximise the empirical generalisability of their findings. Researchers will examine people or settings which are thought to be typical in some way of the aggregate to which they are seeking to generalise. For example, in reviewing an innovative technology, researchers might study its use in a hospital department that is believed to be 'typical' in significant respects of the settings in which it could be applied. They would consciously exclude 'state-of-the-art' centres or locations known to be particularly poorly resourced or staffed. In other cases, though, researchers may deliberately set out to study settings or groups that are in some way atypical. For example, they might choose to study an unusually successful programme in order to identify the characteristics of settings that facilitate achievement. In both cases, the researchers are making principled selection decisions that define the generalisability and utility of their findings. This is not, of course, entirely unproblematic: the validity of purposive sampling is dependent upon the researcher's ability to identify which variables or characteristics are likely to be significant. A ward or clinic which is 'typical' on one dimension may not be typical on another.[45] Nevertheless, purposive sampling makes an important contribution to the generalisability of qualitative research.

Other authors[54–56] suggest that sampling should be directed towards making possible generalisations to theoretical propositions. This approach, sometimes known as theoretical sampling, involves directing case selection towards the testing of some developing theory rather than towards representativeness. Theoretical sampling uses existing theory to make predictions and then seeks out cases which allow the researcher to test the robustness of these predictions under different conditions.[53] As such, it parallels the use of critical experiments in laboratory science.

This approach can be applied at the beginning of the research in identifying the particular settings, groups or individuals to be studied, or in the course of a project, as recurrent decisions are made about who, what and where to study within the setting(s) chosen. A range of sampling techniques can be used, including the study of negative, critical, discrepant and deviant cases, to explore, modify and extend existing theory.[51,53,57]

The relevance of theoretical sampling to research in HTA may be less immediately obvious than approaches that emphasise sample to population inference. However, it allows researchers to take findings that have been established in one context or field and test their applicability in another. Researchers can exploit and build upon existing knowledge from related, or sometimes quite different, fields. Silverman,[35] for example, reports how his observational study of NHS and private oncology clinics was conceived as a test of the generalisability of Strong's findings in paediatric clinics to other medical settings.[58] A study of the general practitioner's role in giving lifestyle advice, reported by Parry and Pill,[59] took theoretical generalisations developed by Bernstein in the context of education and tested them in medical settings.

Qualitative researchers take different views about the relative merits of these sampling approaches, emphasising empirical generalisability or theoretical generalisability. However, these strategies are not incompatible. It is possible, in making sampling decisions, to combine a concern with the empirical generalisability of findings with a commitment to sampling in ways which are theoretically informed and which seek to test, modify and extend existing knowledge. In judging the quality of sampling, the main concern should be with its fitness for the specific purpose of a particular study and the systematicity with which it has been carried out.

JUDGING THE QUALITY OF QUALITATIVE RESEARCH

The contested nature of qualitative research is most clearly evident in debates about its evaluation. Those who adopt the 'two paradigms' approach outlined above, tend to argue that qualitative and quantitative research are so fundamentally different that they cannot be evaluated by the same criteria.[5,29,48,60] In particular, these authors reject the application of conventional criteria such as validity to a research paradigm that, they claim, allows the possibility of multiple and conflicting truths. The alternative position, adopted here, is that all HTA research, whether qualitative or quantitative, should be evaluated in terms of the robustness of its truth claims, on the one hand, and its usefulness in informing policy-making and practice, on the other. If research findings are to inform the development and use of health technologies we must be confident that their findings are sufficiently true for all practical purposes. Their relevance to the concerns identified by commissioners must also be clear.

Whilst it is impossible, in either qualitative or quantitative research, to provide absolute proof of validity, researchers have a number of ways to 'limit the likelihood of error'.[61] The commitment should be to what Dewey has termed 'warranted assertability'.[62] Given the differences between qualitative and quantitative research, in terms both of the problems which each addresses and of their research practices, there will be different means by which warranted assertability and the researchers' success in limiting error can be judged. The ways in which such judgements can be made about qualitative research will now be considered.

It has become fashionable to call for the development of check-lists which can be used to judge the quality of qualitative research reports. These calls often reflect the anxiety of journal editors and systematic reviewers, who are more familiar with the outputs of quantitative research, about their ability to sift wheat from chaff in qualitative research. While the commitment to quality control is commendable, and it is undoubtedly important to clarify the methods of assessing truth claims from qualitative research, the 'check-list' approach seems unlikely to be a profitable strategy. As Hammersley argues, no simple algorithmic criteria can be applied mechanically to establish the quality of qualitative research.[63] The assessment of research always involves judgement and it is impossible to side-step this by means of check-list criteria. Check-lists risk becoming rigid constraints that are an end in themselves, rather than enhancing the validity of a study.[27] The outcome is the research equivalent of defensive medicine in which researchers produce findings which conform to the check-list but are insignificant. Below, we present an alternative to such mechanical check-lists by suggesting a number of questions which evaluators of research findings might reasonably ask in relation to any piece of qualitative research.

Even if a check-list approach to the validity of qualitative research could be established, it is not clear what items it would include. Two frequent candidates are respondent validation and triangulation. However, as Bloor in particular has shown, both of these have substantial problems when used as validity tests.[64]

A number of authors recommend respondent validation (sometimes known as member checking, host recognition or informant validation) as a means of establishing the validity of qualitative research findings.[12,48,65–69] Respondent validation can be carried out in several ways (for details see Bloor[70]), but generally involves the presentation of findings (either orally or in writing) to the researched. If they accept the findings as true, then validity is taken to have been demonstrated.

There are four main difficulties with respondent validation. First, there are practical problems in asking research participants to comment on findings. Participants cannot be relied upon to read or listen to research reports with the critical attention required by this exercise. Researchers who have used the technique report that they have been both criticised and praised for things which their reports do not contain.[71] Second, even where participants have clearly read and fully understood reports, their responses cannot be assumed to represent 'immaculately produced'[70] (p. 171) evaluations of the findings. Responses are inevitably shaped and constrained by the context in which they are produced. Validation interviews are reported to be marked by consensus seeking[64] and deference to the rules of polite behaviour, which normally characterise our social interactions. Participants are reluctant to challenge researchers' findings and eager, as Emerson and Pollner have put it, to 'do friendship' with the researcher rather than to be directly critical of his or her work.[71] Third, participants cannot be assumed to be entirely disinterested evaluators of findings. As members of the setting studied they have their own micro-political agendas. Both of these latter points further exemplify the naivete of treating interview responses as straightforward reproductions of respondents' mental states.[37–39] Finally, as Bloor found, participants' responses may not be consistent either within validation interviews or across time.[64]

Taken together, these problems undermine any claim that respondent validity can be used as a means of establishing the validity of research findings. This procedure might reduce error. Discussions with participants about findings may highlight aspects of the setting that the researcher has overlooked or offer an alternative interpretation of data. In this way, they can contribute additional information that enhances the comprehensiveness of the study. However, they cannot prove or disprove the validity of the findings.[33,63,64,70,71]

The second validation technique often advocated in qualitative research is triangulation. This rests on a metaphor drawn from military, navigational or surveying contexts.[16,72–75] Hammersley and Atkinson[16] describe how triangulation is carried out in surveying:

> For someone wanting to locate their position on a map, a single landmark can only provide the information that they are situated somewhere along a line in a particular direction from that landmark. With two landmarks, however, one's exact position can be pinpointed by taking bearings on both; one is at the point on the map where the two lines cross. (p. 231)

When applied to the evaluation of qualitative research, triangulation involves the combination of two or more methodologies in the study of the same phenomenon.[76,77] This can involve using different methods, data sources, investigators, disciplinary perspectives or theoretical models.[75,76,78] In all these cases, the underlying argument is that where the findings of two or more approaches agree, the validity of findings is confirmed.

Just as with respondent validation, multi-method approaches can enhance the comprehensiveness of a study and reduce the likelihood of error. However, there are again significant problems if triangulation is elevated to the status of a validity test. As Silverman has argued,[35,78] a strength of qualitative method is its recognition of the context-boundedness of data. Used as a test of validity, triangulation involves de-contextualising data, leaving researchers unable to relate their findings to the circumstances of their production. Triangulation encourages researchers to focus on identifying a single reality rather than understanding the way participants use different versions of that reality in different contexts.[79] The resulting limitations are well illustrated by the study of Welsh general practice carried out by Stimson and Webb.[80] They combined participant observation of general practice consultations and interviews with patients. There were striking inconsistencies between patients' reports of their interactions with doctors and the researchers' own observations of such interactions. If Stimson and Webb had used triangulation as a validity check, they would have been forced to adjudicate between their observations and the accounts given by patients in interviews, presumably judging the latter to be invalid. They chose instead to analyse the interviews as data on the ways in which patients represented their interactions with doctors and to consider what this might imply for

the cultural basis of the doctor–patient relationship. Although the particular analysis which they offered has since been a matter of some debate, the methodological lesson has been widely learned.

A fundamental problem with triangulation lies in the asymmetry of the conclusions that can be drawn from it.[64] If we assume that there is one best method of investigating any research topic, triangulation necessarily involves putting the findings of a superior method with those of an inferior. This is not a problem where the findings of the two methods converge, and the findings of the inferior method confirm those of the superior. However, where they diverge, we do not know whether this arises because the findings of the superior method were indeed mistaken or because the inferior method is inadequate. In other words, triangulation can only corroborate findings, it can never refute them. As such it cannot be a validity test.[64,81]

Neither respondent validation nor triangulation can be used mechanically to test the validity of the findings of qualitative research. The same is true of all the other measures that might be proposed for inclusion on a validity check-list. However, this is not to suggest that we must abandon the pursuit of standards in qualitative research. Qualitative research should be subjected to rigorous evaluation, and there are key issues towards which evaluation can appropriately be directed. However, these necessarily involve judgement and cannot be achieved through the simple application of rigid algorithmic criteria. Some of the questions which evaluators might usefully ask are discussed below.

What is the Quality of the Evidence upon which the Researcher's Claims are Based?

The credibility of research findings depends crucially on the nature and quality of the evidence upon which they are based. To judge the extent to which claims are justified, readers require information about the process by which data were collected. Altheide and Johnson have suggested that there is a minimal set of issues that are encountered in almost all studies and should be detailed in research reports, so that readers can assess the likely degree of error.[82] These include: how access was negotiated; how the researchers presented themselves; the role the researchers adopted in the setting or interviews; any 'mistakes' made by the researcher; the types of data collected; and how such data were recorded. On such a basis, readers can exercise what Glaser and Strauss have described as their 'joint responsibility' to judge the evidence alongside the researcher.[83]

By What Process were Conclusions Drawn from the Data Collected?

The adequacy of any analysis depends on the process that is used to organise and interpret data. There has been much criticism of qualitative researchers' failure to clarify the means by which their findings have been derived from the data collected.[5,12,20,46,48,79,83] Calls have been made for the process of analysis to be 'semi-public and not magical'.[56] Concern has centred both on the ways in which data are coded and categorised, and on the way in which conclusions are then drawn.

In quantitative work, researchers are required to operationalise the concepts in which they are interested before the data are collected. The central role of induction[b] in qualitative research means that this is often not appropriate. However, this does not relieve the researcher of the obligation to develop clear definitions of the concepts and categories that are established during the research, so that their meaning and application are clear. In judging a qualitative research report, readers should assess the extent to which key concepts have been defined explicitly and coherently and to which the coding of data has been disciplined by these publicly communicable definitions.

Similarly, researchers can be expected to demonstrate that the conclusions drawn are justified in relation to the data collected. The first requirement here is that the data record should itself be trustworthy. The use of mechanical recording methods[20,51,69,84] and standardised rules for transcribing data help to limit the risk that the data will be misinterpreted at the analysis stage, although it is important not to overestimate the possibility of literal transcription.[85] The use of 'low inference descriptors', such as verbatim accounts and concrete and precise descriptions are recommended.[51,69] To be able to assess the adequacy of an analysis, readers must be able to scrutinise the empirical observations upon which it is based.[86] In particular, sufficient data must be displayed to allow readers to judge whether interpretations are adequately supported by data. Such judgement will depend crucially upon the extent to which researchers have separated out data from analysis in presenting their conclusions.[46] The trustworthiness of researchers' analyses is also enhanced where they demonstrate that they have systematically considered alternative plausible explanations of their data.[27,61,84]

Is the Analysis Sensitive to How the Researcher's Presence and the Analyst's Assumptions Have Shaped the Data and its Analysis?

Quantitative research emphasises the elimination of the researcher's impact on data, primarily through the standardisation of stimuli: qualitative researchers acknowledge that there is 'no way in which we can escape the social world in order to study it'[16] (p. 17). Qualitative research reports can, therefore, be expected to be reflexive, in the sense that they show sensitivity to the ways in which the researcher's presence has contributed to the data collected and their a priori assumptions have shaped the analysis. However, this does not necessarily imply that the data are *solely* an artefact of the researcher's activities and analysis: subtle realism acknowledges that what we see is the result both of the way we look *and* of what is there to be seen. Reflexivity is about the careful consideration of the researcher's role in order better to understand what is left as a description of the world.

Has the Researcher Made the Data Look more Patterned than they Actually Are?

Sandelowski[48] has argued that a major threat to the validity of qualitative research is 'holistic bias' or the tendency to make data look more patterned than they really are. One of the hallmarks of high-quality qualitative research is the conscientious search for, and presentation of, cases that are inconsistent with the emerging analysis.[5,27,46,48,56,78,84,87] Theoretical sampling procedures (see above) facilitate the search for such 'negative cases' and encourage researchers to establish the limits of their findings through the systematic search for disconfirming cases. The careful study of such negative, disconfirming and deviant cases enables researchers to refine their analyses[56] and to show how the analysis can explain such apparent inconsistencies.[87] As in all science, it is the conscientious search for falsifying evidence that adds weight to the truth claims of qualitative research. Whilst such an approach can never guarantee truth, it does support the reduction of error.[61] The credibility of research findings is enhanced where researchers display negative cases in their research reports or, at least, show they have searched carefully for them and can explain their absence.

Does the Research Build upon Existing Knowledge in the Field?

The importance of attention to negative evidence highlights a shortcoming of much current qualitative research.[56] The difficulty of funding large-scale, multi-site studies means that the capacity to search comprehensively for negative evidence within a single study is inevitably constrained. To test the limits of findings emerging from studies in a range of settings and under various conditions, earlier work must be used as a foundation for subsequent studies. Qualitative researchers have been curiously reluctant to work in this way. To some extent this reflects a justifiable concern to avoid imposing 'theories that have dubious fit and working capacity'[88] (p. 4) upon data. It also reflects a widespread misunderstanding of Glaser and Strauss's programme for grounded theory. When this was laid out in the 1960s, there was little to build on, and they emphasised the elements of discovery and theory-creation in qualitative research. In the 1990s, the stress on innovation is less relevant and was greatly modified by Strauss, although not by Glaser.[89] As Strauss's own late work showed, it is certainly possible to avoid the arbitrary imposition of theory while building on what is known from previous work. Our confidence in research findings will always be increased where researchers show how their findings articulate with other studies. A commitment to cumulation increases opportunities for the systematic search for negative evidence that we have already discussed.

Is there Evidence of Partisanship in the Research Report?

The recognition that any phenomenon may be understood from a number of different standpoints has serious implications for the conduct of qualitative research. In particular, researchers should be wary of presenting the perspective of one group as if this defined objective truth about the phenomenon and paying scant regard to other perspectives. This kind of one-sided analysis pervades research in the health field where doctors and senior managers are easily cast in the role of villains.

The debate over partisanship in research has a long history. There are those, such as Becker,[90] who have argued that research is always morally and politically partisan and that the obligation for researchers is not to seek neutrality, but to make a moral decision about 'whose side we are on' (p. 239). This commitment to principled partisanship is characteristic of the work of a range of writers – Marxists, feminists, anti-racists, disability activists, gay and lesbian polemicists, etc. – who have committed themselves to using research as a means of advocacy on behalf of oppressed groups. This 'underdog' perspective has a long, though never unchallenged, history in qualitative research.[35,91]

Research is always and inevitably shaped by values, but this does not *oblige* researchers to adopt a partisan position. In seeking to limit the possibility of error, researchers can plan to include the perspectives of people at different status levels within a group or setting. This commitment to 'fair dealing'[46] means that the perspectives of both the privileged and the less privileged will be incorporated in the data collection and analysis. It is the concern for even-handedness that distinguishes research from sensationalist or investigative journalism.[46,92]

One of the ways in which the truth claims of a research report can be evaluated is the extent to which it offers understanding of the behaviour of people at all levels within an organisation or setting. If the privileged and powerful are presented as mere cardboard cutouts who are either 'misguided or wilfully putting their own interests first'[92] (p. 61) readers should be concerned about the value of the analysis in helping them fully to grasp the complexity of the phenomenon being studied.

WHEN TO USE QUALITATIVE RESEARCH

There are at least four occasions on which HTA research commissioners should consider using qualitative research.

Firstly, qualitative research can be an essential precursor to quantitative work. It is a tool for establishing that the right things are being counted using the right kind of operational definitions. This is particularly important with 'soft technologies' like counselling. One of the reasons why so many trials of counselling, psychotherapy and similar interventions have been so inconclusive is their failure to standardise for the intervention experience itself. The things that are easy to control, like the length of the session, the environment in which it is delivered, or the certification of the counsellor, bear an unknown relationship to what the counsellor actually does. Qualitative work would make it possible to construct more homogeneous and commensurable categories of intervention of the kind required by experimental logic. However, the application of qualitative work does go wider, particularly in understanding the way people interact with 'hard technologies' as much of the work on information technologies has shown.

This spills into the second area, which is where qualitative methods are used to explain unanticipated or inconclusive findings from quantitative studies, or from programme roll-outs. It is not uncommon to find that technologies, which work in the design laboratory or in carefully managed pilots, are far less successful in general use. This is a well-recognised problem in surgery, for instance, where a new technique may be established by its pioneers to the point where its mortality and postoperative morbidity rates fall to acceptable levels, but which then sees a marked jump in risk when it is generally adopted. Although the normal processes of professional trial-and-error will usually correct the problem in time, the application of qualitative methods may help to identify crucial differences between the innovation environment and routine practice. This should reduce the amount of learning from adverse outcomes as opposed to systematic proactive inquiry!

A third area is that of hypothesis generation or need identification. Before mounting a large and expensive RCT to establish whether a technology is an appropriate solution to some problem, it may be useful to get some sense of whether it is reasonable to expect to find an effect and, if so, what would be relevant dimensions to incorporate into a trial design. If, for example, we want to evaluate a new drug for the treatment of schizophrenia, it may be useful to carry out some qualitative studies of small patient groups at an early stage of clinical trialing in order to identify possible areas of impact on interpersonal behaviour and social functioning and to consider whether there are broad variations in response by age, gender or ethnicity. Should these emerge, they may then inform the design of a major trial – for example by suggesting that the costs and benefits for women need to be considered separately from those of men in certain specific ways. In some cases, of course, the hypotheses generated in this way may not be amenable to testing using quantitative methods. In such cases, the researcher may use qualitative methods for hypothesis testing as well as hypothesis generation.

But the most important use of qualitative research is fundamentally to answer the crucial question for any manager, planner or policy-maker – what is going on here? It is not designed to deal with questions of number – how often?, how many?, how much? However, these are a very particular and limited subset of the important questions that anybody working in health technology needs to answer. Qualitative methods are the tools for finding out why this piece of technology is not having the impact it

was supposed to: even more valuably, they are the potential resource for finding out how to improve the chances of implementing the next piece of technology in a way that will achieve its intended impact. How can it be brought into use in ways that work with the grain of an organisation and its stakeholders rather than being imposed in a fashion that invites subversion and misuse? These are problems that are common to all human institutions and where the generic theoretical tools of social science may point to a range of solutions from entirely unexpected quarters.

CONCLUSIONS

Qualitative research has an important contribution to make to HTA. Decisions about whether qualitative or quantitative research (or some combination of the two) are more appropriate for addressing a particular HTA problem should be made in terms of which is most likely to resolve the problem in an efficient and effective manner, rather than on philosophical or ideological grounds.

Qualitative methods are particularly suited to answering 'how does it come to happen?' questions, rather than those concerned with 'how many?', 'how much?' or 'how often?'. They have an important contribution to make wherever the context in which a health technology is applied could be expected to have an impact upon outcome. In some situations, particularly where the groups being researched are involved in sensitive or stigmatised activities, qualitative research may be the only practical, and therefore the preferred, option. In others, a combination of qualitative and quantitative methods will offer the optimum combination.

Given the lack of standardisation in qualitative research, a degree of caution is required from both commissioners and users. Fundamentally different objectives and commitments can drive research on the same substantive topic, using similar research techniques. The products of research carried out by those who are committed primarily to advocacy on behalf of the oppressed are likely to be substantially different from those of researchers committed to the pursuit of warrantable knowledge through scientific rigour. The validity of research findings and their usefulness in informing both policy and practice will depend upon the agenda which the researcher brings to the research, as well as upon the professional judgement, skills, competence and systematicity with which it is carried out.

ACKNOWLEDGEMENTS

This chapter draws on work under contract to the NHS HTA Programme in collaboration with David Greatbatch, Pamela Watson and Susan Parker. We gratefully acknowledge their contribution to the discussions out of which this paper emerged.

NOTES

a. These include Hammersley M, Atkinson P (1995) *Ethnography: Principles in Practice*. London: Routledge, Silverman D (1985) *Qualitative Methodology and Sociology*. 1st edn, Aldershot: Gower, and Silverman D (1993) *Interpreting Qualitative Data: Methods for Analysing Talk, Text and Interaction*. London: Sage.

b. Pointing to the importance of induction in qualitative research does not imply that the logic of qualitative research is exclusively inductive. Rather, qualitative research involves a constant interplay between the logic of induction and the logic of deduction.

REFERENCES

1. Smith J. Social reality as mind-dependent versus mind-independent and the interpretation of test validity. *J. Res. Dev. Education* 1985; **19**: 1–9.
2. Smith J, Heshusius L. Closing down the conversation: the end of the quantitative-qualitative debate among educational inquirers. *Educational Researcher* 1986; **15**: 4–12.
3. Dootson S. An in-depth study of triangulation. *J. Adv. Nursing* 1995; **22**: 183–7.
4. Guba EG, Lincoln YS. Competing paradigms in qualitative research. In: Denzin NK, Lincoln YS (eds). *Handbook of Qualitative Research*. Thousand Oaks: Sage, 1994, pp. 105–17.
5. Lincoln YS, Guba EG. *Naturalistic Inquiry*. Newbury Park: Sage, 1985.
6. Lincoln YS. The making of a constructivist: a remembrance of transformations past. In Guba E (ed.). *The Paradigm Dialog*. Newbury Park: Sage, 1990, pp. 67–87.
7. Smith J. Quantitative versus interpretive: the problem of conducting social inquiry. In: House E (ed.). *Philosophy Evaluation*. San Francisco: Jossey Bass, 1983, pp. 27–51.
8. Smith J. Quantitative versus qualitative research: an attempt to clarify the issue. *Educational Researcher* 1983; **12**: 6–13.
9. Smith J. The problem of criteria for judging interpretive inquiry. *Educational Evaluation and Policy Analysis* 1984; **6**: 379–91.
10. Smith J. *The Nature of Social and Educational Inquiry*. Norwood, NJ: Ablex, 1989.
11. Williams M, May T. *Introduction to the Philosophy of Social Research*. London: UCL, 1996.
12. Guba EG, Lincoln YS. *Fourth Generation Evaluation*. Newbury Park, CA: Sage, 1989.
13. Hammersley M. Ethnography and realism. In: Hammersley M. *What's Wrong with Ethnography?* London: Routledge, 1992, pp. 43–56.
14. Greene J. Qualitative evaluation and scientific citizenship: reflections and refractions. *Evaluation* 1996; **2**: 277–89.
15. Atkinson P, Hammersley M. Ethnography and Participant Observation. In: Denzin N, Lincoln Y (eds). *Handbook of Qualitative Research*. Thousand Oaks: Sage, 1994, pp. 248–61.
16. Hammersley M, Atkinson P. *Ethnography: Principles in Practice*, 2nd edn. London: Routledge, 1995.
17. Campbell D. Can we overcome world-view incommensurability/relativity in trying to understand the other? In: Jessor R, Colby A, Shweder R (eds). *Ethnography and Human Development: Context and Meaning in Social Inquiry*. Chicago: University of Chicago Press, 1994, pp. 153–72.
18. Phillips D. Post-positivistic science: myths and realities. In: Guba E (ed.). *The Paradigm Dialog*. Newbury Park: Sage, 1990, pp. 31–45.
19. Atkinson P. Research design in ethnography. In: DE304 Course Team, *Research Methods in Education and the Social Sciences*. Milton Keynes: Open University Press, 1979, pp. 41–82.
20. Jensen G. Qualitative methods in physical therapy research: a form of disciplined inquiry. *Physical Therapy* 1989; **69**: 492–500.
21. Thomas W, Thomas D. *The Child in America: Behaviour Problems and Programs*. New York: Alfred Knopf, 1927.
22. Wiseman, J. *Stations of the Lost: The Treatment of Skid Row Alcoholics*. Englewood Cliffs, NJ: Prentice-Hall, 1970.
23. Lofland J. *Analyzing Social Settings: A Guide to Qualitative Observation and Analysis*. Belmont, CA: Wadsworth, 1971.
24. Gould L, Walker A, Crane L, Lidz C. *Connections: Notes from the Heroin World*. New Haven: Yale University Press, 1974.
25. Patton MQ. *Qualitative Evaluation Methods*. Newbury Park, CA: Sage, 1980.
26. Duffy M. Designing nursing research: the qualitative-quantitative debate. *J. Adv. Nursing* 1985; **10**: 225–32.
27. Marshall C. Appropriate criteria for the trustworthiness and goodness for qualitative research methods on educational organisations. *Quality and Quantity* 1985; **19**: 353–73.
28. Duffy M. Methodological triangulation: a vehicle for merging quantitative and qualitative research methods. *Image: Journal of Nursing Scholarship* 1987; **19**: 130–3.

29. Henwood K, Pidgeon N. Qualitative research and psychological theorising. *Br. J. Psychol.* 1992; **83**: 97–111.

30. Oiler Boyd C. Combining qualitative and quantitative approaches. In: Munhall PL, Oiler Boyd C (eds). *Nursing Research: a Qualitative Perspective*, 2nd edn. New York: National League for Nursing Press, 1993, pp. 454–75.

31. Lindlof TR. *Qualitative Communication Research Methods*. London: Sage, 1995.

32. Foster P. Unit 12 Observational Research: In DEH313 Course Team, *Principles of Social and Educational Research*. Milton Keynes: The Open University, 1993, pp. 37–73.

33. Emerson R. Observational fieldwork. *Annu. Rev. Sociol.* 1981; **7**: 351–78.

34. Hammersley M. Deconstructing the qualitative-quantitative divide. In: Hammersley M (ed.). *What's Wrong with Ethnography?* London: Routledge, 1992, pp. 159–82.

35. Silverman D. *Interpreting Qualitative Data: Methods for Analysing Talk, Text and Interaction.* London: Sage, 1993.

36. Silverman D, Bor R, Miller R, Goldman E. 'Obviously the advice then is to keep to safe sex': Advice giving and advice reception in AIDS counselling. In: Aggleton P, Davies P, Hart G (eds). *AIDS: Rights, Risks and Reason*. London: Falmer, pp. 174–91.

37. Scott M, Lyman S. Accounts. *American Sociological Review* 1968; **33**: 46–62.

38. Scott M, Lyman S. Accounts, Deviance and the Social Order. In: Douglas J (ed.). *Deviance and Respectability*. New York: Basic Books, 1970, pp. 89–119.

39. Lyman S, Scott M. *A Sociology of the Absurd*, 2nd edn. New York: General Hall Inc., 1989.

40. Smith H. *Strategies of Social Research: The Methodological Imagination*, London: Prentice Hall, 1975.

41. Kennedy M. Generalizing from single case studies. *Evaluation Quarterly* 1979; **3**: 661–78.

42. Miles MB, Huberman MA. *Qualitative Data Analysis: An expanded sourcebook*. 2nd edn. Thousand Oaks, CA: Sage, 1994.

43. Denzin N. Interpretive Interactionism. In Morgan D (ed.). *Beyond Method: Strategies for Social Research*. Beverly Hills: Sage, 1983, pp. 129–46.

44. Stake R. *The Art of Case Study Research*, Thousand Oaks, CA: Sage.

45. Schofield J. Increasing the generalizability of qualitative research. In: Hammersley M (ed.). *Social Research: Philosophy, Politics and Practice.* London: Sage, 1993, pp. 200–25.

46. Dingwall R. Don't mind him – he's from Barcelona: qualitative methods in health studies. In: Daly J, McDonald I, Wilks E (eds). *Researching Health Care*. London: Tavistock/Routledge, 1992, pp. 161–75.

47. Honigman J. Sampling in ethnographic fieldwork. In: Burgess RG (ed.). *Field Research: A Sourcebook and Field Manual*. London: George, Allen and Unwin, 1982, pp. 79–90.

48. Sandelowski M. The problem of rigor in qualitative research. *Ans-Advances in Nursing Science* 1986; **8**: 27–37

49. Johnson J. Selecting ethnographic informants. In: Miller ML, Manning PK, Van Maanen J (eds). *Qualitative Research Methods*. Newbury Park: Sage, 1990.

50. Hammersley M. Some questions about theory in ethnography and history. In: Hammersley M (ed.). *What's Wrong with Ethnography?* London: Routledge, 1992, pp. 32–42.

51. LeCompte M, Preissle J. *Ethnography and Qualitative Design in Educational Research*, 2nd edn. New York: Academic Press Inc., 1993.

52. Hammersley M. The generalisability of ethnography. In: Hammersley M (ed.). *What's Wrong with Ethnography?* London: Routledge, 1992, pp. 85–95.

53. Firestone W. Alternative arguments for generalising from data as applied to qualitative research. *Educational Researcher* 1993; **22**: 16–23.

54. Mitchell JC. Case and situational analysis. *Sociological Rev.* 1983; **31**: 187–211.

55. Bryman A. *Quality and Quantity in Social Research*. London: Unwin Hyman, 1988.

56. Silverman D. Telling convincing stories: a plea for cautious positivism in case studies. In: Glassner B, Moreno JD (eds). *The Qualitative-Quantitative Distinction in the Social Sciences.* Dordrecht: Kluwer Academic Publishers, 1989, pp. 57–77.

57. Gubrium J, Buckholdt D. *Describing Care: Image and Practice in Rehabilitation*. Cambridge MA: Oelgeschlager, Gunn and Hain, 1982.

58. Strong P. *The Ceremonial Order of the Clinic.* London: Routledge and Kegan Paul, 1979.

59. Parry O, Pill R. 'I don't tell him how to live his life': the doctor/patient encounter as an educational context. In: Bloor M, Taraborelli P (eds). *Qualitative Studies in Health and Medicine.* Aldershot: Avebury, 1994, pp. 5–21.

60. Leininger M. Current issues, problems and trends to advance qualitative paradigmatic research methods for the future. *Qual. Health Res.* 1992; **12**: 392–415.

61. Hammersley M. *Reading Ethnographic Research.* New York: Longman, 1990.

62. Phillips D. Validity in qualitative research: why the worry about warrant will not wane. *Education and Urban Society* 1987; **20**: 9–24.

63. Hammersley M. By what criteria should ethnographic research be judged? In: Hammersley M (ed.). *What's Wrong with Ethnography?* London: Routledge, 1992, pp. 57–82.

64. Bloor M. Techniques of validation in qualitative research: a critical commentary. In: Miller G,

Dingwall R (eds). *Context and Method in Qualitative Research*. London: Sage, 1997, pp. 37–50.

65. Frake C. How to ask for a drink in Subanun. *American Anthropologist* 1964; **66**: 127–32.

66. Frake C. How to enter a Yakan house. In: Sanchez M, Blount B (eds). *Socio-cultural Dimensions of Language Use*. New York: Academic, 1975, pp. 25–40.

67. Goodwin L, Goodwin H. Qualitative vs quantitative or qualitative and quantitative research? *Nursing Res.* 1984; **33**: 378–80.

68. Walker M. Analysing qualitative data: ethnography and the evaluation of medical education. *Medical Education* 1989; **23**: 498–503.

69. Beck CT. Qualitative research: the evaluation of its credibility, fittingness and auditability. *West. J. Nurs. Res.* 1993; **15**: 263–6.

70. Bloor M. Notes on member validation. In: Emerson RM (ed.). *Contemporary Field Research: a collection of readings*. Boston: Little, Brown, pp. 156–72.

71. Emerson RM, Pollner M. On members' responses to researchers' accounts. *Human Organization* 1988; **47**: 189–98.

72. Jick TD. Mixing qualitative and quantitative methods: triangulation in action. *Administrative Science Quarterly* 1979; **24**: 602–11.

73. Flick U. Triangulation revisited: strategy of validation or alternative. *J. Theor. Soc. Behav.* 1992; **22**: 175–97.

74. Nolan M, Behi R. Triangulation: the best of all worlds? *Br. J. Nurs.* 1995; **4**: 829–32

75. Janesick V. The dance of qualitative research design: metaphor, methodolatry and meaning. In: Denzin N, Lincoln Y (eds). *A Handbook of Qualitative Research*. Thousand Oaks: Sage, 1994, pp. 209–19.

76. Denzin N. *The Research Act*, 2nd edn. New York: McGraw-Hill, 1978.

77. Krefting L. Rigor in qualitative research: the assessment of trustworthiness. *Am. J. Occup. Ther.* 1991; **45**: 214–22.

78. Silverman D. *Qualitative Methodology and Sociology*. 1st edn. Aldershot: Gower, 1985.

79. Dingwall R. The ethnomethodological movement. In: Payne G, Dingwall R, Payne J, Carter M (eds). *Sociology and Social Research*. London: Croom Helm, 1981, pp. 124–38.

80. Stimson G, Webb B. *Going to See the Doctor*. London: Routledge, 1975.

81. Trend M. On the reconciliation of qualitative and quantitative analyses. In: Reichardt C, Cook T (eds). *Qualitative and Quantitative Methods in Evaluation Research*. Beverly Hills: Sage, 1979, pp. 68–86.

82. Altheide D, Johnson J. Criteria for assessing interpretive validity in qualitative research. In: Denzin N, Lincoln Y (eds). *Handbook of Qualitative Research*. Thousand Oaks: Sage, 1994, pp. 485–99.

83. Glaser BG, Strauss A. The discovery of substantive theory: a basic strategy underlying qualitative research. *The American Behavioural Scientist* 1965; **8**: 5–12.

84. Waitzkin H. On studying the discourse of medical encounters. A critique of quantitative and qualitative methods and a proposal for a reasonable compromise. *Medical Care* 1990; **28**: 473–88.

85. Graffam Walker A. The verbatim record: the myth and the reality. In: Fisher S, Todd A (eds). *Discourse and Institutional Authority: Medicine, Education and the Law*. Norwood, NJ: Ablex, 1986, pp. 205–22.

86. Athens L. Scientific criteria for evaluating qualitative studies. In: Denzin NK (ed.). *Studies in Symbolic Interaction 5*. Greenwich, CT: JAI, 1984, pp. 259–68.

87. Secker J, Wimbush E, Watson J, Milburn K. Qualitative methods in health promotion research: some criteria for quality. *Health Education J.* 1995; **54**: 74–87.

88. Glaser BG, Strauss AL. *The Discovery of Grounded Theory: Strategies for Qualitative Research*. New York: Aldine, 1967.

89. Melia KM. Producing 'plausible stories': interviewing student nurses. In: Miller G, Dingwall R (eds). *Context and Method in Qualitative Research*. London: Sage, 1997, pp. 26–36.

90. Becker HS. Whose side are we on? *Social Problems* 1967; **14**: 239–48.

91. Fielding N. Ethnography. In: Gilbert N (ed.). *Researching Social Life*. London: Sage, 1993, pp. 154–71.

92. Voysey M. *A Constant Burden: the Reconstitution of Family Life*. London: Routledge and Kegan Paul, 1975.

Part III
MEASUREMENT OF BENEFIT AND COST

INTRODUCTION by JOHN BRAZIER

The acquisition of data on the benefits and costs of healthcare interventions forms a core activity in Health Technology Assessment (HTA). Considerable resources are expended on gathering and processing routine administrative data sets and obtaining further data from patients, carers and professionals by questionnaire and other methods. The resulting data form the foundation for any assessment of the clinical or cost-effectiveness of a new healthcare intervention. It is imperative to collect the correct data for the assessment task, and to do so as efficiently as possible.

Assessing the benefits and costs in HTA involves three stages: the *identification* of what benefits and resource costs to measure; the *measurement* of those benefits and the use of resources; and finally, the *valuation* of the benefits and resources. The chapters in this section focus on key aspects of these three stages of assessment: Fitzpatrick and colleagues consider the identification and measurement of benefits from the perspective of the patient; Brazier and colleagues consider the implied values of the patient based measures of health status used in HTA and whether they are suitable for use in economic evaluation; Cairns and van der Pol consider the valuation of health benefits over time, and Johnston the identification and measurement of resource use in clinical trials. McColl reviews the use of questionnaire survey methods for measuring the benefits and costs of healthcare. This is not an exhaustive list, but

represents a key set of methodological questions in the design of HTA studies.

In HTA it has now become widely accepted that conventional clinical measures should be supplemented by more patient-focussed measures. The past 20 years has seen a rapid development of patient based measures of outcome, and a plethora of instruments for collecting data on health-related quality of life. A researcher considering which instruments to use can consult one of the excellent reviews, but these quickly become out of date.[1,2] Furthermore, existing reviews may not address the specific condition or likely outcomes of the intervention being assessed. Researchers may need to undertake their own reviews of instruments. Fitzpatrick and colleagues provide a non-technical and up-to-date review of the key concepts for judging patient based measures.[3] In addition to the usual concerns about the reliability and validity of a measure, they have brought together a range of other criteria in the design of a HTA study, including practicality and interpretability.

It is becoming increasingly common to attempt to undertake economic evaluations alongside clinical studies, since they provide an opportunity to collect patient specific data on resource use and outcomes. This has implications for the type of data to collect. There are currently some excellent texts on the methods of economic evaluation,[4] but there has been rather less written on the practical issues of data collection. One misconception has been the view that an economic evaluation can always be undertaken retrospectively after the trial has been completed. This may be appropriate in some circumstances but often it leaves the analyst without the means to perform an economic evaluation. The precise data requirements of economic evaluation will vary depending on the technology and the decision-making context. What additional data are required on costs and benefits must be carefully considered at the design of HTA studies.

The chapter by Brazier and colleagues examines the use of patient based measures of health status in economic evaluation. Many of these measures have not been designed for the purpose of undertaking economic evaluation, and this review identifies their limited role in economic evaluation. The chapter goes on to review the different economic measures designed to estimate a single index value for health-related quality of life which is used in the estimation of quality adjusted life years (QALYs). The different multi-attribute utility scales and techniques for health state valuation are reviewed, and advice offered to researchers contemplating undertaking an economic evaluation alongside a clinical study. Readers interested in non-QALY economic measures of benefits are referred to an overview by Johannesson et al.[5]

The next chapter examines the somewhat neglected topic of collecting resource use data for costing purposes in clinical trials. It covers many important practical issues often overlooked in the economics literature. Johnston and her colleagues consider what resource items to include, how to measure them, and how to value them. They examine the roles of economic theory and perspective in determining what to measure, and provide practical advice on how to collect data on the economically significant resource items in clinical trials and from routine administrative data sets.

Whether data are being collected for use in a clinical or economic evaluation, an important method of collecting data is the questionnaire survey. There is a very large literature on the conduct and design of questionnaire surveys in the social sciences, much of it outside the field of health. McColl and colleagues supplement existing textbooks (such as Sudman and Bradburn[6]) by bringing together this very diverse literature on the evidence and expert opinion found in more theoretical texts. They

address a range of theoretical and practical questions about the conduct of questionnaire surveys in the health field, not in the ideal, but in the resource constrained world of research studies.

An important area of controversy in HTA has been how to treat benefits which are expected to occur sometime in the future. Previous practice has been to apply the same positive rate of discount to health benefits as to costs (i.e. this assumes that health gains today are preferred to equivalent gains later), but this has been questioned in recent years. The chapter by Cairns and van der Pol reviews the rationale for discounting health benefits,[7] looking at past studies, estimating the appropriate rate for health benefits of saving lives or improving health status, and at the design of a study addressing some of the key questions in estimating time preference rates for use in HTA.

Although these reviews are not comprehensive in their coverage of the issues in measuring the benefits and costs of health technologies, they do provide a unique collection of reviews of a set of fundamental issues in HTA. For an overview of cost and benefit measurement, readers are advised to refer to established text, such as that by Drummond et al.[4]

REFERENCES

1. Bowling, A. *Measuring health: a review of quality of life and measurement scales*. Milton Keynes: Open University Press, 1991.
2. Wilkin D, Hallam L, Doggett MA. *Measures of need and outcome for primary health care*. Oxford: Oxford Medical Press, 1992.
3. Streiner DL, Norman GR. *Health Measurement Scales: a practical guide to their development and use*. Oxford: Oxford University Press, 1989.
4. Drummond MF, O'Brien B, Stoddart GL, Torrance GW. *Methods for the economic evaluation of health care programmes*. Oxford: Oxford Medical Publications, 1997.
5. Johannesson M, Jonsson B, Karlsson G. Outcome measurement in economic evaluation. *Health Economics* 1996; **5**: 279–98.
6. Sudman S, Bradburn N. *Asking questions: a practical guide to questionnaire design*. San Francisco: Jossey-Bass, 1993.
7. Parsonage M, Neuberger H. Discounting and health benefits. *Health Economics* 1992; **1**: 71–6.

11

Criteria for Assessing Patient Based Outcome Measures for Use in Clinical Trials

RAY FITZPATRICK, CLAIRE DAVEY,
MARTIN J. BUXTON and DAVID R. JONES

SUMMARY

Patient based outcome measures in the form of questionnaires or interview schedules are increasingly used in clinical trials to assess outcomes in relation to health status, health-related quality of life and similar constructs. Types of instruments include disease- or condition-specific, dimension-specific, generic, summary items, individualised measures and utility measures. A literature review was undertaken and revised in the light of an expert panel's comments, in order to identify the criteria in terms of which investigators should select patient based outcome measures for use in a clinical trial. Eight criteria for assessing patient based outcome measures are distinguished and briefly described: appropriateness, reliability, validity, responsiveness, precision, interpretability, acceptability and feasibility. These criteria are not precisely or uniformly described in the literature; nor can they be prioritised in terms of importance. Nevertheless, investigators need to consider these criteria in selecting a patient based outcome measure for a trial. Developers of patients based outcome measures need to provide as clear evidence as possible of new instruments in terms of the eight criteria emphasised by this review.

INTRODUCTION

It is increasingly recognised that traditional bio-medically defined outcomes such as clinical and laboratory measures need to be complemented by measures that focus on the patient's concerns in order to evaluate interventions and identify more appropriate forms of healthcare. In the major areas of health service spending, and particularly in areas such as cancer, cardiovascular, neurological and musculoskeletal disease, interventions aim to alleviate symptoms and restore function, with major implications for quality of life. In many new and existing interventions increased attention also has to be given to potentially iatrogenic effects of medical interventions in areas such as well-being and quality of life. Patient based outcome measures provide a feasible and appropriate method for addressing the concerns of patients in the context of controlled clinical trials.

By patient based outcome measures is meant questionnaires or related forms of assessment that patients complete by themselves – or when necessary others complete on their behalf – in order that evidence is obtained of their experiences and concerns in relation to health status, health-related quality of life and the perceived results of treatments received. Although these measures have been developed for a number of other applications, this chapter is concerned with their use in clinical trials. There is now an enormous array of such measures that can be used in clinical trials. The purpose of the chapter is to make clear the criteria investigators should have in mind when they select patient based outcome measures at the stage of designing a clinical trial.

This chapter is based on a structured review carried out for the NHSE R&D programme.[1] The review used a combination of electronic and hand searching. A total of 5621 abstracts and references were identified by initial searches as potentially relevant to the review, but only 404 references were actively used in the final draft review. An initial first draft was written by one of the present authors (R.F.). A second draft, revised in the light of discussion with the other three authors, was then sent out to a panel of ten experts from the fields of clinical medicine, clinical trials, health economics, health services research, psychology, sociology and statistics. They were invited to comment both on broad and strategic aspects of the approach of the review, as well as on whatever specific details they wished. The literature review was then revised considerably in the light of this set of comments. The final draft, of which this is a summary, is a quasi-consensus view of a wide range of experts as to key issues surrounding selection of patient based outcome measures.

Concepts and Definitions

This is a review of a field in which there is no precise definition of or agreement about subject matter. We are concerned with questionnaires and related instruments that ask patients about their health. However, with regard to more precise definitions of what such instruments are intended to assess, there is no agreed terminology, and reviews variously refer to instruments as being concerned with 'quality of life' (QoL), 'health-related quality of life' (HRQoL), 'health status', 'functional status', 'performance status', 'subjective health status', 'disability' and 'functional well-being'. To some extent this diversity reflects real differences of emphasis between instruments. Some questionnaires focus exclusively upon physical function; for example, assessing mobility and activities of daily living without reference to social and psychological factors, and might appropriately be described as functional status instruments. Other instruments may ask simple global questions about the individual's health. Other instruments again are concerned with the impact of health on a broad spectrum of the individual's life, for example, family life and life satisfaction, and might reasonably be considered to assess quality of life. In reality, the various terms such as 'health

status' and 'quality of life' are used interchangeably to such an extent that they lack real descriptive value. The term 'patient based outcome measure' is here used wherever possible as the most all-embracing term to encompass all of the types of instruments conveyed by other terms such as 'health status', or 'quality of life'.

There are circumstances where patients are unable to provide their unique report of their perceptions, due to ill-health, physical or cognitive problems, or some other incapacity. In these cases, proxy reports may be necessary because of the need for some assessment to inform a clinical trial. Because there is consistent evidence of lack of agreement of patients' judgements of their quality of life with assessments made by observers such as health professionals, informal carers, and other so-called proxy judges, this is increasingly considered a second-best solution to be used only when the patient cannot contribute.[2]

The content of the instruments with which we are concerned varies enormously, and in general a researcher will usually be able to find an instrument with questionnaire items that at least approximate to the issues of concern to his or her research question. Every instrument attempts to provide an assessment of at least one dimension of health status, either the respondent's global assessment of health, or more specific dimensions such as mobility, pain or psychological well-being. Instruments range in content from items which are most obviously related to a patient's health status, such as the patient's global view of their health, experiences of symptoms or psychological illness, through to dimensions that increasingly reflect the broader impact of illness on the individual's life such as social function, role activities and impact on paid income.

Types of Instruments

One of the main decisions to be made in selecting an instrument for a clinical trial is to choose among the different kinds of instrument that exist. They differ in content and also in the primary intended purpose.

Disease/condition-specific

As the title implies, these instruments have been developed in order to provide the patient's perception of a specific disease or health problem. An example of such a questionnaire is the Asthma Quality of Life Questionnaire.[3] This contains 32 questions assessing four dimensions (activity limitations, symptoms, emotional function and exposure to environmental stimuli).

Dimension-specific

Dimension-specific instruments assess one specific aspect of health status. By far the most common type of dimension-specific measure is one that assesses aspects of psychological well-being. An example is the Beck Depression Inventory.[4] This contains 21 items that address symptoms of depression, the scores for items being summed to produce a total score. It was largely developed for use in psychiatric patients, but is increasingly used more widely to assess depression as an outcome in physically ill populations.

Generic instruments

Generic instruments are intended to capture a very broad range of aspects of health status and the consequences of illness, and therefore to be relevant to a wide range of patient groups. The content of such questionnaires has been deliberately designed to be widely appropriate. They may provide assessments of the health status of samples of individuals not recruited because they have a specific disease, for example, from primary care or the community as a whole. One of the most widely used of such instruments is the SF-36.[5] This is a 36-item questionnaire which measures health status in eight dimensions: physical functioning, role limitations due to physical problems, role limitations due to emotional problems, social functioning, mental health, energy/vitality, pain and general perceptions of health. Item responses are summed to give a score for each dimension.

Summary items

Single questionnaire items have an important role in healthcare research. They invite respondents to summarise diverse aspects of their health status by means of one or a very small number of questions. The General Household Survey for England and Wales has, in annual surveys since 1974, used two questions that together provide an assessment of chronic illness and disability: 'Do you have any long-standing illness or disability?' and 'Does this illness or disability limit your activities in any way?' A positive answer to the two questions provide an indication of chronic disability.

Individualised Measures

Individualised measures are instruments in which the respondent is allowed to select issues, domains or concerns that are of personal concern that are not predetermined by the investigator's list of questionnaire items. By a variety of means the respondent is encouraged to identify those aspects of life that are personally affected by health, without imposing any standardised list of potential answers. Individualised measures are still in their infancy, but have attracted interest precisely because they appear to offer considerable scope for eliciting respondents' own concerns and perceptions. One example is the Schedule for the Evaluation of Individual Quality of Life (SEIQoL).[6] This is completed in three phases by semi-structured interview in order to produce an overall quality of life score for sick or healthy people. The first stage asks the individual (with structured interviewer prompting when necessary) to list five areas of life most important to their quality of life. Secondly, each of the nominated five areas is rated on a visual–analogue scale from 'as good as it could be' to 'as bad as it could be'. The individual patient also rates overall quality of life. The last stage uses 30 hypothetical case vignettes which vary systematically in terms of the properties respondents have already identified as important to them. Judgement analysis of respondents' ratings of these vignettes allows the investigator to produce weights for the five chosen aspects of life, and an index score is calculated between 0 and 100. This exercise can then be repeated at subsequent assessments.

Utility measures

Utility measures are distinctive because they yield a single number to summarise individuals' overall preferences regarding health status. The most familiar example in Europe is the EuroQol EQ-5D.[7] The part of the EQ-5D questionnaire to elicit health status comprises five questions, each of which has three alternative response categories. The five items assess mobility, self-care, usual activity, pain/discomfort and anxiety/depression. These items can be used by themselves as descriptions of respondents' health states. Responses are also scored by means of weights obtained from the valuations that other samples from the general population have assigned to health states using visual–analogue scales or time–trade-off methods (time–trade-off is discussed in Chapter 12). These weightings combine to provide utilities.

CRITERIA FOR ASSESSING INSTRUMENTS

There are eight issues that need to be examined when selecting a patient based outcome measure for a trial: appropriateness, reliability, validity, responsiveness, precision, interpretability, acceptability and feasibility. These criteria are discussed in turn.

Appropriateness

The first and most fundamental consideration to be faced when selecting a patient based outcome measure is how to identify one that is most appropriate to the aims of the particular trial. This requires careful consideration of the aims of the trial, with reference to the quality of life research questions, i.e. which dimensions will be primary and secondary end-points, the nature of the study intervention and of the patient group, and about the content of possible candidate instruments. For this reason it is particularly difficult to give specific recommendations about what in general makes an outcome measure appropriate to a trial, because this is ultimately a judgement of the fit between investigators' specific trial questions and content of instruments. However, it is clear from a number of reviews already carried out in this field that it is an absolutely fundamental issue.

There have been several previous reviews that have discussed appropriateness of outcome measures in clinical trials in general terms. Some of the early reviews are mainly critical of clinical trials for failing to use *any* kind of patient based outcome measure where the subject matter seemed to indicate that such an approach was needed. Thus, Brook and Kamberg[8] concluded that, from a sample of 73 clinical trials in which they considered health status or quality of life was likely to be a major issue, in only two trials was an appropriate patient based outcome measure used.

A more formal evaluation of outcome measurement in trials is reported by Guyatt and colleagues.[9] In their study, two raters independently examined all clinical trials published in a range of journals in 1986. Of the 75 trials they evaluated, they considered quality of life as crucial or important in 55 (73%) of trials. However, in 44% of this subgroup of trials no effort was made to assess this dimension of outcome. In a further 38% of the 55 trials an untested measure was used that the reviewers considered inappropriate. They concluded that appropriate measures would have considerably strengthened the basis for recommendations emerging from the trial.

Most obviously an instrument needs to fit the purpose of a trial. This purpose needs to be specified as precisely as is reasonable, and outcome measures selected accordingly. The rationale for selection of outcome measures is

often not clear with investigators uncritically inserting questionnaires into their trials without careful consideration of content and relevance to the purpose of the trial.[10]

Reliability

Reliability is concerned with the reproducibility and internal consistency of a measuring instrument. It assesses the extent to which the instrument is free from random error, and may be considered as the proportion of a score that is signal rather than noise. It is a very important property of any patient based outcome measure in a clinical trial because it is essential to establish that any changes observed in a trial are due to the intervention and not to problems in the measuring instrument. As the random error of such a measure increases, so the size of the sample required to obtain a precise estimate of effects in a trial will increase. An unreliable measure may therefore imprecisely estimate the size of benefit obtained from an intervention. The reliability of a particular measure is not a fixed property, but is dependent upon the context and population studied.[11]

In practice, the evaluation of reliability is made in terms of two different aspects of a measure: internal consistency and reproducibility. The two measures derive from classical measurement theory which regards any observation as the sum of two components, a true score and an error term.[12]

Internal consistency

Normally, more than one questionnaire item is used to measure a dimension or construct. This follows from a basic principle of measurement that several related observations will produce a more reliable estimate than one. For this to be true, the items all need to be homogeneous, that is all measuring aspects of a single attribute or construct rather than different constructs.[11] The practical consequence of this expectation is that individual items should highly correlate with each other and with the summed score of the total of items in the same scale.

Internal consistency can be measured in a number of different ways. One approach – split-half reliability – is randomly to divide the items in a scale into two groups and to assess the degree of agreement between the two halves. The two halves should correlate highly. An extension of this principle is Coefficient alpha, usually referred to as Cronbach's alpha, which essentially estimates the average level of agreement of all the possible ways of performing split-half tests.[13] The higher the alpha, the higher the internal consistency. However, it is also possible to increase Cronbach's alpha by increasing the number of items, even if the average level of correlation does not change.[11] Also, if the items of a scale correlate perfectly with each other, it is likely that there is some redundancy among items, and also a possibility that the items together are addressing a rather narrow aspect of an attribute. For these reasons it is suggested that Cronbach's alpha should be above 0.70 but not higher than 0.90.[11,14]

It has been argued that excessive attention to internal reliability can result in the omission of important items, particularly those that reflect the complexity and diversity of a phenomenon.[15] Certainly obtaining the highest possible reliability coefficient should not be the sole objective in developing or selecting an instrument, because the reductio ad absurdum of this principle would be an instrument with high reliability produced by virtually identical items.

Reproducibility

Reproducibility more directly evaluates whether an instrument yields the same results on repeated applications, when respondents have not changed on the domain being measured. This is assessed by test–retest reliability. The degree of agreement is examined between scores at a first assessment and when reassessed. There is no exact agreement about the length of time that should elapse between test and retest; it needs to be a sufficient length of time that respondents are unlikely to recall their previous answers, but not so long that actual changes in the underlying dimension of health have occurred. Streiner and Norman[11] suggest that the usual range of time elapsed between assessments tends to be between 2 and 14 days.

Test–retest reliability is commonly examined by means of a correlation coefficient. This is often the Pearson product moment correlation coefficient. This approach is limited and may exaggerate reproducibility because results from two administrations of a test may correlate highly but be systematically different. The second test may result in every respondent having a lower score than their first response, yet the correlation could be 1.0. For this reason, an intra-class correlation coefficient is advocated. This uses analysis of variance to determine how much of the total variability in scores is due to true differences between individuals and how much due to variability in measurement. Alternatively, Bland and Altman[16] advocate graphically plotting scores for the two administrations of a test, so that, for example, it is possible to identify areas in the range of scores of an instrument which are less reproducible.

Commonly cited minimal standards for reliability coefficients are 0.7 for group data, although some experts set much higher requirements.[17] It can also be argued that absolute minimally acceptable coefficients are not meaningful, since larger sample sizes for a trial permit more measurement error in an instrument.

Validity

The validity of a measure is an assessment of the extent to which it measures what it purports to measure. There are a number of different ways of establishing the validity of a measure. As with reliability, it is not a fixed property of a measure; its validity is assessed in relation to a specific purpose and setting.[14,18] It is therefore meaningless to refer to a validated measure as such; it should be considered a measure validated for use in relation to a specific purpose or set of purposes. For example, a valid measure of disability for patients with arthritis cannot automatically be considered valid for use for patients with multiple sclerosis; a measure considered validated for individuals with mild impairment may not be valid for those with severe impairments.

Some types of validity are not relevant to this field. Criterion validity is concerned with whether a new measure correlates with an existing measure generally accepted as a more accurate or criterion variable. However, in the field of application of health status measures with which we are concerned, as outcome measures in clinical trials, rarely if ever does a perfect 'gold-standard' measure exist against which to test the validity of new health status measure, and a number of different and more indirect approaches are recommended to judge instruments' validity.

Face and content validity

Face, content and (below) construct validity are far the most relevant issues for the use of patient based outcome measures in trials. It is vital to inspect the content of a measure in relation to its intended purpose. This inspection largely involves qualitative matters of judgement that contrast with more statistical criteria that also need to be considered in the context of construct validity. Judgement of the content of an instrument contributes to what has been termed face validity and content validity. The two terms are related but have been distinct. Guyatt and colleagues[19] make the distinction thus: 'Face validity examines whether an instrument appears to be measuring what it is intended to measure, and content validity examines the extent to which the domain of interest is comprehensively sampled by the items, or questions, in the instrument' (p. 624). Together, they address whether items clearly address the intended subject matter and whether the range of aspects are adequately covered. Face validity can overlap with judgements of the interpretability of items, but these aspects are kept separate here.

Another important source of evidence can be obtained from evidence of how the questionnaire was developed in the first place. How extensively did individuals with relevant clinical or health status methodology expertise participate in generating the content?[20] Even more importantly, to what extent did patients with experience of the health problem participate in generating and confirming the content of an instrument?[21] Whilst knowledgeable about an illness, experts such as health professionals cannot substitute completely for the direct experience that patients have of health problems.

Construct validity

A more quantitative form of assessing the validity of an instrument is also necessary. This involves construct validity. A health status measure is intended to assess a postulated underlying construct, such as pain, isolation or disability rather than some directly observable phenomenon. The items of a questionnaire represent something important other than a numerical score but that 'something' is not directly observable. This construct, for example, pain or disability, can be expected to have a set of quantitative relationships with other constructs on the basis of current understanding. Individuals experiencing more severe pain may be expected to take more analgesics; individuals with greater disability to have less range of movement in their environment. Construct validity is examined by quantitatively examining relationships of a construct to a set of other variables. No single observation can prove the construct validity of a new measure; rather it is necessary to build up a picture from a broad pattern of relationships of the new measure with other variables.[22] Patient based outcome measures are sometimes presented as 'validated' because they have been shown to agree with clinical or laboratory evidence of disease severity. Whilst such evidence provides an aspect of construct validity, it is not sufficient. As Streiner and Norman[11] observe (p. 9), 'the burden of evidence in testing construct validity arises not from a single powerful experiment, but from a series of converging experiments'.

Responsiveness

For use in trials, it is essential that a health status questionnaire can detect important changes over time within individuals, that might reflect therapeutic effects.[23] This section addresses sensitivity to change, or responsiveness. The latter term is preferable because 'sensitivity' has a number of more general uses in epidemiology. As it is conceivable for an instrument to be both reliable and valid, but not responsive, this dimension of a health status measure is increasingly essential to evaluate. Guyatt and colleagues[24] define responsiveness as the ability of an instrument to detect clinically important change. They provide illustrative evidence of the importance of this aspect of instruments with data from a controlled trial of chemotherapy for breast cancer. Four health status instruments considered to be validated were completed by women. However, only one of the four instruments showed expected differences over time as well as providing valid evidence of the womens' health status.

Rather like validity, there is no single agreed method of assessing or expressing an instrument's responsiveness, and a variety of statistical approaches have been proposed.

Correlations of change scores

The simplest method to use is to calculate change scores for the instrument over time in a trial or longitudinal study and to examine the correlations of such change scores with changes in other available variables. For example, Meenan and colleagues[25] examined the correlations of changes over time in a health status measure with changes in physiological measures in a trial of patients with arthritis. Correlations were significant, and the health status measure considered responsive. This approach provides important evidence of whether a health status measure provides changes over time that are consistent with other available data. It does not provide a formal statistic of responsiveness.

Effect size

A number of methods, now discussed, have been proposed to provide quantitative expressions of the magnitude and meaning of health status changes. These same approaches may also be considered expressions of the responsiveness of health status instruments. Just as with reliability and validity, the estimates provided for responsiveness are strictly speaking confined to specific uses in particular populations, and are not an inherent property of the instrument.

One common form of standardised expression of responsiveness is the effect size. The basic approach to calculation of the effect size is to calculate the size of change on a measure that occurs to a group between assessments (for example, before and after treatment), compared with the variability of scores of that measure.[26] Most commonly this is calculated as the difference between mean scores at assessments, divided by the standard deviation of baseline scores. The effect size is then expressed in standardised units that permit comparisons between instruments.

Standardised response mean

An alternative measure is the standardised response mean (SRM). This only differs from an effect size in that the denominator is the standard deviation of change scores in the group in order to take account of variability in change rather than baseline scores.[27] Because the denominator in the SRM examines response variance in an instrument, whereas the effect size does not, Katz and colleagues[28] consider that the SRM approach is more informative.

Relative efficiency

Another approach is to compare the responsiveness of health status instruments when used in studies of treatments widely considered to be effective, so that it is very likely that significant changes actually occur. As applied by Liang and colleagues[29] who developed this approach, the performance of different health status instruments is compared to a standard instrument amongst patients who are considered to have experienced substantial change. Thus, they asked patients to complete a number of health status questionnaires before and after total joint replacement surgery. Health status questionnaires that produced the largest paired *t*-test score for pre- and post-surgical assessments were considered most responsive. Liang and colleagues[28] produce a standardised version of the use of *t*-statistics (termed 'relative efficiency'), the square of the ratio of *t*-statistic for two instruments being compared.

In general, these different methods express subtly different aspects of change scores produced by instruments. It is not surprising therefore that when several instruments are compared in terms of their responsiveness, somewhat different impressions can be formed of relative performance depending on which method is used to assess responsiveness.[30,31] Wright and Young[32] found that the rank order of responsiveness of different patient based outcome measures varied according to which of five different methods they used in a sample of patients before and after total hip replacement surgery.

Ceiling and floor effects

The actual form of questionnaire items in an instrument may reduce the likelihood of further improvement or deterioration being recorded beyond a certain point. Put another way, the wording of questionnaire items may not make it possible to report most favourable or worst health states. The terms 'ceiling' and 'floor' effects are usually used to refer to the two forms of this problem. A study administered the MOS-20 scale to patients in hospital at baseline and again six months later.[33] At the follow-up survey respondents also completed a 'transition question' in which they assessed whether their health was better, the same or worse than at baseline assessment. A number of respondents who reported the worst possible scores for the MOS-20 at baseline reported further deterioration in their follow-up assessment in their answers to the transition question. It was clearly not possible for such respondents to report lower scores on the MOS-20 than at baseline.

Precision

An instrument may have high reliability but low precision if it makes only a small number of crude distinctions with regard to a dimension of health. Thus, at the extreme one instrument might distinguish with high reliability only between those who are healthy and those who are ill. For the purposes of a trial such an instrument would not be useful because it is degrees of change within the category of 'unwell' that are likely to be needed to evaluate results of the arms of the trial.

There are a number of ways in which the issue of precision has been raised in relation to patient based outcome measures. This is fairly disparate evidence, and it is reviewed under a number of more specific headings. Precision may sometimes be referred to in the literature as 'discriminative validity'.[23,24]

Precision of response categories

One of the main influences on the precision of an instrument is the format of response categories; i.e. the form in which respondents are able to give their answers. At one extreme, answers may be given by respondents in terms of very basic distinctions, 'yes' or 'no'. Binary response categories have the advantage of simplicity, but there is evidence that they do not allow respondents to report degrees of difficulty or severity that they experience and consider important to distinguish.[15] Many instruments therefore allow for gradations of response, most commonly in the form of a Likert set of response categories such as:

> strongly agree uncertain disagree strongly agree disagree

Alternatively, response categories may require that respondents choose between different options of how frequently a problem occurs.

There is some evidence that there is increased precision from using seven rather than five response categories. A sample of older individuals with heart problems were assigned to questionnaires assessing satisfaction with various domains of life with either five or seven item response categories.[34] The latter showed higher correlations with a criterion measure of quality of life completed by respondents.

The main alternative to Likert format response categories is the visual–analogue scale, which would appear to offer considerably more precision. Respondents can mark any point on a continuous line to represent their experience, and in principle this offers an extensive range of response categories. However, the evidence is not strong that the apparent precision is meaningful. Guyatt and colleagues[35] compared the responsiveness of a health-related quality of life measure for respiratory function, using alternate forms of a Likert and visual–analogue scale. They found no significant advantage for the visual–analogue scale. Similar results were found in a randomised trial setting, showing no advantage in responsiveness for visual–analogue scales.[36] An additional concern is the somewhat lower acceptability of visual–analogue scales as a task.

Scoring methods

Scoring methods that attempt directly to estimate the values of such response categories such as in the Sickness Impact Profile by weighting systems, may appear deceptively precise. Their numerical exactness might lend pseudo-precision to an instrument. For investigators examining the numerical values of instruments, it is sensible to treat all scoring methods as weighted, differing only in how transparent weights are, and to look beyond superficial aspects of precision to examine how weightings have been derived and validated. More pragmatically it is appropriate to ask whether weighting systems make a difference. Sensitivity analysis may reveal that they make no significant difference to results. For example, Jenkinson[37] analysed patterns of change over time in health status for patients with rheumatoid arthritis by means of the Functional Limitations Profile and

Nottingham Health Profile. Sensitivity to change as indicated by a battery of other clinical and laboratory measures was very similar whether weighted or unweighted (items valued as '1' or '0') versions of the instruments were used. Scoring of health status measures for economic evaluations is also extensively considered by Brazier and colleagues in Chapter 12.

Distribution of items over true range

The items and scores of different instruments may vary in how well they capture the full underlying range of problems experienced by patients. It is not easy to examine the relationship between the distinctions made by a measuring instrument and the true distribution of actual experiences, for the obvious reason that one usually does not have access to the true distribution other than through one's measuring instrument.

An illustration of the problematic relationship between items and the 'true' distribution of what is being measured is provided by Stucki and colleagues'[38] analysis of SF-36 physical ability scores in patients undergoing total hip replacement surgery. They showed that many of the items of this scale represent moderate levels of difficulty for patients to perform (e.g. 'bending, kneeling or stooping'); by contrast, there are only a few items that almost everyone could do with no difficulty (e.g. 'bathing and dressing yourself'), and only a few items that were difficult for the majority to perform (e.g. 'walking more than a mile'). A direct consequence of this is that patients passing a difficulty level in the middle of this scale of the SF-36 are more likely to have larger change scores than patients undergoing change at either the top or bottom of the range of difficulty of items, simply because of the larger number of items assessing moderate levels of difficulty.

Interpretability

The issue of the interpretability of scores has only recently received attention in the literature on patient based outcome measures. It has often been commented that patient based outcome measures lack the interpretability that other measures, for example blood pressure or blood sugar levels, have for clinicians.[39] To some extent this may be due to lack of familiarity with use. Researchers have also begun to make efforts to make scores more interpretable. One method used in a trial of antihypertensives was to calibrate change scores on quality of life instruments with the changes for the same instruments that have been found with major life events, such as loss of a job.[40] In this way health status scores could be related to other human experiences that have clear and intuitive meaning.

Another approach to interpreting results is to identify a plausible range within which a minimal clinically important difference (MCID) falls.[41,42] Jaeschke et al. define a MCID as 'the smallest difference in score in the domain of interest which patients perceive as beneficial and which would mandate, in the absence of troublesome side effects and excessive costs, a change in the patient's management' (p. 408). They examined this concept in relation to patients completing at baseline and follow-up either the Chronic Respiratory Questionnaire in a drug trial for asthma or the Chronic Heart Failure Questionnaire in a drug trial for patients with heart failure. Changes between baseline and follow-up were examined in relation to their benchmark for a MCID which was the patient's follow-up assessment in a transition item of whether they were worse, better or the same compared with baseline assessment. They showed that a mean change of 0.5 for a seven-point scale was the minimal change amongst patients reporting a change. Other methods of understanding clinically important changes require the selection of other external benchmarks such as the global judgement of the clinician or laboratory tests or reference to distribution based interpretations, such as using effect size.[27,43]

Acceptability

It is essential that instruments be acceptable to patients. This is clearly desirable to minimise avoidable distress to patients already coping with health problems. It is also essential in order to obtain high response rates to questionnaires in order to make results of trials more easy to interpret, more generalisable, and less prone to bias from non-response. The acceptability of patient based outcome measures has far less frequently been examined than issues such as reliability and validity.

Reasons for non-completion

Patients may either not return a whole assessment, or may omit some items in an assessment. If patients either do not attempt to complete an instrument at all or omit particular items frequently, this is potentially a sign that a questionnaire is difficult to understand, distressing, or in some other way unacceptable. However, there may be other reasons for non-completion such as the method of delivery of the questionnaire. Patients may not receive a mailed questionnaire in the first place or may not have a telephone in order to be contacted in this way.

Patients may also be unable to complete questionnaires because of their health status or other disabilities, particularly cognitive or visual.

More general features of the layout, appearance and legibility of a questionnaire are thought to have a strong influence on acceptability. Some instruments have deliberately included extremely simple and short forms of wording of questions together with pictorial representations to add to ease and acceptability of use. A rare experimental study to test the benefit of pictorial representation in a quality of life study showed that cartoon figures to depict degrees of illness severity improved test–retest reliability compared with responses to conventional formatting.[44]

There is only limited evidence available comparing the response rates of different health status instruments, rather than the method of their administration. In a series of older patients who had undergone total hip replacement surgery, higher completion rates were obtained from a 12-item condition-specific questionnaire compared to a longer generic instrument, the SF-36.[45]

Another form of evidence comes from the differential responses to different subject matters in surveys of health status. Guyatt and colleagues[46] found that a sample of elderly respondents were somewhat more likely to complete the section of a questionnaire concerned with physical rather than with emotional items, suggesting differential acceptability of topics depending on how personal they were. By contrast, in a qualitative study of patients with small-cell lung cancer[47] it was reported that patients found questions about their psychological well-being more tolerable than questions about tumour-related symptoms.

Time to complete

It is often assumed that one aspect or determinant of the acceptability of a questionnaire is its length; the longer it takes to complete, the less acceptable is the instrument. Many instruments are published with claims by their developers about the length of time required to complete them. Far less commonly is this property independently assessed or instruments' time to complete measured comparatively. Amongst instruments requiring the least time to complete are the self-completed COOP charts which have been estimated to take 2–3 min.[48] Similarly, Wolfe and colleagues[49] directly assessed the mean length of time required to complete one of the most commonly used of instruments for arthritis – the Health Assessment Questionnaire (HAQ) – as 3 min. Most health status instruments are longer than these two examples, and probably require more time to complete. Aaronson and colleagues[50] directly measured time to complete the EORTC QLQ-C30 on two separate occasions, before and during active treatment (12 and 11 min, respectively). The time required may depend upon the characteristics of respondents.

A smaller number of studies have examined comparatively the time required for various instruments or methods of administration. Weinberger and colleagues[51] assessed the time required for SF-36 to be completed by two different methods of administration; when self-completed, the instrument required 12.7 min, compared to 9.6 min for face-to-face interviews. In an elderly group of patients the SF-36 took 14 min by personal interview and 10.2 min by telephone administration.[52] Read and colleagues[53] compared the time to administer of the General Health Rating Index, the Quality of Well-Being Scale and the Sickness Impact Profile, which required 11.4, 18.2 and 22.4 min, respectively. Generally such evidence is not available. In a comparative study of health status measures of outcomes, Bombardier and colleagues[54] estimated that the HAQ required 5 min to complete, compared to three different utility measures that required administration by interview and between 30 and 60 min to complete. Independent assessment of timing is important because developers of instruments may be overoptimistic in their estimates.

It is increasingly argued that, if there are no or minimal costs in terms of validity, responsiveness and other key components of instruments, then instruments should be reduced in terms of length and number of items in order to increase acceptability.[55] Some comparative studies have shown no loss of responsiveness when such shorter instruments are used.[28,56]

Evidence of difficulties with an instrument is provided by Guyatt and colleagues,[35] who compared the measurement properties of Likert and visual–analogue forms of response categories to a health-related quality of life instrument. In explaining the two forms of task to patients they found that patients viewed visual–analogue scales as harder to understand. In specific terms, they report that it took up to twice as long to explain.

Direct assessment of acceptability

It is preferable directly to assess patients' views about a new questionnaire. Sprangers and colleagues[57] argue that patients' views should be obtained at the pre-testing phase prior to formal tests for reliability, etc., by means of a structured interview in which they are asked whether they found any questionnaire items difficult, annoying or distressing, or whether issues were omitted. When the EORTC QLQ-C30 was assessed in this way, 10% of patients reported one or more items was confusing or difficult to answer, and less than 3% that an item was upsetting, whilst more generally patients welcomed the opportunity to report their experiences.[50] Another formal evaluation of acceptability of a questionnaire found that 89% enjoyed the task of completing the COOP instrument, and 97% reported understanding the questions.[48]

In general, users should expect to see evidence of acceptability being examined at the design stage. Subsequently, the most direct and easy to assess evidence are the length and response rates of questionnaires.

Translation and cultural applicability

One basic way in which a questionnaire may fail to be acceptable is if it is expressed in a language unfamiliar to respondents. This issue has received a large amount of attention in recent literature on patient based outcomes, mainly because of the increasing need for clinical trials incorporating quality of life measures to be conducted on a multi-national basis, especially in Europe.[58,59] As a result there are quite elaborate guidelines available intended to ensure high standards of translation of questionnaires.[60,61] Amongst procedures to improve translation, according to such guidelines, are: use of several independent translations that are compared; back-translation; testing of the acceptability of translations to respondents. Less attention has been to cultural and linguistic variations within national boundaries, but it would seem that similar principles could be applied to increase cultural applicability. Presently, few patient based outcome measures have been translated into the languages of ethnic minorities in the UK.

Feasibility

In addition to patient burden and acceptability, it is important to evaluate the impact of different patient based outcome measures upon staff and researchers in collecting and processing information.[62,63] Data from patients for clinical trials are often gathered in the context of regular clinical patient care, and excessive burden to staff may jeopardise trial conduct and disrupt clinical care. An obvious example is the additional staff effort and costs involved in personally administering questionnaires compared to postal delivery. To a lesser extent the length and complexity of instrument are an additional component. Certainly it may require additional staff time to assist and explain how more complex questionnaires are to be filled out by patients. The simplest of instruments such as the nine-item COOP charts require a minimum of time and effort to process.[48] Their brevity (one item per domain) and pictorial representation mean that they require less staff supervision than most alternatives. A related component of feasibility is time required to train staff to use an instrument, with questionnaires designed for self-completion imposing the least burden in this respect. Where instruments do require interviewer administration, training needs can vary according to the complexity of the tasks. Read and colleagues[53] compared the training times required for three health status instruments and found that they varied from 1–2 hours for the easiest to 1–2 weeks for the most complex instrument.

OVERALL SUMMARY AND RECOMMENDATIONS

The rapid expansion of efforts to assess outcomes of healthcare from the patient's perspective has resulted in hundreds of instruments that have in common that they purport to provide standardised assessments of matters of importance to patients such as functional status, subjective health and broader aspects of health-related quality of life.

There are substantial areas of uncertainty and dispute regarding outcome measurement. Over a number of issues, gaps and limitations of concepts and measurement have been acknowledged in the literature. This chapter has built on and attempted to integrate previous efforts to identify desirable properties of patient based outcome measures. It is very encouraging that authors from three disciplines of social science (R.F.), health economics (M.B.) and medical statistics (D.J.) can agree to this document; this is itself an important step in progress to define the field. Broad assent to the principles of the review was also obtained from a wide range of disciplines and expertise relevant to health technology assessment and health services research: comments on a draft were sought from those with expertise in clinical medicine and clinical trials, health economics, health service research, psychology, sociology and statistics. Every effort was made to respond to and integrate expert advisers' suggestions. We feel that the resulting document presents views based on substantial consensus about issues.

We recommend that, on grounds stated as explicitly as possible, and making use of available evidence about instruments, outcome measures for clinical trials should be chosen by evaluating evidence about instruments in relation to the following eight criteria: appropriateness,

reliability, validity, responsiveness, precision, interpretability, acceptability and feasibility.

The selection of instruments on the basis of our criteria cannot, given the present state of the field, be a straightforward or mechanical one. This is partly because there is only a moderate level of consensus about what exactly is meant by some criteria. The literature does not provide unambiguous definitions and advice regarding the issues we have reviewed. The evidence for any given instrument will be partial and complex to assimilate. Above all, the criteria themselves cannot be weighted or prioritised given the current state of knowledge.

Investigators need to think of the desirable properties of outcome measures for a specific use in a specific trial question. Instruments do not have properties of being reliable, valid and so on in some universal sense; they are properties in relation to a specific use. This makes selection of instruments a complex process. Investigators need to select outcomes appropriate to the question addressed by a trial. Ideally, each instrument should be optimally appropriate, valid, reliable and so on, although, in reality, trials may include combinations of outcome measures that together have optimal measurement properties.

To encourage more appropriate use of outcome measures, those who develop such instruments need to provide as clear evidence as possible of the available evidence of new instruments in terms of the eight criteria emphasised by this review.

To facilitate appropriate selection of instruments for clinical trials, two types of further research are needed. In trials and observational studies, the performance of patient based outcome measures should be directly compared. It will then be possible to address questions such as whether disease-specific, generic or other types of instruments are more responsive in various clinical contexts. Secondly, researchers and clinicians in specific areas, oncology, rheumatology, psychiatry and so on, should carry out assessments of evidence for the comparative performance generally of the more widely used of outcome measures in their field. This process has begun to happen in some specialities, and publication of such consensus views would further promote awareness of the role of patient based outcomes in clinical trials.

By identifying a set of criteria and making some attempt to be more explicit about their meaning, this chapter and its accompanying larger review are intended to progress the appropriate use of such methods in order to facilitate the conduct of clinical trials taking full account of patients' judgements about their health and healthcare.

REFERENCES

1. Fitzpatrick R, Davey C, Buxton M, Jones D. *Evaluating patient-based outcome measures for use in clinical trials.* NHS HTA Programme. Monograph, 1998.
2. Sprangers MA, Aaronson NK. The role of health care providers and significant others in evaluating the quality of life of patients with chronic disease: a review. *J. Clin. Epidemiol.* 1992; **45**: 743–60.
3. Juniper EF, Guyatt GH, Willan A, Griffith LE. Determining a minimal important change in a disease-specific Quality of Life Questionnaire. *J. Clin. Epidemiol.* 1994; **47**: 81–7.
4. Beck A, Ward C, Medelson M, Mock J, Erbaugh J. An inventory for measuring depression. *Arch. Gen. Psychiatry* 1961; **4**: 561–71.
5. Ware J, Sherbourne CD. The MOS 36-item short-form health survey (SF-36). I. Conceptual framework and item selection. *Med. Care* 1992; **30**: 473–83.
6. O'Boyle CA, McGee H, Hickey AM, O'Malley K, Joyce CR. Individual quality of life in patients undergoing hip replacement. *Lancet* 1992; **339**: 1088–91.
7. Brooks RH and with the EuroQol Group. Euro-Qol: the current state of play. *Health Policy* 1996; **37**: 53–72.
8. Brook R, Kamberg CJ. General health status measures and outcome measurement: a commentary on measuring functional status. *J. Chron. Dis.* 1987; **40**: 131S–136S.
9. Guyatt GH, Veldhuyzen Van Zanten SJ, Feeny FH, Patrick DL. Measuring quality of life in clinical trials: a taxonomy and review. *Can. Med. Assoc. J.* 1989; **140**: 1441–8.
10. Editorial. Quality of life and clinical trials. *Lancet* 1995; **346**: 1–2.
11. Streiner DL, Norman GR. *Health Measurement Scales: A Practical Guide to their Development and Use.* 2nd edn. Oxford University Press, Oxford, 1995.
12. Bravo G, Potvin L. Estimating the reliability of continuous measures with Cronbach's alpha or the intraclass correlation coefficient: toward the integration of two traditions. *J. Clin. Epidemiol.* 1991; **44**: 381–90.
13. Cronbach L. Coefficient alpha and the internal structure of tests. *Psychometrica* 1951; **16**: 287–334.
14. Nunnally J, Bernstein JC. *Psychometric Theory*, 3rd edn. McGraw-Hill, New York, 1994.
15. Donovan JL, Frankel SJ, Eyles JD. Assessing the need for health status measures. *J. Epidemiol. Community Health* 1993; **47**: 158–62.
16. Bland JM, Altman DG. Statistical methods for assessing agreement between two methods of clinical measurement. *Lancet* 1986; **1**: 307–10.
17. Scientific Advisory Committee of the Medical Outcomes Trust. Instrument Review Criteria. *Medical Outcomes Trust Bulletin* 1995; **3**: I–IV (Abstract).
18. Jenkinson C. Evaluating the efficacy of medical treatment: possibilities and limitations. *Soc. Sci. Med.* 1995; **41**: 1395–401.
19. Guyatt GH, Feeny DH, Patrick DL. Measuring health-related quality of life. *Ann. Intern. Med.* 1993; **118**: 622–9.
20. Guyatt GH, Cook DJ. Health status, quality of life, and the individual. *JAMA* 1994; **272**: 630–1.
21. Lomas J, Pickard L, Mohide A. Patient versus clinician item generation for quality-of-life measures. The case of language-disabled adults. *Med. Care* 1987; **25**: 764–9.
22. Bergner M, Rothman ML. Health status measures: an overview and guide for selection. *Annu. Rev. Public Health* 1987; **8**: 191–210.
23. Kirshner B, Guyatt GH. A methodological framework for assessing health indices. *J. Chronic. Dis.* 1985; **38**: 27–36.
24. Guyatt GH, Deyo RA, Charlson M, Levine MN, Mitchell A. Responsiveness and validity in health status measurement: a clarification. *J. Clin. Epidemiol.* 1989; **42**: 403–8.
25. Meenan RF, Anderson JJ, Kazis LE, et al. Outcome assessment in clinical trials. Evidence for the sensitivity of a health status measure. *Arthritis Rheum.* 1984; **27**: 1344–52.
26. Kazis LE, Anderson JJ, Meenan RF. Effect sizes for interpreting changes in health status. *Med. Care* 1989; **27**: S178–89.
27. Lydick E, Epstein RS. Interpretation of quality of life changes. *Qual. Life Res.* 1993; **2**: 221–6.
28. Katz JN, Larson MG, Phillips CB, Fossel AH, Liang MH. Comparative measurement sensitivity of short and longer health status instruments. *Med. Care* 1992; **30**: 917–25.
29. Liang MH, Fossel AH, Larson MG. Comparisons of five health status instruments for orthopedic evaluation. *Med. Care* 1990; **28**: 632–42.
30. Deyo RA, Centor RM. Assessing the responsiveness of functional scales to clinical change: an analogy to diagnostic test performance. *J. Chronic. Dis.* 1986; **39**: 897–906.
31. Liang MH, Larson MG, Cullen KE, Schwartz JA. Comparative measurement efficiency and sensitivity of five health status instruments for arthritis research. *Arthritis Rheum.* 1985; **28**: 542–7.
32. Wright JG, Young NL. A comparison of different indices of responsiveness. *J. Clin. Epidemiol.* 1997; **50**: 239–46.
33. Bindman AB, Keane D, Lurie N. Measuring health changes among severely ill patients. The floor phenomenon. *Med. Care* 1990; **28**: 1142–52.
34. Avis NE, Smith KW. Conceptual and methodological issues in selecting and developing quality of life measures. In: Fitzpatrick R (ed.). *Advances*

in Medical Sociology. JAI Press Inc.: London, 1994, pp. 255–80.

35. Guyatt GH, Townsend M, Berman LB, Keller JL. A comparison of Likert and visual analogue scales for measuring change in function. *J. Chronic. Dis.* 1987; **40**: 1129–33.

36. Jaeschke R, Singer J, Guyatt GH. A comparison of seven-point and visual analogue scales. Data from a randomized trial. *Controlled Clinical Trials* 1990; **11**: 43–51.

37. Jenkinson C. Why are we weighting? A critical examination of the use of item weights in a health status measure. *Soc. Sci. Med.* 1991; **32**: 1413–16.

38. Stucki G, Daltroy L, Katz JN, Johannesson M, and Liang MH. Interpretation of change scores in ordinal clinical scales and health status measures: the whole may not equal the sum of the parts. *J. Clin. Epidemiol.* 1996; **49**: 711–17.

39. Deyo RA, Patrick D L. Barriers to the use of health status measures in clinical investigation, patient care, and policy research. *Med. Care* 1989; **27**: S254–68.

40. Testa MA, Anderson RB, Nackley JF, Hollenberg NK. Quality of life and antihypertensive therapy in men. A comparison of captopril with enalapril. The Quality-of-Life Hypertension Study Group. *N. Engl. J. Med.* 1993; **328**: 907–13.

41. Jaeschke R, Singer J, Guyatt GH. Measurement of health status. Ascertaining the minimal clinically important difference. *Controlled Clinical Trials* 1989; **10**: 407–15.

42. Jaeschke R, Guyatt GH, Keller JL, and Singer J. Interpreting changes in quality-of-life score in n of 1 randomized trials. *Controlled Clinical Trials* 1991; **12**: 226S–233S.

43. Deyo RA, Patrick DL. The significance of treatment effects: the clinical perspective. *Med. Care* 1995; **33**: AS286–91.

44. Hadorn DC, Hays RD, Uebersax J, Hauber T. Improving task comprehension in the measurement of health state preferences. A trial of informational cartoon figures and a paired-comparison task. *J. Clin. Epidemiol.* 1992; **45**: 233–43.

45. Dawson J, Fitzpatrick R, Murray D, Carr A. Comparison of measures to assess outcomes in total hip replacement surgery. *Qual. Health Care* 1996; **5**: 81–8.

46. Guyatt GH, Eagle DJ, Sackett B, Willan A, Griffith LE, McIlroy W, Patterson CJ, Turpie I. Measuring quality of life in the frail elderly. *J. Clin. Epidemiol.* 1993; **46**: 1433–44.

47. Bernhard J, Gusset H, Hurny C. Quality-of-life assessment in cancer clinical trials: an intervention by itself? *Support. Care Cancer* 1995; **3**: 66–71.

48. Nelson EC, Landgraf JM, Hays RD, Wasson JH, Kirk JW. The functional status of patients. How can it be measured in physicians' offices? *Med. Care* 1990; **28**: 1111–26.

49. Wolfe F, Kleinheksel SM, Cathey MA, Hawley DJ, Spitz PW, Fries JF. The clinical value of the Stanford Health Assessment Questionnaire Functional Disability Index in patients with rheumatoid arthritis. *J. Rheumatol.* 1988; **15**: 1480–8.

50. Aaronson NK, Ahmedzai S, Bergman B, et al. The European Organization for Research and Treatment of Cancer QLQ-C30: a quality-of-life instrument for use in international clinical trials in oncology. *J. Natl Cancer Inst.* 1993; **85**: 365–76.

51. Weinberger M, Oddone EZ, Samsa GP, Landsman PB. Are health-related quality-of-life measures affected by the mode of administration? *J. Clin. Epidemiol.* 1996; **49**: 135–40.

52. Weinberger M, Nagle B, Hanlon JT, Samsa GP, Schmader K, Landsman PB, Uttech KM, Cowper PA, Cohen HJ, Feussner JR. Assessing health-related quality of life in elderly outpatients: telephone versus face-to-face administration. *J. Am. Geriatr. Soc.* 1994; **42**: 1295–99.

53. Read JL, Quinn RJ, Hoefer MA. Measuring overall health: an evaluation of three important approaches. *J. Chron. Dis.* 1987; **40**(Suppl. 1): 7S–26S.

54. Bombardier C, Raboud J and The Auranofin Cooperating Group. A comparison of health-related quality-of-life measures for rheumatoid arthritis research. *Controlled Clinical Trials* 1991; **12**: 243S–256S.

55. Burisch M. You don't always get what you pay for: measuring depression with short and simple versus long and sophisticated scales. *J. Res. Personality* 1984; **18**: 81–98.

56. Fitzpatrick R, Newman S, Lamb R, Shipley M. A comparison of measures of health status in rheumatoid arthritis. *Br. J. Rheumatol.* 1989; **28**: 201–6.

57. Sprangers MA, Cull A, Bjordal K, Groenvold M, Aaronson NK. The European Organization for Research and Treatment of Cancer. Approach to quality of life assessment: guidelines for developing questionnaire modules. EORTC Study Group on Quality of Life. *Qual. Life Res.* 1993; **2**: 287–95.

58. Orley J, Kuyken W. *Quality of Life Assessment: International Perspectives.* Springer-Verlag, Berlin, 1994.

59. Shumaker S, Berzon RA. *The International Assessment of Health-Related Quality of Life: Theory, Translation, Measurement and Analysis.* Rapid Communications of Oxford, Oxford, 1995.

60. Bullinger M, Anderson R, Cella D, Aaronson N. Developing and evaluating cross-cultural instruments from minimum requirements to optimal models. *Qual. Life Res.* 1993; **2**: 451–9.

61. Leplege A, Verdier A. The adaptation of health status measures: methodological aspects of the translation procedure. In: Shumaker S, Berzon R

(eds). *The International Assessment of Health-Related Quality of Life: Theory, Translation, Measurement and Analysis*. Rapid Communications of Oxford: Oxford, 1995, pp. 93–101.

62. Aaronson NK. Assessing the quality of life of patients in cancer clinical trials: common problems and common sense solutions. *Eur. J. Cancer* 1992; **28A**: 1304–7.

63. Erickson P, Taeuber RC, Scott J. Operational aspects of quality-of-life assessment: choosing the right instrument: review article. *Pharmaco-Economics* 1995; **7**: 39–48.

12

The Use of Health Status Measures in Economic Evaluation

JOHN BRAZIER, MARK DEVERILL and COLIN GREEN

SUMMARY

This chapter presents a review of the use of measures of health status in the assessment of benefits in economic evaluation, whether or not they were designed for the purpose.[1]

The topics addressed in this chapter are as follows: how to judge the appropriateness of a health status measure for use in economic evaluation; a comparison of techniques for valuing health states; a comparison of five preference based measures of health status, known as multi-attribute utility scales; the limitations of non-preference based measures of health status in economic evaluation; and a review of the use of health status measures in economic evaluations in studies published in 1995.

These topics were addressed by conducting reviews of the literature based on systematic searches which identified over 3000 papers, of which 632 were found to be relevant. The purpose of these reviews was to be comprehensive and to present an accurate reflection of evidence and opinion in the literature.

Considerable inadequacies in the current practice of using health state measures in economic evaluation were identified. This chapter provides a set of recommendations for improving practice including: a check-list of questions for selecting a measure for use in economic evaluation; a list of circumstances when non-preference based measures of health status can be used to assess relative efficiency; and recommendations surrounding the use of health state valuation techniques and multi-attribute utility scales. These recommendations should help to identify poor economic evaluations and hence guard against inefficient conclusions being drawn regarding the provision of healthcare. Finally, a future research agenda is proposed for this important and developing field.

CONTEXT

Measures of Health Status

Health status measures are standardised questionnaires used to assess patient health across broad areas including symptoms, physical functioning, work and social activities, and mental well-being[2] (see for example the SF-36 health survey in Table 1). They consist of items covering one or more dimensions of health. Health status measures are either administered directly to patients, often by self-completion, or less commonly through a third party (such as their doctor). Responses to items are combined into either a single index or a profile of several subindices of scores using a scoring algorithm. For most measures, scoring is typically a simple summation of coded responses to the items. The SF-36 physical functioning dimension, for example, has 10 items, to which the patient can make one of three responses: 'limited a lot', 'limited a little' or 'not limited at all'.[3] These responses are coded 1, 2 and 3, respectively and the 10 coded responses summed to produce a score from 10 to 30 (for the SF-36 these raw scores are then transformed onto a 0 to 100 scale). A measure can be specific to a condition,

Table 1   *An example of a measure of health status – the SF-36 health survey*[3]

Dimension	No. of items	Summary of content	No. of response choices	Range of response choice
Physical functioning	10	Extent to which health limits physical activities such as self-care, walking, climbing stairs, bending, lifting, and moderate and vigorous exercises	3	'Yes limited a lot' to 'no, not limited at all'
Role limitations – physical	4	Extent to which physical health interferes with work or other daily activities, including accomplishing less than wanted, limitations in the kind of activities, or difficulty in performing activities	2	Yes/No
Bodily pain	2	Intensity of pain and effect of pain on normal work, both inside and outside the home	5 and 6	'None' to 'very severe' and 'not at all' to 'extremely'
General health	5	Personal evaluation of health, including current health, health outlook, and resistance to illness	5	'All of the time' to 'none of the time'
Vitality	4	Feeling energetic and full of life versus feeling tired and worn out	6	'All of the time' to 'none of the time'
Social functioning	2	Extent to which physical health or emotional problems interfere with normal social activities	5	'Not at all' to 'extremely' and 'All of the time' to 'none of the time'
Role limitations – emotional	3	Extent to which emotional problems interfere with work or other daily activities, including decreased time spent on activities, accomplishing less and not working as carefully as usual	2	Yes/No
Mental health	5	General mental health, including depression, anxiety, behavioural-emotional control, general positive effect	6	'All of the time' to 'none of the time'

such as the chronic respiratory questionnaire,[4] or more generic, such as the SF-36.

The patient focus of these measures has made them popular amongst health services researchers and clinicians in clinical research (see Chapter 11). One of the questions addressed in this chapter is whether such measures can be used in economic evaluation even if they have not been designed for the purpose.

A small subset of health status measures have been specially developed for use in economic evaluation known as multi-attribute utility scales. They comprise a health state classification system with multi-level dimensions or attributes (e.g. the EQ-5D). Health states are constructed from these classifications by selecting one level from each dimension (and in this way it is possible to define 243 health states with the EQ-5D). A special feature of multi-attribute utility scales is that a single index score is calculated for each state of health using preference weights. Each health state has a value from 0 to 1, where death is equivalent to 0 and full health is 1. States of health regarded as worse than death can have a value of less than 0. These single index scores, sometimes referred to by economists as health state utilities, are used to adjust survival to calculate quality adjusted life years (QALYs).[5] The five most widely used multi-attribute utility scales are reviewed in this chapter.

Health Status Measures in Economic Evaluation

Economic evaluation is the comparative assessment of the costs and benefits of alternative healthcare interventions. The measure of benefit is the key feature that distinguishes the different techniques of economic evaluation.[5]

Measures of health status are not used in cost-effectiveness analysis, which typically employs 'natural' units such as life years or cancer cases detected, or cost–benefit analysis, where all the benefits of an intervention are valued in monetary terms.

A technique of economic evaluation which does use measures of health status is cost–utility analysis, where benefits are measured in terms of health gain.[6] The most widely used measure is years in full health or the QALY. The number of QALYs is calculated by multiplying the value of each health state, which can be obtained by using multi-attribute utility scales, by the length of time spent in each health state. QALYs can be used to undertake comparisons between healthcare interventions in terms of cost per QALY at the margin.

Beyond the usual suite of economic evaluation techniques is cost–consequences analysis, where there is no attempt to combine multiple outcomes into a single indicator of value (such as the QALYs or £s).[7] The decision-maker is left with the task of weighing-up the costs and the multiple outcomes, which may include measures of health status such as the SF-36. There is no formal theoretical basis for the outcome measures used, and cost–consequences analysis is not strictly one of the techniques of economic evaluation but it retains the discipline of the framework of economic evaluation.

Scope of the Reviews

The scope of the reviews reported in this chapter is limited to the use of health status measures in economic evaluation. These measures are not used in CEA and CBA, and hence these techniques of economic evaluation are excluded from this review. The review also excludes a number of wider issues. For example, there have been criticisms of using the QALY as a measure of benefit, since it makes a number of limiting assumptions about people's preferences for health, including the assumption that health state values are independent of how long they last, when they occur and their context (e.g. whether they occur at the start or the end of a poor sequence of states).[8,9] This review also excludes consideration of the important debate about whose values to elicit in the valuation of health states. There are also other methods of measuring benefit, including health year equivalents, willingness to pay and conjoint analysis. These too are excluded.

This leaves a large area of issues and controversies to be tackled by this review. These were identified at the start of the project and include the following:

1 *How to judge the appropriateness of health status measures for use in economic evaluation.* There have been a number of published reviews of measures of health status.[2,10–12] The absence of economic considerations from these criteria has often resulted in economic measures of health-related quality of life being neglected and portrayed as 'invalid' or irrelevant in the assessment of health benefits. This is an important omission given the role of assessing efficiency in modern health services research. We have developed, therefore, a check-list for judging the merits of health status measures for use in economic evaluation by adapting the criteria used by psychometricians to judge the performance of non-preference based measures of health status.

2 *A comparison of the techniques for valuing health states.* The relative merits of these techniques has been a subject for debate for many years. There have been a number of informative reviews of the techniques,[6,13–15] and our review builds upon this earlier work, in particular using a review by Froberg and Kane[13] published in 1989 as a point of departure. It focuses on the following techniques for the elicitation of preferences (or quality weights) for use in the valuation of health states: standard gamble (SG), time trade-off (TTO), visual–analogue or rating scales (VAS), magnitude estimation (ME) and person trade-off (PTO).

3 *A comparison of multi-attribute utility scales.* This review examines the five most widely used multi-attribute utility scales: Quality of Well-Being (QWB) scale,[16] Rosser's disability/distress classification,[17] the Health Utility Index versions one, two and three (HUI-I, HUI-II and HUI-III),[18] the EQ-5D[19] and the 15D.[20] These multi-attribute utility scales are reviewed against the criteria of practicality, reliability and validity using the check-list developed in the first review.

4 *The use of non-preference based measures in economic evaluation.* Non-preference based measures of health status, such as the SF-36, are used in clinical trials to assess the efficacy and benefits of healthcare interventions in terms of patient-perceived health. These measures may be intended to assess patient-perceived health, but there are considerable doubts as to whether the scoring systems they employ reflect patient's views. They have been used in economic evaluations[21,22] and are likely to continue to be so.[23] This review examines the use and abuse of these measures in economic evaluation.

5 *The practice of using health status measures in economic evaluations in studies published*

in 1995. This final review uses the criteria developed in reviews one and four to assess the appropriateness of the measures of health status measures used in these published studies, and whether they are correctly employed in the economic evaluation.

We provide here an overview of these reviews of the use of health status measures in economic evaluation. Detailed findings have been reported elsewhere.[1]

METHODS

Data Sources

Literature searches were undertaken on the five topics identified. The core databases used were Medline, EMBASE, Science Citation Index (BIDS) and Social Citation Index (BIDS). In addition, the general economics databases ECONLIT (Silverplatter) and IBIS (British Library Political and Economic Science) were searched. However, the additional yield from the latter two databases was minimal. The NHS Economic Evaluations Database (NEED) was not appropriate for the methodological components of the review, but was searched for practical instances of economic evaluation. Bibliographic searching was supplemented by citation searching, review of references from the bibliographies of relevant articles, and by manual searching of an extensive personal collection of relevant reprints.

Time Period

Medline was searched back to 1966 (its inception). However, pragmatic cut-off dates varied according to the development of each scale or concept (e.g. EuroQol). Science Citation Index and Social Science Citation Index were followed back to 1981, whilst EMBASE covers the period from 1980 onwards. The two general economics databases cover the literature back to the mid-1980s (exact dates vary according to type of material). This gives adequate coverage of the period from which the majority of papers originate.

Searches

The purpose of the five searches was be comprehensive. The search strategies used resulted

from a collaboration between economists (J.B., M.D. and C.G.) and an expert in searching literature databases and are fully documented in the main report.[1]

Issues in using health status measures in economic evaluation

This search yielded over 1300 papers, of which 154 were found to be relevant for the review.

Health state valuation techniques

In total, 1581 references were found across the five techniques, which were narrowed to 285 papers, following the application of review criteria and further bibliographic searching.

Comparisons of non-preference health status measures and preference measures

We updated an earlier review of studies using health status measures alongside preference measures by Revicki and Kaplan[24] to the end of 1995. Overall, there were 19 studies identified.

The five multi-attribute utility scales

A total of 163 papers was found: QWB ($n = 56$), EQ-5D ($n = 44$), Rosser ($n = 34$), the different versions of the HUI ($n = 21$), and 15-D ($n = 9$). These papers were divided into methodology ($n = 92$) and empirical, which were papers reporting the results of administering the scale to patients ($n = 71$).

Economic evaluations published in 1995 using health status measures

The search strategy produced a total of 1659 papers. Only 11 of these met the criteria for an economic evaluation alongside a clinical trial.

Reviews

The papers were not systematically reviewed in the conventional sense of applying quality criteria, since such a method of grading does not exist for this type of literature, other than via the peer review system used by journal editors. Nor is there a quantitative method for synthesising opinion. The aim was to be comprehensive and to present an accurate balance of opinion, where it exists, and to reflect a range of opinion, including disagreement, where evidence is not definitive.

Judging the Appropriateness of Health Status Measures for Use in Economic Evaluation

Psychometric criteria: what can economists learn?

The psychometric criteria of practicality and reliability (in terms of stability) are relevant for any measure (see Chapter 11).[10] The main differences between psychometric and economic criteria arise with the concept of validity. Psychometricians in the field of health status measurement are concerned with the ability of an instrument to measure or numerically describe patient health. However, what economists want to know is the *relative value* patients and others place on aspects of health in order to undertake more than the most rudimentary form of economic evaluation.[25,26] The value of any given improvement in health will be related to a change in the score of a health status measure, but these two concepts will not be perfectly correlated. For example, someone may regard a large improvement in health, such as the ability to walk upstairs, as being of little or no benefit if they live in a bungalow. Conversely, an apparently small reduction in pain may be highly valued by the patient.

Towards an economic understanding of validity

The gold standard or criterion test of the validity of a measure intended to reflect preferences would be the extent to which it was able to predict those preferences *revealed* from actual decisions. However, revealed preference (RP) methods have not been applied in the healthcare field due to the well-documented features of this commodity.[27–29] RP methods require the consumer to be sovereign, but in healthcare the consumer is often ignorant of the outcomes of care. Furthermore, the doctor can act as the patient's agent in the consumption of healthcare, but the level of ignorance is such that the patient cannot be sure their doctor is being a perfect agent.

For this reason economists have often been sceptical about the value of trying to prove validity at all. Williams[30] suggested that '. . . searching for "validity" in this field, at this stage in the history of QOL measurement, is like chasing will o' the wisp, and probably equally unproductive'. Other health economists have focused on establishing the economic basis of the measure with Gafni and Birch, for example,

arguing:[9] 'In economics the validity of the instrument stems from the validity of the theory which the instrument is derived from. Thus instead of determining the validity of the instrument itself (the typical case when one uses the classical psychometric approach) one has to establish the validity of the underlying theory'. According to this view, the assumptions underlying a measure must be shown empirically to reflect individuals' preferences for the benefits of healthcare. Others have argued that any measure should be meaningful to decision-makers,[14] and that for informing social resource allocation decisions, measures should reflect *social* rather than individual level valuation of health states.[31] These differences of opinion have implications for the chosen test of validity.

We believe it is important to consider explicitly the validity of preference based measures of health in designing, conducting and reviewing an economic evaluation. We have, therefore, developed a three-part approach to examining the validity of preference based measures from the economics literature. The first part is to examine the validity of the description of health, and second is to examine the way in which items and dimensions of health are scored or valued. The descriptive validity of a measure concerns the comprehensiveness of its content, its suitability and its sensitivity. The conventional psychometric tests for health status measure, such as construct validation (see Chapter 11) are also relevant. The scoring of questionnaire items should, however, be based on the values people place on health rather than some arbitrary, if convenient, assumption of equal weighting. Economists have used a number of preference elicitation techniques for obtaining these weights, and these are reviewed in the next section.

A critical assessment of the descriptive validity and the methods of valuation should help in understanding the extent to which a measure is able to be a valid measure of preferences. However, it is also important not to lose sight of empirical validity, and this forms the third part of the approach. Empirical validity can be tested indirectly in terms of convergence with stated preferences, but this raises the question of whose stated preference and this depends on the perspective being adopted. The conventional welfare economic perspective is to use the views of the gainers and losers. One test of this individually based perspective would be the views of patients on the relative desirability of one state they have experienced versus another. A less satisfactory test would be for the researcher to assume a set of hypothetical orderings between health states, such as different illness

Table 2 *Check-list for judging the merits of preference-based measures of health*

	Components
Practicality	• how long does the instrument take to complete? • what is the response rate to the instrument? • what is the rate of completion?
Reliability	• what is the test–re-test reliability? • what are the implications for sample size? • what is the inter-rater reliability? • what is the reliability between places of administration?

Validity
  Description
	• content validity:
	  – does the instrument cover all dimensions of health of interest?
	  – do the items appear sensitive enough?
	• face validity:
	  – are the items relevant and appropriate for the population?
	• construct validity:
	  – can the unscored classification of the instrument detect known or expected differences or changes in health?

Valuation	• whose values have been used?
	• assumptions about preferences
	  – what is the model of preferences being assumed?
	  – what are the main assumptions of this model?
	  – how well are the preferences of the patients/general population/decision-makers likely to conform to these assumptions (see examples in text)?
	• technique of valuation
	  – is it choice based?
	  – which choice based method has been used?
	• quality of data
	  – are the background characteristics of the respondents to the valuation survey representative of the population?
	  – what was the degree of variation in the valuation survey?
	  – was there evidence of the respondents' understanding of the task
	  – what was the method of estimation (where relevant)

Empirical	• is there any evidence for the empirical validity of the instrument?
	  – revealed preferences?
	  – stated preferences?
	  – hypothesised preferences?

severity levels, and see whether the scales are able to reproduce the orderings. Some economists believe social values are different from individually based ones and hence would want a different test. Nord et al.[31] have proposed that '. . . the validity of the values obtained from different scaling techniques may be tested by asking whether the people from whom the values were elicited actually agree with the consequences in terms of the implied priorities for different health programs'. Different perspectives imply different tests of validity.

A check-list

We have developed a check-list of questions for examining these three aspects of validity, along with reliability and practicality, which

researchers are recommended to use when selecting a measure for use in economic evaluation (Table 2).

Techniques for Health State Valuation

Visual–analogue scale (VAS)

The VAS (sometimes referred to as the category rating scale or just rating scale) is simply a line, usually with well-defined end-points, on which respondents are asked to indicate the desirability of a health state. There are many variants of the technique. The lines can vary in length, be vertical or horizontal, and may or may not have intervals marked out with different numbers. An example is shown in Figure 1 (i.e. the

To help people say how good or bad their health is, we have drawn a scale (rather like a thermometer) on which the best state you can imagine is marked by 100 and the worst state you can imagine is marked by 0.

We would like you to indicate on this scale how good or bad is your own health today, in your opinion. Please do this by drawing a line from the box below to whichever point on the scale indicates how good or bad your current health state is.

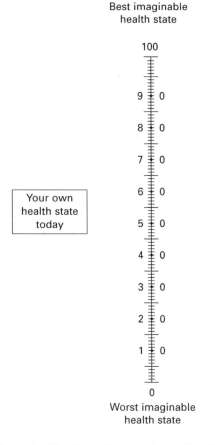

Figure 1   *Visual–analogue scale used by the EuroQol group.*

'thermometer rating scale' used by the EuroQol Group[32]).

Magnitude estimation (ME)

ME asks subjects to provide the ratio of undesirability of pairs of health states. For example, subjects may say that state A is x times better than state B. Therefore, the undesirability (disutility) of state A is x times as great as that of state B. By asking a series of questions, all states can be related to each other on the undesirability scale.[6]

Standard gamble (SG)

The SG asks respondents to make a choice between alternative outcomes, where one of them involves uncertainty (Figure 2). They are asked how much in terms of risk of death, or some other outcome worse than the one being valued, they are prepared to trade in order to avoid the certainty of the health state being valued. This technique is based on the Expected Utility Theory (EUT) of decision-making under uncertainty developed by von Neumann and Morgenstern.[33]

Time trade-off (TTO)

The TTO technique was developed as an alternative to SG, and was designed to overcome the problems of explaining probabilities to respondents.[34] The choice is between two alternatives, both with certain prospects, i.e. years in full health (x) and years (t) in the health state being valued (Figure 3). The respondent is directly asked to consider trading a reduction in their length of life for a health improvement. The health state valuation is the fraction of healthy years equivalent to a year in a given health state, i.e. x/t.

Person trade-off (PTO)

The PTO asks the respondent to make a choice in the context of a decision involving other people rather than themselves. For example: 'If there are x people in adverse health situation A, and y people in adverse health situation B, and if you can only help (cure) one group (for example, due to limited time or limited resources), which group would you choose to help?' One of the numbers, x or y, can then be varied until the subject finds the two groups equivalent in terms of needing or deserving help; then the undesirability (desirability) of condition B is x/y times as great as that of condition A. By asking a series of such questions, all conditions can be related to each other on the undesirability scale.[6]

Criteria for Reviewing Performance

These valuation techniques are reviewed against the criteria of practicality, reliability, and validity. For this review, validity has been examined as follows.

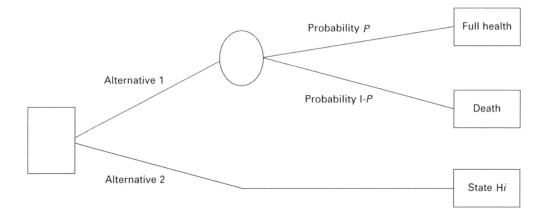

The subject is offered two alternatives. Alternative 1 is a treatment with two possible outcomes: either the patient is returned to normal health and lives for an additional *t* years (probability *P*), or the patient dies immediately (probability 1-*P*). Alternative 2 has the certain outcome of chronic state *i* for life (*t* years). Probability *P* is varied until the respondent is indifferent between the two alternatives, at which point the required preference value for state *i* is simply *P*; that is H*i* = *P*.[5]

Figure 2   *Standard gamble.*

Theoretical validity

Understanding the basis of the valuation techniques in economic theory is important. This review examines the validity of any such theoretical basis, by examining both contributions to the literature surrounding theoretical underpinnings and the subsequent literature which seeks empirically to test the extent to which the assumptions underlying the different techniques correctly describe individual preferences.

Empirical validity

As we have highlighted earlier, it is not possible to test the valuation techniques against revealed preferences, due to an absence of revealed preference data in the healthcare field. Therefore, we review the evidence for the extent to which techniques are able to correctly describe individual preferences against stated preferences (stated ordinal preferences and convergence with other valuation techniques) and hypothetical preferences (such as consistency with multi-attribute utility scales descriptive orderings).

Comparison of Health State Valuation Techniques

Practicality

Although, the five techniques have been reported to be practical and acceptable,[13] we found a lack

of empirical evidence to demonstrate the acceptability of ME and PTO. The evidence supported the acceptability of SG, TTO and VAS methods. This in part reflects the development of props, training of interviewers and other aspects of good quality in the administration of the techniques.[6] VAS was often found to be slightly better in terms of response rate and cost, whilst TTO out performed SG by a small margin.[15,35,36]

Reliability

Froberg and Kane report a general lack of evidence surrounding the reliability of techniques.[13] They present data to support an acceptable level of intra-rater reliability for all five of the techniques, and good to moderate levels of inter-rater reliability for RS, ME and PTO (Equivalence). Ten years on we have found that there is still a scarcity of evidence.

There is a lack of evidence surrounding the test–retest reliability of PTO and ME techniques. SG, TTO and VAS techniques have all demonstrated an acceptable level of reliability, with only small differences between the three techniques. There is little to choose between the three techniques on the grounds of reliability.

Theoretical validity

Although some commentators argue in favour of VAS techniques as a means of eliciting a measurable value function,[37] such a theoretical basis is not widely accepted in health economics.[38,39]

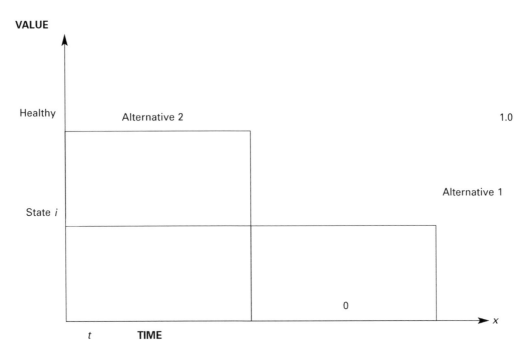

The subject is offered two alternatives – alternative 1: state *i* for time *t* (life expectancy of an individual with the chronic condition) followed by death; and alternative 2: healthy for time *x<t* followed by death. Time *x* is varied until the respondent is indifferent between the two alternatives, at which point the required preference value for state *i* is given by $Hi = x/t$.[6, a]

Figure 3 *Time trade-off.*

VAS techniques do not present respondents with a choice, they have no element of sacrifice or opportunity cost, and hence have no basis in economic theory. With respect to ME, assumptions surrounding the ratio level properties of the technique remain unsupported and it is not related to economic theory.

PTO is a choice-based technique, but it relates to social choice and the opportunity cost is not directly borne by the individual; therefore, consumer theory is not applicable. However, the PTO is intuitively appealing and its approach is considered by some to be more meaningful to decision-makers.[14] The TTO technique has merit, in that it is a choice based technique, but its theoretical underpinnings are not well developed.[15,40] Of all the techniques, SG has the most rigorous theoretical foundation. SG is supported by expected utility theory which has been the dominant theory of decision-making under uncertainty since the 1950s. Through its association with expected utility theory, SG has often been referred to as the 'gold standard', or reference method, of health state valuation.[6,41]

However, there are theoretical arguments against the preferred use of SG in health state valuation[14] and limited empirical support for assumptions underpinning expected utility theory;[8] therefore we are unable to support the 'gold standard' status which some attach to the SG.

The empirical literature to inform on the extent to which the assumptions underlying the different techniques correctly describe individual preferences is not extensive. We find that PTO and ME lack theoretical support; therefore, we do not comment further on theoretical validity in terms of empirical evidence. When considering VAS, TTO and SG, the empirical evidence casts doubt on the theoretical basis of all of these techniques.

In consideration of the theoretical support offered for VAS,[37] we find evidence to suggest that a measurable value function does not underlie the technique, and that VAS health state valuations are influenced by the severity of the other health states being valued and a spreading effect.[41–44] Empirical evidence has shown that duration and time preference have an impact on the elicitation of TTO values.[45,46] Given the absence of risk in the TTO, it is possible to adjust TTO-elicited values to incorporate uncertainty, yet this is rarely done in practice.[47,48] The SG is the only technique with clear theoretical foundations, but the evidence suggests that SG values can be strongly influenced by the outcomes used in the task and by the manner in which the task is presented.[49,50] There is also evidence to suggest that attitude to risk is not constant.[8,51] Further to such findings, there is evidence that respondents systematically violate the axioms of expected utility theory in the health context[15,52] and more generally.[53,54]

On the basis of theoretical validity, we conclude that only choice based techniques should be used. The comparison between SG, TTO and PTO depends on the perspective employed. The debate surrounding SG versus TTO is unresolved and depends on ones belief in the empirical support for expected utility theory *or* its normative basis.

Empirical validity

There is not a large literature reporting on the empirical validity of valuation techniques. We find evidence reported of a poor to moderate correlation between VAS and the choice based valuation techniques.[36,55–57] These findings, together with significant evidence to suggest a strong correlation between VAS and non-preference based measures of health status[24] raise further concerns over the ability of VAS methods to elicit strength of preference for health states. Such concerns are also supported by qualitative data reported in the study undertaken by Robinson and colleagues,[58] where respondents indicated that their VAS responses were not intended to reflect their preferences.

There is empirical evidence which reports that SG and TTO values correlate reasonably well with one another.[6,59] Whilst we have found no direct evidence to inform on the performance of SG against stated ordered preferences, TTO mean values have been found to be consistent with respondent rank ordering of health states,[60] and Robinson et al.[58] present qualitative evidence to indicate TTO responses are intended to reflect the preferences of individuals.

SG, TTO and VAS have demonstrated good levels of consistency with hypothesised preferences,[15,61] whilst a lack of evidence surrounding PTO and ME leaves the consistency of these methods unproven. A number of studies have reported the performance of SG and TTO against hypothesised (or expected) preferences[15,50,62] offering some positive insights to their empirical validity. In terms of consistency with multiattribute utility scales findings, the evidence

marginally favours TTO. However, there is not sufficient evidence to say that one technique is more valid than another on empirical grounds.

Mapping from VAS to SG or TTO Valuations

There would be significant practical advantages to being able to map from VAS to one of the choice based techniques. Studies mapping the relationship between VAS and the choice based methods have used regression analyses. Some use aggregate level data sets, where the regression analyses have been undertaken on mean health state values, and others have used individual level data.

The amount of evidence available to address the question was limited. There were only seven studies in total reporting estimated relationships.[35,47,63–67] At both levels of analyses the relationships were not stable between studies in terms of the form of the relationship and size of model parameters. At the individual level, there were also significant misspecification problems. The models performed better at the group level, and were able to explain a majority of the variation, but existing studies were based on small numbers in some instances, and none reported diagnostic test results for evaluating the appropriateness of different specifications. There has also been no attempt to test the ability of these models to predict directly obtained mean SG values on an independent data set. This lack of evidence would seem to provide an insecure foundation on which to conclude that there is a unique and stable relationship between VAS and SG or TTO.

Review of Five Multi-Attribute Utility Scales

The five multi-attribute utility scales differ considerably in terms of the characteristics of their health state classification and methods of valuation (Table 3). There is little guidance in the literature on which multi-attribute utility scale to use and to the best of our knowledge, there has been no systematic review undertaken of existing scales.

Practicality

There is little to choose between the questionnaires on the basis of practicality except in so far as the QWB does not have an accepted method of self-completion. The other four use a reasonably brief self-completed questionnaire. The QWB has an interview schedule involving

Table 3 *Characteristics of multi-attribute utility scales*

	Descriptive characteristics			Valuation characteristics			
Scale	Dimension	Levels	Health states	Valuation technique	Method of extrapolation	Sample	Country
Rosser	Disability	8	29	1) ME	None	70 (selected)	UK
	Distress	4		2) Synthesis of ME, VAS, TTO	None	140 (rep.)	(London) UK (York)
QWB	Mobility, physical activity, social functioning 27 symptoms/problems	3 2	1170	VAS	Modelling	866 (rep.)	USA (San Diego)
HUI-II	Sensory, Mobility, Emotion Cognitive, Self-care, Pain Fertility	4–5 3	24 000	VAS transformed into SG	Algebraic	203 (parents)	Canada (Hamilton)
HUI-III	Vision, Hearing, Speech Ambulation, Dexterity Emotion, Cognition, Pain	5-6	972 000	Ditto	Ditto	504 (rep.)	Canada (Hamilton)
EQ-5D	Mobility, Self-care, Usual Activities, Pain/discomfort Anxiety/depression	3	243	MVH-TTO and VAS	Modelling	3395 (rep.)	UK
15-D	Mobility, vision, hearing, breathing, sleeping, eating, speech, elimination, usual activities, mental function, discomfort/symptoms, depression, distress, vitality, sexual activity	4–5	Billions	VAS	Algebraic		Finland

detailed probing of the respondents taking up to 20 min.[68] All multi-attribute utility scales have achieved high levels of response and completion.

Reliability

There is evidence of differences between the assessment by patients of their own health compared to that of health professionals using the Rosser[69] and HUI.[70,71] This implies that the method of administering these instruments must be standardised. There is evidence for the test–re-test reliability in patient populations of the EQ-5D[72,73] and 15-D,[20] but this property has not been adequately investigated in any of the five measures.

Descriptive validity

The dimensions and their items were selected from reviews of the literature on health status measures for the QWB, EQ-5D, HUIs and 15-D. Items for the Rosser were based on interviews with professionals. The HUIs and 15-D enhanced their expert approach to item generation with surveys of patients.

The scales do not cover the same aspects of health. They all include physical functioning, but there are differences in whether the concept is described in terms of capacity (e.g. HUI) or actual behaviour and performance (e.g. QWB). The coverage of symptoms, mental health and social health is variable. The QWB explicitly excludes mental health as a separate dimension, but has a long list of symptoms and problems. The HUI-III covers many of the symptoms or health problems, but does not examine role or social function, since these are regarded as 'out of skin' and not appropriate in a measure of individual health preferences. The EQ-5D has dimensions for role and social function, and pain and mood, but not for many other symptoms and health problems.

The Rosser disability and distress classification is inferior to the others in terms of coverage. The choice from the remaining four will depend on what aspects of health the potential user wishes to cover. Their relevance may therefore vary depending on the disease group and age of the patients being evaluated. The HUI measures (particularly HUI-II) may be better suited to a younger population than the EQ-5D, for example, though this has not been empirically demonstrated. There are also issues about perspective and whether or not social health is relevant.

There is evidence that all measures can detect differences in group comparisons and the scores were significantly correlated with other measures of the health. However, it is difficult to compare their performance owing to the absence of studies using the measures on the same populations. Most of the evidence on the QWB scale was limited to correlations with related health status measures,[74] with very little detailed scrutiny of the descriptive classification, whereas evidence for the HUI-II was limited to survivors of childhood cancer.[75] There was some suggestion of insensitivity in all measures,[71,72,76,77] except the 15D where there had been insufficient published studies at the time of the review.

Valuation

The QWB, Rosser and the 15D can be regarded as inferior to the other two multi-attribute utility scales owing to their use of VAS and ME to value the health descriptions. HUI-II and III might be preferred to the EQ-5D by those who regard the SG as the 'gold standard'. However, the SG utilities for the HUIs have been derived from VAS values using a power transformation criticised earlier in this chapter. The valuation of the HUI has also been obtained from a smaller and less representative sample of the general population than the MVH survey.

A further difference between them is in the methods of estimating values for scoring the states defined by the EQ-5D and HUIs. The HUIs use multi-attribute utility theory which substantially reduces the valuation task by making simplifying assumptions about the relationship between dimensions and health state values. The simple additive functional form assumes dimensions to be independent and hence permits no interaction. The multiplicative function permits a very limited form of interaction between dimensions which assume the inter-dependency to be the same between all dimensions and for all levels of each dimension. To apply this approach, respondents are asked to value the level of each dimension separately to estimate single attribute utility functions, and then a sample of (multi-attribute) health states. The overall function is calculated by solving a system of simultaneous functions. By contrast, the EQ-5D TTO tariffs were estimated by multivariate statistical techniques. A simple additive model was chosen which contains decrements for each of the moderate and severe dysfunctional categories of the five dimensions, a constant for any kind of dysfunction and the term 'N3' for whenever any of the dimensions are severe. This last term was a crude way of allowing for interactions, since it implies that the impact of a severe problem is less if it is a second or subsequent severe problem. The ability of these two estimation procedures to predict health state values has not been compared, and hence there is no means of determining which is best.

Empirical validity

Evidence on empirical validity was found to be very limited from both an individual and a social perspective. The QWB has been shown to correlate with direct preference elicitation from patients,[78] but such evidence has not been published for the EQ-5D and HUI-I. There is evidence of the EQ-5D correlating with patient perception of health change in one study,[79] but not another,[72] whilst no evidence was found of the correlation of the HUIs scores with individual stated preferences. The scores were also found to reflect hypothesised preferences between patient groups,[75,80–82] but the evidence was too limited to draw firm conclusions.

Nord and his colleagues[31] compared the values generated by the QWB and HUI-I, and Rosser with stated social preferences according to the person trade-off method. The Rosser approach was found to reflect social preference better than the other two, but this study was too crude to come to any definite conclusions.[1]

The Use of Non-Preference Based Measures of Health in Economic Evaluation

Economic criticisms of non-preference based measures

The simple scoring algorithms used by most of these measures assume equal intervals between the response choices, and that the items are of equal importance.[26] The SF-36 physical functioning dimension, for example, assumes that being limited in walking has the same importance as being limited in climbing flights of stairs, but there is no reason for this to be the case. The theoretical concerns with simple aggregation has been confirmed by the evidence. Studies found in the search reported only low to moderate correlations between health status measures than preference based measures. A small minority of measures have used weights obtained from patients or professionals using VAS,[83] but these are also unlikely to reflect cardinal preferences given the criticisms presented above.

For measures presenting results as a profile, there are additional problems with conflicts between the dimensions, such as in a study

Table 4 *Assessing the relative efficiency of two interventions given different cost and health outcome scenarios*

Scenario	Cost	Health status measure	Can relative efficiency be evaluated?
1	Lower	Better in at least one dimension and no worse on any other	Yes, by dominance[a]
2	Same	Better in at least one dimension and no worse on any other	Yes[a]
3	Lower	Same across all dimensions	Yes, by cost-minimisation[a]
4	Lower	Better on some dimensions and worse on others	No
5	Same	Better on some dimensions and worse on others	No
6	Higher	Better in at least one dimension and no worse on any other	No
7	Higher	Better on some dimensions and worse on others	No

[a] Given the provisos about the ordinality of the scales.

comparing surgical with non-invasive interventions, where surgery may be more effective at reducing symptoms but is associated with a range of complications. These measures also do not incorporate death as an outcome measure, and hence there is no easy solution where there is a conflict between the impact on survival and health related quality between different interventions (see Chapter 20).

The use and abuse of health status measures in economic evaluation

The usefulness of health status measures in assessing the relative efficiency of interventions depends on the results of the study. In Table 4 we present seven scenarios of costs and outcomes in a comparison of two interventions, and consider whether it is possible to assess their relative efficiency. The first scenario is a case of dominance where one treatment is cheaper *and* better on at least one of the dimensions of the health status measures, whilst being no worse on any other. In the second scenario it is also straightforward to assess relative efficiency, since it is simply a question of choosing the treatment with the better health status measure scores, as the two have been found to cost the same. The third scenario is the same across all dimensions of the health status measures and hence is a *cost-minimisation analysis*. Even for these three scenarios it is necessary to demonstrate the ordinality of the scale of the health status measure scores in relation to preferences.

The result is less straightforward for scenarios 4 to 7. In scenarios 4 and 5, one treatment performs better on same dimensions but worse on others, and hence one treatment could have a lower cost per unit of health gain on some dimensions but higher on others. Even where one treatment is apparently more cost-effective across all the health dimensions, care must be

taken in the interpretation. Our review of the evidence found that health status measures do not possess the interval properties required to undertake such comparisons. Furthermore, it is the incremental cost-effectiveness ratio which is important for resource allocation purposes. Therefore, where the least cost-effective intervention costs more and yields a higher benefit, then the greater benefit could be worth the extra cost.

For multiple outcomes, the recommended approach is to present the costs and benefits of the alternatives in a cost consequences analysis.[7] This type of presentation uses an economic framework, but is unlikely to be helpful since health status measures scores have no obvious intuitive meaning. Score differences cannot be compared between dimensions, nor can health status measures scores be compared to other outcomes, such as survival, or cost. Non-preference based health status measures cannot be used to assess the efficiency of interventions in such circumstances.

Developing non-preference based measures for use in economic evaluation

There are four methods for developing non-preference based measures of health status measures. One is to assign responses to the non-preference based measures of health to the classification of a multi-attribute utility scale, but this is difficult and often arbitrary in practice.[69,84] Furthermore, the predictive ability of any explicit mapping rules have not been tested. Another is to derive exchange rates between health status measures and preferences, but this does not look promising given the weak relationship. A more radical way forward is to obtain preference weights using preference elicitation techniques, which has been successfully undertaken on the SF-36,[85] but this is a complex and expensive task and is only likely to be undertaken on the most widely used measure. A final way is to generate health scenarios from the data, but there were no examples of this in the literature.

The Use of QALY and Non-QALY Measures of Health Status: Assessing the State of Art in 1995

The literature

To be included in the review each paper had to meet the following criteria:

1 The study had to be a 'full' economic evaluation: this implies the following:
 (a) the technology in question had to have a comparator (before and after studies were thus excluded);
 (b) both costs and consequences (outcomes) of the technology had to be identified and primary data gathered accordingly.
2 The outcomes or consequences of technologies had to be assessed using a recognised QALY or non-preference based health status measures.

A total of 42 papers (approximately 2.5% of the original number) was initially identified as economic evaluations in terms of using either QALY-type measures (hence cost–utility analyses) or non-QALY based health status measures (hence 'cost–consequences' analyses). On receipt of the 42 papers the inclusion criteria outlined above were once again strictly applied. It was found that 31/42 (74%) could not be included; the main reason for such a high exclusion rate was an inability at the abstract stage to apply the inclusion criteria. Just 11 papers met our strict entry criteria, and these are reported on below.

Questions to be applied to published economic evaluations

1 Did the paper discuss or address the issue of the validity and/or suitability of a health status measures for the particular study question?
2 Was the health status measures compatible with the method of economic evaluation chosen?
3 Given the health status measures and economic evaluation framework used, were any conclusions presented in the paper legitimate?

Studies using QALY measures

Four studies were identified using QALY measures and which met our inclusion criteria. Table 5 summarises the performance of these in terms of the three questions outlined above. Two of the studies failed against the first criteria.[86,88] Kennedy et al.[87] make no attempt to qualify their use of the TTO method within their analysis, relying on general references relating to health state valuation. Mark et al.[89] do not address issues of validity or suitability with respect to their use of the TTO method in their calculation of QALYs.

For question 2, some ambiguity is present. Whilst the health status measures and form of evaluation can be seen as compatible, the way in which the health status measures are used to obtain QALY values casts doubt on the 'study-specific compatibility'. In Kerridge et al.[88] the QALY values used in the analysis are determined through an assessed survival effect linked with valuations from the Rosser Matrix. Gournay et al.[86] derived QALY values by mapping patient characteristics onto the Rosser matrix. Mark et al.[89] used the TTO technique only at year 1 post-treatment, they did not use it to generate both pre- and post-treatment values.

For question 3, there is initial support for a positive response in two studies,[87,88] but there

Table 5 *Cost–utility analyses*

			Responses to key questions (see above)		
Article authors	Clinical area	Health status measure	Q1 (Validity/ Suitability)	Q2 (Compatability)	Q3 (Legitimacy)
Gournay et al.[86]	Mental health	QALY:Rosser GHQ & BDI	✓	✓ – ✗	✗
Kennedy et al.[87]	Lung cancer	QALY:TTO	✗	✓	✓
Kerridge et al.[88]	Intensive care	QALY:Rosser	✓	✓ – ✗	✓
Mark et al.[89]	Thrombolytic therapy	QALY:TTO	✗	✓ – ✗	✓ – ✗

BDI = Beck Depression Inventory; GHQ = General Health Questionnaire; TTO = time trade-off.

Table 6   *Cost–consequences analyses*

| | | | Responses to key questions (see above) | | |
Article authors	Clinical area	Health status measure	Q1 (Validity/ Suitability)	Q2 (Compatability)	Q3 (Legitimacy)
Cottrell et al.[90]	Respiratory tract	SIP	✘	✓	✓
Johnson et al.[91]	Limb ischaemia	HADS, Barthel, FAI	✓	✓	✓
Knobbe et al.[92]	Mental illness	RLI, SNLAF	✓	✓	✓ – ✘
Lawrence et al.[93]	Hernia repair	SF-36,EQ-5D (VAS only)	✘	✓	✓
Prince et al.[94]	Tetraplegic care/ rehabilitation	RAND-36, LSI-A, Chart	✓	✓	✓
Uyl de Groot et al.[95]	Chemotherapy Non-Hodgkin lymphoma	NHP, RSC, KPI	✘	✓	✓
Wimo et al.[96]	Mental illness	GDS, IWB	✘	✓ – ✘	✓ – ✘

CES-D = Centre for Epidemiological Studies Depression Scale; CHART = Craig Handicap Assessment and Reporting Technique; FAI = Frenchay Activities Index; GDS = Global Deterioration Scale; HADS = Hospital Anxiety and Depression Scale; IWB = Index of Well Being; KPI = Karnofsky Performance Index; LSI = Life Satisfaction Index-A; NHP = Nottingham Health Profile; RLI = Resident Lifestyle Inventory; MOS SF GHS & RAND-36 = Medical Outcomes Study Short Form General Health Survey; RSC = Rotterdam Symptom Checklist; SIP = Sickness Impact Profile; SNLAF = Social Network Lifestyle Analysis Form.

are some problems. In Kennedy et al.[87] the results of the TTO came from a small sample ($n = 9$) of clinicians. In Kerridge et al.[88] expert opinion was used to gauge the survival effect of intensive care. The conclusions from the remaining two studies[86,89] are in more doubt. Gournay et al.[86] used data covering absence from work as a proxy for health status; thus they only loosely address the valuation of the benefits attributable to the intervention being assessed consequently. Although Mark et al.[89] present a cost per QALY ratio in their study, the methods employed in determining such a ratio would not substantiate their findings. They do not present their conclusions in a cost per QALY framework, relying instead on 'cost per life year saved' in their conclusions.

Studies using non-preference based measures

Three of the seven studies reviewed included little detail on the validity and/or suitability of the health status measures used (Table 6).[91,92,94] Six of the studies used the health status measures correctly within the cost consequences analysis framework.[90–95] Wimo et al.[96] mapped Index of Well Being (IWB) values from the Global Deterioration Scale (GDS) but had not presented any cost per QALY calculations. The UK NHS Centre for Reviews and Dissemination database entry for this study commented that the actual process of mapping GDS values onto the IWB was of dubious merit. It can be said,

however, that the GDS was suitable for a cost–consequences analysis.

For the third question there are problems in three papers. In the paper by Johnson et al.,[91] surgery for limb-threatening ischaemia, the authors failed to ascertain the quality of life scores prior to the onset of limb-threatening ischaemia, whilst then claiming that limb salvage 'can be the most cost-effective way of managing limb-threatening ischaemia'. This is doubtful given that limb salvage does not appear to dominate the alternative (limb revascularisation) on all the health status dimensions recorded. Knobbe et al.[92] failed to state the health status measures values found in the study, thus making the paper difficult to use in any form of decision-making. Wimo et al.[96] presented disaggregated cost and outcome results but wisely (considering the mapping of GDS values) made no attempt at presenting a cost per QALY result.

RECOMMENDATIONS ON USING HEALTH STATUS MEASURES IN ECONOMIC EVALUATION

Selection of Health Status Measure

We recommend that researchers planning to conduct economic evaluations alongside clinical trials pay careful attention to the check-list in Table 2 when selecting health status measures. The purpose of the check-list approach is to provide guidance rather than rules, and to acknowledge disagreements where they exist. The precedent in health economics is the widely used check-list for economic evaluation developed by Drummond et al.,[5] which was compiled despite areas of disagreement in the literature. The check-list we propose is likely to need updating given further theoretical development and the accumulation of more evidence.

Selection of Valuation Technique

We recommend only choice based techniques, either SG or TTO, be used to value health states. SG and TTO values should be obtained directly, rather than estimating them from VAS values via a mapping function.

Selection of Multi-Attribute Utility Scales

We conclude that, at the present time, the best of the five multi-attribute utility scales reviewed are the EQ-5D and HUI-II and III. The HUI-II is recommended for children, but in the absence of published weights for HUI-III, the EQ-5D is preferred for adult patients. This will have to be re-appraised when (Canadian) weights become available for the HUI-III.

Using Non-Preference Based Health Status Measures In Economic Evaluation

We recommend that researchers recognise the limitations of non-preference based health status measures at the design stage of a study. It is not possible to use such measures to assess efficiency when trade-offs must be made between dimensions of health and/or cost. The usability of health status measures in economic evaluation depends on the results of the study, but it is usually not possible to predict the results of a study in advance. Therefore, we recommend a multi-attribute utility scale be used in all economic evaluations alongside clinical trials

Future Research Agenda

Valuation techniques   Research evidence is required on the theoretical assumptions underlying each technique and comparative evidence on their empirical validity as measures of strength of preference.

Comparing the performance of EQ-5D and HUI-III   Research is required to compare the EQ-5D and HUI-III head-to-head in terms of the criteria in the check-list in Table 2.

Studies to re-value existing multi-attribute utility scales   There is a strong case for obtaining weights in other countries for the HUI-II and the HUI-III if the HUI-III is found to perform well against the EQ-5D. There could also be a case for obtaining weights for the QWB using a choice based technique if this continues to be widely used.

The development of new multi-attribute utility scales   The EQ-5D and HUI may not be suitable for many patient groups, and hence another measure, perhaps based on a more sensitive classification, may be required. This could either be done by: (i) developing new multi-attribute utility scales *de novo*, such as the Australian quality of life measure;[97] or (ii) estimating preference weights for an existing measure of health status such as the SF-36,[85] though this latter option is only advisable for the most widely used measures.

The valuation of scenarios constructed from health status measures data   This approach has the advantage of being able to focus on those aspects of health most relevant to the treatment being evaluated. It is also possible to incorporate the time profile of health, with timing, duration and sequence of states. The methodology for constructing the vignettes from the potentially large volume of health status measures (and other) data needs to be developed.

Conclusions

There is considerable scope for improving current practice in the use of health status measures in economic evaluation. The quality of published studies would be significantly improved if journals adopted the recommendations presented in this chapter in their peer review process. There are also important implications for policymakers who are considering whether or not to support the adoption of a new health care technology. These recommendations should help to identify poor studies, and hence guard against inefficient recommendations · regarding new technologies. There are also important implications for policy-makers in countries with guidelines on the conduct of economic evaluations of pharmaceuticals and other new technologies, such as Canada[98] and Australia,[99] or those countries intending to do so (including the UK[100]). Our findings would indicate that it is premature to recommend any one measure of health (such as the EQ-5D) for use in economic evaluation.

ACKNOWLEDGEMENTS

We would like to thank Andrew Booth and Rosemary Harper for their help in the literature searches. This research project was funded by the NHS HTA programme.

NOTE

a. TTO and SG have been adapted for valuing health states regarded as worse than death. For TTO alternative 1 involves dying immediately. Alternative 2 involves x years in the health states regarded as worse than death followed by $(t - x)$ years in perfect health. Again, duration x is varied until the respondent is indifferent between the two alternatives. The formula for calculating the health state value becomes $-X/(t - x)$.

REFERENCES

1. Brazier JE, Deverill M, Green C, Harper R, Booth A. A review of the use of health status measures in economic evaluation. *NHS Health Technology Assessment* 1999; **3**(9).
2. Bowling A. *Measuring health: a review of quality of life and measurement scales*. Milton Keynes: Open University Press, 1991.
3. Ware JE, Snow KK, Kolinski M, Gandeck B. *SF-36 Health Survey manual and interpretation guide*. Boston: The Health Institute, New England Medical Centre, Boston, MA, 1993.
4. Guyatt GH, Thompson PJ, Bernam LB, et al. How should we measure function in patients with chronic lung disease? *J. Chron. Dis.* 1985; **38**: 517–24.
5. Drummond MF, Stoddart GL, Torrance GW. *Methods for the economic evaluation of health care programmes*. Oxford: Oxford Medical Publications, 1987.
6. Torrance GW. Measurement of health state utilities for economic appraisal: a review. *J. Health Econ.* 1986; **5**: 1–30.
7. Drummond MF. *Economic analysis alongside controlled trials*. London: Department of Health, 1994.
8. Loomes G, McKenzie L. The use of QALYs in health care decision making. *Soc. Sci. Med.* 1989; **28**: 299–308.
9. Gafni A, Birch S. Preferences for outcomes in economic evaluation: an economic approach to addressing economic problems. *Soc. Sci. Med.* 1995; **40**: 767–76.
10. Streiner DL, Norman GR. *Health Measurement Scales: a practical guide to their development and use*. Oxford: Oxford University Press, 1989.
11. McDowell I, Newell C. *Measuring Health: A Guide to rating scales and questionnaire*. Oxford: Oxford University Press, 1996.
12. Wilkin D, Hallam L, Doggett MA. *Measures of need and outcome for primary health care*. Oxford: Oxford Medical Press, 1992.
13. Froberg DG, Kane RL. Methodology for measuring health-state preferences. II: Scaling methods. *J. Clin. Epidemiol.* 1989; **42**: 459–71.
14. Richardson J. Cost–utility analysis – what should be measured. *Soc. Sci. Med.* 1994; **39**: 7–21.
15. Dolan P, Gudex C, Kind P, Williams A. Valuing health states: a comparison of methods. *J. Health Econ.* 1996; **15**: 209–31.
16. Kaplan RM, Anderson JP. A general health policy model: update and application. *Health Services Research* 1988; **23**: 203–35.
17. Kind P, Rosser R, Williams A. Valuation of Quality of Life: Some Psychometric Evidence. In: Jones-Lee MW (ed.). *The Value of Life and Safety*. North Holland, 1982.
18. Torrance GW, Furlong W, Feeny D, Boyle M. Multi-attribute preference functions. Health Utilities Index. *PharmacoEconomics* 1995; **7**: 503–20.
19. Dolan P, Gudex C, Kind P, Williams A. *A social tariff for Euroqol: Results from a UK general population survey*, Centre for Health Economics Discussion Paper 138, University of York, 1995.
20. Sintonen H. *The 15D measure of HRQoL: reliability, validity, and the sensitivity of it's health state descriptive system*. NCFPE Working paper 41, Monash University/The University of Melbourne, 1994.
21. Buxton M, Acheson R, et al. *Costs and Benefits of the Heart Transplant programmes at Harefield and Papworth hospitals*, DHSS Office of the Chief Scientist Research Report No. 12, London: HMSO, 1985.
22. Nicholl J, Brazier JE, Milner PC, et al. Randomised controlled trial of cost-effectiveness of lithotripsy and open cholecystectomy as treatments for gallbladder stones. *Lancet* 1992; **340**: 801–7.
23. Drummond MF, Davies L. Economic Analysis alongside clinical trials: Revisiting the methodological issues. *Int. J. Technol. Assess. Health Care* 1991; **7**: 561–73.
24. Revicki DA, Kaplan RM. Relationship between psychometric and utility-based approaches to the measurement of health-related quality of life. *Quality in Life Research* 1993; **2**: 477–87.

25. Williams A. Measuring functioning and well-being, by Stewart and Ware. Review article. *Health Economics* 1992; **1**: 255–8.

26. Culyer AJ. *Measuring Health: Lessons for Ontario*. Toronto, University of Toronto Press, 1978.

27. Arrow KJ. Uncertainty and the Welfare Economics of Medical Care. *American Economic Review* 1963; **53**: 941–73.

28. Culyer AJ. The nature of the commodity health care and its efficient allocation. *Oxford Economic Papers* 1971; **24**: 189–211.

29. Donaldson C, Gerard K. *Economics of Health Care Financing: the Visible Hand*. Macmillan, London, 1993.

30. Williams A. *The role of the Euroqol instrument in QALY calculations*. Discussion paper 130. Centre for Health Economics, University of York, 1995.

31. Nord E, Richardson J, Macarounds-Kichnamm K. Social evaluation of health care versus personal evaluation of health states: evidence on the validity of four health-state instruments using Norwegian and Australian surveys. *Int. J. Technol. Assess. Health Care* 1993; **9**: 463–78.

32. Euroqol group Euroqol – a new facility for the measurement of health-related quality-of-life. *Health Policy* 1990; **16**: 199–208.

33. von Neumann J, Morgenstern O. *Theory of Games and Economic Behaviour*. Princeton: Princeton University Press, 1944.

34. Torrance GW, Thomas WH, Sackett DL. A utility maximisation model for evaluation of health care programmes. *Health Services Research* 1972; **7**: 118–33.

35. Reed WW, Herbers JE, Jr, Noel GL. Cholesterol-lowering therapy: what patients expect in return. *J. Gen. Intern. Med.* 1993; **8**: 591–6.

36. van der Donk J, Levendag PC, Kuijpers AJ, Roest FH, Habbema JD, Meeuwis CA, Schmitz PI. Patient participation in clinical decision-making for treatment of T3 laryngeal cancer: a comparison of state and process utilities. *J. Clin. Oncol.* 1995; **13**: 2369–78.

37. Dyer JS, Sarin RK. Relative risk aversion. *Management Science* 1982; **28**: 875–86.

38. Bleichrodt H, Johannesson M. An experimental test of a theoretical foundation for rating-scale valuations. *Med. Decis. Making* 1997; **17**: 208–16.

39. Loomes G, Jones M, Lee M, Robinson A. *What do visual analogue scales actually mean?* Paper presented to HESG Conference, Newcastle, 1994.

40. Johannesson M. QALYs, HYEs and individual preferences – a graphical illustration. *Soc. Sci. Med.* 1994; **39**: 1623–32.

41. Gafni A. The standard gamble method: what is being measured and how it is interpreted. *Health Serv. Res.* 1994; **29**: 207–24.

42. Parducci A, Carterette E, Friedman M (eds). *Handbook of Perception, Vol II. Contextual effects. A range-frequency analysis*. New York: Academic Press, 1974.

43. Nord E. The validity of a visual analogue scale in determining social utility weights for health states. *Int. J. Health Policy Management* 1991; **6**: 234–42.

44. Kuppermann M, Shiboski S, Feeny D, Elkin EP, Washington AE. Can preference scores for discrete states be used to derive preference scores for an entire path of events? An application to prenatal diagnosis. *Med. Decision Making* 1997; **17**: 42–55.

45. Sutherland HJ, Llewellyn TH, Boyd D, Till JE. Attitudes towards quality of survival: The concept of maximum endurable time. *Med. Decision Making* 1982; **2**: 299–309.

46. Dolan P, Gudex C. Time preference, duration and health state valuations. *Health Econ.* 1995; **4**: 289–99.

47. Stiggelbout AM, Kiebert GM, Kievit J, Leer JW, Stoter G, de Haes JC. Utility assessment in cancer patients: adjustment of time tradeoff scores for the utility of life years and comparison with standard gamble scores. *Med. Decision Making* 1994; **14**: 82–90.

48. Cher DJ, Miyamoto J, Lenert LA. Incorporating risk attitude into Markov-process decision models: Importance for individual decision making. *Med. Decision Making* 1997; **17**: 340–50.

49. Llewellyn Thomas H, Sutherland HJ, Tibshirani R, Ciampi A, Till JE, Boyd NF. The measurement of patients' values in medicine. *Med. Decision Making* 1982; **2**: 449–62.

50. Gage BF, Cardinalli AB, Owens DK. The effect of stroke and stroke prophylaxis with aspirin or warfarin on quality of life. *Arch. Intern. Med.* 1996; **156**: 1829–36.

51. Kahneman D, Tversky A. Prospect theory: an analysis of decision under risk. *Econometrica* 1979; **47**: 263–91.

52. Read JL, Quinn RJ, Berwick DM, Fineberg HV, Weinstein MC. Preferences for health outcomes. Comparison of assessment methods. *Med. Decision Making* 1984; **4**: 315–29.

53. Hershey JC, Kunrather HG, Schoemaker PJH. Sources of bias in assessment procedures for utility functions. *Management Science* 1981; **28**: 936–54.

54. Schoemaker PJH. The expected utility model: its variants, purposes, evidence and limitations. *J. Econ. Lit.* 1982; 529–63.

55. Rutten van Molken MP, Bakker CH, van Doorslaer EK, van der Linden S. Methodological issues of patient utility measurement.

Experience from two clinical trials. *Med. Care* 1995; **33**: 922–37.

56. Clarke AE, Goldstein MK, Michelson D, Garber AM, Lenert LA. The effect of assessment method and respondent population on utilities elicited for Gaucher disease. *Qual. Life Res.* 1997; **6**: 169–84.

57. Zug KA, Littenberg B, Baughman RD, et al. Assessing the preferences of patients with psoriasis. A quantitative, utility approach. *Arch. Dermatol.* 1995; **131**: 561–8.

58. Robinson A, Dolan P, Williams A. Valuing health states using VAS and TTO: what lies behind the numbers? *Soc. Sci. Med.* 1997; **45**: 1289–97.

59. Dolan P, Gudex C, Kind P, Williams A. The time trade-off method: results from a general population study. *Health Econ.* 1996; **5**: 141–54.

60. Ashby J, O'Hanlon M, Buxton MJ. The time trade-off technique: how do the valuations of breast cancer patients compare to those of other groups? *Qual. Life Res.* 1994; **3**: 257–65.

61. Gudex C, Dolan P, Kind P, Williams A. Health state valuations from the general public using the visual analogue scale. *Qual. Life Res.* 1996; **5**: 521–31.

62. Churchill DN, Torrance GW, Taylor DW, Barnes CC, Ludwin D, Shimizu A, Smith EK. Measurement of quality of life in end-stage renal disease: the time trade-off approach. *Clin. Invest. Med.* 1987; **10**: 14–20.

63. Torrance GW, Zhang Y, Feeny D, Furlong W, Barr R. *Multi-attribute preference functions for a comprehensive health status classification system.* Hamilton, Ontario: Centre for Health Economics and Policy Analysis, McMaster University, 1992.

64. Bombardier C, Wolfson AD, Sinclair AJ, et al. *Choices in Health Care: Decision Making and Evaluation of Effectiveness. Comparison of three measurement technologies in the evaluation of a functional status index.* Toronto: University of Toronto, 1982.

65. Torrance GW, Feeny DH, Furlong WJ, Barr RD, Zhang Y, Wang Q. Multiattribute utility function for a comprehensive health status classification system. Health Utilities Index Mark 2. *Med. Care* 1996; **34**: 702–22.

66. Dolan P, Sutton M. Mapping visual analogue scale health state valuations onto standard gamble and time trade-off values. *Soc. Sci. Med.* 1997; **44**: 1519–30.

67. Torrance GW. Social preferences for health states: an empirical evaluation of three measurement techniques. *Socio-Econ. Plan. Sci.* 1976; **10**: 129–36.

68. Bombardier C, Ware J, Russell I, Larson MG, Chalmers A, Leighton Read J. Auranofin therapy and quality of life in patients with rheumatoid arthritis. *Am. J. Med.* 1986; **81**: 565–78.

69. Bryan S, Parkin D, Donaldson C. Chiropody and the QALY – a case-study in assigning categories of disability and distress to patients. *Health Policy* 1991; **18**: 169–85.

70. Feeny D, Leiper A, Barr RD, Furlong W, Torrance GW, Rosenbaum P, Weitzman S. The comprehensive assessment of health status in survivors of childhood cancer: application to high-risk acute lymphoblastic leukaemia. *Br. J. Cancer* 1993; **67**: 1047–52.

71. Barr RD, Pai MKR, Weitzman S, Feeny D, Furlong W, Rosenbaum P, Torrance GW. A multi-attribute approach to health status measurement and clinical management – illustrated by an application to brain tumors in childhood. *Int. J. Oncol.* 1994; **4**: 639–48.

72. Harper R, Brazier JE, Waterhouse JC, Walters S, Jones N, Howard P. A comparison of outcome measures for patients with chronic obstructive pulmonary disease in an outpatient setting. *Thorax* 1997; **52**: 879–87.

73. Hurst NP, Jobanputra P, Hunter M, Lambert M, Lochhead A, Brown H. Validity of Euroqol – a generic health status instrument – in patients with rheumatoid arthritis. Economic and Health Outcomes Research Group. *Br. J. Rheumatol* 1994; **33**: 655–62.

74. Kaplan RM, Anderson JP, Patterson TL, et al. Validity of the Quality of Well-Being Scale for persons with human immunodeficiency virus infection. HNRC Group. HIV Neurobehavioral Research Center. *Psychosom. Med.* 1995; **57**: 138–47.

75. Feeny D, Furlong W, Boyle M, Torrance GW. Multi-attribute health status classification systems. Health Utilities Index. *Pharmaco-Economics* 1995; **7**: 490–502.

76. Hollingworth W, Mackenzie R, Todd CJ, Dixon AK. Measuring changes in quality-of-life following magnetic-resonance-imaging of the knee – SF-36, Euroqol or Rosser index. *Qual. Life Res.* 1995; **4**: 325–34.

77. Liang MH, Fossel AH, Larson MG. Comparisons of five health status instruments for orthopaedic evaluation. *Medical Care* 1990; **28**: 632–42.

78. Fryback DG, Dasbach EJ, Klein R, Klein BE, Dorn N, Peterson K, Martin PA. The Beaver Dam Health Outcomes Study: initial catalog of health-state quality factors. *Med. Decision Making* 1993; **13**: 89–102.

79. Hurst NP, Kind P, Ruta D, Hunter M, Stubbings A. Measuring health-related quality of life in rheumatoid arthritis: validity, responsiveness and reliability of EuroQol (EQ-5D). *Br. J. Rheumatol.* 1997; **36**: 551–9.

80. Kallis P, Unsworth White J, Munsch C, et al. Disability and distress following cardiac surgery

in patients over 70 years of age. *Eur. J. Cardio-thorac. Surg.* 1993; **7**: 306–11.

81. Rissanen P, Aro S, Slatis P, Sintonen H, Paavolainen P. Health and quality of life before and after hip or knee arthroplasty. *J. Arthroplasty* 1995; **10**: 169–75.

82. Essink-Bot ML, Vanroyen L, Krabbe P, Bonsel GJ, Rutten FFH. The impact of migraine on health-status. *Headache* 1995; **35**: 200–6.

83. Jones PW. Quality of life measurement for patients with diseases of the airways. *Thorax* 1991; **46**: 676–89.

84. Coast J. Reprocessing data to form QALYs. *Br. Med. J.* 1992; **305**: 87–90.

85. Brazier JE, Usherwood TP, Harper R, Jones NMB, Thomas K. Deriving a preference based single index measure for health from the SF-36. *J. Clinical Epidemiol.* 1998; **51**: 1115–28.

86. Gournay K, Brooking J. The community psychiatric nurse in primary care: an economic analysis. *J. Advanced Nursing* 1995; **22**: 769–78.

87. Kennedy W, Reinharz D, Tessier G, et al. Cost utility of chemotherapy and best supportive care in non-small cell lung cancer. *Pharmaco-Economics* 1995; **8**: 316–23.

88. Kerridge RK, Glasziou PP, Hillman KM. The use of 'quality-adjusted life years' (qalys) to evaluate treatment in intensive care. *Anaesth. Intensive Care* 1995; **23**: 322–31.

89. Mark DB, Hlatky MA, Califf RM, et al. Cost effectiveness of thrombolytic therapy with tissue plasminogen activator as compared with streptokinase for acute myocardial infarction. *N. Engl. J. Med.* 1995; **332**: 1418–24.

90. Cottrell JJ, Openbrier D, Lave JR, Paul C, Garland JL. Home oxygen therapy: a comparison of 2- vs. 6-month patient reevaluation. *Chest* 1995; **107**: 358–61.

91. Johnson BF, Evans L, Drury R, Datta D, Morris-Jones W, Beard JD. Surgery for limb threatening ischaemia: a reappraisal of the costs and benefits. *Eur. J. Vasc. Endovasc. Surg.* 1995; **9**: 181–8.

92. Knobbe CA, Carey SP, Rhodes L, Horner RH. Benefit-cost analysis of community residential versus institutional services for adults with severe mental retardation and challenging behaviors. *Am. J. Ment. Retard.* 1995; **99**: 533–41.

93. Lawrence K, McWhinnie D, Goodwin A, Doll H, Gordon A, Gray A, Britton J, Collin J. Randomised controlled trial of laparoscopic versus open repair of inguinal hernia: early results. *Br. Med. J.* 1995; **311**: 981–5.

94. Prince JM, Manley MS, Whiteneck GG. Self-managed versus agency-provided personal assistance care for individuals with high level tetraplegia. *Arch. Phys. Med. Rehab.* 1995; **76**: 919–23.

95. Uyl de Groot CA, Hagenbeek A, Verdonck LF, Lowenberg B, Rutten FFH. Cost-effectiveness of abmt in comparison with chop chemotherapy in patients with intermediate- and high-grade malignant non-Hodgkin's lymphoma (nhl). *Bone Marrow Transplantation* 1995; **16**: 463–70.

96. Wimo A, Mattson B, Krakau I, Eriksson T, Nelvig A, Karlsson G. Cost-utility analysis of group living in dementia care. *Int. J. Technol. Assess. Health Care* 1995; **11**: 49–65.

97. Hawthorne G, Richardson J, Osborne R, McNeil H. *The Australian Quality of Life (AQoL) Instrument.* Monash University Working Paper 66, 1997.

98. Ministry of Health (Ontario) *Ontario guidelines for the economic evaluation of pharmaceutical products.* Toronto: Ministry of Health, 1994.

99. Commonwealth Department of Health, Housing and Community Service *Guidelines for the pharmaceutical industry on the submission to the pharmaceutical benefits advisory committee.* Canberra: Australian Government Publishing Service, 1992.

100. Department of Health and the Association of the British Pharmaceutical Industry *Guidelines for the economic evaluation of pharmaceuticals* [Press release]. London: Department of Health, 1994.

13

Collecting Resource Use Data for Costing in Clinical Trials

KATHARINE JOHNSTON, MARTIN J. BUXTON,
DAVID R. JONES and RAY FITZPATRICK

SUMMARY

The recent increase in the number of economic evaluations being conducted alongside, or as an integral part of, clinical trials has provided the opportunity to collect and analyse patient-specific resource use (and hence cost) data. These opportunities have in turn focused attention on a range of important methodological issues concerning the collection of resource use data for costing purposes. This chapter identifies and discusses these methodological issues in order to establish how more informed and appropriate choices could be made in the future about the design, conduct and analysis of data for costing in clinical trials.

This chapter considers the different types of costs and the factors influencing the choice of which types to include in a costing, including the role of economic theory and perspective, and the methods for measuring resource use, including sampling strategies and obtaining data alongside and outside of clinical trials. The review identifies where economists are in agreement and where there is disagreement and identifies a research agenda around those issues of disagreement which can be resolved by further research.

CONTEXT

The relatively recent growth of serious interest in formal economic evaluation of health tech-nologies has led to the recognition that higher and more consistent methodological standards are required to ensure that results available to decision-makers are appropriate, reliable and comparable. In particular, as economic analyses are increasingly being proposed or required alongside or in relation to clinical trials, a range of issues arise, both of methodological principle and of best practice, for the process of obtaining and analysing resource use and cost data. As the collection of economic data alongside clinical trials becomes routine, and decisions about data collection are made by investigators designing trials who may not themselves have experience or formal training in health economics, the importance of clarifying and, if possible, resolving these issues increases.

The advantage of using clinical trials as a framework for economic evaluation is that they provide an opportunity to collect and analyse patient-specific resource use data. In principle, this allows comprehensive and detailed data to be collected for each patient, but in practice there is a legitimate concern not to overburden the trial data collection process. Consequently, the choice of resource use items for data collection and the methods used need to be very carefully considered.

METHODS

This chapter is based on a systematic review of the methodological issues to be addressed when assessing the costs of healthcare technologies.[1]

The literature was reviewed with the aim of identifying methodological principles and issues of method relating to the collection and analysis of cost data within the context of clinical trials. Although the focus of the review was on costing alongside clinical trials, the methodological issues were derived from five strands of relevant literature. Firstly, reviews of the specific topic (costing alongside clinical trials) were included, as well as review papers addressing single methodological issues. Secondly, empirical papers conducting economic evaluations alongside clinical trials were included as they might raise additional methodological issues. Thirdly, the literature on costing methods in economic evaluation in other contexts was included, since this forms the basis for the design of many economic evaluations. Fourthly, guidelines recently produced for various countries which attempt to standardise methodologies employed for economic evaluation were also included, since they make recommendations about methods. Finally, guidelines for authors intending to publish economic evaluations in peer-reviewed journals were also included in the review since, by implication, they comment on methodological issues.

The initial stages of the review consisted of: a definition of inclusion criteria; a search of in-house bibliographic data bases; and a manual search of key journals. As a result of this the the search strategy and inclusion criteria were refined. This was then followed by electronic searches; issue-specific searches; citation searches of key articles; and searches of reference lists of the identified literature. Finally, experts commenting on the review were asked to identify any relevant literature that they felt were missing. The aim was not to record the frequencies with which issues were raised, but to be comprehensive in identifying the methodological issues. The final literature included therefore covers all the issues rather than all papers discussing all the issues. The number of papers retrieved at each stage is reported in Table 1.

From this literature, this chapter identifies and comments on the various issues that commonly arise in designing studies such as the types of cost for inclusion; determining the sampling approach and sample size; how to measure resource use data; how to analyse cost data; and how to present results.

Nature of Evidence

The evidence can be classified into three broad categories:

1 Statements of method for conducting economic evaluation both in general, and in relation to clinical trials.[2–11] This category also includes context-specific guidelines.[12–15] All these works were important as statements of agreed principle and as highlighting points of current disagreement, but did not readily provide practical advice to those designing clinical trials to provide economic information.

2 Published studies on economic evaluations alongside clinical trials, of which there are a growing number.[16–24] These studies often adopted, developed and justified a particular strategy relating to these methodological issues.

3 Experimental studies testing the relative performance of different methods. Overall, the review found few examples of this type. It appears from the review that the need to improve our understanding of, for example, the relative merits of alternative methods of data collection, have largely been ignored in the literature. Thus, the relative merits of many of the approaches to handling methodological issues remain untested.

Methodological Issues

Study Design

Types of cost

Cost is the product of two elements, the quantity of resources consumed, and the unit cost of the resources. Thus when estimating costs, the correct approach is to identify and measure separately these two elements. Traditionally, costs were classified into direct and indirect but recently, partly as a result of the confusion regarding the interpretation of indirect costs,

Table 1   *Number of papers retrieved at each stage*

Stage	Number of papers identified	Number of papers included
In-house search	174	24
Manual search	n/a	81
Main electronic search	397	76
Issue searches (all)	143	18
Citation searches (all)	161	16
Reference lists	n/a	24
Experts	n/a	14
Total		253

n/a, not applicable.

Table 2   *Types of cost*

Health service costs
Direct costs of the whole intervention
General illness costs
Trial costs
Future costs
Non-health service costs
Costs incurred by other public sector budgets
Informal care costs
Patients' travel costs
Other out-of-pocket expenses incurred by the patient
Patients' time costs incurred in receiving treatment
Productivity costs
Future costs (food and shelter costs)
Non-resource costs
Transfer payments

there has been a move away from this dichotomous classification.[2,4] A more useful approach is to classify costs into three broad categories: health service costs; non-health service costs; and non-resource costs and within each category to include a more detailed categorisation of costs (Table 2).

Health service costs   These include the direct costs of the whole intervention such as hospital resources, for example, the number of treatments, bed days, as well as out-patient, GP and nurse visits. They include resource use associated with the main intervention, as well as any resource use arising from treatment of complications or side-effects. They also include the use of buildings, other capital and equipment, and overheads, such as heating and lighting, arising from the health service intervention.[2,6] The term 'whole intervention' is used to stress the fact that the costs of the intervention should include the broader health service costs.

General illness costs are the costs of being treated for other illnesses whilst being treated for the intervention in question. These may be either illnesses arising from the intervention or may be illnesses unrelated to the intervention.[2,4] Whether a cost is attributable to an intervention is discussed below. General illness costs occur during the trial period rather than in the future.

A particular issue concerns trial costs which, as well as referring to the costs of doing the research, are the costs of procedures in the trial protocol that are required solely for the purposes of the trial.[25-27] These types of event may arise because patients are more closely monitored in the trial, or because of the necessity to preserve blinding.[9] The more pragmatic the trial design, the more the resource use estimates are likely to reflect actual practice. A related type of cost is protocol-driven costs, which usually refer to

events for which the timing (and/or frequency) is set by the trial protocol and hence does not vary between the arms of the trial, but in a real world situation may be required to vary. Trial costs should only be ignored if the resource use they represent does not affect outcome. Trial costs can be addressed, for example, by collecting additional information on the number of tests or visits carried out in usual practice and re-analysing the costs accordingly.

Future health service costs are the additional costs of treatment for diseases occurring either in life years gained because of the initial intervention or in years of life that would have been lived anyway.[4,28] These costs can be further classified by whether they are related or unrelated diseases or treatments.[4,28] Future costs in years of life lived anyway are similar to general illness costs introduced above, except that they occur in the future periods rather than current periods. Future costs in years of life gained occur commonly in prevention programmes where costs arise in the years gained from the prevention programme. It is usual to include all the future effects of the prevention programme in the economic evaluation and therefore, for consistency, it could be argued that future costs should be included.[2] There is no consensus in the literature, however, as to whether all types of future costs should be included, and there is particular disagreement about whether future costs – particularly in life years gained – should be included. Given the disagreement concerning how to handle future health service costs, analysts should consider the impact on the results of the inclusion or exclusion of future costs through methods such as sensitivity analysis.[4]

An applied example of the different types of health service cost is presented in Table 3 and illustrates their complex nature.

Non-health service costs   These include the costs incurred by other public sector budgets, such as social service costs.[5] The sector incurring costs may change as budgetary arrangements change. If it is unclear which budget costs fall under, the implication is that cost shifting may be possible; that is, costs incurred by one sector may be shifted to another. This is a strong argument for including these costs in a study. Informal care costs are the costs incurred by family or friends in caring for patients, usually unpaid. These costs include the financial outlays incurred by the carer, but also the time spent by the informal carer in providing care. Studies attempting to include these costs have used inconsistent methodologies.[29] Again, it is important to include this type of cost if an intervention has the potential to shift the burden of costs to informal carers.

Table 3   *Applied example of types of Health Service cost*

Study context:
   A randomised cardiovascular screening and intervention programme led by practice nurses aims to achieve
   a reduction in blood pressure, cholesterol concentration and smoking prevalence among subjects in the
   intervention arm and thus reduce subsequent heart disease and stroke. Examples of the different types of
   health service cost in this context are:

1.   Direct costs of the whole intervention
     Programme costs (nurse time, consumables, buildings costs); drug costs; broader health service costs (GP
     health checks, other health checks); hospitalisations due to heart disease.

2.   General illness costs
     (a) Costs of treating other illnesses arising from the intervention: For example, where a visit to a practice
     nurse identified other illnesses, such as hypertension, for which treatment was required.
     (b) Costs of treating other illnesses unrelated to the intervention: For example, in-patient costs for an
     unrelated accident.

3.   Future costs
     (a) Related costs arising in years of life lived anyway: The costs associated with treatment of coronary
     events without the intervention.
     (b) Related costs arising in life years gained: The costs of treating all coronary events in the life years
     gained from the intervention.
     (c) Unrelated costs arising in years of life lived anyway: The costs of treating non-coronary events in life
     years lived without the intervention.
     (d) Unrelated costs arising in life years gained: The costs of treating non-coronary events in the life years
     gained. For example, costs of treatment for colorectal cancer.

4.   Trial costs
     Costs of the research team and the costs of any tests undertaken only for the purposes of the trial, for
     example extra visits to the GP.

Patients may incur non-health service costs including travel costs, other out-of-pocket expenses, and the time costs they incur when receiving treatment or attending for screening.[30,31] The opportunity cost of patients' time associated with receiving treatment is a further type of non-health service cost. These time costs have often, confusingly, been referred to as 'indirect' costs.[3] If a societal perspective is adopted, time costs incurred by individuals in receiving treatment reflect the loss of production to society. Unlike the productivity costs associated with morbidity discussed below, there is agreement that patient's time costs associated with treatment should be included in the numerator (costs) of a cost–effectiveness ratio.

Productivity costs may also be incurred by society, and these include the costs (in terms of time and lost production) associated with the patient taking time off work. Productivity costs may be separated into three phases: treatment (as just discussed); morbidity (incurred as a result of patients being ill); and mortality (incurred as a result of death).[4] There are several methodological issues surrounding productivity costs, including the scope of their measurement; whether they should be included as a cost or an effect; and how they should be valued. Several authors have rehearsed these issues.[32–36] The

issues surrounding productivity costs is an area of costing where there is little consensus.

A final type of non-health service cost is future costs incurred, for example food and shelter costs, as a result of additional life years added because of the intervention.[4] As with productivity costs discussed above, future non-health service costs may be excluded if the measure of effect is restricted to health outcomes.

Non-resource costs   These include transfer payments which are flows of money from one group in society to another, such as social security benefits. They are a loss to the payer and a gain to the recipient, and since they involve no resource consumption they are usually excluded.[2,4]

Factors influencing the types of cost included

For each type of cost, a decision has to be made as to whether its inclusion is appropriate and this should be based on the factors listed in Table 4. Feasibility of measurement should not be a criterion for deciding whether costs should be included,[4] although it does have implications for the methods of resource use measurement.

Table 4   *Summary of potential factors influencing costs for inclusion*

Economic welfare theory
Perspective
Form of economic evaluation
Double counting
Quantitative importance
Attribution
Time horizon

Economic welfare theory   Some economists argue that economic welfare theory alone should dictate which costs are included, which implies all costs except transfer payments.[37–39] If economic welfare theory is the criterion for inclusion, it becomes the sole criterion and thus the remaining criteria discussed in this section become irrelevant.

Perspective   The alternative, extra-welfarist position, is that the perspective of the decision-maker should influence the costs included.[2,40] Possible perspectives of the study include the patient, the health service or society. A health service perspective implies that only healthcare costs are included; a societal perspective implies that productivity costs should be included. A societal perspective therefore reduces the likelihood of cost shifting since, for example, the non-health service costs borne by others, such as the patient or social services, are included.

The form of economic evaluation   The form of economic evaluation to be conducted, such as cost–effectiveness analysis, or cost–utility analysis, also determines the costs included. These techniques restrict the effects measured to health, and thus the argument is there should be consistency between the breadth of measurement of costs and effects.[41] This implies that the costs included should relate only to health and thus, for example, productivity costs would not be included. This then relates back to the issue of perspective.

Double counting   Double counting, that is, counting the same cost twice or including an item both as a cost and as an effect, should be avoided. The potential for double counting is greatest in cost–utility analysis since some individuals may take account of cost when answering quality of life questions.[42] For example, a change in leisure time may be captured in the quality of life measure. The potential for double counting therefore depends on how healthcare and income losses resulting from disease are financed, and how the questions assessing quality of life are phrased.[42]

Quantitative importance   The expected quantitative importance of a type of cost should influence whether it is included. For particular health service interventions, certain types of costs will be more quantitatively important than others. For example, if evaluating preventive programmes, then future costs may be particularly relevant. In principle, quantitative importance should be defined as a cost large enough to have an impact on the cost–effectiveness ratio.[4] This may arise either from resource use with a low unit cost occurring frequently or from resource use with a high unit cost occurring infrequently.[43] If there is no expected difference in the magnitude of a particular type of cost between the two interventions being compared, then the cost could be excluded since it does not affect the choice between the interventions. It is important to relate the magnitude of cost differences to the magnitude of effect differences since, in cost–effectiveness terms, small differences in cost are important if there are small differences in effect. Pretrial modelling can be used to establish expected quantitative effects of particular costs,[44] but what is regarded as quantitatively important is subjective, particularly when the magnitude of clinical difference is not known.

Attribution   A factor sometimes overlooked in the decision as to which costs to include is attribution: that is, whether resource use is attributable to the intervention. The issue is whether to include all resource use or only that related to the disease.[45] Establishing whether or not resource use is related is often a subjective decision, and depends on whether its use can be attributed to the disease. Determining attribution involves having an understanding of the reasons why resources are consumed, and having clearly defined criteria for attribution. A pragmatic approach is to present all costs, as well as attempting to determine their attribution. Defining attribution according to the underlying clinical reasons for resource use is often arbitrary,[46] and thus further research on the implications of alternative criteria for attribution is required.

Time horizon   The time horizon – the period of time for which costs and effects are measured – influences which costs are included. If a short time horizon is chosen then future costs are not included. The time horizon chosen for the study also has implications for resource measurement, since if resource use changes over time or if new resource items are consumed, this will ultimately affect the direction and magnitude of cost differences. Limiting the costs of analysis to a fixed time period after the intervention may introduce bias into the cost comparison, especially if a disproportionate amount of resource consumption is made near death.[47] This is particularly relevant in advanced cancer clinical trials where, generally, high costs are incurred during the terminal phase of the illness.[11] Rather than collecting data over a longer period, an alternative approach is to model results beyond the end-point of the trial.[48]

Measuring resource use

Cost-generating events   Once the decision as to the types of cost to be included has been taken, it is necessary to identify the specific items, or cost-generating events, for which data collection is required. Examples of cost-generating events are a day in hospital or a GP visit. If the key cost-generating events can be established in advance, then it is possible to limit data collection to these.[49,50]

Cost-generating events can be considered key where: the frequency of the event varies between arms of the trial or between patients within arms; or the event has a large expected impact on total cost or the cost-effectiveness ratio.[4,9] Key cost-generating events can be identified from previous studies or pretrial data collection; from pilot studies, models or expert opinion.[9,49,51,52] All methods require having access to existing knowledge in the form of published studies or best available data.

Relating resource use to valuation   Resource use quantities can be defined in a number of ways. For example, health service resource use is usually measured in physical units, such as hours of staff time, or doses of a drug, but could also be measured at a more crude level, for example whether a patient has received a drug. Thus, it is important to consider the intensity of resource use measurement as well as the quantity.[53] The measurement of resource use quantities is also relevant when considering the variability in cost data. If the measurement is intensive, this may affect the variability in cost data and have implications for sample sizes. This is discussed further below.

Unit costs are attached to resource quantities to estimate costs. Therefore the definition of appropriate resource quantities must relate to the unit costs available. For example, if measuring high-dependency bed days, then this requires an appropriate unit cost. The resource quantities measured will therefore affect the level of detail at which the unit costs have to be measured and there is a spectrum of detail (or precision of measurement) of unit cost data.[2,14] The ends of the spectrum have been described as gross costing and micro costing.[4] Gross costing is where resources are identified at an aggregated level

and a unit cost attached. For example, the number of hospital days could be measured and valued by the unit cost of a hospital day. Micro costing is where resource use is identified at a detailed level and a unit cost attached to each resource. For example, staff time administering a drug could be measured and valued by a staff cost per hour.

The timing of resource use measurement   This is driven by: when the cost-generating events occur; when other data, such as quality of life, are to be collected; or when the trial protocol events occur.[54] The intervals of data collection depend on the assumptions made about accurate recall and the time cycle of the disease.[53]

Sampling strategy

Sample size calculations require a judgement about the economically important difference to detect between the two interventions in terms of cost–effectiveness, costs or resource use (see Chapter 19). Existing information on the distribution and variability of cost-effectiveness, cost or resource data is then required.[54-57] Ideally, sample sizes are calculated to estimate or test for differences in cost–effectiveness, but this is technically difficult since it requires that the distinct features of the incremental cost–effectiveness ratio are taken into account[58] (see Chapter 18). These features include that it is a ratio of two variables, with separate and non-independent variances, and that the numerator of the ratio comprises multiple cost-generating events multiplied by the unit cost of the events, and summed.[58,59]

Instead, sample sizes can be calculated to estimate or test differences between costs alone. Separate sample size calculations are required if the aim is to detect differences between groups for different types of costs, such as health service costs and patients travel costs.[55] If data are unavailable to calculate sample sizes on costs, then sample sizes can be based on estimating or testing differences in an individual resource type, for example, hospital days or GP consultations. The variability (or dispersion) in cost-generating events should also be considered at the design stage, since over-dispersion of events may require larger sample sizes[43] and ultimately variability will depend both on the units of resource measurement used and the number of events measured.

The ability to conduct sample size calculations will depend on prior knowledge of the variability of resource use or costs. Data from previous studies can be used to inform sample sizes and if data are unavailable, pilot studies can be performed.[11,57] There are, however, limitations of using pilot studies to determine sample sizes such as their limited length of follow-up, small sample sizes and low power, and these need to be recognised and understood.[60]

Beyond sample size, there are additional sampling issues. One is that it may not be necessary to collect all resource use data from all patients and that some resource use data could be collected from a subsample of patients only. Another is that, in multi-centre studies, the selection of centres is important. Differences among centres (heterogeneity) may exist and be considerable.[11,58] Heterogeneity in resource use arises because of different practices and policies, whilst heterogeneity in unit cost data is a result of different cost structures at centres.[11] The choice of centres for inclusion are often determined by the investigators on the basis of where data are easiest to collect, and the representativeness of the sample. Disagreement exists as to the extent to which unit cost data need be collected from all centres or countries participating in a multi-centre trial.[18,61] The use of centre-specific unit cost data may conceal differences in resource use; use of a single set of unit cost estimates may not reflect the true range in unit costs. The former approach is preferred but this is an issue that can be addressed with sensitivity analysis, and is discussed below.

Data required from outside the trial

Data from outside the trial are usually required to perform the economic evaluation.[62] Firstly, unit cost estimates are required to value resource use and special unit costing studies are usually required, particularly in order to match the unit cost data with the resource use quantities. The quality of the unit cost data is important, and biases in unit cost measurement exist including centre selection bias, methods bias and case-mix bias.[61] In practice, unit costs of healthcare resources can be estimated from, for example, data from local hospital finance departments. For some resource use, published unit cost data is available. The sources of unit cost data in the UK differ from other countries, in particular the USA, where charge data are readily available and valuation issues focus on the relationship between costs and charges. In the UK, most hospitals have extra contractual referral (ECR) tariffs which might be seen as corresponding to US charges, but do not always reflect the costs of the bulk of patients covered under large contracts. There is also a growing database of costs per HRG (healthcare resource group) in the UK.[63] The preferred approach to unit cost estimation is to perform specific unit cost studies for the key resources, supplementing them with published unit cost estimates for non-key resources. The uncertainty in unit cost estimates can be addressed using sensitivity analysis.

Secondly, a commonly cited limitation of clinical trials is their low external validity. Although this usually refers to the distinction between efficacy and effectiveness, it applies equally to cost data. Factors limiting external validity include the fact that the clinical outcomes realised in a non-trial setting may be different due to different locations, differences between the trial protocol and routine practice and atypical patient compliance within clinical trials.[9] Additional data are therefore required to generalise results. Information can be collected on normal clinical practice at the trial site so that the user of the study can translate results to their own circumstances.[27]

Thirdly, clinical trials are usually conducted for a limited period of time, yet the real interest may be in examining the costs and benefits over a longer period.[52] Consequently, some form of modelling may be required to extrapolate beyond the end-point of the clinical trial and to adjust or supplement the original data.[2,48] There are several methods available to address this, including Markov models and survival analysis.[48]

Analysis plan

An analysis plan for costing is useful in finalising study design. Analysis plans should include details of the descriptive and multi-variate analyses planned and the modelling approach, if any, to be adopted.[64] They should also explain how resource use and unit cost data are to be synthesised and how missing data are to be handled.[57] It is not always possible to predetermine the precise form of economic analysis to be conducted in the analysis plan, since the final form of analysis is conditional on whether the clinical effect is the same, better or worse.[2,65] The criteria used to choose between the forms of economic evaluation should, however, be stated in the analysis plan.

Data Collection

Patient-specific resource use from patients

Patient-specific resource use data can be collected from patients by one of the following methods: interviews; questionnaires; case record forms; diary cards; or standardised instruments. Interviews are usually face to face, but can also be carried out by telephone.[66] Questionnaires are administered by post or given to patients to complete when they attend their appointments. Postal questionnaires are a cheaper method data collection compared to interviews, but may result in a low response rate.[67] Patient's travel and time costs are often collected by questionnaire,[30,31] but there is no standardised, validated questionnaire available to use to collect these costs. Case record forms are often used in clinical trials to collect clinical data, and can be adapted to include both resource use and quality of life questions. Adding questions into case record forms may, however, lead to lower overall completion rates as a result of increased burden.

Diary cards can also be used to collect patient-specific resource use data. For example, patients are asked to record resource use in a diary at home when care is received, or returned on a daily or weekly basis.[64] Two important considerations when using diary cards are whether patients fill them in at the time of receiving care, or whether they wait to fill them in immediately prior to the return date. These design aspects will affect the validity of the method. A disadvantage of using diary cards is that patients may fail to complete them, although this can be overcome through reminder telephone calls.[64] The costs of data collection by diary card increases if researchers are required to motivate patients to complete diary cards and to monitor diary completion.

Investigators often design a new data collection instrument for each study, as noted above for questionnaires determining travel and time costs. This results in wide variation in both the information collected and its accuracy. These instruments or adaptations are rarely tested for validity and reliability. This increases flexibility but results in wide variations in the information collected and limits comparability with other studies. In order to increase the comparability of resource use estimates, some researchers have developed standard instruments for collecting resource use data. An American modular instrument, the Resource Utilisation Survey (RUS), has been developed for use in clinical trials.[68] In the UK, the Client Service Receipt Interview (CSRI) has been developed to gather retrospective information on health and social services resource use within a community/mental health context.[69] If service provision has changed since the instrument was developed, however, standardised instruments are unable to detect any changes in resource use associated with the change in service delivery.[53]

The above data collection methods could be completed by those other than the patient, such as staff at the hospital.[70,71] If this approach is adopted, then guidelines on how to complete the forms should be provided in order to maximise the quality of the data.[64]

In selecting a method of data collection from patients, potential sources of bias to be addressed are non-response bias, evasive answer bias, selection bias, question format and recall bias. Bias may be in either direction. There is no clear evidence regarding the appropriate recall interval, and recall has been shown to depend on the level of utilisation of resources, the frequency of use, type of resource and severity of the illness.[72,73]

Patient-specific resource use from existing records and administrative databases

It is possible to derive patient-specific resource use information from routine health service records, such as patient notes, hospital records, GP records or laboratory records (see Chapter 9). Computer linkage systems are a further type of secondary dataset, where available.

Health records include clinical records, and patient notes. If detailed resource use information is required, records have been suggested as a better source of data than burdening the patient with detailed data collection.[64] Even when records exist, however, they are often incomplete and difficult to access or retrieve.[53] An important practical issue is how easy existing records will be to access or retrieve. This may also include issues regarding patient consenting for investigators to access their records. As with data collection methods directly from patients, the type of resource use affects the validity of the method.[74,75]

Administrative databases can be used to derive resource use estimates.[76] In the USA, these administrative databases relate to clinical and claims databases which are less common in the UK. The advantages of administrative databases are that they are inexpensive to use compared to primary data collection.[58] There are several factors to be addressed when considering using administrative databases to derive patient-specific resource use. Firstly, missing data are likely to be a problem since databases may not have been designed to record all relevant information for research purposes. Secondly, extraction of health record data is also subject to problems relating to level of coder training and amount of interpretation necessary.[77] Thirdly, measurement error occurs since there is a risk that the data in such a database could be an artefact of the way the data were collected.[78] Accuracy of the data is also related to the intended purpose of the database.[79] Differences between patients may reflect measurement error rather than any real differences. Finally, databases become dated and irrelevant as time goes on.

Non-patient-specific resource use methods

Where cost-generating events are not considered key, it is sufficient to measure them on a non-patient-specific basis. Existing records and databases are also used to derive non-patient-specific resource use data, for example, length of stay may be derived from HRG data. The general limitations of administrative databases are discussed above, but their use as estimates of non-patient-specific resource use raises further issues. For example, sample selection bias may occur, that is, the population coverage of the database is not representative of the population at large.[80]

Estimates of resource use can also be derived using consensus gathering techniques from experts (see Chapter 24), although this method is unlikely to form the main mode of data collection. Evans[81] reviewed consensus gathering methods and found that the criteria for selecting experts and the baseline information provided to the panel are important aspects of designing panel studies. Expert panels have been used in several studies,[82–84] the advantage of this being that it is an inexpensive, quick and easy method for estimating resource use, particularly in economic evaluations that are performed after the clinical trial has ended. The limitations of basing resource use on expert panel estimates is that it may be an inaccurate method if recollection is poor and if estimates relate to the ideal service rather than what happens in practice.[27]

Mixed modes of data collection

Often, mixed modes of data collection will be used to collect data for different types of resource use. Patient self-report and records are often used together either sequentially, in a two-step process, or concurrently.[64] An example of a two-step process is where patients report the number of events and investigators follow-up on the detail of those events through records. Since the problem of defining a gold standard method of data collection remains, multiple sources of data can be used for the same information in order to test for validity.[53]

Organisation of data collection

Piloting of data collection methods is an important aspect of data collection design and activities, such as data monitoring, are important organisational aspects.[57,64] Steps to assess quality assurance, such as visits to each centre, and maintaining contact between site visits are also important.[85] Further organisational aspects relate to quality control issues, such as training staff

involved in the trial and having clear procedures for data entry.

Data Analysis

Summarising cost data

Once resource use and unit cost data have been collected, a cost per patient can be calculated. For each resource item, the resource quantity used by each patient is multiplied by the unit cost of the resource item. These costs are then summed for each intervention, or arm of the trial, to give the total cost per intervention, or per arm of the trial. At its simplest, the mean total cost for each intervention or arm of the trial, is calculated by dividing the total cost by the number of patients in each arm. Costs should be measured in a specific base year and hence adjusted for the effects of inflation and discounted to convert the future costs into present values.[2,4] An indication of uncertainty, or variability, should also be reported, such as standard deviation around a mean total cost.

Missing and censored data   Certain features, such as missing and censored data, complicate this summarising process and need to be addressed.[2,86] It is important to know why data are missing and what implications missing data may have.[58] Data may be missing because patients did not return or complete the data collection instruments. Data are seldom missing at random, and therefore the analytical method used in the presence of missing data has implications for the results.[87] Missing data may be handled by imputing mean values, but this may artificially reduce the variability in total cost. Missing data may also arise because of loss to follow-up, and these are termed censored data. If patients have not been followed for the entire duration of the trial, then their costs are unknown.

Statistical approaches used to handle censored clinical data have been adapted for use with economic data. Non-parametric methods, such as Kaplan–Meier survival analysis and life-table analysis, have been suggested.[86] In using this approach, costs, rather than survival time, are used as the dependent variable and are treated as right censored. It has been argued, however, that this approach is only valid if the additional cost per period is constant over time and a preferred method is therefore to partition the survival curve over a number of intervals.[88]

Synthesising costs and effects   Incremental cost–effectiveness ratios are only calculated for interventions that are more costly and produce greater effects than the intervention being used in comparison. If more than one strategy is being compared, strategies can be ranked in terms of increasing effectiveness and dominated strategies omitted from further consideration. Strategies or interventions are dominated if an intervention is less effective and more costly than an alternative; if an intervention is less costly and more effective then the treatment dominates.[89]

Handling uncertainty

Uncertainty arises from a number of sources. These include the data inputs, methods and assumptions as well as from the extrapolation or generalisability of results.[90] Uncertainty exists with respect to the parameters used as data inputs, such as the unit costs or discount rate. Uncertainty relates to the methods used, such as the data collection methods or model, as well as to the assumptions made by the investigator.[4] The generalisability of results to other settings is a further source of uncertainty.[90]

The two main methods for analysing uncertainty are statistical analysis and sensitivity analysis, and these two forms of analysis have complementary roles.[4] Uncertainty in resource use and cost differences can be examined using confidence intervals or by performing statistical tests of difference, depending on whether the interest is in estimation or hypothesis testing. An estimation approach is often preferred since estimation of a relevant quantity is more informative than significance value. With either approach, examining the distribution of cost data is important, since a relatively small number of high-cost events can skew the distribution of total cost (see Chapter 18). The implications of skewed data are that the mean cost and the variance around the mean are disproportionately affected, and the ability to detect significant differences between patient groups is perhaps reduced.[9] There are several options in such a situation: use non-parametric tests; transform the data and continue to use parametric tests, assuming the transformation produces a normal distribution;[91] or use bootstrapping to construct a confidence interval empirically. The latter two approaches are preferred since the aim is usually to determine a mean difference and an associated confidence interval since, unlike the median, the mean cost can be related back to total cost. Examining uncertainty in the cost–effectiveness ratio requires more complex statistical methods which are still in development[58] (see Chapter 18).

Confidence intervals should be presented around point estimates to indicate significant differences. The uncertainty in cost-generating events and total costs can be explored by using measures of variability such as a standard deviation or variance, and these should be presented around the mean cost differences. Variability in cost-generating events can also be examined by calculating the variance/mean ratio (or over-dispersion) of events.[43] If the variance equals the mean, there is no over-dispersion. Variability in costs can be examined by calculating the co-efficient of variation which expresses the standard deviation of a cost-generating event as a percentage of the mean.[16] This measure allows the variability between different types of cost to be compared.

Sensitivity analysis involves the systematic investigation of how changes in the selected assumptions affect the costs and cost–effectiveness. It can be used to examine the impact of changes in, for example, length of stay, on total costs or cost–effectiveness. It can also be used to generalise results.[92] The parameters to be varied and the amount of variation (or ranges) to be imputed are selected. The specification of ranges across which to vary parameters is a key component of sensitivity analysis, and justification for the ranges imputed should be given.[90] Ranges are based on clinically meaningful ranges; 95% confidence intervals for parameters; or highest and lowest ranges possible.[4] The amount of change in base results that is acceptable or constitutes a robust finding also has to be specified. All the stages of sensitivity analysis thus involve subjective elements.

Presentation and Reporting of Results

The emphasis on reporting of studies should be on transparency. The methods used should be made transparent and therefore a description of the costing methods used, including the type of costs included should be given and the reasons for adopting methods reported.[14] Sample size calculations and assumptions should also be reported,[93] along with the reasoning behind centre selection. The data collection instruments used and evidence on their validity and reliability should be reported. Reporting of cost information should include sources of resource use and unit cost estimates, price bases and discount rates. The methods used to handle missing and censored data should be reported. Costs should be presented with some information on their variability. Mean, rather than median costs, convey more useful information. The cost–effectiveness results can be presented graphically, for example, using the cost–effectiveness plane.[94]

Disaggregation of results can aid transparency.[2] Results can be disaggregated in a number of ways. For example, costs can be disaggregated into resource use and unit costs; total costs can be disaggregated into components; productivity costs can be disaggregated into resource quantities and valuation; the ratio can be disaggregated into total costs and total effects; and costs and effects can be disaggregated according to the groups affected.

Reporting styles are influenced by the objectives of the study and the perspective of the analysis. Despite differences in objectives, there is some common agreement as to reporting styles.[2] A common reporting format for economic evaluations increases the transparency of methods and results, and facilitates comparison across studies.[2] This common format should include the reporting of: research objectives; description of comparators; perspective; time horizon of study; patient characteristics; and centre characteristics.[2,4,14]

KEY ISSUES AND CONTROVERSIES

The methodological issues described above can be classified into those where there is agreement as to how to handle them, and those where there is disagreement. Given, however, that methodological approaches to the collection and analysis of resource use data for costing are still developing, recommendations may impose rigid standards and constrain further methodological development and debate. Clearly, there are some methodological issues where there is agreement. There are other issues, however, where disagreement about how to handle them is the inevitable consequence of needing different methods to answer different economic questions, or the same question in different health service contexts. Furthermore, resolutions of many of the design decisions in costing, and in economic evaluation more generally, are fundamentally dependent on the theoretical perspective of the analyst, and the perspective of the study. Such issues can only be resolved once there is a decision about the appropriate value system, viewpoint or theoretical standpoint for a particular study.

Consequently, in discussing the status of current methodological issues, issues are separated into those where there is general agreement and those where there is disagreement. The latter are further divided into those which reflect legitimate differences in values and perspective and those, often more practical issues, that are amenable to further elucidation by empirical research.

Issues of Agreement

Issues where there is agreement are shown in Table 5. Agreed methodological issues include the need to identify the perspective of the study in order to determine the appropriate types of costs for inclusion and the separate identification and measurement of resource use and unit costs. The need to measure all the direct health service costs of an intervention is generally agreed. In the context of clinical trials, the potential advantages of using existing information to inform the design of data collection is recognised. Analysis of uncertainty and the use of discounting are also accepted methodological conventions. The importance of generalising results are recognised, but the methods for doing so require further development. In terms of the reporting of methods and results, transparency is important, and so the separate reporting of, for example, resource use and unit cost data, can aid transparency.

Issues of Disagreement

There are several key methodological issues that remain open because they depend upon the perspective and values adopted in the study: choice of perspective, adoption of a welfare theoretical approach and use of hypothesis testing or estimation (as shown in Table 5). These issues can only be resolved by agreement as to what are the appropriate values and perspective in the context of a particular study or programme of research. These could of course legitimately be determined by a funder or user of such studies prescribing what values that body wishes to see reflected in studies undertaken for it, or with its funding. This indeed has been the case with the context-specific guidelines produced for example in Australia[12] or Ontario[15] for economic evaluations required to support submissions to have new drugs reimbursed within those publicly funded healthcare systems. As discussed above, there is disagreement about the scope of measurement of productivity costs and future costs. Resolution of these issues requires more considered arguments about the basis upon which they should be included or excluded.

The other category of issue of disagreement is shown in Table 5 and includes study design, data collection, data analysis and presentation issues. Many of them concern the more detailed methodological issues, for example, the sources of information, levels of necessary detail, the frequency of collecting data, modes of data

Table 5   *Status of methodological issues*

Agreement	Disagreement: Remaining open	Disagreement: Requiring further empirical research
Identifying perspective of study	Which perspective to adopt	Measuring productivity costs
Measure units of resource use and apply appropriate unit cost	Whether to base choices on economic welfare theory	Implications of alternative criteria for attribution of costs
Measurement of health service costs of the whole intervention	Whether to adopt a hypothesis testing or estimation approach	Exploring optimal sampling approaches
Need to use existing information or pretrial study to inform study design	Which productivity costs should be included?	Issues surrounding multi-centre clinical trials and handling centre effects
Need to calculate sample sizes for costs/cost-effectiveness	Which future costs should be included?	Sample sizes for cost–effectiveness
Analysis of uncertainty		Determining appropriate recall periods for data collection
Use of discounting		Determining the validity and reliability of resource use data collection instruments
Importance of generalising results		Development of a standard questionnaires for patient costs
Transparency in methods and results		Investigation of methods of handling censored data
		Identifying methods of generalising or adjusting results from clinical trials
		Exploring uncertainty in cost–effectiveness results (linking costs and effects)
		Development of a common reporting format for economic evaluations

collection, and so on. In principle, for such issues it should be possible to make specific or, at least context-specific, recommendations based on past experience. Unfortunately, whilst there are successful studies that can be drawn on as examples of seemingly good practice, there are few experimental studies to test the relative performance of different methods. Hence it is probably premature to offer firm recommendations on methods for handling even these methodological issues. These issues could, and should, be resolved by formal empirical testing of alternative methods and thus form part of a future research agenda.

IMPLICATIONS FOR PRACTITIONERS OF HTA

There are several implications for practitioners arising from this review:

1   Practitioners should adhere to the methodological issues of agreement (Table 5).
2   In undertaking studies, practitioners should consider, in a systematic way, the options for resource use data collection and ensure that the rationale for the chosen design is made explicit and transparent.
3   Practitioners should also ensure that, in determining the design, full use is made of existing evidence relating to costs of the technologies or treatments under study in order to aid the design of well-focused data collection. In doing so, investigators may be able to draw on data archives, if such are established.
4   If, when designing studies, practitioners confront methodological issues of disagreement that could be resolved by further empirical research, they should consider whether these could be formally tested within the applied study. This would contribute to the reduction in uncertainty surrounding the relative merits of alternative approaches.
5   In order to aid transparency of results, practitioners should aim to ensure that details of their data collection methods and instruments are readily available and ensure that they report results in such a way that analysis is repeatable by other investigators.
6   Practitioners should also be willing to share data from previous studies with other researchers designing costing studies in similar areas. They should be prepared to deposit work in data archives if such are set up and, in so doing, contribute to the critical appraisal of the usefulness of such archives.

CONCLUSION

This chapter has drawn on the existing methodological literature on conducting economic evaluation alongside clinical trials, identifying the main methodological issues associated with costing data collection and analysis, and establishing whether these issues can be resolved by reference to the theory underlying economic evaluation or the practical experience of undertaking such studies.

Methodological issues where there is general agreement include identifying perspective; measuring units of resource use and applying appropriate unit cost. Methodological issues remaining open because of legitimate differences in values or perspectives are which perspective to adopt, and whether to base decision on economic welfare theory. Finally, methodological issues requiring further empirical research include: exploring optimal sampling approaches; issues surrounding multi-centre clinical trials; testing the validity and reliability of resource use data collection methods; and methods used to generalise results. By presenting issues in this way, the review recognises the inevitability of some issues remaining unresolved, whilst at the same time allowing the specification of a future research agenda.

ACKNOWLEDGEMENTS

We would like to thank Mike Drummond for advice throughout the project; Ann Raven for assistance in the early stages of the project; Claire Davey for help in developing methods of the review. We thank Martin Backhouse, Ray Churnside, Doug Coyle, Linda Davies, Cam Donaldson, Miranda Mugford, Max Parmar, Kevin Schulman and Ken Wright for comments made on the main systematic review. The views expressed, and any errors remaining are, however, those of the authors.

REFERENCES

1. Johnston K, Buxton MJ, Jones DR, Fitzpatrick R. Assessing the costs of health technologies in clinical trials. *Health Technology Assessment* 1999; **3**: 6.
2. Drummond MF, O'Brien B, Stoddart GL, Torrance GW. *Methods for the economic evaluation of health care programmes*. Oxford, Oxford University Press, 1997.
3. Luce BR, Elixhauser A. Estimating costs in the economic evaluation of medical technologies. *Int. J. Technol. Assess. Health Care* 1990; **6**: 57–75.
4. Gold MR, Siegel JE, Russell LB, Weinstein MC. *Cost-effectiveness in health and medicine*. New York: Oxford University Press, 1996.
5. Donaldson C, Shackley P. Economic evaluation. In: Detels R, Holland WW, McEwen J, Omenn GS (eds). *Oxford Textbook of Public Health*, 3rd edn. Oxford: Oxford University Press, 1997.
6. Donaldson C. The state of the art of costing health care for economic evaluation. *Community Health Studies* 1990; **14**: 341–56.
7. Evans DB. Principles involved in costing. *Med. J. Aust.* 1990; **153**: S10–S12.
8. Johannesson M. The concept of cost in the economic evaluation of health care. *Int. J. Technol. Assess. Health Care* 1994; **10**: 675–82.
9. Drummond MF, Davies L. Economic analysis alongside clinical trials: Revisiting the methodological issues. *Int. J. Technol. Assess. Health Care* 1991; **7**: 561–73.
10. Adams M, McCall N, Gray D, Orza M, Chalmers T. Economic analysis in randomized control trials. *Med. Care* 1992; **30**: 231–43.
11. Bonsel G, Rutten F, Uyl de Groot C. Economic evaluation alongside cancer trials: methodological and practical aspects. *Eur. J. Cancer* 1993; **29A**: S10–S14.
12. Commonwealth of Australia. Guidelines for the pharmaceutical industry on preparations of submissions to the Pharmaceutical Benefits Advisory Committee (including submissions involving economic analyses. Canberra, Australian Government Print Office, 1995.
13. ABPI (Association of the British Pharmaceutical Industry). *Pharmaceutical industry and Department of Health agree guidelines for the economic analysis of medicines*, 1994.
14. CCOHTA (Canadian Coordinating Office for Health Technology Assessment). *Guidelines for economic evaluation of pharmaceuticals*. Canada, 1994.
15. Ministry of Health. *Ontario guidelines for economic analysis of pharmaceutical products*, 1994.
16. Gray AM, Marshall M, Lockwood A, Morris J. Problems in conducting economic evaluations alongside clinical trials: lessons from a study of case management for people with mental disorders. *Br. J. Psychiatry* 1997; **170**: 47–52.
17. Hlatky MA, Boothroyd DB, Johnstone IM, et al. Long-term cost-effectiveness of alternative management strategies for patients with life-threatening ventricular arrhythmias. *J. Clin. Epidemiol.* 1997; **50**: 185–93.
18. Menzin J, Oster G, Davies L, et al. A multinational economic evaluation of rhDNase in the treatment of cystic fibrosis. *Int. J. Technol. Assess. Health Care* 1996; **12**: 52–61.
19. Nicholl JP, Brazier JE, Milner PC, et al. Randomised controlled trial of cost-effectiveness of lithotripsy and open cholecystectomy as treatments for gallbladder stones. *Lancet* 1992; **340**: 801–7.

20. Rutten-Van Molken MPMH, Van Doorslaer EKA, Jansen MCC, Kerstijens HAM, Rutten FFH. Costs and effects of inhaled corticosteroids and bronchodilators in asthma and chronic obstructive pulmonary disease. *Am. J. Respir. Crit. Care Med.* 1995; **151**: 975–82.

21. Schulman KA, Buxton M, Glick H, et al. Results of the economic evaluation of the first study: a multinational prospective economic evaluation. *Int. J. Technol. Assess. Health Care* 1996; **12**: 698–713.

22. Sculpher MJ, Dwyer N, Byford S, Stirrat G. Randomised trial comparing hysterectomy and transcervical endometrial resection: effect on health related quality of life and costs two years after surgery. *Br. J. Obstet. Gynaecol.* 1996; **103**: 142–9.

23. van Bergen PFMM. Costs and effects of long-term oral anticoagulant treatment after myocardial infarction. *JAMA* 1995; **273**: 925–8.

24. Wonderling D, McDermott C, Buxton M, et al. Costs and cost effectiveness of cardiovascular screening and intervention: the British family heart study. *Br. Med. J.* 1996; **312**: 1269–73.

25. Rittenhouse B. *Uses of models in economic evaluations of medicines and other health technologies.* London: Office of Health Economics, 1996.

26. Langham S, Thorogood M, Normand C, Muir J, Jones L, Fowler G. Costs and cost effectiveness of health checks conducted by nurses in primary care: the Oxcheck study. *Br. Med. J.* 1996; **312**: 1265–8.

27. Drummond MF, Jefferson TO, on behalf of the BMJ economic evaluation working party. Guidelines for authors and peer reviewers of economic submissions to the BMJ. *Br. Med. J.* 1996; **313**: 275–83.

28. Meltzer D. Accounting for future costs in medical cost-effectiveness analysis. *J. Health Economics* 1997; **16**: 33–64.

29. Smith K, Wright K. Informal care and economic appraisal: a discussion of possible methodological approaches. *Health Economics* 1994; **3**: 137–48.

30. Bryan S, Buxton M, McKenna M, Ashton H, Scott A. Private costs associated with abdominal aortic aneurysm screening: the importance of private travel and time costs. *J. Med. Screening* 1995; **2**: 62–6.

31. Sculpher MJ, Buxton MJ. The private costs incurred when patients visit screening clinics: the cases of screening for breast cancer and for diabetic retinopathy. Health Economics Research Group Discussion Paper, Brunel University, Uxbridge, 1993.

32. Weinstein MC, Siegel JE, Garber AM, et al. Productivity costs, time costs and health-related quality of life: a response to the Erasmus group. *Health Economics* 1997; **6**: 505–10.

33. Brouwer WBF, Koopmanschap MA, Rutten FFH. Productivity costs measurement through quality

34. Koopmanschap MA, Rutten FFH. Indirect costs in economic studies: confronting the confusion. *PharmacoEconomics* 1993; **4**: 446–54.

35. van Roijen L, Essink-Bot ML, Koopmanschap MA, Bonsel G, Rutten FFH. Labor and health status in economic evaluation of health care: the health and labor questionnaire. *Int. J. Technol. Assess. Health Care* 1996; **12**: 405–15.

36. Koopmanschap MA, Rutten FFH. A practical guide for calculating indirect costs of disease. *PharmacoEconomics* 1996; **10**: 460–6.

37. Garber AM, Phelps CE. Economic foundations of cost-effectiveness analysis. *J. Health Economics* 1997; **16**: 1–31.

38. Weinstein MC, Manning WG. Theoretical issues in cost-effectiveness analysis. *J. Health Economics* 1997; **16**: 121–8.

39. Birch S, Gafni A. Cost-effectiveness ratios: in a league of their own. *Health Policy* 1994; **28**: 133–41.

40. Davidoff A, Powe NR. The role of perspective in defining measures for the economic evaluation of medical technology. *Int. J. Technol. Assess. Health Care* 1996; **12**: 9–21.

41. Gerard K, Mooney G. QALY league tables: Handle with care. *Health Economics* 1993; **2**: 59–64.

42. Johannesson M. Avoiding double-counting in pharmacoeconomics studies. *PharmacoEconomics* 1997; **11**: 385–8.

43. Spiegelhalter DJ, Jones DR, Parmar MKB, Gore SM, Fitzpatrick R, Cox DR. Being economical with the costs. Department of Epidemiology and Public Health Technical Paper 96-06, University of Leicester, 1996.

44. Sculpher M, Drummond M, Buxton M. The iterative use of economic evaluation as part of the process of health technology assessment. *J. Health Services Res. Policy* 1997; **2**: 26–30.

45. Jonsson B, Weinstein MC. Economic evaluation alongside multinational clinical trials: study considerations for GUSTO 11b. *Int. J. Technol. Assess. Health Care* 1997; **13**: 49–58.

46. Hurley SF, Bond LM, Carlin JB, Evans DB, Kaldor JM. A method for estimating baseline health care costs. *J. Epidemiol. Community Health* 1995; **49**: 525–31.

47. Dranove D. Measuring costs. In: Sloan FA (ed.) *Valuing health care: cost, benefits and effectiveness of pharmaceuticals and other medical technologies.* Cambridge; Cambridge University Press, 1995.

48. Buxton MJ, Drummond MF, Van Hout BA, et al. Modelling in economic evaluation: an unavoidable fact of life. *Health Economics* 1997; **6**: 217–27.

of life? A response to the recommendation of the Washington panel. *Health Economics* 1997; **6**: 253–9.

49. Morris J, Goddard M. Economic evaluation and quality of life assessments in cancer clinical trials: the CHART trial. *Eur. J. Cancer* 1992; **29A**: 766–70.

50. Knapp M, Beecham J. Reduced list costings: examination of an informed short cut in mental health research. *Health Economics* 1993; **2**: 313–22.

51. Backhouse M, Mauskopf JA, Jones D, Wold DE. Economics outcomes of colfosceril palmitate rescue therapy in infants weighing 1250g or more with respiratory distress syndrome. *Pharmaco-Economics* 1994; **6**: 358–69.

52. Sheldon TA. Problems of using modelling in the economic evaluation of health care. *Health Economics* 1996; **5**: 1–11.

53. Clark RE, Teague GB, Ricketts SK, et al. Measuring resource use in economic evaluations: determining the social costs of mental illness. *J. Mental Health Admin.* 1994; **21**: 32–41.

54. O'Brien BJ, Drummond MF, Labelle RJ, Willan A. In search of power and significance: issues in the design and analysis of stochastic cost-effectiveness studies in health care. *Medical Care* 1994; **32**: 150–63.

55. Drummond M, O'Brien B. Clinical importance, statistical significance and the assessment of economic and quality-of-life outcomes. *Health Economics* 1993; **2**: 205–12.

56. Torgerson DJ, Ryan M, Ratcliffe J. Economics in sample size determination for clinical trials. *Q. J. Med.* 1995; **88**: 517–21.

57. Coyle D, Davies L, Drummond M. Trials and tribulations: Emerging issues in designing economic evaluations alongside clinical trials. *Int. J. Technol. Assess. Health Care* 1998; **14**: 135–44.

58. Mullahy J, Manning W. Statistical issues in cost-effectiveness analysis. In: Sloan FA (ed.) *Valuing health care: costs benefits and effectiveness of pharmaceutical and other medical technologies.* Cambridge; Cambridge University Press, 1995.

59. Mullahy J. What you don't know can't hurt you? Statistical issues and standards for medical technology evaluation. *Medical Care* 1996; **34**: DS124–DS135.

60. Wittes J, Brittain E. The role of internal pilot studies in increasing the efficiency of clinical trials. *Stat. Med.* 1990; **9**: 65–72.

61. Jacobs P, Baladi JF. Biases in cost measurement for economic evaluation studies in health care. *Health Economics* 1996; **5**: 525–9.

62. Rittenhouse B. Exorcising protocol-induced spirits: making the clinical trial relevant for economics. *Medical Decision Making* 1997; **17**: 331–9.

63. CHKS. *Acute Care 1996: Healthcare resource groups national statistics 1995/1996.* Warwickshire: CHKS, 1996.

64. Mauskopf J, Schulman K, Bell L, Glick H. A strategy for collecting pharmacoeconomic data during phase II/III clinical trials. *Pharmaco-Economics* 1996; **9**: 264–77.

65. Donaldson C, Hundley V, McIntosh E. Using economics alongside clinical trials: why we cannot choose the evaluation technique in advance. *Health Economics* 1996; **5**: 267–9.

66. Anie KA, Jones PW, Hilton SR, Anderson HR. A computer-assisted telephone interview technique for assessment of asthma morbidity and drug use in adult asthma. *J. Clin. Epidemiol.* 1996; **49**: 653–6.

67. Streiner DL, Norman GR. Health measurement scales: A practical guide to their development and use. Oxford: Oxford University Press, 1989.

68. Copley-Merriman C, Egbuonu-Davis L, Kotsanos JG, Conforti P, Franson T, Gordon G. Clinical economics: a method for prospective health resource data collection. *PharmacoEconomics* 1992; **1**: 370–6.

69. Beecham J. Collecting information: The client service receipt interview. *Mental Health Res. Rev.* 1994; **1**: 6–8.

70. Hundley VA, Donaldson C, Lang GD, et al. Costs of intrapartum care in a midwife- managed delivery unit and a consultant led labour ward. *Midwifery* 1995; **11**: 103–9.

71. Hughes J, Ryan M, Hinshaw K, Henshaw R, Rispin R, Templeton A. The costs of treating miscarriage: a comparison of medical and surgical management. *Br. J. Obstet. Gynaecol.* 1996; **103**: 1217–21.

72. Brown JB, Adams ME. Patients as reliable reporters of medical care process: recall of ambulatory encounter events. *Medical Care* 1992; **30**: 400–11.

73. Revicki DA, Irwin D, Reblando J, Simon GE. The accuracy of self-reported disability days. *Medical Care* 1994; **32**: 401–4.

74. Boyer GS, Templin DW, Goring WP et al. Discrepancies between patient recall and the medical record. *Arch. Intern. Med.* 1995; **155**: 1868–72.

75. Linet MS, Harlow SD, McLaughlin JK, McCaffrey LD. A comparison of interview data and medical records for previous medical conditions and surgery. *J. Clin. Epidemiol.* 1989; **42**: 1207–13.

76. Lave JR, Pashos CL, Anderson GF, et al. Costing medical care: Using medicare administrative data. *Medical Care* 1994; **32**: JS77–JS89.

77. Aaronson LS, Burman ME. Focus on Psychometrics. Use of health records in research: reliability and validity issues. *Research in Nursing and Health* 1994; **17**: 67–73.

78. Safran C. Using routinely collected data for clinical research. *Stat. Med.* 1991; **10**: 559–64.

79. Wolff N, Helminiak TW. Nonsampling measurement error in administrative data: implications for economic evaluations. *Health Economics* 1996; **5**: 501–12.

80. Kuykendall DH, Johnson ML. Administrative databases, case-mix adjustments and hospital resource use: the appropriateness of controlling patient characteristics. *J. Clin. Epidemiol.* 1995; **48**: 423–30.

81. Evans C. The use of consensus methods and expert panels in pharmacoeconomic studies. Practical applications and methodological shortcomings. *PharmacoEconomics* 1997; **12**: 121–9.

82. Phillips K, Lowe E, Kahn J. The cost-effectiveness of HIV testing of physicians and dentists in the United States. *JAMA* 1994; **271**: 851–8.

83. Jonsson B, Bebbington PE. What price depression? The cost of depression and the cost-effectiveness of pharmacological treatment. *Br. J. Psychiatry* 1994; **164**: 665–73.

84. O'Brien B, Goeree R, Mohamed AH, Hunt R. Cost-effectiveness of helicobacter pylori eradication for the long-term management of duodenal ulcer in Canada. *Arch. Intern. Med.* 1995; **155**: 1958–64.

85. Morris J, Goddard M, Coyle D, Drummond M. Measuring cost and quality of life in radiotherapy trial treatments. Centre for Health Economics, discussion paper 112 ,1993.

86. Fenn P, McGuire A, Phillips V, Backhouse M, Jones D. The analysis of censored treatment cost data in economic evaluation. *Medical Care* 1995; **33**: 851–63.

87. Crawford SL, Tennstedt SL, McKinlay JB. A comparison of analytic methods for non-random missingness of outcome data. *J. Clin. Epidemiol.* 1995; **48**: 209–19.

88. Lin DY, Feuer EJ, Etzioni R, Wax Y. Estimating medical costs from incomplete follow-up data. *Biometrics* 1997; **53**: 419–34.

89. Karlsson G, Johanesson M. The decision rules of cost-effectiveness analysis. *PharmacoEconomics* 1996; **9**: 113–20.

90. Briggs A, Sculpher M, Buxton M. Uncertainty in the economic evaluation of health care technologies: the role of sensitivity analysis. *Health Economics* 1994; **3**: 95–104.

91. Coyle D. Statistical analysis in pharmacoeconomic studies. *PharmacoEconomics* 1996; **9**: 506–16.

92. Sculpher MJ, Michaels J, McKenna M, Minor J. A cost-utility analysis of laser assisted angioplasty for peripheral arterial occlusions. *Int. J. Technol. Assess. Health Care* 1996; **12**: 104–25.

93. Mason J, Drummond M. Reporting guidelines for economic studies. *Health Economics* 1995; **4**: 85–94.

94. Black WC. The cost-effectiveness plane: a graphic representation of cost-effectiveness. *Medical Decision Making* 1990; **10**: 212–15.

14

Eliciting Time Preferences for Health

JOHN CAIRNS and MARJON VAN DER POL

SUMMARY

This chapter reviews the stated preference approach to the elicitation of inter-temporal preferences for future health events and presents an outline of a project to establish the nature of individual preferences. Research in this area is important for two reasons: (i) discounting practices often play a central role in determining the relative cost–effectiveness of different interventions; and (ii) an understanding of how individuals view future costs and benefits is valuable with respect to the design of policies for the promotion of health. Despite the growing number of empirical studies, there is a need for further research to add to the understanding of time preferences and ultimately to lead to better informed decision-making with respect to discounting practice. This chapter reports on a project designed to address many of these outstanding issues.

The specific objectives for the TEMPUS project are: to derive implied discount rates for future health benefits for a sample of the general public in the UK; to establish whether individual inter-temporal preferences with respect to their own health differ from those with respect to the health of others; to investigate the effect of different ways of asking questions on apparent inter-temporal preferences; and to establish whether individuals value future health benefits in line with the traditional discounted utility model and to investigate alternative discounting models. There are many choices and issues with respect to the elicitation of time preferences for health. These are made explicit in this chapter, including their relative advantages and disadvantages. The methods chosen in this study are open-ended and closed-ended (discrete choice modelling) stated preference methods, and the data are collected with postal questionnaires. In order to meet all objectives four different questionnaires are designed. The methods and questionnaires are discussed in detail, including the econometric issues arising, and some preliminary results are reported.

INTRODUCTION

Generally, individuals would prefer to receive a benefit today rather than in the future and to incur a cost later rather than sooner. Economists call these time preferences. Such preferences are relevant in two ways in the context of healthcare. Firstly, how individuals view future costs and benefits influences health-affecting behaviour such as smoking, exercising and following dietary restrictions. Information on individuals' time preferences could therefore be valuable with respect to the design of policies for the promotion of health. Secondly, methods are required to take into account the timing of costs and benefits when undertaking economic evaluation of healthcare interventions. This is achieved by discounting future costs and benefits to present values whereby smaller and smaller weights are attached to future events the further in the future they occur. These declining weights or discount factors are equal to $(1 + r)^{-t}$ where r is the discount rate and t is the year in which the event occurs.

It is conventional to explain the practice of discounting either in terms of social choices or in terms of individual preferences. As an economy it is possible to defer consumption and undertake investment so that a higher level of future consumption can be enjoyed. Thus, the opportunity cost of current consumption is some higher level of future consumption, and the discount factor is a formal recognition of this opportunity cost. At the individual level it is suggested that most individuals have time preferences; that is, they are not indifferent with respect to the timing of future events. The reasons suggested for this include: that individuals cannot be sure that they will be alive at any particular point in the future; that they anticipate being better off and will as a result attach less weight to further increments to their wealth or income; and what Pigou famously described as a defective telescopic faculty.

Discounting practices often play a central role in determining the relative cost–effectiveness of different interventions. If evaluations are undertaken on an incorrect basis the quality of decision-making will suffer and health service efficiency will be reduced. Moreover, confusion or lack of agreement over standard discounting practice potentially undermines the credibility and value of economic evaluation. Different rates are applied in different jurisdictions but they are generally between 0.03 and 0.06. The impact of discounting is especially marked when considering projects where some of the effects are fairly far in the future. For example, the discount factor applied to costs arising in 20 years time would be 0.31 at the currently recommended UK rate ($r = 0.06$).

Despite the potential importance of individuals' preferences for future health events, current knowledge regarding the nature of these preferences is poor. Systematic investigation of, the influence of type of choice on apparent time preferences, the characteristics of different methods of eliciting preferences, and the underlying models of time preferences for analysing responses, is required.

AIMS OF THE CHAPTER

This chapter has the following aims:

1   To review the stated preference approach to the elicitation of inter-temporal preferences.
2   To outline *The Estimation of Marginal time Preference in a UK-wide Sample* (TEMPUS) project and explain the choice of methods used.
3   To report some preliminary findings.

THE ESTIMATION OF TIME PREFERENCES

Two broad approaches have been used to estimate time preference rates – revealed preference

and stated preference. The distinction is that the former involves observing actual behaviour, specifically inter-temporal decisions, whereas the latter involves asking individuals what they would do in particular hypothetical circumstances. Despite a predisposition in favour of revealed preference, economists have in recent years shown an increasing willingness to explore the stated preference approach. There are still concerns about the validity of the information generated, and the ideal corroborating evidence remains observed behaviour.

A wide range of behaviour has been studied including: the purchase of consumer durables;[1-4] educational investment decisions;[5] food consumption;[6] and labour market wage-risk choices.[7-9] These studies generally are based on larger sample sizes than those used in applications of the stated preference approach. Also, the estimation of discount rates is relatively indirect and quite complicated. This results partly from the difficulty of using data collected primarily for some other purpose and the many more factors outwith the researchers control (as compared to an experimental approach).

The stated preference approach has also been applied in a wide range of settings. These have included: financial choices;[10-13] purchases of consumer durables;[14,15] saving lives; and non-fatal changes in health. The last two groups of studies are of course of particular relevance.

Underlying both of these approaches has been a reliance on the Discounted Utility (DU) model which has dominated economic thought with respect to inter-temporal choice for over 50 years. The most important assumption of the model is that individuals discount future events at a constant rate. Loewenstein and Prelec[16] identify four inter-temporal choice anomalies that run counter to the predictions of the model. They describe these as: (i) the common difference effect; (ii) the absolute magnitude effect; (iii) the gain-loss asymmetry; and (iv) the delay–speedup asymmetry. The last three are self-explanatory. The DU model assumes that the discount rate applied will not be related to the magnitude of the event which is subject to discounting, nor to whether the event represents a gain or a loss, nor to whether it is being brought forward or delayed. The common difference effect refers to the impact on choice between two delayed outcomes of a change in the delay applied equally to both outcomes. The DU model assumes that the choice depends only on the absolute interval between the two outcomes.

These anomalies are explained by Loewenstein and Prelec in general terms with reference to future consumption, and supported by evidence from monetary choices. However, there is no reason to suppose that they are any less in evidence when the outcomes are in terms of health.

Is Health Different?

Before outlining the work done on the estimation of time preferences for health it is worth addressing the basic question – is health different? There are at least two ways in which this question can be addressed: as a practical issue arising in economic evaluation; and at a more methodological level. The practical question is whether or not future health effects should be discounted at the same rate as future costs. This question has generated considerable interest in recent years, and much of the empirical work that has been undertaken has aimed to inform this debate.

Parsonage and Neuberger[17] claim that '. . . in practice, for most purposes, it is appropriate to use a zero discount rate for future health benefits' (p. 72). They argue that the traditional sources of time preference are unimportant in the context of future health benefits. Whether or not monetary costs and non-monetary benefits should be discounted at the same rate can be viewed as largely an empirical question.[18] Is the sum of *undiscounted* health benefits a better or a poorer approximation to the true value of a stream of future benefits than the sum of the *discounted* health benefits? The answer would appear to depend on the social valuation of the health benefits and how it changes over time. The greater the increase in social valuation over time the closer will the undiscounted sum approximate the true value. The smaller the increase in social valuation, the closer the approximation provided by the discounted sum.

Currently the only jurisdiction where formal guidance encourages the differential discounting of monetary costs and non-monetary benefits is England and Wales, where 6% is recommended for financial values and 1.5–2% for health effects quantified in physical units.[19] Such advice is at odds with that elsewhere, for example, Canada[20] and the USA[21] (5% and 3% respectively applied to all costs and benefits).

The methodological issue concerns whether or not it is possible to identify individuals' rates of time preference with respect to future health effects and is rather more important in the context of this chapter. Gafni and Torrance[22] hint at the potential difficulties in doing so, and Gafni[23] develops the argument more fully. Gafni and Torrance relate attitude towards risk in health to three distinct effects: a quantity effect; a time preference effect; and a gambling effect. It is interesting to note that Gafni and Torrance

suggest that '. . . time preference is measured by asking conventional time preference questions . . . but cast in the health, as opposed to financial domain.' (p. 449). Also they claim that it is not necessary to speculate on the nature of time preference '. . . since it is empirically determinable' (p. 449). However, drawing on Loewenstein and Prelec,[24] which highlighted the importance of another class of effects – sequence effects, Gafni[23] argues robustly that no measurement technique allows pure time preference to be distinguished, and the best that can be achieved is a measure of time preference for a given sequence of events. This may be true of preferences over one's own future health states; however, it is less clear that the sequence of events will be an important influence when considering preferences over life-saving profiles.

A further way in which some health benefits may be different arises when the change in health is measured in terms of QALYs. Krahn and Gafni[25] argue that, because of the methods sometimes used to measure QALYs, time preferences may already have been taken into account. As a result further discounting of the QALYs might represent a form of double counting.

Using Stated Preference to Estimate Time Preferences for Health

As noted above, a distinction can be drawn between those studies with respect to life saving and those with respect to non-fatal changes in health. Table 1 provides a brief overview of this literature.

Saving lives

The first studies of time preferences with respect to life saving[26–29] adopted fairly similar approaches. Horowitz and Carson[26] offered respondents dichotomous choices between a programme saving lives for the next 15 years and a programme saving lives for 10 years, starting in 5 years time. Cropper et al.[28] asked two linked dichotomous questions offering a context-free choice between programmes saving lives now and various times in the future. Both then used econometric methods to identify median implied time preferences rates for the sample interviewed. A broadly similar approach was followed in a recent Swedish study[30] of intergenerational choices.

Later studies by Olsen,[31] Cairns[32] and Cairns and van der Pol[33,34] used variants of an open-ended approach where the data were collected with a self-completed questionnaire. Through this approach the identification of rates of time

Table 1 *Summary of empirical time preference literature in health*

Study	Median r	Mean r	Type	Delay	Sample
Cairns[37]	–	−0.001 to 0.030	Health states	10 to 28 years	29 economics undergraduates
Chapman, Elstein[38]	0.360 and 1.000	0.640 and 1.240	Health states	1 to 12 years	104 psychology undergraduates
Dolan, Gudex[42]	0.000	−0.029 to 0.014	Health states	9 years	39 members of general public
Lipscomb[36]	–	–	Health states	1 to 25 years	52 undergraduate students
MacKeigan et al.[41]	–	–	Health states	1 week to 1 year	108 members of university staff and hospital volunteers
Redelmeier, Heller[40]	–	0.023 to 0.041	Health states	1 day to 10 years	121 medical students, house officers and physicians
Cairns, van der Pol[33,34]	0.160 to 0.410	0.140 to 0.450	Lives	2 to 19 years	473 members of general public
Cairns[32]	0.160 to 0.380	0.140 to 0.370	Lives	4 to 19 years	223 members of general public
Cropper et al.[27]	–	0.027 to 0.086	Lives	25 to 100 years	1600 members of general public
Cropper et al.[28]	0.038 to 0.168	–	Lives	25 to 100 years	3200 members of general public
Enemark et al.[35]	0.104	0.102	Lives	≈ 10 years	25 vascular surgeons
Horowitz, Carson[26]	0.045	–	Lives	5 years	75 economics undergraduates
Johannesson, Johansson[30]	0.080 to 0.250	–	Lives	20 to 100 years	850 members of general public
Olsen[31]	0.058 to 0.229	0.066 to 0.233	Lives and health state	4 to 19 years	250 members of general public and 77 health planners

preference can be made on an individual basis through simple manipulation of the responses. The price of this advantage may be increased problems with respect to framing effects and related biases.

A third approach followed by Enemark et al.[35] differs in that it is not concerned with choices between saving differing numbers of statistical lives at different times in the future. It concerns the choice between watchful waiting and surgery for abdominal aortic aneurysms for a hypothetical cohort. In a classification between life-saving and non-fatal changes in health it is probably appropriate to put it with the life-saving studies, but it is rather different from the rest of the literature and as such may offer a new line of enquiry.

Non-fatal changes in health

The first significant study of time preferences for non-fatal changes in health was by Lipscomb.[36] His approach requires subjects to classify 96 scenarios on a 0 to 10 category scale. Regression analysis is then used to explain these scores using the characteristics of the health state. Lipscomb suggests that time preference '. . . be regarded as operationally equivalent to the (marginal) influence of the delay-of-onset variable on preference scores' (p. S243). Notwithstanding the practical difficulties of applying the approach (such as the demands on individual respondents), it represents an attractive means of determining the impact of delay on the valuation of an outcome.

In the report by Cairns,[37] implied discount rates are calculated directly from the duration of ill health which renders the respondent indifferent between being ill in the further future and in the near future. A broadly similar approach has been followed by Chapman and Elstein[38] and Chapman[39] in which subjects indicated what period of relief from ill health at a specified point in the future would make them indifferent between relief from ill health for a specified period now.

Redelmeier and Heller[40] used the standard gamble and categorical scaling to elicit preferences for a number of different health states, one aspect of which was the timing of onset of ill health. MacKeigan et al.[41] also used a categorical rating scale to elicit preferences for different health states with different delays of onset. They examined the effect of duration of health gain *and* health loss, and delay before health change, on the valuation of health states, but did not estimate the implied discount rates. Finally, Dolan and Gudex[42] estimate time preference rates using time trade-off valuations for two

health profiles which differ only in the timing of the period of ill-health.

Research Issues Addressed by the TEMPUS Project

Despite the growing number of empirical studies there are numerous opportunities for further research to add to the understanding of time preferences, and ultimately lead to better informed decision-making with respect to discounting practice. This listing does not seek to be comprehensive but rather highlights three areas explored in the TEMPUS project.

Different methods of eliciting time preferences

Little is known about the influence on estimates of implied discount rates of different methods of eliciting preferences. A major issue in the field of contingent valuation has been the use of closed-ended (are you willing to pay £100?) versus open-ended questions (how much are you willing to pay?). With respect to the elicitation of time preferences, open-ended methods[31–34,37–39] have proved more popular to date than closed-ended,[26–30] particularly if those studies adopting a more indirect approach (via the valuation of different health outcomes[35,36,40–42]) are classified as open-ended. No studies have been published which explicitly compare different methods of eliciting time preferences.

Further issues concern the use of self-completed questionnaires versus interviews (face-to-face and telephonic), and the presence and impact of framing effects. Both of these have yet to be systematically investigated. Whilst there are undoubtedly lessons to be learned from work in other fields, such as contingent valuation, there is clearly considerable scope for designing time preference studies to address these issues directly.

Nature of the inter-temporal choice

An important question on which little is known is the extent and nature of differences between time preferences with respect to one's own health and others' health. The studies with respect to saving statistical lives clearly refer to the health of others.[26–34] Generally, questions with respect to non-fatal changes in health have been posed in terms of the respondents' *own* health,[37–42] although MacKeigan et al.,[41] whilst inviting respondents to consider their own health, asked respondents to imagine that they were 50 years old and married with children (none of whom lived with them). The exceptions are: Lipscomb,[36] whose scenarios start 'A person in your community is now 25 years old'; and part of the Olsen[31] life-saving study in which the life-saving questions were repeated substituting '. . . a programme which improves the health of people in a chronic state of dysfunction and distress' for '. . . a programme which saves human lives'; and a study of vascular surgeons time preferences for their patients' future health.[35] The distinction between own and others' health is important because time preferences with respect to own health are likely to be more relevant to explaining health-affecting behaviour, whereas preferences with respect to others' health are potentially more important if the focus is on the evaluation of publicly funded healthcare programmes.

Further issues concern: the nature and extent of differences between time preferences for saving lives and those for non-fatal changes in health; and whether time preferences are to some extent health state-specific. Loewenstein claims '. . . the dependence of discounting on the characteristics of awaited consumption means that discount rates estimated in specific contexts . . . cannot be generalised beyond the domain of behaviour in which they were derived'.[43] Although this remark was made with respect to a comparison of the purchase of consumer durables and savings behaviour, it does raise the issue of whether implied discount rates are similar within the health domain. The health states examined to date have included: an arthritic condition; a strangulated internal hernia; a depressive illness; and temporary blindness.

Underlying model of time preferences

Harvey[44] has emphasised the distinction between constant and decreasing timing aversion. Most, but not all, studies[36,41] have assumed constant timing aversion, whereas the empirical evidence suggests that decreasing timing aversion might represent individuals' inter-temporal preferences more accurately. Preferences are defined as *constant timing averse* where an individual is indifferent between (x, s) and (y, t), and between $(x, s + \Delta)$ and $(y, t + \Delta)$, where x and y are benefits accruing at times s and t and $0 < x < y$ and $s < t$. Preferences are defined as *decreasing timing averse* where an individual is indifferent between (x, s) and (y, t) and prefers $(y, t + \Delta)$ to $(x, s + \Delta)$. That is, less importance is attached to a fixed difference $t - s$ between two times s and t the farther into the future these times are moved. Proportional discounting models[44] and hyperbolic discounting models[45] are examples of

models which allow for decreasing timing aversion. However, there has been little investigation of alternative models.[27,33,34]

The TEMPUS Project

The specific objectives of the TEMPUS study are:

1 To derive implied discount rates for future health benefits for a sample of the general public in the UK.
2 To establish whether individual inter-temporal preferences with respect to their own health differ from those with respect to the health of others.
3 To investigate the effect of different ways of asking questions on apparent inter-temporal preferences (specifically closed-ended and open-ended methods are compared).
4 To establish whether individuals value future health benefits in line with the traditional discounted utility model and to investigate in addition how well the hyperbolic and proportional discounting models explain individual responses.

DESIGN AND METHODS

Stated preference techniques comprising a series of health-related choices are used to elicit the time preferences of a random sample of adults. In order to meet the specific objectives of the TEMPUS project, both open-ended and closed-ended questions were used. There are several choices to be made when designing either open-ended or closed-ended time preference questions. Most are relevant to both types of questionnaire but some are specific to one or other question type.

The following are potentially relevant to both types of question:

(a) Number of points in time: respondents can be asked to consider two points in time or they can be presented with a profile. The standard approach has been the former, with only two studies comparing profiles.[26,35]
(b) Base health state: the base health state can be full-health and respondents make choices with respect to the consumption of ill-health,[37,40,41] or the base health state is ill-health and respondents make choices with respect to the consumption of full-health.[38,39,41]
(c) Number of ill-health states considered: one ill-health state[37–39,41] can be considered or more than one ill-health state[36,40,42] can be considered.

(d) Single or mix of health states: respondents could be invited to imagine being in only one health state in a year or experiencing several different health states in a year (all studies to date have used single health states).

(e) Time period considered: a limited time period can be considered[37-41] (for instance 5 years), or a scenario can describe remaining life.[36,42]

Open-ended questions must in addition consider whether respondents are asked about: the *timing* of a given change in health; or the *magnitude* to be experienced at a certain point of time; or possibly the health-related *quality of life* to be experienced. Studies to date have asked individuals to specify the magnitude of the health benefit to be enjoyed at a particular point in the future (either in terms of lives saved[31-34] or duration of health state[37-39]). No study has asked individuals to specify timing or quality.

With respect to closed-ended questions, an additional issue would be which method to use: dichotomous choice; dichotomous choice with follow-up; conjoint analysis, etc. The studies to date involve choosing between two options.[26-30]

There are a number of criteria which are relevant when making these choices: (i) how difficult the questions are to answer; (ii) degree of realism; (iii) possibility of computation of discount factor; and (iv) degree of influence of factors other than time preference on response. The first two are clearly relevant because of the impact that they might have on response rates and on the meaningfulness of responses. Other things equal the more straightforward the computation of implied discount factors the better. Similarly, methods which are less likely to be influenced by factors other than time preferences are to be preferred.

Appendix 1 shows how the various options perform with respect to these four criteria. There appears to be a trade-off between realism and how easy it is to answer, and between accuracy and how easy it is to answer. The specific approach adopted to elicit time preferences will have implications for the sample size required, the estimation methods to be used, and the methods of data collection employed. The determination of the specific approaches to be adopted is clearly a matter of judgement. Most of the decisions made were in line with those generally adopted in the literature. Thus comparisons were between points in time rather than profiles; departures from full health rather than from ill health were considered; choices involved a single ill-health state; and a limited period of time. In the open-ended questions individuals were asked to choose durations of ill-health.

Health State

The health state selected (which is used in both the open-ended and closed-ended approach) is based on the Euroqol descriptive system which has five dimensions: mobility; self-care; usual activities; pain/discomfort; and anxiety/depression. Each dimension has three severity levels. Individual's inter-temporal preferences are expected to differ according to the severity of the selected health state. Individuals might have a tendency to minimise duration for very serious health states, and to maximise delay for very minor health states. The aim is to select a health state that is not too severe but is generally regarded as serious enough. The following health state is selected: no problems in walking about; no problems with self-care; some problems with performing my usual activities; moderate pain or discomfort and not anxious or depressed. The tariff for this Euroqol state (11221) is 0.773 assuming a 1-month duration.[46] Individuals were asked to rate the health state using a visual–analogue scale. This gives some insight into how serious they regard the chosen health state. It permits some limited testing of the hypothesised relationship between inter-temporal preferences and perceived severity of the health state.

In the case of own health, individuals are asked to imagine being ill as described by the Euroqol health state. The case of others' health is more complicated. If respondents are asked to imagine a person of the same age and gender as themselves there is a danger that they might answer the questions as if they concerned their own health. This could be a problem even when nothing is specified about the individual. In order to reduce the likelihood of this happening the question is formulated in terms of a group of middle-aged patients rather than in terms of an individual patient. Their approximate age was stated because time preference is expected to be a function of age.

Open-Ended Method

Each open-ended question asks the respondent to imagine being ill at a point in the future, and offers the opportunity for this spell of ill health to be delayed (as a result of treatment). Individuals have to identify a maximum number of days of future ill health at which it would still be worthwhile receiving this treatment (see Appendix 2 for an example).

Investigation of different discounting models requires a relatively wide range of delays and several observations per respondent. In this study six observations are obtained from each individual. Two different years are chosen for the initial point at which ill health will be experienced if treatment is not received. Having more than two starting points might make the questions too difficult to answer, whereas having a common starting point for all six questions might result in respondents getting bored.

The periods of delay chosen range from 2 to 13 years from the starting point. The range of delays were selected on the pragmatic grounds that if the delay was too short, factors other than time preference would have a major influence on the responses, and if it was too long, some respondents might have difficulties imagining it (particularly older respondents). Each subject is asked six questions: three with a starting point 2 years in the future; and three with a starting point 3 years in the future. Each questionnaire contains three different delays for each starting point: a short-term delay (2–5 years); a medium-term delay (6–9 years); and a long-term delay (10–13 years). Also the difference between the short- and medium-term delay and between the medium- and long-term delay is not the same in any questionnaire (for each starting point). Table 2 shows four different versions of the questionnaire (A, B, C, and D) which have these properties. The purpose of this somewhat complex design is to collect data for a wide range of delays, and to ensure that the questions do not appear to conform to any pattern in case respondents think that they are expected to respond in a certain way.

Derivation of implied discount rates is straightforward with such data. The individual chooses a duration of ill-health x such that if it were experienced y years in the future it would be equivalent to 20 days experienced 2 years in the future. Letting $b = 1/(1 + r)$ the respondent's choice implies that $20b^2 = xb^{y-2}$ and

$$r = \left(\frac{x}{20}\right)^{\frac{1}{y-2}} - 1 \qquad (1)$$

Table 2   *The four versions of the questionnaire (A–D)*

| Starting point | Years before delayed ill health | | | |
	A	B	C	D
2 years	2	3	4	5
2 years	7	9	6	8
2 years	10	11	12	13
3 years	3	5	2	4
3 years	6	7	8	9
3 years	10	11	12	13

Closed-Ended Method: Discrete Choice Modelling

The basic underlying idea is that individuals' time preferences are revealed by how much longer they are willing to be ill for in exchange for a delay in the onset of that ill-health. In order to establish the relative importance of duration of a selected ill-health state and the relative importance of the year in which the spell of ill-health occurs, these two attributes are included. The Euroqol health state 11221 used in the open-ended study was also used in the discrete choice modelling.

The choice of attribute levels (for duration of ill-health and year in which the ill-health occurs) is to some extent arbitrary. It is important that the options are plausible and that they are informative, in the sense that it is not always obvious which choice will be made. The levels chosen for the year in which the spell of ill-health occurs are: 2, 7 and 15 years in the future. The levels chosen for the duration of the health state are: 20, 24, 26, 33 and 38 days.

These attributes and levels give rise to 15 possible scenarios ($3^1 \times 5^1$). A discrete choice method is used where individuals are asked to choose between pairs of scenarios. Each pairwise comparison implies a particular discount rate. Two sets of eight pairwise choices are selected based on the following criteria: (i) inclusion of all 15 scenarios; (ii) a wide range of implied discount rates; and (iii) one pairwise comparison representing a negative discount rate. Table 3 shows the selected pairwise comparisons.

The design of the questionnaire has to place the pairwise choices in a realistic context, and has to minimise the number and the effect of possible biases. Generally, individuals themselves cannot delay their ill-health. In order to make it as realistic as possible the respondent is asked to imagine that s/he will be ill and that two alternative treatments are available. The effects of the alternative treatments vary with regard to when the illness occurs and how long it lasts. They are then asked to indicate which treatment they prefer. (See Appendix 3 for an example.)

A relationship must be specified between the attributes and utility. The difference in utility between option B and A can be expressed as:

$$\Delta U = \beta_3 Days_B + \beta_4 Year_B - \beta_1 Days_A - \beta_2 Year_A + \varepsilon_3 \qquad (2)$$

where U = utility or preference score; $Days$ = the number of days in the selected health state; $Year$ = the year in which the spell of ill-health occurs; ε = random error term.

Table 3 *Selected pairwise comparisons*

Choices	Year option A	Days option A	Year option B	Days option B	Discount rate
Version 1					
1	7	33	2	26	0.05
2	2	33	15	38	0.01
3	2	20	7	38	0.14
4	15	38	7	20	0.08
5	2	38	7	33	−0.03
6	7	20	15	26	0.03
7	7	33	2	20	0.11
8	7	20	15	24	0.02
Version 2					
1	15	38	7	24	0.06
2	2	33	15	38	0.01
3	7	38	2	20	0.14
4	7	20	15	38	0.08
5	15	20	7	24	−0.02
6	2	26	15	33	0.03
7	2	20	7	33	0.11
8	7	26	2	24	0.02

The ratio of the coefficients of *Days* and *Year* represent the marginal rate of substitution between duration and year, in other words how much longer individuals are willing to be ill for a delay in the onset of that ill-health. The ratios β_2/β_1 and β_4/β_3 can be used to identify (year, duration) pairs between which the individual would be indifferent. From this the implied discount rate can be estimated.

$$r = \frac{\beta_2}{\beta_1 Days_n} \text{ or } r = \frac{\beta_4}{\beta_3 Days_n} \quad (3)$$

The β coefficients are estimated using a random effects ordered probit model.[47] This technique is preferred to ordinary least squares because of the ordinal nature of the dependent variable (prefer A, no preference, prefer B) and because multiple observations are obtained from each individual.

General Questions

Individuals are also asked to indicate how they perceive the Euroqol health state 11221 on a visual–analogue scale (ranging from worst to best imaginable health). The perception of the ill-health state might have an effect on inter-temporal preferences for that health state. Questions about year of birth, gender, perception of current long-term health, how many cigarettes per day they smoke, and education are also included in the questionnaire.

The Four Questionnaires

The different type of questions that are required with respect to both own and others' health are: six open-ended questions (four versions); and eight discrete choices (two versions). In order to avoid overburdening respondents there are four different types of questionnaires:

1 Six open-ended questions with respect to *own* health;
2 Six open-ended questions with respect to *others'* health;
3 Eight discrete choices with respect to *own* health;
4 Eight discrete choices with respect to *others'* health.

The comparisons that are made using these four distinct questionnaires are summarised in Figure 1.

Meeting the Four Objectives

Derivation of discount rates

Individual implied discount rates are derived from the open-ended questions assuming the traditional discounted utility model. Six open-ended questions are asked, which provides six discount rates for each individual. Median and mean discount rates are estimated. These discount rates are also regressed on the duration of the delay and characteristics of the individual

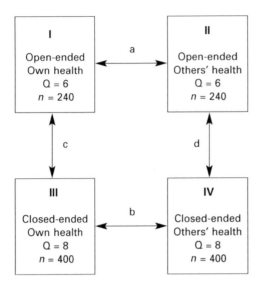

Figure 1   *The four questionnaires.*

(age, gender, health, education, smoking status). Average discount rates for the whole sample are estimated from the closed-ended questions. Depending on the model it might be possible to estimate average discount rates for specific groups (for example, age–gender groups).

Comparison of inter-temporal preferences for own and others' health

The questions with respect to own and others' health are in separate questionnaires (sent to different subsamples). The inter-temporal preferences for own versus others' health are therefore compared on a group basis [using both closed-ended and open-ended questions (comparisons *a* and *b* in Figure 1)]. If the distribution of discount factors is normal, an independent sample *t*-test can be used to test whether there is a statistically significant difference in the mean discount factors between the groups. If the distribution is non-normal, a non-parametric two-sample median test is used to determine whether the difference in the median discount factor of the groups is statistically significant.

Comparison of closed-ended and open-ended approach

The open-ended questions and the discrete choices are in separate questionnaires. The discount factors estimated from these approaches are compared on a group basis (comparisons *c* and *d* in Figure 1).

Investigation of different models of time preferences

Testing the hypothesis of constant timing aversion If individuals' preferences are constant timing averse, the implied discount rate *r* should not be a function of the period of delay of the benefit or loss. The implied discount rates are regressed on period of delay, and if the estimated coefficient for delay is statistically significantly the hypothesis of constant timing aversion is rejected and the hypothesis of decreasing timing aversion is supported.

Testing the hypothesis of decreasing timing aversion Particular models of proportional and hyperbolic discounting are selected. Since six observations per respondent are too few to estimate a particular proportional and hyperbolic functional form for each individual, age gender groups are used instead. The goodness of fit of the selected proportional and hyperbolic models are assessed and compared to that of the constant discounting model.

DATA

Data were collected in six urban and rural areas in Scotland, England and Wales (Edinburgh, Caithness, Manchester, Norfolk, Cardiff, and Pembrokeshire). In previous studies[32,33] it was found that higher socio-economic status areas had a higher response rate, so wards were selected with a high percentage home ownership (using 1991 Census data). The sample is therefore not representative for the UK population, but representativeness is not of primary importance since the aim of the study is to explore the nature of individuals' time preferences and not to identify the mean or median population discount rates. For these wards, 5120 names were randomly selected from the electoral register. In total, 1162 questionnaires were received, including 54 questionnaires without the time preference questions being attempted. Forty-three questionnaires were returned by the Post Office for a variety of reasons. Table 4 shows the response rate by questionnaire and area. The questionnaires returned without the time preference questions being attempted are not counted as a response. The overall response rate and the response rate for each of the four questionnaires is lower than the expected 25%. The response rates for the open-ended questionnaires are lower than for the closed-ended questionnaires. This is perhaps not surprising, since the open-ended questions are harder to answer. The response rates vary by area.

Table 4 *Response rate by questionnaire and area*

	I	II	III	IV
Caithness	0.152	0.158	0.268	0.219
Edinburgh	0.220	0.210	0.286	0.331
Norfolk	0.146	0.169	0.275	0.273
Manchester	0.157	0.131	0.231	0.190
Pembrokeshire	0.176	0.144	0.189	0.188
Cardiff	0.189	0.169	0.269	0.268
Overall	0.173	0.163	0.252	0.244
Overall (I–IV)		0.218		

PRELIMINARY RESULTS

Because of the limitations of space it is only possible to report a subset of the results of the analyses undertaken as part of the TEMPUS project. First, the sample is described and the age–gender structure of the sample is compared to that of the population. Then results regarding the four objectives are presented, but only for the overall sample and not on a subgroup basis.

Table 5 shows some descriptive statistics for the overall sample. There are slightly more females in the sample. Most respondents describe their current long-term health as good and do not smoke. A high percentage of respondents have either a professional or technical qualification or

Table 5 *Descriptive statistics*

		n	%
Gender	Male	516	46.6
	Female	589	53.2
	Missing value	3	0.3
Health	Good	803	72.5
	Fair	250	22.6
	Poor	53	4.8
	Missing value	2	0.2
Smoke	None	946	85.4
	1–5 cigarettes	39	3.5
	6+ cigarettes	121	10.9
	Missing value	2	0.2
Education	Secondary school	328	29.6
	Other professional or technical qualification	442	39.9
	University degree	321	29.0
	Missing value	17	1.5

		Mean	Range
Age		49.9	17–95
	Missing value	6	
Health state		54.6	0–100
	Missing value	124	

a university degree. The average age of the sample is 49.9 years, with a minimum of 17 and a maximum of 95. The ill-health state was valued at 54.6 on the visual–analogue scale.

Table 6 shows how the sample compares with the population in terms of age, gender and education. The age–gender structure of the sample seems fairly representative for the population. However, the younger age group (<30 years) tends to be under-represented. A higher percentage of respondents have a university degree compared to the population.

Derivation of Discount Rates

Table 7 shows the median discount rates (*r*). The median discount rates for the open-ended questions are 0.054 and 0.060. The median discount rate estimated from the discrete choice modelling ranges from 0.031 to 0.039 depending on the delay of the ill-health.

Comparison of Inter-Temporal Preferences for Own and Others' Health

The implied discount rates for own health appear to be very similar to those for others' health. This is the case for both the open-ended and the closed-ended approach. The median is only 0.006 higher in the case of the open-ended questions and 0.000/0.004 in the case of the discrete choice modelling.

Comparison of Closed-Ended and Open-Ended Approach

The median discount rate is higher when using the open-ended approach. The implied median discount rate estimated from the open-ended questions is about 0.021 higher in the case of own health, and about 0.025 higher in the case of others' health.

Investigation of Different Models of Time Preferences

The coefficient of delay in regressions using the open-ended data are statistically significant -0.009 ($t = 4.83$) for own health and -0.006 ($t = 3.69$) for others' health. In other words, as delay increases by 5 years the discount rate falls by 4.5% in the case of own health. The hypothesis of the constant discounting model can therefore be rejected. The next step is to

Table 6　Age, gender and education of sample and population

	Caithness		Edinburgh		Norfolk	
	% sample	Census	% sample	Census	% sample	Census
Age (years)						
<30	13.6	23.6	9.6	20.8	11.8	20.9
30–44	28.4	25.9	31.3	25.0	24.1	27.8
45–64	42.6	30.6	32.2	31.0	43.6	31.6
>64	14.8	19.9	26.5	23.2	20.0	19.8
Gender						
Male	44.3	48.6	49.6	46.2	41.0	49.4
Female	55.7	51.4	50.0	53.8	58.5	50.6
Education						
University	17.6	5.8	27.4	10.4	21.5	7.2
	Manchester		Cardiff		Pembrokeshire	
Age (years)						
<30	28.7	28.9	14.6	17.8	13.2	20.3
30–44	26.8	27.4	22.1	24.4	25.2	25.3
45–64	20.4	24.0	30.7	30.5	37.7	31.4
>64	23.6	19.7	32.2	27.3	23.2	23.0
Gender						
Male	45.2	47.3	47.2	46.1	52.3	48.6
Female	54.8	52.7	52.3	53.9	47.7	51.4
Education						
University	49.0	16.9	34.7	16.6	25.8	7.4

Table 7　Estimated median implied discount rates

	Own health Median r	Others' health Median r
Open-ended questions	0.054	0.060
Discrete choice modelling	0.031–0.035	0.031–0.039

investigate functional forms for alternative discounting models, but this is not reported in this chapter.[48]

CONCLUSIONS

This chapter has reviewed the stated preference approach to the elicitation of inter-temporal preferences for health events. Several important research issues which remain to be addressed were identified. Three issues, in particular, were addressed by the TEMPUS project. Firstly, whether individual inter-temporal preferences with respect to own health differ from those with respect to the health of others. Secondly, the impact of different methods of eliciting preferences on apparent inter-temporal preferences. Thirdly, whether or not individuals value future health events in line with the traditional discounted utility model. The design of the

TEMPUS study and the methods used were described, after which some preliminary results were reported.

The implied discount rates elicited in this study should not be over-emphasised because of the unrepresentativeness of the study sample. In particular, the respondents were markedly better educated than the population as a whole. This is not surprising given the deliberate policy of sampling in more socio-economically advantaged areas. However, it is notable how close the estimated median rates are to the rates advocated for use in economic evaluation in a range of countries (for example, 3% in the US, 5% in Australia and Canada). Also the degree of convergence between rates for own and others' health and between the open-ended and closed-ended approach is striking.

The over-representation of more highly educated groups is of less concern when considering the three main research issues addressed by

TEMPUS. Implied discount rates with respect to own health and others' health were shown to be similar. An open-ended method elicited higher discount rates than a closed-ended method. Finally, some preliminary evidence for decreasing timing aversion was presented, specifically that implied discount rates are a function of the period of delay.

There are limitations inherent in the stated preference approach – specifically there are concerns over the validity of responses compared to values derived from observing behaviour. However, it is difficult to observe inter-temporal choices in a healthcare context and then to control for the large number of potential influences. The use of postal questionnaires was driven largely by the desire to obtain reasonably large sample sizes. Such an approach offers less opportunity to establish whether or not the respondent understands the question; moreover, the questions are pre-determined and do not give an opportunity for the questions to be responsive to the previous answers.

Regarding future research, the topics identified above remain relevant. A single, albeit multifaceted, project such as TEMPUS can add significantly to our understanding, but cannot by itself resolve the outstanding research issues. Thus the three themes addressed in this paper: the influence on estimates of implied discount rates of different methods of eliciting preferences; the nature of the inter-temporal choice; and the underlying model of time preferences, all require further investigation. Further issues concern the use of self-completed questionnaires versus interviews (face-to-face and telephonic), and the presence and impact of framing effects. Also, there is considerable scope for the investigation of the nature and extent of differences between time preferences for saving lives and those for non-fatal changes in health; and whether time preferences are to some extent health state-specific. The empirical investigation of alternative models of time preference, in particular, models which allow for decreasing timing aversion, such as proportional and hyperbolic discounting models, is at an early stage in the economics literature.

ACKNOWLEDGEMENTS

HERU is funded by the Chief Scientist Office of the Scottish Executive Health Department (SEHD). The views expressed in this paper are those of the authors and not SEHD. This study received financial support from the NHS R&D Health Technology Assessment Programme (project 94/35/1).

REFERENCES

1. Hausman JA. Individual discount rates and the purchase and utilisation of energy-using durables. *Bell J. Economics* 1979; **10**: 33–54.
2. Gately D. Individual discount rates and the purchase and utilisation of energy-using durables: comment. *Bell J. Economics* 1980; **11**: 373–4.
3. Dreyfus MK, Viscusi WK. Rates of time preference and consumer valuations of automobile safety and fuel efficiency. *J. Law Economics* 1995; **38**: 79–105.
4. Kooreman P. Individual discounting, energy conservation, and household demand for lighting. *Resource and Energy Economics* 1996; **18**: 103–14.
5. Lang K, Ruud PA. Returns to schooling, implicit discount rates and black-white wage differentials. *Rev. Economics Statist.* 1986; **69**: 41–7.
6. Lawrance EC. Poverty and the rate of time preference: evidence from panel data. *J. Political Economy* 1991; **99**: 54–77.
7. Viscusi WK, Moore MJ. Rates of time preference and valuations of the duration of life. *J. Public Economics* 1989; **38**: 297–317.
8. Moore MJ, Viscusi WK. The quantity-adjusted value of life. *Economic Inquiry* 1988; **26**: 369–88.
9. Moore MJ, Viscusi WK. Discounting environmental health risks: new evidence and policy implications. *J. Environ. Economics Management* 1990; **18**: S51–S62.
10. Thaler R. Some empirical evidence on dynamic inconsistencies. *Economics Lett.* 1981; **8**: 201–7.
11. Fuchs VR. Time preference and health: an exploratory study. In: Fuchs VR (ed.). *Economic Aspects of Health.* Chicago: The University of Chicago Press, 1982.
12. Benzion U, Rapoport A, Yagil J. Discount rates inferred from decisions: an experimental study. *Management Science* 1989; **35**: 270–84.
13. Myerson J, Green L. Discounting of delayed rewards: models of individual choice. *J. Exp. Anal. Behav.* 1995; **64**: 263–76.
14. Houston DA. Implicit discount rates and the purchase of untried, energy-saving durable goods. *J. Consumer Res.* 1983; **10**: 236–46.
15. Sultan F, Winer RS. Time preferences for products and attributes and the adoption of technology-driven consumer durable innovations. *J. Economic Psychol.* 1993; **14**: 587–613.
16. Loewenstein GF, Prelec D. Anomalies in inter-temporal choice: evidence and an interpretation. *Q. J. Economics* 1992; **107**: 573–97.
17. Parsonage M, Neuberger H. Discounting and health benefits. *Health Economics* 1992; **1**: 71–6.

18. Cairns JA. Discounting and health benefits: another perspective. *Health Economics* 1992; **1**: 76–9.

19. Department of Health. *Policy Appraisal and Health*. London: HMSO, 1995.

20. Torrance GW, Blaker D, Detsky A, Kennedy W, Schubert F, Menon D, Tugwell P, Konchak R, Hubbard E, Firestone T. Canadian guidelines for economic evaluation of pharmaceuticals. *PharmacoEconomics* 1996; **9**: 535–59.

21. Gold MR, Siegel JE, Russell LB, Weinstein MC. *Cost-effectiveness in health and medicine*. Oxford: Oxford University Press, 1996.

22. Gafni A, Torrance GW. Risk attitude and time preference in health. *Management Science* 1984; **30**: 440–51.

23. Gafni A. Time in health: can we measure individuals' pure time preferences? *Medical Decision Making* 1995; **15**: 31–7.

24. Loewenstein GF, Prelec D. Preferences for sequences of outcomes. *Psychol. Rev.* 1993; **100**: 91–108.

25. Krahn M, Gafni A. Discounting in the economic evaluation of health care interventions. *Medical Care* 1993; **31**: 403–18.

26. Horowitz JK, Carson RT. Discounting statistical lives. *J. Risk Uncertainty* 1990; **3**: 403–13.

27. Cropper ML, Aydede SK, Portney PR. Discounting human lives. *Am. J. Agric. Economics* 1991; **73**: 1410–15.

28. Cropper ML, Aydede SK, Portney PR. Rates of time preference for saving lives. *Am. Economic Rev.* 1993; **82**: 469–72.

29. Cropper ML, Aydede SK, Portney PR. Preferences for life saving programs: how the public discount time and age. *J. Risk Uncertainty* 1994; **8**: 243–65.

30. Johannesson M, Johansson P-O. The discounting of lives saved in future generations – some empirical results. *Health Economics* 1996; **5**: 329–32.

31. Olsen JA. Time preferences for health gains: an empirical investigation. *Health Economics* 1993; **2**: 257–65.

32. Cairns JA. Valuing future benefits. *Health Economics* 1994; **3**: 221–9.

33. Cairns JA, van der Pol M. Saving future lives: a comparison of three discounting models. *Health Economics*, 1997; **6**: 341–50.

34. Cairns JA, van der Pol M. Constant and decreasing timing aversion for saving lives. *Soc. Sci. Med.* 1997; **45**: 1653–9.

35. Enemark U, Lyttkens CH, Tröeng T, Weibull H, Ranstam J. Time preferences of vascular surgeons. *Medical Decision Making* 1998; **18**: 168–77.

36. Lipscomb J. The preference for health in cost-effectiveness analysis. *Medical Care*, 1989; **27**: S233–S253.

37. Cairns JA. Health, wealth and time preference. *Project Appraisal*, 1992; **7**: 31–40.

38. Chapman GB, Elstein AS. Valuing the future: temporal discounting of health and money. *Medical Decision Making* 1995; **15**: 373–86.

39. Chapman GB. Temporal discounting and utility for health and money. *J. Exp. Psychol. [Learn., Mem. Cogn.]* 1996; **22**: 771–91.

40. Redelmeier DA, Heller DM. Time preference in medical decision making and cost effectiveness analysis. *Medical Decision Making* 1993; **13**: 212–17.

41. MacKeigan LD, Larson LN, Draugalis JR, Bootman JL, Burns LR. Preferences for health gains versus health losses. *PharmacoEconomics* 1993; **3**: 374–86.

42. Dolan P, Gudex C. Time preference, duration and health state valuations. *Health Economics* 1995; **4**: 289–99.

43. Loewenstein G. Anticipation and the valuation of delayed consumption. *Economic J.* 1987; **97**: 666–84.

44. Harvey, CM. The reasonableness of non-constant discounting. *J. Public Economics* 1994; **53**: 31–51.

45. Ainslie, G. Derivation of rational economic behaviour from hyperbolic discount rates. *Am. Economic Rev.* 1991; **81**: 334–40.

46. Dolan P. Modelling valuations for health states: the effect of duration. *Health Policy* 1996; **38**: 189–203.

47. McKelvey R., Zaviona W. Statistical Model for the Analysis of Ordinal Level Dependent Variables. *J. Math. Sociol.* 1975; **4**: 103–20.

48. van der Pol M, Cairns JA. The discounted utility model versus a hyperbolic discounting model. Paper presented at the Health Economists' Study Group Meeting, University of Birmingham 6–8th January, 1999.

Appendix 1 *Options and criteria*

	Degree of difficulty to answer	Degree of realism	Computation of discount factor	Other factors than time preference influence response
Number of points in time Two points Profile	Having to consider only two points in time is easier.	A profile is more realistic whereby ill-health is spread over a couple of years instead of being concentrated in one particular year.	Discount factors are more easily computed when only two points in time are considered. Discount factors can, in some case, not be computed from profiles.	
Timing versus quantity Timing Quantity	It is easier to choose when something takes place than to choose how much health or ill-health has to be consumed at a certain time.	Choosing how ill or how healthy is less realistic. Timing is more realistic (treatments can for instance postpone a certain disease taking place)	The choice of timing versus quantity does not have an influence on how difficult or whether a discount factor can be calculated	With giving a choice of timing it is more likely that other factors will influence the response. Certainly so in the short term (respondents might have things planned) but also in the long run.
Basic health state Full-health Ill-health	Since majority will be healthy it is easier to imagine full-health.	Majority of people will be healthy so full health as basic health state appears more realistic; on the other hand choosing when or how much to be ill is less realistic	Choice of basic health state does not have an influence on how to compute the discount factor.	People are averse to ill-health. When having to choose ill-health other factors might influence the response such as fear of being ill.
Number of ill-health states One ill-health state More than one	Considering two or more ill-health states will make the question more complex.	It is more realistic to be in more than one ill-health state when you have a spell of ill-health (for instance going from being ill to being less severely ill to healthy)	If two or more ill-health states are used, these have to be valued first before a discount factor can be computed.	
Single or mix of health states in a year Single health state Mix of health states	Being in a single health state is easier because only one health state has to be considered for each year	Being in one single health state during a whole year is less realistic unless it is a chronic condition.	It is probably easier to compute a discount factor when only one health state is used in a year.	
Time period considered Limited time period Remaining life	Respondents might have difficulty imagining remaining life if they have to consider a long time period which makes it more difficult.	Especially for older respondents a long remaining life scenario is less realistic	The choice between a limited period and remaining life does not influence whether a discount factor can be calculated but a limited period is less complex.	Age has more of an influence on the responses when considering remaining life. Older respondents might not be able or willing to consider a long remaining life.

Appendix 2   *Example of open-ended question*

Imagine the following ill-health: You have some problems with performing your usual activities (e.g. work, study, housework, family or leisure activities) and you have moderate pain or discomfort. You have no problems in walking about, nor with washing and dressing yourself, and you are not anxious or depressed.

Imagine that you will be ill, as described above, starting **2** years from now for **20** days. There is a minor one-off treatment available that will postpone this spell of ill-health to a point further in the future. For instance, the treatment could have the following effects: your period of ill-health would start **9** years from now instead of **2** years from now; and you would then be ill for **30** days instead of **20** days.

You might think this treatment is a good idea: the advantage of postponing the ill-health outweighs the disadvantage of being ill for a longer period. Or you might think the treatment is not worthwhile: you do value the postponement but the advantage of this is outweighed by the disadvantage of being ill for a longer period; or you might simply prefer to be ill 2 years from now instead of 9 years from now. Imagine again that you will be ill starting **2** years from now for **20** days, and that treatment is again available that will postpone this spell of ill-health.

We will now ask you to state the maximum number of days of ill-health that would still make the treatment worthwhile for you. For example, say that the treatment can postpone the period of ill-health to **6** years in the future. If the number of days of ill-health in that year would be zero everyone would probably choose the treatment. As the number of days of ill-health in that year increases individuals would at some point no longer prefer to be treated. What we are interested in is the *maximum number* of days of ill-health at which you would still choose to be treated.

If the ill-health would then start 4 years from now, what is the maximum number of days of ill-health that would still make the treatment worthwhile?

Appendix 3   *Example of closed-ended question*

Imagine the following ill-health:

> You have some problems with performing your usual activities (e.g. work, study, housework, family or leisure activities) and you have moderate pain or discomfort. You have no problems in walking about, nor with washing and dressing yourself and you are not anxious or depressed.

Imagine that you will be ill (as described in the box above). There are two *alternative* treatments (A and B) available. The effects of the alternative treatments vary with regard to *when* the illness will occur and *how long* you will be ill for (you cannot be cured completely). Below is an example of how they can vary. With treatment A you will be ill starting *2* years from now for *20* days, and with treatment B you will be ill starting *6* years from now for *48* days. Assuming everything else about the treatments is the same (i.e. severity of the treatment, side-effects, costs), which treatment would you prefer?

- Example

	When you are ill	How long for	*Which treatment would you prefer?*
Treatment A	in 2 years time	for 20 days	
Treatment B	in 6 years time	for 48 days	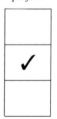
		No preference	

15

The Conduct and Design of Questionnaire Surveys in Healthcare Research

ELAINE McCOLL, ANN JACOBY, LOIS THOMAS,
JENNIFER SOUTTER, CLAIRE BAMFORD,
NICK STEEN, ROGER THOMAS, EMMA HARVEY,
ANDREW GARRATT and JOHN BOND

SUMMARY

Our aim in carrying out this literature review was to provide guidelines for best practice in the design and conduct of questionnaire surveys, especially on health-related topics. Identifying best practice involved a review of expert opinion as expressed in classic texts on survey methods and in theoretical papers on respondent behaviour, as well as synthesising empirical evidence from experiments on questionnaire design and administration. The primary objective in survey research is the collection of valid and reliable data from as many of the targeted individuals, and as representative a sample, as possible. However, limited resources often dictate a trade-off between the ideal and the optimal. No single mode of questionnaire administration is universally superior. Similarly, in wording and ordering questions and response categories, designing the physical appearance of the questionnaire, and administering the survey, the particular characteristics, needs and motivations of the target audience should be taken into account.

from patients and healthcare professionals. The aim is to gather valid and reliable data from a representative sample of respondents. These data must be capable of one or more of: discriminating between groups and individuals at a given point in time; detecting change over time; and predicting future behaviour or needs.

Good questionnaire design and careful survey administration can reduce errors and bias in data collection. However, those carrying out surveys typically rely on tradition and 'conventional wisdom', rather than on sound theories of respondent behaviour and evidence from empirical studies. A number of the classic texts on questionnaire development, commonly used by survey researchers, are now quite dated.[1–4] Moreover, many of these texts draw primarily on the accumulated experience and opinions of the expert authors, despite the caution from Bradburn and colleagues[5] that, in their experiments with questionnaire wording and administration, there were 'just enough surprises to warn us that we should not rely entirely on our own experience but should check things out empirically whenever possible'.

WHY THIS REVIEW WAS NEEDED

Questionnaire surveys are frequently the method of choice for gathering primary quantitative data

The Readership for this Review

This review of best practice in questionnaire design and survey administration is aimed primarily at researchers and practitioners using questionnaires in the evaluation of health technologies, that is '. . . all the methods used by health professionals to promote health, to prevent and treat disease, and to improve rehabilitation and long-term care'.[6] We recognise that questionnaires are also widely used in other fields of healthcare research and in research on topics unrelated to health. Our findings and recommendations will be of general interest to all researchers for whom questionnaire surveys are the chosen method of data collection. Nonetheless, in synthesising the findings and making recommendations, we distinguished between evidence from studies on health-related topics and those on other subjects. We did this because there is empirical evidence that patterns of response to surveys on topics perceived to be important and relevant to respondents (such as health) are significantly different from those for surveys of general populations, or on topics perceived as less personally relevant.[7,8] There are also likely to be ethical concerns particular to health surveys.

METHODS OF THE REVIEW

Objectives

Our principal objectives in carrying out this literature review were:

1   To identify current 'best practice' (informed by expert opinion, sound theory and empirical evidence from well-designed studies) with respect to the design and conduct of questionnaire surveys.
2   To identify, analyse and synthesise evidence of methods to improve the quality of survey data (particularly response rates, validity and reliability) by attention to aspects of questionnaire design and survey conduct. ['Validity' refers to whether a data collection instrument truly measures what it purports to measure. 'Reliability' refers to whether 'the measure is consistent and minimises random error'.[9]]
3   To identify practical issues (for example, ethical concerns, resource implications) surrounding the design and administration of questionnaires.
4   To evaluate the extent to which approaches from other disciplines are likely to be transferable to a health-specific context.
5   To identify gaps in current knowledge and to recommend topics for further research.

Defining the Scope of the Review

An operational definition of 'questionnaire'

We defined 'questionnaire' as 'a structured schedule used to elicit predominantly quantitative information, by means of direct questions, from respondents, either by self-completion or via interview'. We chose this deliberately broad definition because we recognised that interviewer administration may be the most appropriate mode of data collection in certain circumstances. However, we also accepted that, because of resource constraints, self-completion questionnaires are likely to be the method of choice in many health surveys. Our review therefore commenced with an examination of the relative strengths and weaknesses of interviewer administration and self-report. Throughout the review, in synthesising and interpreting evidence from primary studies and from previous reviews of the literature, we distinguished between different modes of administration and sought to highlight the extent to which findings from one mode can be extrapolated to another.

Focus of the review

We decided to focus on those important aspects of the survey process which we judged to be most amenable to generalisation, namely:

(a)   mode of survey administration;
(b)   question wording, response format, and question sequencing;
(c)   questionnaire appearance; and
(d)   aspects of survey administration intended to enhance response rates and reduce threats of bias, with particular emphasis on postal surveys.

For guidance on aspects of survey research beyond the scope of this review, such as definition of data requirements, sampling, data coding and analysis, we refer readers to the many comprehensive texts available.[1,9–14]

Gathering the Evidence

Sources of evidence

We took as the starting point for our review 'expert opinion' as expressed in key texts on survey methods.[1,3–5,11,12,15] We then looked for support for the recommendations made by these experts, either from theories of respondent behaviour or in the form of empirical evidence (in particular from well-designed experimental studies in which some aspect of questionnaire design or administration was manipulated).

Resource constraints precluded an exhaustive systematic review of all the published literature on the subject of survey methodology. We therefore imposed arbitrary cut-off dates of 1975–96, and carried out a keyword search of two databases (Medline and PsycLit), using the search terms (MeSH headings and Thesaurus terms respectively) 'surveys', 'questionnaires' and 'interviews'; we restricted our search to journal articles in English. Medline was chosen because of its health-related focus, whilst PsycLit was selected because we were aware that many innovative and experimental studies on questionnaire design and administration, as well as papers on theories of respondent behaviour, are published in the market research, social research and psychological journals indexed on that database.

In abstracting and synthesising evidence from primary research, we focused principally on randomised controlled trials (RCTs) and other quasi-experimental designs which met specified methodological criteria, in particular regarding group size, method of allocation to groups and baseline comparability. However, we also drew on the findings from previous literature reviews of methods of questionnaire design and administration, especially where there was a lack of evidence from primary empirical studies.

Framework for presentation and appraisal of evidence

The primary objective in survey research is the collection of valid and reliable data from as many of the targeted individuals, and as representative a sample, as possible. At each stage in the survey process, threats to validity arise and there is the potential for bias; Sackett,[16] following Murphy,[17] defines bias as 'any process at any stage of inference which tends to produce results or conclusions that differ systematically from the truth'. Similarly, at each stage in the process, targeted individuals may decide not to participate in the survey[18] to the detriment of response rates.

In synthesising and interpreting the evidence yielded by primary empirical studies, we therefore looked for the effects on response rates and on the quality of the data yielded, in particular the validity of those data. However, people carrying out surveys generally have limited time, money and other resources, and operate within ethical constraints. As a result, a trade-off is often required between what is optimal in terms of data quality, and what is practicable in the face of such constraints. Therefore, in drawing conclusions from the evidence and in making recommendations for 'good practice' we also highlighted issues of timeliness, cost and other resource implications.

THE QUALITY AND DEPTH OF EVIDENCE

The electronic search described above yielded 478 papers from Medline and 4851 from PsycLit, with significant overlap in the coverage of the two databases. We initially scanned the titles and abstracts against explicit inclusion and exclusion criteria. Hard copies of 663 papers identified in this way as 'definitely' or 'possibly' relevant to our review were obtained. The full text of these papers was further reviewed against the inclusion and exclusion criteria; 230 papers were rejected at this stage. Of the remaining 433 papers, 143 were reports of high-grade primary empirical studies (high-quality RCTs or quasi-experimental studies on some aspect of questionnaire design or survey administration). These 143 studies, of which 56 were from surveys on health topics, provided the empirical evidence base for our review.

Although there was a wealth of evidence on some aspects of questionnaire design, other areas were less well researched. In particular, we found a lack of a theoretical basis for[19] and of empirical studies on questionnaire format and layout.

The reasons behind this lack of critical investigation are unclear. Some aspects of questionnaire design and survey administration do not lend themselves readily to experimental manipulation. In other cases, 'expert opinion'[1–5,11,12,15] may have become so enshrined in current practice as to remain unchallenged.

The majority of the empirical studies we identified, and opinions of many experts, were concerned with surveys on non-health-related topics and were often of general populations. Caution needs be exercised in generalising the findings and recommendations to health surveys.

The heterogeneity of identified studies led to considerable problems in comparing and interpreting the evidence. For instance, comparisons of response rates across studies in which the use of incentives was manipulated were hampered by lack of comparability with respect to the nature and magnitude of the incentive and to other aspects of questionnaire design and administration known to affect response rates, such as length of questionnaire and number of reminders sent[7,8] and by differences in study populations.

Few researchers exactly replicated the methods of previous studies in a new setting, to see whether findings were generalisable or whether they were context- or mode-specific; for example, whether the effects of personalisation were the same in surveys of general and special populations, or whether methods shown to stimulate response rates to self-completion questionnaires were also effective in interviewer-administered surveys.

In designing some experiments, scant attention was paid to the complexity of the survey process, in particular the way in which a number of factors interact to influence respondent behaviour.[18] Ignoring likely interactions led, in some cases, to inappropriate and unrealistic experiments (such as a highly personalised letter with an assurance of anonymity!).

In their experiments, many researchers considered only single measures of 'success', typically overall response rates. Other important indicators of the quality of the data yielded, such as item response rates or the validity of the information provided, were frequently ignored. It is possible that factors shown to be successful in bringing about high response rates have a detrimental effect on the quality of response (for instance, induce bias).

We recognised ethical barriers to applying some of the techniques shown to be effective in other sectors. For example, Hornik[20] demonstrated that deceiving respondents regarding the time required for questionnaire completion improved response rates; deliberately misleading respondents in this way may be unethical, at least in health surveys. Similarly, although the provision of incentives has been shown to be a powerful means of stimulating response, paying survey respondents is generally unacceptable in health-related research.[9]

We also identified practical barriers in applying some of the techniques recommended. For example, Dillman[3] strongly advocated that covering letters should be individually signed by hand. In a large health survey, this would usually be unfeasible. It appeared to us that some of the recommendations previously made in the literature were based purely on considerations of effectiveness, and did not take resource implications into account. For example, emphasis was placed on response rates rather than on the cost per response; few asked whether the additional costs of resource-intensive methods (for instance multiple reminders) outweighed the marginal benefits in terms of increased response. Indeed, only in a minority of identified studies did the authors consider and report resource implications.

Finally, the technologies available to survey researchers are constantly evolving and the world in which surveys are carried out is ever changing. Computer-assisted interviewing and computer-readable questionnaires are growing in popularity. At the same time, there are increasingly negative attitudes towards surveys among both the public and professionals, reflected in a downwards trend in response rates for health professionals.[21] Without doubt, recommendations made on the basis of which methods of questionnaire design and administration are effective today will need to be reviewed in the future to take account of these changes.

KEY ISSUES IN SURVEY DESIGN AND ADMINISTRATION

Expert opinion, encapsulated in key texts[1,3–5,11,12,15] has highlighted a range of key issues in questionnaire design and survey administration. The authors, drawing on their accumulated experience, in some cases backed by experimental studies, have made the observations and recommendations summarised below.

Response Rates

Surveys with a low response rate have low precision; the confidence intervals around any estimates of population parameters (for example mean age or percentage holding a particular opinion) are wide. Poor response rates are also likely to be a source of bias, since non-respondents tend to differ from respondents in important and systematic ways. The most consistent finding[8] is that respondents tend to be better educated. In interview surveys, participation rates (assuming initial contact has been made) are generally positively correlated with socio-economic status and negatively correlated with age.[22] In health surveys of general populations and specific patient groups, non-respondents tend to be older, of lower socio-economic status, from minority groups and to have poorer health status.[23] In surveys of health professionals, relatively lower response rates have been observed amongst older doctors, those with poorer qualifications and with non-university appointments.[24] Experts suggest that a response rate in excess of 70% is desirable;[25,26] by these standards, response rates to postal surveys published in the medical literature are low.[27]

The five main sources of non-response in surveys are: those unsuitable for inclusion (for example, in self-completion surveys, those who are illiterate); people who have moved from their listed address; those away from home for the duration of the survey; those not at home when an interviewer tries to make contact; and refusals.[1] The relative importance of each of

Table 1   *Means of achieving objectives in maximising response rates (After Dillman[3])*

Minimising cost of responding	Maximising rewards of responding	Establishing trust

Making questionnaire clear and concise
 attention to issues of question
   wording and sequencing
	Making questionnaire interesting to respondent
	 choice of topic
	 addition of 'interesting'
	   questions
		Establishment of benefit of participation
		 statement of how results will be
		   used to benefit respondents/others
		 promise to send results of research

Making questionnaire (appear) to be simple to complete
 attention to issues of
   questionnaire appearance
	Expression of positive regard for respondent as an individual
	 stating importance of
	   individual's contribution
	 individual salutation
	 hand-written signature
	 individually typed letter
	 stamped (not franked) mail
		Establishment of credentials of researchers
		 use of headed notepaper
		 naming of researchers

Reduction of mental/physical effort required for completion and of feelings of anxiety/inadequacy
 simple questions
 clear instructions
 sensitive handling of potentially
   embarrassing questions
	Expression of verbal appreciation
	 statement of thanks in all
	   communications
	 statement of thanks on
	   questionnaire
	 follow-up 'thank you' letter
	   or card
		Building on other exchange relationships
		 endorsement by well-regarded
		   organisation/individual

Avoidance of subordination of respondent to researcher	*Support of respondent's values* appeal to personal utility appeal to altruism/social utility	

Reduction of direct monetary costs of responding
 provision of pre-paid envelopes
   for return of postal
   questionnaires
	Incentives
	 monetary or material
	   incentive at time of response
	 provision of results of
	   research	

these sources will depend on a range of factors, including the mode of administration and the sampling frame (the list or source of population members from which the sample is drawn).

Appropriate methods for ensuring adequate response rates depend on the likely sources of non-response. The theory of social exchange[28–30] provides a useful framework for understanding respondent behaviour and addressing the threat of non-response due to refusals. This theory suggests that respondents will only participate in a survey if the anticipated rewards of doing so are at least equal to the costs of responding. It was used by Dillman[3] to construct a framework for maximising response rates (Table 1). Brown and colleagues[18] further developed this framework into a four-stage task–analysis model of respondent decision-making (Table 2). The decision to proceed to each successive step is influenced by many factors, including aspects of questionnaire design and survey administration.

Achieving a Representative Sample

Achieving a sample that is representative of the underlying population is, in part, a function of the adequacy of the sampling frame. For example, telephone surveys in which the telephone directory is used to select the sample are biased against those without phones (about 4% of households in the UK, in particular the young, those on lower incomes, minority groups and recent movers) and those who are ex-directory (about 30% of households in the UK).

The extent to which a representative sample is achieved is also a function of the mode of questionnaire administration and of techniques used to enhance response rates (for example, sample composition bias may occur if the appeal of incentives varies across sample members). In this respect, however, no mode of administration has been found to be unequivocally superior to another (Table 3).

Table 2   *Task-analysis model of respondent decision-making (After Brown et al.[18])*

Stage 1 Interest in task	Stage 2 Evaluation of task	Stage 3 Initiation and monitoring of task	Stage 4 Completion of task
Personal contact personalisation of letter personalisation of envelope class of mail	*Time and effort required* length of questionnaire size of pages supply of addressed return envelope supply of stamped return envelope	*Actual difficulty encountered* clarity of question wording clarity of instructions complexity of questions	*Provision of SAE*
Questionnaire appearance cover illustration colour of cover layout and format quality/clarity of type	*Cursory evaluation of difficulty* number of questions complexity of questions	*Sensitivity of requests* number and nature of sensitive questions	*Reminders to return*
Topic questionnaire title cover illustration content of cover letter timeliness relevance/salience		*Actual time required*	
Source credibility/trust image of sponsor credentials of individual investigator message in cover letter			
Reward for participation tangible rewards; monetary and other incentives intangible rewards; appeals to altruism, self-interest, etc.			
Persistence of source follow-up procedures			

Finally, ensuring that the target respondent, and not a relative or carer, actually completes the questionnaire may also be a problem, particularly in postal surveys.

Volume, Complexity and Nature of Data Collected

The desired volume, complexity and nature of data to be collected will vary from survey to survey. It has been asserted[11] that the largest volume of data can be collected in face-to-face interviews (since the burden of recording responses falls on the interviewer rather than the respondent). The downside is the temptation to collect more data than is strictly necessary, which wastes resources and may be unethical.

Data of greater complexity can also be gathered in face-to-face interviews, because visual aids can be used and the interviewer can more readily provide explanations and probe and prompt for additional information. However, self-completion questionnaires are generally held to be superior to telephone surveys for collecting complex data. For example, questions involving the ranking of several items, or those using multiple response categories (for instance, a seven-point scale of satisfaction) are difficult to use in telephone surveys because there is no visual stimulus; instead, the respondent must mentally retain and process the items or categories.

Table 3 *Advantages and disadvantages of modes of questionnaire administration (Adapted from De Vaus[161], after Dillman[3])*

	Face-to-face interviews	Telephone interviews	Postal questionnaires
Response rates			
General samples	Good	Good	Poor to Good
Specialised samples	Good	Good	Satisfactory to Good
Representative samples			
Avoidance of refusal bias	Good	Good	Poor
Control over who completes the questionnaire	Good	Satisfactory	Satisfactory to Good
Gaining access to the selected person	Satisfactory	Good	Good
Locating the selected person	Satisfactory	Good	Good
Ability to handle:			
Long questionnaires	Good	Satisfactory	Satisfactory
Complex questions	Good	Poor	Satisfactory
Boring questions	Good	Satisfactory	Poor
Item non-response	Good	Good	Satisfactory
Filter questions	Good	Good	Satisfactory
Question sequence control	Good	Good	Poor
Open-ended questions	Good	Good	Poor
Quality of answers			
Minimise social desirability responses	Poor	Satisfactory	Good
Ability to avoid distortion due to:			
Interviewer characteristics	Poor	Satisfactory	Good
Interviewer's opinions	Satisfactory	Satisfactory	Good
Influence of other people	Satisfactory	Good	Poor
Allows opportunities to consult	Satisfactory	Poor	Good
Avoids subversion	Poor	Satisfactory	Good
Implementing the survey			
Ease of finding suitable staff	Poor	Good	Good
Speed	Poor	Good	Satisfactory
Cost	Poor	Satisfactory	Good

Interviews facilitate the use of open-ended questions or open-ended probes, where the interviewer can record verbatim the answers given by respondents. This may generate richer and more spontaneous information than would be possible using self-completion questionnaires. Although open-ended questions can be used in self-completion questionnaires, responses are typically less detailed since respondents tend to be less expansive in writing than in speaking.

Collecting data on 'boring' topics is easier in interviewer-administered surveys; interviewers can engage subjects' attention and interest and can use their powers of persuasion to maximise participation.[31] By contrast, response rates to postal surveys on topics perceived to be unimportant or lacking in relevance are generally low.[32]

Response Bias

Response bias occurs when the answers provided by respondents are invalid – in other words, they do not reflect their true experiences

or attitudes. Response bias can arise in a number of ways. 'Social desirability' bias is particularly likely in respect of questions on sensitive topics, and occurs when respondents conceal their true behaviour or attitudes and instead give an answer that shows them in a good light, or is perceived to be socially acceptable. Related to this is 'sponsorship' bias, by which respondents' answers differ according to who is conducting the survey. 'Memory' bias occurs in questions involving recall of past events or behaviour and can include omission and telescoping (misplacing an event in time). Biases can also arise from the respondent mishearing or misunderstanding the question or accompanying instructions.

The relative threat of different types of response bias depends in part on the mode of administration. In surveys using mixed modes of administration, care is needed in interpreting findings; observed differences between respondents may be attributable to the methods of data collection, rather than to true underlying differences in experiences and attitudes. The greater anonymity afforded by a postal questionnaire, and to a lesser extent by a telephone interview, may mean that patients are more likely to report truthfully on potentially embarrassing behaviour or experiences (for example, mental health problems). Social desirability bias is more likely in interviewer-administered surveys, since respondents may wish to 'save face'. By contrast, other forms of deception can be minimised by interviews, because some responses can be verified by observation.

Questionnaire wording and design can also induce response bias, for example through question sequencing effects (where the response given to a particular question differs according to the placement of that question relative to others), and the labelling and ordering of response categories.

Other Sources of Bias

A significant disadvantage of interviewer-administered surveys is that the interviewers themselves can introduce errors both in a random and a systematic way.[11] Random errors are more likely to be due to interviewer inaccuracy, for example recording answers incorrectly or altering the wording of a question by mistake. Examples of systematic effects are: selective recording of subjects' responses; differences in the extent to which interviewers probe for a substantive response or accept 'don't know' answers; and consistent re-wording of questions. Systematic bias can occur even when there is only one interviewer, if the interviewer does not accurately record the respondent's answers, but instead is consistently selective in what he or she records. It is an even greater problem where a survey requires multiple interviewers; observed differences across respondents may be an artefact of the way in which different interviewers have posed questions or recorded answers, rather than an indication of true underlying differences between respondents. The advent of computer-assisted personal interviewing (CAPI) may prevent routine errors and omissions, but at present requires prohibitively high levels of investment for many survey researchers.

Personal characteristics of the interviewer, such as age, gender, social class, race or level of experience and training may also affect both response rates and the nature of the responses given. Similarly, the setting in which data is collected may affect responses. For example, it has been shown that responses to physical function items on a health status measure may be confounded by place of administration, with higher scores for hospital in-patients resulting

from restrictions caused by the hospital regime rather than by impaired health.[33]

Practicalities

Interviewer-administered surveys are generally held to be more expensive than postal surveys.[11,12] The additional expense derives mainly from the costs of training and paying interviewers and of their travel costs. Face-to-face interviews also generally require an initial contact (by letter, telephone or in person) to set up an appointment for the interview; multiple contacts may be needed to agree a convenient time. Although multiple contacts may also be required to achieve a telephone interview, the elimination of travel costs and time can mean that they are a low cost and speedy method of data collection.[11,34] However, costs increase with the number of attempts required to contact subjects who are not available at the first call, and with the number of long-distance calls required. Whilst the costs of all interview surveys increase significantly with geographical dispersal of sample members, postal surveys can cover scattered populations without increasing survey costs. Similarly, in 'captive audience' self-completion surveys (for example, administered to a group of patients in a waiting room), data can be collected simultaneously from a large number of respondents. Telephone interviews[31] and postal surveys allow survey researchers to access areas where safety might be compromised, such as inner cities.

Interviewer-administered surveys are generally more appropriate when a large number of open-ended questions are required. However, coding responses to such open-ended questions can be both time-consuming and costly. As a result, interviewer-administered surveys may take longer to produce results than postal surveys. Balanced against this, however, there is no need to wait for questionnaires to be returned through the post; if two rounds of reminders are used, the interval between dispatch and return of questionnaires can be as much as 12–16 weeks. In interviewer-administered surveys, the speed with which data are available for analysis can be increased by the use of computer-assisted techniques, which minimise the need for subsequent data entry and checking.

Face-to-face interviews generally require highly trained and motivated interviewers, since they must work autonomously. Less experienced interviewers may be used in telephone surveys, since stricter control and closer supervision is possible.[31] This greater control can also reduce inter-interviewer variability. Postal surveys require the fewest personnel and need minimal equipment.

Mode of Administration

Telephone interviews versus postal surveys

In three identified studies, all on health-related topics,[35–37] higher response rates were obtained for telephone surveys; in a fourth[38] (also health-related), overall response rates to the postal survey were significantly higher. In this latter study, however, rates of item non-response (question omission) were higher for postal administration. These studies demonstrated no consistent advantage of one approach over the other with respect to non-response bias, quality of response, anonymity or cost. It is, however, important to note that all the identified studies were carried out in the USA, where telephone ownership rates are higher. In the UK, telephone surveys may suffer from non-response bias against the young, poor, ethnic minorities and the domestically mobile, since these groups are most likely to be among the 4% of the population who do not have a telephone.

Face-to-face interviews versus self-completion questionnaires

We identified six relevant studies,[35,39–43] five of which were on health-related topics. Evidence from two studies[35,42] supported expert views that face-to-face interviews tend to yield higher response rates. Evidence from a single study[39] suggested that respondents may be more likely to give no answer or to say 'don't know' in an interview. However, there was no unequivocal evidence to support the view that postal surveys yield more truthful responses to sensitive questions or elicit more critical or less socially acceptable responses.

Telephone versus face-to-face interviews

Four comparative studies were identified,[44–47] three of which were on health topics. Although one non-health study[45] found telephone interviews to be quicker, there was no consistent evidence of the relative superiority of either mode in terms of overall response rates, item non-response rates or the elicitation of sensitive information.

Computer-assisted versus self-completion questionnaires

Four comparative studies were found;[48–51] generalisability is limited by the fact that all were on non-health topics. Findings with respect to response rates, response quality and answers to sensitive questions were equivocal. However, evidence from a single study[48] suggested that respondents to computerised questionnaires may use a wider range on rating scales. Quicker responses may also be obtained using computer-assisted questionnaires.[48]

Computer-assisted telephone interviewing (CATI) versus conventional telephone interviewing

We identified one health-related study on this topic.[52] Response rates for the non-CATI group were significantly higher, and the time taken to complete a CATI was longer. On most of the criteria measured, only small differences were found between the two approaches, but there was some evidence of less interviewer variability in CATI.

Question Wording and Sequencing

Some caution is required in interpreting the available evidence on the effects of questionnaire wording and sequencing, and on the presentation of response categories, in terms of the validity and quality of the data obtained. Both theory and limited empirical evidence suggest that these effects may vary with mode of administration, but the majority of empirical studies involve interview approaches. Furthermore, few identified studies were in the context of health surveys; those that were health-related are highlighted below.

Question wording

Schuman and colleagues[53] found that open-ended questions produce more non-common responses than closed questions, but most additional response categories are small and miscellaneous. Therefore, use of either question form will ordinarily lead to similar conclusions. However, open-ended questions are preferable in development stages and pilot studies, to generate appropriate response categories for closed questions.

Bishop and co-workers[54] compared the effects of presenting one versus two sides of an issue in survey questions and demonstrated that giving a second substantive choice on attitude questions increased the likelihood of respondents expressing an opinion.

Researchers have shown that survey respondents employ a wide range of cognitive processes in formulating responses to behavioural frequency questions, including both episodic enumeration (recalling and counting specific instances on which the behaviour occurred) and rate processing (aggregating from the 'normal' rate at which the behaviour takes place in a unit of time, such as a week). Task conditions, such as time-framing, have been shown to influence the processes employed, both in health-related[55] and other surveys.[56]

One form of response bias is the acquiescence effect (the tendency to agree with questions presented in the form of statements); this is most common amongst less-educated respondents.[54] Conventional wisdom suggests that presenting a mixture of positively and negatively phrased statements will control or offset acquiescence tendencies; however, the actual effect of mixing statements in this way may be to reduce response validity.[57]

The wording of filter questions, asking whether the respondent has knowledge of or has thought about an issue, can significantly affect the percentages of 'don't know' responses elicited at a subsequent substantive question, particularly for topics less familiar to the respondent. Conversely, the content of the question can have an important independent effect on 'don't know' responses, regardless of the filter wording. The use of filter questions can thus alter the conclusions drawn.[58,59]

Interpretation of questions that include prestige names is complicated by the fact that subjects respond not only on the basis of the content of issues but also on the basis of the names.[60]

Question sequencing

Question order effects may influence overall response rates; they may also be a significant source of response bias. The direction and strength of these effects can vary with survey topic, the context in which the questions are presented and the study population. Context effects appear to be especially likely when researchers attempt to summarise complex issues in a single general item.[61] It seems that question order effects are consistent across gender and education levels, and so are as much of a concern in surveys of restricted populations as in those of general populations.[62]

Ordering effects may bias estimates of the prevalence of attitudes and behaviour. If otherwise identical questions are posed in a different order or a different context across surveys, apparent differences in response patterns may reflect these context effects rather than true differences between settings or over time.[62]

It has been argued that question order effects are less common in self-completion questionnaires than in interviewer-administered surveys.[63] This may be the result of reduced serial-order constraints (for example, in interviewer-administered surveys, respondents may wish to present a consistent image to the interviewer[64]). Moreover, in self-completion questionnaires, respondents have the opportunity to read all the questions before responding, and thus have a better feel for the relationship between questions; they are not forced by time constraints to give 'top-of-the-head' responses.[65] However, research[64] which tested whether specific question order effects, previously observed in interview surveys, occurred also in postal surveys was inconclusive.

The content of opening items may influence subjects' motivation to complete a questionnaire; the more interesting and relevant these items are, the greater the likelihood of response.[66] Findings by Jones and Lang[67] also suggested that topic ordering within a questionnaire may differentially affect response rates amongst groups holding different attitudes, thus increasing non-response bias.

It is usually recommended[4,68] that general questions should precede more specific ones, since specific questions may create a 'saliency' effect which influences responses to more general questions.[68] Empirical evidence supports this view. Prior items in a questionnaire have been shown to exert a 'carry-over' effect by priming respondents about their beliefs/attitudes towards a particular topic.[69,70] Similarly, the meaning of a potentially ambiguous question may be clarified by the wording of a preceding question, through a 'contrast' effect,[62] as demonstrated by Colasanto and colleagues[71] in a study on beliefs about transmission of AIDS and HIV.

Expert opinion on the relative placement of questions on related topics varies. Moser and Kalton[1] equivocate and suggest that questionnaires may be designed so that earlier questions (or groups thereof) set the context for later ones, or conversely so that responses to later questions are not influenced by those preceding them. By contrast, Sudman and Bradburn[4] recommend that all questions on one topic should be completed before embarking on a new topic. The view that questions should be grouped by topic, and topics ordered so that related ones are adjacent to one another, ignores the issue of context effects; yet empirical evidence suggests that such effects are common. However, evidence from studies on both health-related[72] and other topics[69,70] indicates that 'buffering' (interposing unrelated items between questions known or thought likely to influence one another) is not guaranteed to completely eliminate context effects. Researchers therefore need to balance the risk of context effects with the desirability of coherence and continuity.

Response categories

Sudman and Bradburn[4] suggest that the distinction between question wording and response format is to some extent artificial, since the form of the question often dictates the most appropriate response format.

Nonetheless, the question of whether to include or exclude 'no opinion', 'don't know' or middle response categories is one which has been considerably debated. It has been argued that inclusion of such options, especially in self-completion questionnaires, may lead respondents to take the easy way out rather than spending time formulating an opinion or recording factual details, thereby yielding invalid data. The counter-argument is that their exclusion encourages respondents to make wild guesses or to omit the question altogether, presenting different threats to data completeness and quality. Empirical evidence,[59,64,73,74] including findings from one health-related study,[75] suggests that response distributions vary according to whether or not middle alternatives and explicit 'don't know' response categories are included. It appears that offering such response options is generally preferable for attitudinal questions. Providing respondents with an explicit opportunity to have no opinion may also avoid spurious representativeness.[59,73] Middle alternatives and 'don't know' response categories may be less important for factual questions.

The order of response alternatives may affect both distribution of responses to individual items and associations between these and other items. Israel and Taylor[76] have shown this effect to be particularly marked in respect of questions prone to social desirability bias; the percentage endorsing the 'socially acceptable' response was significantly higher when this was presented first.

Two specific types of response order effects are 'primacy' effects (the tendency to select the first response category presented) and 'recency' effects (the tendency to choose the last response option). Schuman and Presser[62] assert that primacy effects are more common in self-completion questionnaires (a view supported by empirical evidence[64]) and that recency effects are more usual in interviews.

In pre-coded (closed) questions, the 'codes' or 'labels' attached to each response category may also be seen as part of the question–response stimulus. One identified study[77] compared numerical and verbal labelling of response categories and showed no significant differences. However, findings by the same authors suggested that fully defined scales (labelling all scale points) may act as a check on leniency errors (the tendency to bias ratings in an upward direction). In another study,[78] however, there was no significant differences in response patterns to scales in which only the end-points were explicitly labelled and those in which all scale points were labelled to indicate equal spacing. These conflicting findings suggest that the wording of response alternatives may be as critical as question wording.

Response formats

Most experts[3,4,19,79] recommend a vertical answer format (Figure 1) for multiple choice questions, except in respect of rating scales. In the latter case, they favour a horizontal format (Figure 2), both to save space and to avoid the erroneous impression that each category is independent of each other.[80]

---

1. Do you take a daily dose of aspirin?
   *(Please **circle the number** that describes you)*

   Yes, got on prescription 1

   Yes, bought over the counter 2
   (e.g. in a chemist or supermarket)

   No, I don't take daily aspirin 3

Figure 1 *Example of vertical format for factual questions.*

1. In the **past month**, on how many **days** have you been **short of breath during exercise** (for example going upstairs, walking up hill, gardening, taking part in sports)?

Never	On one or a few days	On several days	On most days	Every day
1	2	3	4	5

Figure 2 *Example of horizontal format for rating scale.*

In a health-related survey, differences in response rates or response quality between a 'tick the box' format and a 'circle the number' format have not been shown to be significant, though the former required time-consuming and expensive coding on receipt of completed questionnaires, because the boxes were not pre-numbered.[23] In a non-health-related study, we found some evidence that the positioning of response categories relative to the corresponding question stem can affect responses; Stem and colleagues[81] showed that 'remote' placement (showing a rating scale only at the top of the page or the beginning of a set of questions) elicited more neutral responses than did placing the response categories alongside each individual question.

Questionnaire Appearance

Expert opinion, as well as common-sense, indicates that attention to the appearance of a questionnaire, including its length and layout, is important. As Sudman and Bradburn[4] noted, in interview surveys, a well-designed questionnaire can simplify the tasks of both interviewers and data processors. Good design can reduce the risk of errors in posing questions, and coding responses and can minimise potential variability between interviewers. The influence of aspects of questionnaire appearance on response rates is also well recognised[3,18] (Tables 1 and 2). Nonetheless, this is perhaps the least well researched aspect of survey research, especially in relation to health surveys. Furthermore, there have been 'few systematic efforts . . . to derive principles for designing self-administered questionnaires from relevant psychological or sociological principles'.[19]

Jenkins and Dillman[19] have drawn on theories of cognition, perception and pattern recognition and processing to derive a set of principles for the design of self-completion questionnaires, as shown in Figure 3.

It is often asserted that questionnaire response rates are inversely related to the amount of data sought. A 'Survey of Surveys'[82] provided some weak evidence that lower response rates were obtained in respect of longer interviews. Cannell and Kahn[83] postulate that motivation may decline when the interview extends beyond some optimal (unspecified) length. However, Bradburn[84] argues that, where the survey is perceived to be important or interesting to respondents, the questionnaire can be quite long without having a detrimental effect on the rate or quality of response. There is some empirical support for this view, though comparison of findings across studies is difficult because of wide variation in the definition of 'long' and 'short'. In previous literature reviews[7,8] an interaction between saliency (relevance and interest) and length has been demonstrated. Evidence from primary research studies has shown no significant effect of length on response rates for two surveys on health topics,[85,86] but lower response rates were obtained for longer questionnaires on other topics;[87–89] this contrast is probably due to the higher saliency of the health surveys.

Sudman and Bradburn[4] suggest that bias in favour of individuals with strong opinions is likely to occur in respect of long questionnaires. There is also the potential for response bias, due to fatigue or carelessness, in the latter part of long questionnaires, particularly with respect to answers to 'item sets' (series of questions on a related topic and usually with the same response format throughout); we found weak evidence from one non-health study[90] in support of this view.

In another non-health study, the colour of paper on which questionnaires are printed has

---

Principle 1: Use the visual elements of brightness, colour, shape and location in a consistent manner to define the desired navigational path for respondents to follow when answering the questionnaire.

Principle 2: When established format conventions are changed in the midst of a questionnaire, use prominent visual guides to re-orient respondents.

Principle 3: Place instruction and directions where they are to be used and where they can be seen.

Principle 4: Present information in a manner that does not require respondents to connect information from separate locations in order to comprehend it.

Principle 5: Ask people to answer only one question at a time.

Figure 3   *Jenkins and Dillman's[19] principles for the design of self-administered questionnaires.*

not been shown to have a significant impact on response rates.[91] However, guidelines on enhancing the readability of documents, produced by the United Kingdom based Basic Skills Agency (whose remit is assisting those with literacy problems) and the Royal National Association for the Blind, indicate that dark backgrounds (particularly shades of blue and purple) should be avoided; black type on a white or yellow background provides the best contrast. These organisations recommend the use of a clear and distinct type face, with a minimum font size of 12 points (larger if readers are likely to have visual impairment). They advise against excessive use of upper-case letters, suggesting that emphasis is more appropriately provided by underlining or emboldening; such formatting may also be used to distinguish questions, answers and instructions from each other.

Enhancing Response Rates

Factors influencing survey response rates may be conveniently divided into mechanical and perceptual factors (timing of survey; number, timing and method of contacts; postage rates and types); general motivational factors (anonymity and confidentiality; personalisation; nature of appeal; other aspects of covering letters; sponsorship; saliency); and financial and other incentives.

Mechanical and perceptual factors

Evidence from a single, health-related, study of day of posting[92] found no significant effect on response rates. Expert advice[3] and evidence from a series of non-health surveys[18] suggest that month of posting may affect response rates (in particular, December should be avoided); however, it is unclear whether this effect is universal or is population- or topic-specific.

One of the most potent ways of enhancing response rates is through multiple contacts.[32,67,93] Both pre-notification and follow-up contacts (reminders) have been found to be effective.[7,94,95]

We found one non-health study which suggested that a letter may be more effective than a telephone call in pre-notifying subjects.[96] However, the findings from three studies (one on a health-related topic) with respect to 'high involvement' methods of pre-notification (such as 'foot-in-door' approaches, whereby subjects are first asked to comply with a small task, in the hope that they will continue to comply with the larger task of survey participation) were equivocal.[87,97,98]

Nor did we find any conclusive evidence from three identified studies (one health-related) that a 'threat' in the reminder letter of further follow-

ups enhances response rates.[99–101] Including a duplicate questionnaire with the first reminder does not appear to have a significant impact, but inclusion of a replacement questionnaire with a second reminder appears to be effective.[102] Contrary to the recommendations of Dillman[3] and the conclusions from an earlier review,[32] we found no conclusive evidence that special mailing techniques for final reminders are superior to standard mailing.[103,104] One health-related study suggested that postcard reminders appear to be as effective as letters and are generally cheaper.[105]

Findings both from primary studies[94,95,104,106–113] and from previous reviews[7,8,27,32,114,115] show no consistent advantage of class of mail, or of stamped envelopes over franked or reply-paid envelopes, either for outgoing or return mail.

General motivational factors

Anonymity and confidentiality are frequently confused by survey researchers, but they are not equivalent.[116] Under conditions of anonymity, no identification appears on the questionnaire, and it is not possible to link individual responses to a specific named person. As a result, reminders cannot be targeted specifically to initial non-respondents. Under conditions of confidentiality, an identification code (usually a number) appears on the questionnaire; researchers can link this code to a named individual, but individual responses cannot be attributed to a specific person by anyone who does not have access to the link between code and name. Ethical principles also require that respondents' answers are not revealed to a third party without their explicit permission, and that results are presented in such a way that individual respondents cannot be identified. Evidence from the five studies (one on a health-related topic) we identified[117–121] failed to provide consistent evidence of the effects of anonymity and confidentiality on response rates or data quality.

Despite Dillman's[3] recommendation regarding the personalisation of covering letters 'to show regard for respondents', only two (both non-health)[104,122] out of 11 studies[94,95,104,108,119,122–128] showed a significant positive effect of personalisation on response rates; in neither health-related study[123,128] did personalisation significantly enhance response rates. However, it appears that personalisation may interact with such factors as the nature of the appeal made in the covering letter and assurances of confidentiality.[129]

We found some evidence[130] that traditional-style letters are more effective than novel approaches. However, only one[108] out of three identified studies[108,131,132] suggested that the characteristics of the signatory affect response rates. Nor does response rate appear to be positively related to hand-written signatures[131] or colour of ink.[132] Although a 'social utility' appeal in the covering letter (emphasising the value of the response to society in general) has been advocated,[3] empirical evidence from ten studies (four of which were health-related) indicates that no single type of appeal offers a consistent advantage;[67,107,113,123,124,131,133–136] it seems that the appeal should be matched to the anticipated motivations of the recipients.

Specifying that the questionnaire will only take a short time to complete has been shown to be effective in stimulating responses.[20] However, although specification of a deadline for responding appears to increase the speed of response (and thereby reduce the number of reminders needed), it may have no effect on overall response rates.[99,123]

A 'salient' topic is generally effective in enhancing response rates.[32,137,138] The impact of sponsorship appears to be situation- and location-specific.[67,86,107,117,139]

Incentives

In general surveys, incentives are usually a highly effective means of increasing response rates.[109,135,140–145] However, the benefit of incentives in health surveys (where response rates are typically higher in any case) is less clearcut.[133,146–152] Financial incentives may be more effective than non-monetary incentives of similar value.[140] Regardless of setting and topic, enclosed incentives generally generate higher response rates than promised incentives.[141,142,146,151,153–155] Findings on the effects of different sizes of incentive were equivocal.[141,152]

Although a number of experts[3,156,157] have recommended offering survey participants a copy of the results, we found little evidence that such an offer has a significant effect on response rates, at least in general surveys.[88,122,137,158]

Finally, it appears that personal drop-off of questionnaires for self-completion may offer some advantages, but the cost–effectiveness of this approach may be situation-specific.[159]

RECOMMENDATIONS FOR USERS OF QUESTIONNAIRE SURVEYS

In so far as possible, the recommendations we make below are based on empirical evidence from the primary research studies identified in our review. However, for some aspects of the design and conduct of surveys, there was little such evidence. In these cases, we have drawn on the recommendations of survey experts and on our own extensive experience of conducting surveys. Where recommendations are not evidence based, we highlight this fact.

Mode of Administration

Empirical evidence[35–52] does not demonstrate any consistent advantage of any single method of questionnaire administration over all others. The choice of mode of administration should therefore be made on a survey-by-survey basis, taking into account: study population; survey topic; sampling frame and method; volume and complexity of data to be collected; and resources available.

Question Wording and Sequencing

Theories of respondent behaviour[4,5,62] and findings from empirical studies[53–56] suggest that researchers aiming to increase the validity and reliability of respondents' answers should consider the range of cognitive processes involved in response formulation and the potential impact of task variables such as: the likely salience and temporal regularity of events; method of survey administration; and question design issues such as time-frame.

In the absence of any strong evidence to the contrary, general principles of questionnaire wording (Figure 4) should be maintained. Moreover, Sudman and Bradburn's[4] guidelines for the wording of specific types of questions, the presentation of response categories and question ordering (Figures 5–10) have stood the test of time and, in many instances, are supported by empirical evidence.[53–78] Avoid the use of questions involving prestige names[60] wherever possible.

Caution should be exercised in the use of negatively phrased attitudinal items, specifically in using a mix of positive and negative items in the hope of reducing acquiescence bias.[57]

Consider carefully the implications of including or excluding filter questions on response distributions. Filter questions may be appropriate to identify which respondents should answer subsequent questions (for example, to avoid asking questions about smoking behaviour of lifetime non-smokers). Filters can also be used to avoid 'spurious representativeness'[58,59] resulting from trying to elicit opinions from those who have no views on the subject. Bear in mind also that filter questions and skip instructions are less well-handled by respondents to self-completion questionnaires than they are by trained interviewers

Although the potential for question order effects may be reduced in postal surveys,[63] it is

- Use simple language; avoid acronyms, abbreviations, jargon and technical terms

- Keep the question short (sentence of less than 20 words approximately)

- Avoid questions which are insufficiently specific

- Avoid ambiguity

- Avoid vague words and those with more than one meaning (for example, 'dinner')

- Avoid double-barrelled questions (those with an 'and' or an 'or' in the wording)

- Avoid double negatives (for instance, a negative statement followed by a 'disagree' response)

- Avoid proverbs and clichés when measuring attitudes

- Avoid leading questions (for example, 'Do you agree that the NHS is under-funded?')

- Beware loaded words and concepts (those implying a value judgement)

- Beware of presuming questions (for example, those which assume that a respondent has indulged in a specific type of behaviour)

- Be cautious in use of hypothetical questions

- Do not over-tax respondents' memories (for example, by asking for detailed recall of trivial issues)

Figure 4   *General principles of question wording (After Moser and Kalton[1] and Oppenheim[11]).*

- Make all questions as specific as possible

- Include all reasonable response alternatives

- Relate the time-frame to how salient or memorable the topic is

- Consider the use of aided recall procedures and memory cues

- If appropriate, give permission to consult documentary sources (such as diaries or records)

Figure 5   *Guidelines for presenting non-threatening questions about behaviour (Sudman and Bradburn[4]).*

unlikely to be eliminated entirely; general principles of question ordering should therefore be adhered to regardless of mode of administration. As experts[4] suggest, the questionnaire should open with interesting but non-threatening questions. If respondents are expected to have stronger opinions on some survey topics than others, the questionnaire should be assembled to reflect these priorities.[66] General questions should precede specific ones.[68–70] Since evidence from primary research studies[69,70,72] suggests that 'buffering' questions are unlikely to eliminate context effects, the conventional wisdom of grouping questions by topic should be adhered to. In situations where researchers are uncertain about the impact of question order

on results, the order should be randomised. Because they may be potentially sensitive, demographic questions should be placed at the end of the questionnaire, as Sudman and Bradburn recommend.[4]

Follow expert advice[4] and use open-ended questions sparingly, particularly in self-completion questionnaires. However, in piloting and pre-testing, open-ended questions should be used to ensure that the response categories subsequently used for closed questions adequately represent the likely range of responses. As recommended in key texts,[10,12] response categories for closed questions should be mutually exclusive (unambiguous, not overlapping) and collectively exhaustive (all contingencies catered

- Use long introductions

- Use open-ended questions

- Use familiar or colloquial words

- Use an appropriate time-frame for questions about behaviour

- Deliberately load the question by:

  ⇨ indicating that the behaviour is very common (for example, 'Most people occasionally go to bed without cleaning their teeth. How many times in the last week have you done this?')

  ⇨ assuming the behaviour and asking merely about frequency or other details (for example, 'How many cigarettes do you smoke each day?', with the option of responding 'None')

  ⇨ citing authority to justify behaviour (for example, 'Many doctors now say that drinking red wine reduces the risk of heart disease. Have you drunk any red wine in the past month?')

- Embed the threatening topic within a list of more and less threatening subjects to reduce its perceived importance

- Use techniques such as card sorting and randomised response (whereby respondents throw a dice or pick a coloured counter; the outcome determines whether they answer the sensitive question or an innocuous question with a known probability of a positive response – for example 'Were you born in January?'; statistical techniques are applied to infer the percentage answering the sensitive question in a positive manner)

Figure 6   *Guidelines for obtaining accurate responses to threatening questions (Sudman and Bradburn[4]).*

- Use filter questions to screen out respondents who lack sufficient information

- Include a 'don't know' response category to reduce the perceived threat

- In interviews, ask open-ended questions even if numerical answers are required and recorded (to counter the tendency to choose the mid-point)

- Use pictures and other non-verbal procedures as well as standard questions

- Ask several questions on the same topic to reduce the likelihood of successful guessing especially where 'yes/no' responses are required

Figure 7   *Guidelines for optimising responses to knowledge questions (Sudman and Bradburn[4]).*

- Avoid double-barrelled questions

- Standardise the stimulus question by explicit specification of the alternatives

- Include a middle response category unless there are persuasive reasons not to do so

- Since they seem more susceptible to ordering effects, ask general questions before specific ones

- If measuring changes in attitudes over time, ask exactly the same questions at each time point

Figure 8   *Guidelines for presenting attitude questions (Sudman and Bradburn[4]).*

- Place easy, salient and non-threatening questions first in a questionnaire

- Place demographic questions last (since they can be seen as threatening), unless they are required to determine respondent's eligibility to complete the remainder of the questionnaire

- Use funnelling procedures to minimise question order effects, starting with the general and moving to the specific

- Complete questions on one topic before embarking on a new topic

- Use transitional phrases and instructions when switching topics

- Order filter questions (those intended to establish who should answer what questions) in such a way to cover all contingencies and encourage complete responses

Figure 9   *Guidelines for question ordering (Sudman and Bradburn[4]).*

- Use open-ended questions sparingly (because they are more resource-intensive and are more subject to inter-interviewer variability)

- Start with the least socially desirable option

- Limit rating scales to not more than five points when written descriptors are attached

- For more than five response categories, use numerical scales

- Consider analogues such as ladders, clocks or thermometers for numerical scales with many points

- Ask respondents to respond to every item in a list rather than indicating only those that apply (that is, to respond 'yes/no' or 'applies/does not apply' to each item rather than simply complying with the instruction 'circle as many as apply')

Figure 10   *Guidelines for presenting response categories (Sudman and Bradburn[4]).*

for, if necessary by the inclusion of an option of 'Other, please specify').

Since the middle response category on attitude/opinion questions does not necessarily represent a position of neutrality, it should be included.[59,64,73-75] However, for factual questions, the 'don't know' response can be omitted. Since the evidence is inconsistent,[77,78] it is preferable to label all response categories rather than only the endpoints.

Experts[3,4,19,79] recommend a vertical response format (Figure 1) for multiple-choice questions, except for rating scales. Empirical evidence and expert opinion[19,80] suggests that a horizontal response format (Figure 2) is more appropriate for item sets involving the same response categories throughout, and in rating scales. Consider natural reading style (left to right, and horizontally oriented) in placing headings and codes for responses. If a 'remote scale' format is used, the scale should be repeated after every three or four questions to minimise the rate of inappropriate neutral responses.[81] To reduce

subsequent data coding and editing time and costs, a 'circle the number' format is preferable to a 'tick the box' format, since evidence indicates no difference in response rates or data quality.[23]

Questionnaire Appearance

In the absence of empirical evidence, a good deal of expert opinion makes sound sense and is supported by theories of cognition, perception and pattern recognition.[19] The principles shown in Figure 3 provide appropriate guidelines. Although we did not identify any literature on the topic, computer-readable questionnaires (optical character recognition) are likely to assume greater importance in the future. Their design should take into account the hardware and software to be used. In health surveys, it is likely that a significant proportion of the sample will have some degree of visual impairment. Their needs should be borne in mind in designing self-completion questionnaires.

The 'optimal' length of questionnaire will depend upon data requirements, mode of administration, survey topic and study population. Although we did not find any evidence of lower response rates in longer questionnaires on health-related topics,[85,86] it would be rash to conclude that there is no upper limit to the length of questionnaire feasible in health surveys. Principles of design[19] and empirical evidence[160] indicate that it is desirable to avoid crowding questions or reducing 'white space' in an effort to reduce apparent length.

As Dillman[3] suggests, a booklet format with double-sided printing presents a more professional image. To facilitate use of standard stationery and to avoid excessive production costs, use standard-sized paper (A4 folded to A5 booklet or A3 folded to A4 booklet, as dictated by length of questionnaire).

White paper or a light tint enhance legibility. However, coloured covers can facilitate questionnaire identification. Dillman[3] recommends that the front cover should contain the title of the survey, the identity of the organisation carrying it out and, for self-completion questionnaires, a neutral graphic illustration. The back cover should provide some blank space for respondents' open comments, and should specify the address of the organisation conducting the survey (if not on the front cover) and say 'thank you' to the respondent.

A font size of at least 12 points should be used; a larger font size (up to 14 or 16 points, depending on type face) is desirable if respondents may have some visual impairment. Choose a distinct type face. Emboldening, italicisation and underlining should be used to distinguish questions, response categories and instructions.

Maintain a consistent format throughout the questionnaire. As Dillman[3] advocates, respondents should not be asked to do two things (for example, rating and ranking) in the one question. Avoid splitting a question, its associated response categories and instructions for answering over two pages. In questions where the list of response categories is too long to fit on a single page, continue the response categories on a facing page if possible; otherwise repeat the question on the subsequent page. Where one question is logically dependent upon another, every effort should be made to place both on the same page. Avoid placing a short question at the foot of a page, especially if preceded by a long question with a number of subparts.

When open-ended questions are used, sufficient space should be left to record responses; respondents take the amount of space provided as indicative of the level of detail required. Do not use lines for open-ended questions, unless only a short response (a number or a few words) is required.

Follow sound design principles[19] and use elements of brightness, colour, shape and location, as well as verbal indicators, to 'steer' respondents through the questionnaire. Graphical means, for example arrows and boxes, help to indicate skip patterns. Place instructions and directions at the point where they are required; if a series of questions involves turning a page, it may be necessary to repeat instructions on the new page.

Enhancing Response Rates

The choice of techniques for enhancing response rates should be informed by consideration of the likely barriers and motivational factors for each particular survey topic and study population. The frameworks presented by Dillman[3] and Brown and colleagues[18] (Tables 1 and 2) form a useful basis for deliberation. In assessing potential methods, consider the potential for sample composition bias, response bias, item non-response effects, and resource implications, as well as the likely impact on response rates. The marginal benefits of intensive approaches to enhancing response rates may be outweighed by the marginal costs. Manipulation of a single factor is unlikely to prove fruitful.[18] Instead, consideration should be given to the total 'package' of: questionnaire wording; questionnaire appearance; general motivational factors; mechanical and perceptual factors; and financial and other incentives. The possibility of interactions between factors should be taken into count and care should be exercised to avoid apparent mismatches.

Expert opinion[3] and empirical evidence[18] suggest that, if possible, the month of December should be avoided in conducting postal surveys. Depending on the survey topic and the study population, avoidance of the peak holiday months (July and August) may also be advisable.

Evidence from primary studies and previous reviews[32,67,93] suggest that multiple contacts are a potent means of enhancing response. If resources allow, consider pre-notification,[7,94,95] preferably by letter,[96] to alert target respondents to the arrival of the questionnaire. However, if resource constraints limit the number of contacts which can be made, put resources into follow-ups rather than pre-notification. Regardless of whether subjects have been pre-notified, at least one reminder should be sent to non-respondents.[7,94,95] No one style of reminder is universally appropriate;[99–101] match the appeal in the reminder letter to the perceived motivations of the study population. A consensual approach (stressing how many people have already responded) may be appropriate to some groups, while an indication of the likelihood of further follow-up in the absence of a response may be more effective with others. Our own experience leads us to recommend the inclusion of a duplicate questionnaire with at least one reminder, if initial non-response is believed to be related to non-delivery or mislaying of the original. If multiple reminders are used, it may be appropriate to wait until the second or subsequent reminder to enclose the duplicate.[102] Choose a mode of contact appropriate to the survey topic and study population. Intensive techniques, such as certified or recorded-delivery mailing, have not been conclusively demonstrated[103,104] to have an advantage over standard mailing and may be considered by target respondents, or by ethical committees, to be overly intrusive or unduly coercive. Whilst postcard reminders may be cost-effective,[105] concerns regarding confidentiality may preclude their use in surveys on health-related topics.

Respondents should not have to bear the cost of returning the questionnaire; a pre-paid and addressed return envelope should always be provided. Since evidence from empirical studies[94,95,104,106–115] and previous reviews[7,8,27,32,114,115] shows no consistent effect of type of postage, for convenience use franking rather than postage stamps for out-going mail, and use business reply envelopes for return of questionnaires. The choice between first-class and second-class mail should involve consideration of the relative costs, the speed with which results are required, and whether it is anticipated that respondents will be aware of or influenced by the class of mail.

In general, total anonymity is not appropriate since it precludes targeting reminders and linking questionnaire responses with other data sources (such as medical records). Moreover, empirical evidence does not provide any clear support for a totally anonymous approach.[117–121] We therefore recommend the use of coded (numbered and therefore identifiable) questionnaires. It is appropriate to be explicit in a covering letter or information sheet about how the code number will be used (to keep a check on who has responded and thereby to allow non-respondents to be followed-up). Provide appropriate assurances of confidentiality, clarifying what this means (generally that only the research team will be able to link the numbered questionnaire to a named individual and that individual responses will not be revealed to a third party without the explicit permission of the respondent concerned).

In surveys of general populations, the balance of evidence[94,95,104,108,119,122–128] suggests that personalisation may offer no significant advantage. However, personalisation is probably appropriate if the message in the letter suggests personal knowledge of the circumstances of the recipient or uses a self-interest appeal. We also favour personalisation when the target respondents are in fact personally or professionally known to the surveyor.

A traditional letter format, using headed notepaper, is most appropriate.[130] Keep the covering letter short and use language appropriate to the target recipients. If extensive or detailed information needs to be given, consider including a separate information sheet. In most circumstances, a facsimile signature is likely to be adequate.[131] However, care should be taken to match the style of signature to the degree of personalisation of the body of the letter. No single type of cover letter appeal is universally appropriate.[67,107,113,123,124,131,133–136] Rather, the nature of the appeal should be based on the perceived motivations of the study population and should be ethically sound. Consider including a realistic indication of the time required for completion of the questionnaire.[20] A deadline for questionnaire return may also be specified, especially if a timely response is of the essence.[99,123]

If ethical and practical constraints permit, choose a study 'sponsor' appropriate to the survey topic and study population;[67,86,117,139] manipulate the covering letter and return address appropriately. In surveys on health-related topics, response rates may be enhanced if the covering letter purports to come from the recipients' healthcare provider.[86,139] However, consideration should be given to whether this approach may induce response bias, and to whether it is practicable.

In as far as possible, ensure the relevance and interest of the survey topic to the study population.[8,32,137,138] Fortunately, surveys on health-related topics are generally perceived to be highly salient!

If ethical and budgetary constraints allow, consider the use of enclosed, financial incentives,[109,135,140–146,151,153–155] though their impact may be less in health surveys.[133,146–152] In making the choice, the most relevant cost to consider is the projected cost per returned questionnaire; will the likely additional yield in responses outweigh the additional cost of providing the incentive? Note also that incentives are often regarded as unethical in health research, and grant-awarding bodies tend to disapprove of the practice.[9] Providing feedback to study respondents is probably unnecessary in surveys of the general public or of patients,[88,122,137,158] but may be appropriate in surveys of health professionals.

PRIORITIES FOR FUTURE RESEARCH

As we have already noted, many of the identified studies were of surveys on non-health topics, thus potentially limiting their generalisability to design and conduct of health surveys. We recommend further research to test whether the findings from other sectors are replicated in health-related surveys. In particular, we recommend further investigation of: the effect of mode of administration in collecting data of a sensitive and personal nature; the effect on acquiescence bias of mixing positive and negative statements in scales to measure attitudes; the impact of various types of appeal in covering letters (in particular the comparison of self-interest and social utility appeals) on response rates and data quality; the effectiveness and cost–effectiveness of the number and mode of contacts (pre-notification and reminders) in postal surveys.

Particularly in relation to question wording and sequencing, much of the current evidence has been derived from interview surveys. It has been postulated[63] that these effects are minimised in postal surveys, but there is little empirical evidence to back this assertion. We therefore recommend further investigation of question ordering effects in self-completion questionnaires. Of particular interest in the context of health surveys is whether the relative placement of entire scales (such as generic versus condition-specific health status measures) affects response rates and scale scores. We identified one study on this topic,[162] which indicated no ordering effect. However, we concur with the authors of that study, who emphasise the need for larger studies in other disease groups to determine whether their results are generalisable.

Rather than designing and implementing studies specifically to investigate methodological aspects of survey design and administration, we recommend incorporating such experiments into surveys which are being carried out anyway. For example, a split-half design, examining the impact of different styles of reminder letter on response rates and response quality, could be easily included in many studies.

Finally, we recommend that all reports of survey research should include methodological details (for example, length of questionnaire; mode of administration; number, timing and mode of administration). Such data would facilitate further reviews and meta-analyses.

REFERENCES

1. Moser CA, Kalton G. *Survey methods in social investigation*. 2nd edn. Aldershot: Gower, 1971.
2. Bennett AE, Ritchie R. *Questionnaires in medicine: a guide to their design and use*. London: Oxford University Press, 1975.
3. Dillman DA. *Mail and telephone surveys: The total design method*. New York: John Wiley and Sons, Inc., 1978.
4. Sudman S, Bradburn N. *Asking questions: a practical guide to questionnaire design*. San Francisco: Jossey-Bass, 1982.
5. Bradburn N, Sudman S and Associates. *Improving interview method and questionnaire design*. San Francisco: Jossey Bass, 1979.
6. Advisory Group on Health Technology Assessment. *Assessing the effects of health technologies*. London: Department of Health, 1993.
7. Linsky AS. Stimulating responses to mailed questionnaires: a review. *Public Opinion Quarterly* 1975; **39**: 82–101.
8. Kanuk L, Berenson C. Mail surveys and response rates: A literature review. *J. Marketing Res.* 1975; **12**: 440–53.
9. Bowling A. *Research methods in health: Investigating health and health services*. Buckingham: Open University Press, 1997.
10. Abramson JH. *Survey methods in community medicine*. Edinburgh: Churchill Livingstone, 1990.
11. Oppenheim AN. *Questionnaire design, interviewing and attitude measurement*. 2nd edn. London: Pinter Publishers, 1992.
12. Fink A. *The survey kit*. Thousand Oaks: Sage Publications, 1995.
13. Crombie IK, Davies HTO. *Research in health care: design, conduct and interpretation of health services research*. Chichester: John Wiley and Sons, 1996.
14. Øvretveit J. *Evaluating health interventions*. Buckingham: Open University Press, 1998.
15. Czaja R, Blair J. *Designing surveys: a guide to decisions and procedures*. Thousand Oaks: Pine Forge Press, 1995.
16. Sackett DL. Bias in analytic research. *J. Chron. Dis.* 1979; **32**: 51–63.
17. Murphy EA. *The logic of medicine*. Baltimore: Johns Hopkins University Press, 1976.
18. Brown TL, Decker DJ, Connelly NA. Response to mail surveys on resource-based recreation topics: A behavioral model and an empirical analysis. *Leisure Sciences* 1989; **11**: 99–110.
19. Jenkins CR, Dillman DA. Towards a theory of self-administered questionnaire design. In:

Lyberg L, Biemer P, Collins M, et al (eds). *Survey measurement and process quality.* New York: John Wiley & Sons Inc, 1997; pp. 165–96.

20. Hornik J. Time cue and time perception effect on response to mail surveys. *J. Marketing Res.* 1981; **18**: 243–8.

21. McAvoy BR, Kaner EFS. General practice postal surveys: a questionnaire too far? *Br. Med. J.* 1996; **313**: 732–3.

22. Goyder J. *The silent minority: Nonrespondents on sample surveys.* Cambridge: Polity Press, 1987.

23. Cartwright A. Some experiments with factors that might affect the response of mothers to a postal questionnaire. *Stat. Med.* 1986; **5**: 607–17.

24. Cartwright A. Professionals as responders: variations in and effects of response rates to questionnaires, 1961–77. *Br. Med. J.* 1978; **2**: 1419–21.

25. Fowler FJ. *Survey research methods.* Beverly Hills, CA: Sage, 1984.

26. Borg WR, Gall MD. *Educational research: an introduction.* New York: Longman, 1983.

27. Asch DA, Jedrziewski K, Christiakis NA. Response rates to mail surveys published in medical journals. *J. Clin. Epidemiol.* 1997; **50**: 1129–36.

28. Thibaut JW, Kelley HH. *The social psychology of groups.* New York: Wiley, 1959.

29. Homans GC. *Social behavior: Its elementary forms.* New York: Harcourt, Brace and World, 1961.

30. Blau PM. *Exchange and power in social life.* New York: Wiley, 1964.

31. Morton Williams J. *Interviewer approaches.* Aldershot: Dartmouth Publishing Company Limited, 1993.

32. Heberlein TA, Baumgartner R. Factors affecting response rates to mailed questionnaires: A quantitative analysis of the published literature. *Am. Sociol. Rev.* 1978; **43**: 447–62.

33. Jenkinson C, Ziebland S, Fitzpatrick R, Mowat A, Mowat A. Hospitalisation and its influence upon results from health status questionnaires. *Int. J. Health Sci.* 1993; **4**: 13–19.

34. Frey JH; Oishi SM. *How to conduct interviews by telephone and in person.* Thousand Oaks: Sage Publications, 1995.

35. Hinkle AL, King GD. A comparison of three survey methods to obtain data for community mental health program planning. *Am. J. Community Psychol.* 1978; **6**: 389–97.

36. Talley JE, Barrow JC, Fulkerson KF, Moore CA. Conducting a needs assessment of university psychological services: A campaign of telephone and mail strategies. *J. Am. Coll. Health* 1983; **32**: 101–3.

37. Pederson LL, Baskerville JC, Ashley MJ, Lefcoe NM. Comparison of mail questionnaire and telephone interview as data gathering strategies in a survey of attitudes toward restrictions on cigarette smoking. *Can. J. Public Health* 1994; **76**: 179–82.

38. McHorney CA, Kosinski M, Ware JE, Jr. Comparisons of the costs and quality of norms for the SF–36 health survey collected by mail versus telephone interview: results from a national survey. *Medical Care* 1994; **32**: 551–67.

39. Newton RR, Prensky D, Schuessler K. Form effect in the measurement of feeling states. *Soc. Sci. Res.* 1982; **11**: 301–17.

40. Nederhof AJ. Visibility of response as a mediating factor in equity research. *J. Soc. Psychol.* 1984; **122**: 211–15.

41. Oei TI, Zwart FM. The assessment of life events: self-administered questionnaire versus interview. *J. Affect. Disord.* 1986; **10**: 185–90.

42. Cartwright A. Interviews or postal questionnaires? Comparisons of data about women's experiences with maternity services. *Milbank Q.* 1988; **66**: 172–89.

43. Boekeloo BO, Schiavo L, Rabin DL, Conlon RT, Jordan CS, Mundt DJ. Self-reports of HIV risk factors by patients at a sexually transmitted disease clinic: audio vs written questionnaires. *Am. J. Public Health* 1994; **84**: 754–60.

44. Jordon LA, Marcus AC, Reeder LG. Response styles in telephone and household interviewing: A field experiment. *Public Opinion Q.* 1980; **44**: 210–22.

45. Quinn RP, Gutek BA, Walsh JT. Telephone interviewing: A reappraisal and a field experiment. *Basic Appl. Soc. Psychol.* 1980; **1**: 127–53.

46. Aneshensel CS, Frerichs RR, Clark VA, Yokopenic PA. Telephone versus in person surveys of community health status. *Am. J. Public Health* 1982; **72**: 1017–21.

47. Fenig S, Levav I, Kohn R, Yelin N. Telephone vs face-to-face interviewing in a community psychiatric survey. *Am. J. Public Health* 1993; **83**: 896–8.

48. Allen DF. Computers versus scanners: An experiment in nontraditional forms of survey administration. *J. Coll. Student Personnel* 1987; **28**: 266–73.

49. Higgins CA, Dimnik TP, Greenwood HP. The DISKQ survey method. Special Issue: Political opinion polling. *J. Market Research Soc.* 1987; **29**: 437–45.

50. Liefeld JP. Response effects in computer-administered questioning. *J. Marketing Res.* 1988; **25**: 405–9.

51. Helgeson JG, Ursic ML. The decision process equivalency of electronic versus pencil-and-paper data collection methods. *Soc. Sci. Computer Rev.* 1989; **7**: 296–310.

52. Groves RM, Mathiowetz NA. Computer assisted telephone interviewing: Effects on interviewers and respondents. *Public Opin. Q.* 1984; **48**: 356–69.

53. Schuman H, Ludwig J, Krosnick JA. The perceived threat of nuclear war, salience, and open questions. *Public Opin. Q.* 1986; **50**: 519–36.

54. Bishop GF, Oldendick RW, Tuchfarber AJ. Effects of presenting one versus two sides of an issue in survey questions. *Public Opin. Q.* 1982; **46**: 69–85.

55. Larsen JD, Mascharka C, Toronski C. Does the wording of the question change the number of headaches people report on a health questionnaire? *Psychol. Record* 1987; **37**: 423–7.

56. Blair E, Burton S. Cognitive processes used by survey respondents to answer behavioral frequency questions. *J. Consumer Research* 1987; **14**: 280–8.

57. Schriesheim CA, Hill KD. Controlling acquiescence response bias by item reversals: The effect on questionnaire validity. *Educational and Psychological Measurement* 1981; **41**: 1101–14.

58. Bishop GF, Oldendick RW, Tuchfarber AJ. Effects of filter questions in public opinion surveys. *Public Opin. Q.* 1983; **47**: 528–46.

59. Bishop GF, Tuchfarber AJ, Oldendick RW. Opinions on fictitious issues: the pressure to answer survey questions. *Public Opin. Q.* 1986; **50**: 240–50.

60. Smith ER, Squire P. The effects of prestige names in question wording. *Public Opin. Q.* 1990; **54**: 97–116.

61. Schuman H, Presser S, Ludwig J. Context effects on survey responses to questions about abortion. *Public Opin. Q.* 1981; **45**: 216–23.

62. Schuman H, Presser S. *Questions and answers in attitude surveys: experiments on question form, wording and content.* New York: Academic Press, 1981.

63. Smith TW. *Condition order effects: GSS technical report No. 33.* Chicago: National Opinion Research Centre, 1982.

64. Ayidiya SA, McClendon MJ. Response effects in mail surveys. *Public Opin. Q.* 1990; **54**: 229–47.

65. Hippler H-J, Schwarz N. Response effects in surveys. In: Hippler H-J, Schwarz N, Sudman S (eds). *Social information processing and survey methodology.* New York: Springer-Verlag, 1987.

66. Roberson MT, Sundstrom E. Questionnaire design, return rates, and response favorableness in an employee attitude questionnaire. *J. Appl. Psychol.* 1990; **75**: 354–7.

67. Jones WH, Lang JR. Sample composition bias and response bias in a mail survey: A comparison of inducement methods. *J. Marketing Res.* 1980; **17**: 69–76.

68. Bradburn NM, Mason WM. The effect of question order on response. *J. Marketing Res.* 1964; **1**: 61

69. Tourangeau R, Rasinski KA, Bradburn N, D'Andrade R. Belief accessibility and context effects in attitude measurement. *J. Exp. Soc. Psychol.* 1989; **25**: 401–21.

70. Tourangeau R, Rasinski KA, Bradburn N, D'Andrade R. Carryover effects in attitude surveys. *Public Opin. Q.* 1989; **53**: 495–524.

71. Colasanto D, Singer E, Rogers TF. Context effects on responses to questions about AIDS. *Public Opin. Q.* 1992; **56**: 515–18.

72. Schuman H, Kalton G, Ludwig J. Context and contiguity in survey questionnaires. *Public Opin. Q.* 1983; **47**: 112–15.

73. Hawkins DI, Coney KA. Uninformed response error in survey research. *J. Marketing Res.* 1981; **18**: 370–4.

74. Wandzilak T, Ansorge CJ, Potter G. Utilizing 'undecided' option with Likert items: Associated measurement problems. *Int. J. Sport Psychol.* 1987; **18**: 51–8.

75. Poe GS, Seeman I, McLaughlin J, Mehl E. 'Don't know' boxes in factual questions in a mail questionnaire: Effects on level and quality of response. *Public Opin. Q.* 1988; **52**: 212–22.

76. Israel GD, Taylor CL. Can response order bias evaluations? *Evaluation and Program Planning* 1990; **13**: 365–71.

77. Frisbie DA, Brandenburg DC. Equivalence of questionnaire items with varying response formats. *J. Educational Measurement* 1979; **16**: 43–8.

78. Lam TC, Klockars AJ. Anchor point effects on the equivalence of questionnaire items. *J. Educational Measurement* 1982; **19**: 317–22.

79. Bourque LB, Fielder EP. *How to conduct self-administered and mail surveys.* Thousand Oaks: Sage, 1995.

80. Gaskell GD, O'Muircheartaigh CA, Wright DB. Survey questions about vaguely defined events: the effects of response alternatives. *Public Opin. Q.* 1994; **58**: 241–54.

81. Stem DE, Lamb CW, MacLachlan DL. Remote versus adjacent scale questionnaire designs. *J. Market Res. Soc.* 1978; **20**: 3–13.

82. Market Research Society R&DC. Report of the Second Working Party on Respondent Co-operation: 1977–80. *J. Market Res. Soc.* 1981; **23**: 3–25.

83. Cannell CF, Kahn RL. Interviewing. In: Lindzey G, Aronson E. (eds). *The handbook of social psychology – volume II.* Reading: Addison-Wesley, 1968;

84. US Department of Health, Education and Welfare and National Centre for Health Services Research. *Health survey methods – respondent*

burden. 1977; Proceedings from the 2nd Biennial Conference.

85. Cartwright A. Who responds to postal questionnaires? *J. Epidemiol. Community Health* 1986; **40**: 267–73.

86. Jacoby A. Possible factors affecting response to postal questionnaires: findings from a study of general practitioner services. *J. Public Health Med.* 1990; **12**: 131–5.

87. Hansen RA, Robinson LM. Testing the effectiveness of alternative foot-in-the-door manipulations. *J. Marketing Res.* 1980; **17**: 359–64.

88. Powers DE, Alderman DL. Feedback as an incentive for responding to a mail questionnaire. *Res. Higher Education* 1982; **17**: 207–11.

89. Roszkowski MJ, Bean AG. Believe it or not – Longer questionnaires have lower response rates. *J. Business Psychol.* 1990; **4**: 495–509.

90. Herzog AR, Bachman JG. Effects of questionnaire length on response quality. *Public Opin. Q.* 1981; **45**: 549–59.

91. Jobber D, Sanderson S. The effects of a prior letter and coloured questionnaire paper on mail survey response rates. *J. Market Res. Soc.* 1983; **25**: 339–49.

92. Olivarius NdF, Andreasen AH. Day-of-the-week effect on doctors' response to a postal questionnaire. *Scand. J. Primary Health Care* 1995; **13**: 65–7.

93. Peterson RA, Albaum G, Kerin RA. A note on alternative contact strategies in mail surveys. *J. Market Res. Soc.* 1989; **31**: 409–18.

94. Martin WS, Duncan WJ, Powers TL, Sawyer JC. Costs and benefits of selected response inducement techniques in mail survey research. *J. Business Res.* 1989; **19**: 67–79.

95. Martin WS, Duncan WJ, Sawyer JC. The interactive effects of four response rate inducements in mail questionnaires. *College Student J.* 1984; **18**: 143–9.

96. Faria AJ, Dickinson JR, Filipic TV. The effect of telephone versus letter prenotification on mail survey response rate, speed, quality and cost. *J. Market Res. Soc.* 1990; **32**: 551–68.

97. Allen CT, Schewe CD, Wijk G. More on self-perception theory's foot technique in the pre-call/mail survey setting. *J. Marketing Res.* 1980; **17**: 498–502.

98. Kamins MA. The enhancement of response rates to a mail survey through a labelled probe foot-in-the-door approach. *J. Market Res. Soc.* 1989; **31**: 273–83.

99. Nevin JR, Ford NM. Effects of a deadline and a veiled threat on mail survey responses. *J. Appl. Psychol.* 1976; **61**: 116–18.

100. Blass T, Leichtman SR, Brown RA. The effect of perceived consensus and implied threat upon responses to mail surveys. *J. Soc. Psychol.* 1981; **113**: 213–16.

101. Dommeyer CJ. The effects of negative cover letter appeals on mail survey response. Special Issue: political opinion polling. *J. Market Res. Soc.* 1987; **29**: 445–51.

102. Swan JE, Epley DE, Burns WL. Can follow-up response rates to a mail survey be increased by including another copy of the questionnaire? *Psychological Reports* 1980; **47**: 103–6.

103. Gitelson RJ, Drogin EB. An experiment on the efficacy of a certified final mailing. *J. Leisure Res.* 1992; **24**: 72–8.

104. Kahle LR, Sales BD. Personalization of the outside envelope in mail surveys. *Public Opin. Q.* 1978; **42**: 547–50.

105. Roberts H, Pearson JCG, Dengler R. Impact of a postcard versus a questionnaire as a first reminder in a postal lifestyle survey. *J. Epidemiol. Community Health* 1993; **47**: 334–5.

106. Harris JR, Guffey HJ. Questionnaire returns: Stamps versus business reply envelopes revisited. *J. Marketing Res.* 1978; **15**: 290–3.

107. Jones WH, Linda G. Multiple criteria effects in a mail survey experiment. *J. Marketing Res.* 1978; **15**: 280–4.

108. Labrecque DP. A response rate experiment using mail questionnaires. *J. Marketing* 1978; **42**: 82–3.

109. Hopkins KD, Podolak J. Class-of-mail and the effects of monetary gratuity on the response rates of mailed questionnaires. *J. Exp. Education* 1983; **51**: 169–70.

110. Corcoran KJ. Enhancing the response rate in survey research. *Social Work Research and Abstracts* 1985; **21**: 2.

111. Elkind M, Tryon GS, de Vito AJ. Effects of type of postage and covering envelope on response rates in a mail survey. *Psychological Rep.* 1986; **59**: 279–83.

112. Harvey L. A research note on the impact of class-of-mail on response rates to mailed questionnaires. *J. Market Res. Soc.* 1986; **28**: 299–300.

113. Cartwright A, Windsor J. Some further experiments with factors that might affect the response to postal questionnaires. *Survey Methodology Bulletin* 1989; **25**: 11–15.

114. Duncan W. Mail questionnaires in survey research: A review of respondent inducement techniques. *J. Management* 1979; **5**: 39–55.

115. Armstrong JS, Lusk EJ. Return postage in mail surveys: A meta-analysis. *Public Opin. Q.* 1987; **51**: 233–48.

116. Zeinio RN. Data collection techniques: mail questionnaires. *Am. J. Hosp. Pharmacy* 1980; **37**: 1113–19.

117. Jones WH. Generalizing mail survey inducement methods: Population interactions with anonymity and sponsorship. *Public Opin. Q.* 1979; **43**: 102–11.

118. McDaniel SW, Rao CP. An investigation of respondent anonymity's effect on mailed questionnaire response rate and quality. *J. Market Res. Soc.* 1981; **23**: 150–60.

119. Childers TL, Skinner SJ. Theoretical and empirical issues in the identification of survey respondents. *J. Market Res. Soc.* 1985; **27**: 39–53.

120. Campbell MJ, Waters WE. Does anonymity increase response rate in postal questionnaire surveys about sensitive subjects? A randomised trial. *J. Epidemiol. Community Health* 1990; **44**: 75–6.

121. McKee DO. The effect of using a questionnaire identification code and message about non-response follow-up plans on mail survey response characteristics. *J. Market Res. Soc.* 1992; **34**: 179–91.

122. Green KE, Kvidahl RF. Personalization and offers of results: Effects on response rates. *J. Exp. Education* 1989; **57**: 263–70.

123. Roberts RE, McCrory OF, Forthofer RN. Further evidence on using a deadline to stimulate responses to a mail survey. *Public Opin. Q.* 1978; **42**: 407–10.

124. Childers TL, Pride WM, Ferrell OC. A reassessment of the effects of appeals on response to mail surveys. *J. Marketing Res.* 1980; **17**: 365–70.

125. Woodward JM, McKelvie SJ. Effects of topical interest and mode of address on response to mail survey. *Psychological Rep.* 1985; **57**: 929–30.

126. Worthen BR, Valcarce RW. Relative effectiveness of personalized and form covering letters in initial and follow-up mail surveys. *Psychological Rep.* 1985; **57**: 735–44.

127. Green KE, Stager SF. The effects of personalization, sex, locale, and level taught on educators' responses to a mail survey. *J. Exp. Education* 1986; **54**: 203–6.

128. Wunder GC, Wynn GW. The effects of address personalization on mailed questionnaires response rate, time and quality. *J. Market Res. Soc.* 1988; **30**: 95–101.

129. Wiseman F. A reassessment of the effects of personalization on response patterns in mail surveys. *J. Marketing Res.* 1976; **13**: 110–11.

130. Wagner WG, O'Toole WM. The effects of cover letter format on faculty response rate in mail survey research. *Educational Psychol. Res.* 1985; **5**: 29–37.

131. Dodd DK, Boswell DL, Litwin WJ. Survey response rate as a function of number of signatures, signature ink color, and postscript on covering letter. *Psychological Rep.* 1988; **63**: 538.

132. Dodd DK, Markwiese BJ. Survey response rate as a function of personalized signature on cover letter. *J. Soc. Psychol.* 1987; **127**: 97–8.

133. Salomone PR, Miller GC. Increasing the response rates of rehabilitation counselors to mailed questionnaires. *Rehabilitation Counseling Bulletin* 1978; **22**: 138–41.

134. McKillip J, Lockhart DC. The effectiveness of cover-letter appeals. *J. Soc. Psychol.* 1984; **122**: 85–91.

135. Biner PM. Effects of cover letter appeal and monetary incentives on survey response: A reactance theory application. *Basic Appl. Soc. Psychol.* 1988; **9**: 99–106.

136. Biner PM, Barton DL. Justifying the enclosure of monetary incentives in mail survey cover letters. *Psychol. Marketing* 1990; **7**: 153–62.

137. Dommeyer CJ. Does response to an offer of mail survey results interact with questionnaire interest? *J. Market Res. Soc.* 1985; **27**: 27–38.

138. Hovland EJ, Romberg E, Moreland EF. Non-response bias to mail survey questionnaires within a professional population. *J. Dental Education* 1980; **44**: 270–4.

139. Smith WC, Crombie IK, Campion PD, Knox JD. Comparison of response rates to a postal questionnaire from a general practice and a research unit. *Br. Med. J.* 1994; **1985**: 1483–5.

140. Hansen RA. A self-perception interpretation of the effect of monetary and nonmonetary incentives on mail survey respondent behavior. *J. Marketing Res.* 1980; **17**: 77–83.

141. Furse DH, Stewart DW. Monetary incentives versus promised contribution to charity: new evidence on mail survey response. *J. Marketing Res.* 1982; **19**: 375–80.

142. Paolillo JG, Lorenzi P. Monetary incentives and mail questionnaire response rates. *J. Advertising* 1984; **13**: 46–8.

143. Blythe BJ. Increasing mailed survey responses with a lottery. *Social Work Research and Abstracts* 1986; **22**: 18–19.

144. Trice AD. Maximizing participation in surveys: hotel ratings VII. *J. Soc. Behav. Personality* 1986; **1**: 137–41.

145. Brennan M. The effect of a monetary incentive on mail survey response rates: new data. *J. Market Res. Soc.* 1992; **34**: 173–7.

146. Little RE, Davis AK. Effectiveness of various methods of contact and reimbursement on response rates of pregnant women to a mail questionnaire. *Am. J. Epidemiol.* 1984; **120**: 161–3.

147. Cook JR, Schoeps N, Kim S. Program responses to mail surveys as a function of monetary incentives. *Psychol. Rep.* 1985; **57**: 366.

148. Mortagy AK, Howell JB, Waters WE. A useless raffle. *J. Epidemiol. Community Health* 1985; **39**: 183–4.

149. Woodward A, Douglas B, Miles H. Chance of free dinner increases response to mail questionnaire [letter]. *Int. J. Epidemiol.* 1985; **14**: 641–2.

150. Weltzien RT, McIntyre TJ, Ernst JA, Walsh JA. Crossvalidation of some psychometric properties

of the CSQ and its differential return rate as a function of token financial incentive. *Community Mental Health J.* 1986; **22**: 49–55.

151. Berry SH, Kanouse DE. Physician response to a mailed survey: An experiment in timing of payment. *Public Opin. Q.* 1987; **51**: 102–14.

152. Fiset L, Milgrom P, Tarnai J. Dentists' response to financial incentives in a mail survey of malpractice liability experience. *J. Public Health Dentistry* 1994; **54**: 68–72.

153. Hubbard R, Little EL. Promised contributions to charity and mail survey responses: replication with extension. *Public Opin. Q.* 1988; **52**: 223–30.

154. Gajraj AM, Faria AJ, Dickinson JR. A comparison of the effect of promised and provided lotteries, monetary and gift incentives on mail survey response rate, speed and cost. *J. Market Res. Soc.* 1990; **32**: 141–62.

155. Dommeyer CJ. How form of the monetary incentive affects mail survey response. *J. Market Res. Soc.* 1988; **30**: 379–85.

156. Erdos PL, Morgan AJ. *Professional mail surveys.* New York: McGraw-Hill, 1970.

157. Sudman S. Mail surveys of reluctant professionals. *Evaluation Rev.* 1985; **9**: 349–60.

158. Dommeyer CJ. Offering mail survey results in a lift letter. *J. Market Res. Soc.* 1989; **31**: 399–408.

159. Lovelock CH, Stiff R, Cullwick D, Kaufman IM. An evaluation of the effectiveness of dropoff questionnaire delivery. *J. Marketing Res.* 1976; **13**: 358–64.

160. Layne BH, Thompson DN. Questionnaire page length and return rate. *J. Soc. Psychol.* 1981; **113**: 291–2.

161. de Vaus DA. *Surveys in social research.* 3rd edn. London: UCL Press Ltd, 1991.

162. Barry MJ, Walker-Corkery E, Chang Y, Tyll LT, Cherkin DC, Fowler FJ. Measurement of overall and disease specific health status: does order of the questionnaires make a difference. *J. Health Services Research and Policy* 1996; **1**: 20–7.

Part IV
ANALYTICAL METHODS

INTRODUCTION by KEITH R. ABRAMS

This section of the book considers developments in analytical methodology. Over the past 5–10 years, these have predominantly been concentrated in four separate, but linked areas: Bayesian methods; hierarchical modelling; quality of life research; and economic evaluation.

Bayesian methods, first advocated by the Reverend Thomas Bayes in the 1700s, and for much of the 20th century thought controversial by many statisticians, have developed rapidly in recent years. This development has been fuelled by computational advances and a realisation that such methods, now that they can be applied relatively easily, can make a major contribution in a number of key areas in health services, technology and policy research,[1,2] for example monitoring and interpreting clinical trials and in meta-analysis. The key distinction between the Bayesian approach to statistical inference and the 'classical' approach, is that evidence external to the current study, either in the form of evidence from other studies or as subjective judgements, can be – and is – formally incorporated into the analysis.

The other area of rapid development over approximately the same time period has been that of hierarchical modelling.[3] As in the development of Bayesian methods, the foundations of hierarchical modelling had been laid many years previously – in the early part of the 20th century by Fisher and colleagues working in agricultural research. Again, it has only been with computational advances that such methods can now be applied to problems in healthcare research – an area which does not benefit from the same level of experimental control as agricultural research.

Hierarchical modelling enables proper allowance to be made for the often natural nesting or clustering that occurs in much healthcare research. For example, repeated observations are nested within patients, who themselves are nested within healthcare units. Ignoring such clustering can lead to biased estimation, whilst modelling it often specifically addresses questions of interest, for example identifying where the largest source of variation is.

Quality of life research has over the past decade become an integral part of almost every evaluation of a health technology. In terms of methodological development to date, much work has been undertaken on the development, validation and choice of specific instruments, as has been discussed in Chapter 11 by Fitzpatrick et al. and by Bowling (1996).[4] By comparison, relatively little work has been done on either specific design issues for studies that contain a quality of life element or in the development of appropriate methods of analysis.[5] The widespread use of quality of life measures in both randomised and non-randomised studies and across a diverse range of clinical and service/care delivery settings makes consideration of methods for the design and analysis of such studies particularly timely.

Economic evaluation concerns the systematic evaluation of alternative courses of action in terms of both costs and health outcomes.[6] Whilst economic evaluation within a health technology context has previously not been quite as prolific as the use of quality of life measures, it is quickly reaching a stage where it is almost mandatory that any evaluative study comprises *both* a quality of life and an economic element. During the 1980s much of health economics literature addressed the question of the relevance and justification of economic evaluation within a health context, but by the 1990s the literature had started to consider what the most appropriate approaches and methods are for such evaluations – for example whether it was necessary for them to be conducted *within* a randomised controlled trial. In terms of methodological development, one of the key – if not the overriding – questions is how can uncertainty, in terms of both methodology *and* costs/outcomes, be taken into account in any analysis. In addressing this question a dialogue is developing between methodologists regarding the merits or otherwise of the various possible approaches, and in particular as regards the use of sensitivity analyses compared with stochastic or probabilistic modelling.[7]

Whilst a methodological health technology literature is beginning to be established in all four fields, they will all undoubtedly be active areas of methodological research over the next 5–10 years. This section of the book is organised into five chapters which specifically consider the use of Bayesian methods, design and analysis issues in quality of life research, the evaluation of area-wide technologies, and uncertainty in economic evaluation. Spiegelhalter and colleagues consider the use of Bayesian methods in Health Technology Assessment (HTA). They explain what Bayesian methods are, and consider the advantages and disadvantages of using such methods. Campbell and colleagues and Billingham and colleagues consider different aspects of designing and analysing studies in which quality of life is a primary outcome measure. Whilst Campbell looks at issues concerning the design, and in particular the issue of how large such studies should be, Billingham addresses the problem of how studies in which *both* quality *and* quantity of life are primary outcome measures should be analysed, and the methods currently available for doing so. Gulliford and colleagues consider the design and analysis of studies which evaluate area-wide interventions. The very nature of such evaluative studies means that explicit account must be taken of the hierarchical or clustered nature of the data both in the design, because subjects within the same interventional unit will be more similar than those in different units, and in the analysis. Gray and Briggs consider the issue of uncertainty in economic evaluation; both the extent to which, and the means by which, it is taken into account in the healthcare research literature. In addition they consider issues surrounding the distribution of cost data in economic evaluations.

REFERENCES

1. Berry DA, Stangl DK. *Bayesian Biostatistics*. New York: Marcel Dekker, 1996.
2. Gilks WR, Richardson S, Spiegelhalter DJ. *Markov Chain Monte Carlo in Practice*. London: Chapman & Hall, 1996.
3. Goldstein H. *Multilevel Statistical Models*. 2nd edn. London: Edward Arnold, 1995.
4. Bowling A. *Measuring disease: a review of disease-specific quality of life measurement scales*. Buckingham: Open University Press, 1996.
5. Cox DR, Fitzpatrick R, Fletcher AE, Gore SM, Spiegelhalter DJ, Jones DR. Quality-of-life assessment: can we keep it simple? *Journal of the Royal Statistical Society* 1992; **155**: 353–93.
6. Drummond MF, O'Brien B, Stoddart GL, Torrence G. *Methods for the economic evaluation of health care programmes*. 2nd edn. Oxford: Oxford University Press, 1997.
7. Briggs A, Sculpher M, Buxton M. Uncertainty in the economic evaluation of health care technologies: the role of sensitivity analysis. *Health Analysis* 1994; **3**: 95–104.

16

Bayesian Methods

DAVID J. SPIEGELHALTER, JONATHAN P. MYLES,
DAVID R. JONES and KEITH R. ABRAMS

SUMMARY

Bayesian methods allow the explicit incorporation of external evidence and judgement into the analysis and interpretation of a health technology assessment, and extend naturally to making predictions, designing studies, and analysing policy decisions. We review the literature concerning Bayesian ideas in general, and as specifically applied to randomised controlled trials, observational studies and evidence synthesis. Contrast is made with conventional statistical methods, and suggestions made for the future assimilation of the ideas into health technology assessment.

WHAT THIS CHAPTER IS ABOUT

Much of the standard statistical methodology used in health technology assessment (HTA) revolves around that for the classical randomised controlled trial: these include power calculations at the design stage, methods for controlling Type I errors within sequential monitoring, calculation of P-values and confidence intervals at the final analysis, and meta-analytic techniques for pooling the results of multiple studies. Such methods have served the medical research community well.

The increasing sophistication of HTA studies is, however, highlighting the limitations of these traditional methods. For example, the many sources of evidence and judgement available before a trial may be inadequately summarised by a single 'alternative hypothesis', monitoring may be complicated by simultaneous publication of related studies, multiple subgroups may need to be analysed and reported, and finally the results of the trial may need to be combined with other evidence and formally incorporated within a policy decision. These and other concerns have led many researchers to consider an alternative, Bayesian, basis for statistical methodology.

The basic idea of Bayesian analysis can be illustrated by a simple example and, although we shall try to keep mathematical notation to a minimum in this chapter, it will be very helpful if we are allowed one Greek letter θ (theta) to denote a currently unknown quantity of primary interest. Suppose our quantity θ is the median life-years gained by using an innovative rather than a standard therapy on a defined group of patients. A clinical trial is carried out, following which conventional statistical analysis of the results would typically produce a P-value, an estimate and a confidence interval as summaries of what this particular trial tells us about θ. A Bayesian analysis supplements this by focusing on the question: 'how should this trial change our opinion about θ?' This perspective forces the analyst to explicitly state

(a) a reasonable opinion concerning θ *excluding* the evidence from the trial (known as the prior distribution);
(b) the support for different values of θ based *solely* on data from the trial (known as the likelihood);

and to combine these two sources to produce

(c) a final opinion about θ (known as the posterior distribution).

The final combination is done using a rule in probability theory known as Bayes' theorem, thus giving rise to the 'Bayesian' label. This chapter attempts to provide a guide to the diverse literature on the ramifications of this apparently straightforward idea.

What, then, is a Bayesian approach to HTA? We have defined it[1] as 'the explicit quantitative use of external evidence in the design, monitoring, analysis, interpretation and reporting of a health technology assessment study'.

After describing the methods used in searching and summarising the literature, we provide a brief critique of conventional statistical approaches, and then outline the main features of a general Bayesian philosophy as applied in the context of HTA. Sections then deal in more detail with the source of the prior distribution, randomised trials, observational studies, evidence synthesis and policy making, and finally we provide some suggestions for future research. Mathematical and computational methods will be barely mentioned, and details should be sought in the references provided. The chapter is therefore structured by context rather than methods, although some methodological themes inevitably run throughout; for example, what form of prior distribution is appropriate, how can the posterior distributions be presented, and what is the contrast to traditional methods?

It will be clear that Bayesian methods are a controversial topic in that they may involve the explicit use of subjective judgements in what is supposed to be a rigorous scientific exercise in HTA. We should therefore be quite explicit as to our own subjective biases, which will doubtless be apparent from the organisation and text of this chapter. We favour the Bayesian philosophy, would like to see its use extended in HTA, but feel that this should be carried out cautiously and in parallel with the currently accepted methods.

METHODS USED IN THIS REVIEW

In common with all such methodological reviews, it is essential to define what we mean by 'systematic'. In our full report[2] we have only attempted a comprehensive review (i.e. all references) of 'proper' Bayesian HTA studies, which we define as those in which an informative prior distribution has been given to the quantity of interest. In this chapter we have necessarily been more selective, and so use 'systematic' in the sense of identifying the major issues and references.

We also emphasise that our definition of 'Bayesian' may be more restrictive than that of other researchers, in that we are only concerned with revision of beliefs after evidence, and do not particularly focus on decision-making or decision analysis. We are also not concerned with using Bayes' theorem for prognostic or diagnostic statements.

Our initial electronic search yielded over 4000 papers on 'Bayesian' methods between 1990 and 1998, and all of the abstracts were hand-searched for relevant material. Forward and backward searches, personal collections and hand-searching of recent journals provided additional references, and a subjective judgement as to their relative importance led to the selection in this chapter. The references provided are by no means exhaustive, but should form a convenient starting point for the literature.

THE 'CLASSICAL' STATISTICAL APPROACH IN HTA

It would be misleading to dichotomise statistical methods as either 'classical' or 'Bayesian', since both terms cover a bewildering range of techniques. It is a little more fair to divide conventional statistics into two broad schools: Fisherian and Neyman–Pearson.

1   The Fisherian approach to inference on an unknown intervention effect θ is based on the likelihood function mentioned earlier, which gives rise to an estimate comprising the 'most-likely' value for θ, intervals based on the range of values of θ supported by the data, and the evidence against specified null hypotheses summarised by *P*-values (the chance of getting a result as extreme as that observed were the null hypothesis true).

2   The Neyman–Pearson approach is focused on the chances of making various types of error, so that clinical trials are designed to have a fixed Type I error (the chance of incorrectly rejecting the null hypothesis), usually 5%, and fixed power (one minus the Type II error, the chance of not detecting the alternative hypothesis), often 80% or 90%. The situation is made more complex if a sequential design is used, in which the data are periodically analysed and the trial stopped if sufficiently convincing results obtained. Repeated analysis of the data has a strong effect on the Type I error, since there are many opportunities to obtain a false positive result, and thus the *P*-value and

the confidence interval need adjusting[3] (although this rarely appears to be carried out in the published report of the trial). Such sequential analysis is just one example of a problem of 'multiplicity', in which adjustments need to be made due to multiple analyses being carried out simultaneously. A standard example is the use of Bonferroni adjustments when estimating treatment effects in multiple subsets.

Clinical trials are generally designed from a Neyman–Pearson standpoint, but analysed from a Fisherian perspective.[4] Methods for observational methods and evidence synthesis are generally Fisherian in their perspective, although there is continued disagreement about the need for adjustments for multiple comparisons.[5,6]

Critique

Some Bayesian criticisms apply to both of the conventional approaches outlined above. In particular, *P*-values (and hence confidence intervals, since these are just hypotheses that cannot be rejected) are explicitly concerned with the chance of observing the data (or something more extreme) given certain values of the unknown quantity θ, and use an inverse (and frequently misunderstood) argument for deriving statements about θ. In contrast, the Bayesian perspective directly applies the probability statement to the quantity of interest, and answers the question: what is it reasonable to believe about θ given the data? The other primary criticism of conventional statistical analysis is that it fails to incorporate formally the inevitable background information that is available both at design and analysis.

An Overview of the Bayesian Philosophy in the Context of HTA

In this section we give an overview of some of the generic features of the Bayesian philosophy that find application in HTA. Limited references to the literature are given at this stage, but relevant sections within randomised trials, observational studies and evidence synthesis are identified. We shall use a simple running example to illustrate the general issues: the GREAT trial[7] of early thrombolytic treatment for myocardial infarction, which reported a 49% reduction in mortality (23/148 deaths on control versus 13/163 deaths on active treatment).

Bayes' Theorem

Bayesian analysis is named after the Reverend Thomas Bayes, a non-conformist minister from Tunbridge Wells, England, whose posthumous publication[8] established Bayes' theorem as a fundamental result in probability theory. Suppose θ is some quantity that is currently unknown, for example a specific patient's true diagnosis or the true success rate of a new therapy, and let $p(\theta)$ denote the probability of each possible value of θ (where for the moment we do not concern ourselves with the source of that probability). Suppose we have some observed evidence *y* whose likelihood of occurrence depends on θ, for example a diagnostic test or the results of a clinical trial. This dependence is formalised by a probability $p(y|\theta)$, which is the (conditional) probability of *y* for each possible value of θ. We would like to obtain the new probability for different values of θ, taking account of the evidence *y*; this probability has the conditioning reversed and is denoted $p(\theta|y)$. Bayes' theorem simply says

$$p(\theta|y) \propto p(y|\theta) \times p(\theta).$$

(The proportionality is made into an equality by making probabilities for all possible values of θ add to 1.) The usual term for $p(\theta)$ is the *prior*, for $p(y|\theta)$ the *likelihood*, and for $p(\theta|y)$ the *posterior*, and hence Bayes' theorem simply says that the posterior distribution is proportional to the product of the prior times the likelihood.

Pocock and Spiegelhalter[9] discuss the GREAT trial, in which the unknown quantity θ is the true percentage change in risk of mortality from using home thrombolytic therapy. They obtained a prior distribution for θ expressing belief that 'a 15–20% reduction in mortality is highly plausible, while the extremes of no benefit and a 40% reduction are both unlikely'. This prior is shown in Figure 1(a), while Figure 1(b) shows the likelihood expressing the support by the data for various values of θ. In contrast to the prior distribution, there is strong support for value of θ representing a 40–60% risk reduction.

Figure 1(c) shows the posterior distribution, obtained by multiplying the prior and likelihood together and then making the total area under the curve be equal to one (i.e. 'certainty'). The evidence in the likelihood has been pulled back towards the prior distribution – a formal representation of the belief that the results were 'too good to be true'. The posterior distribution provides an easily interpretable summary of the evidence, and probabilities for hypotheses of interest can then be read off the graph by calculating the relevant areas under the curve. For example, the most likely benefit is around a 24% risk reduction (half that observed in the

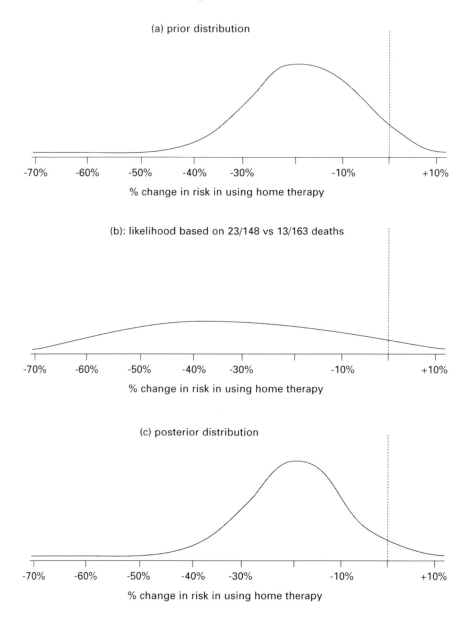

(a) prior distribution

% change in risk in using home therapy

(b): likelihood based on 23/148 vs 13/163 deaths

% change in risk in using home therapy

(c) posterior distribution

% change in risk in using home therapy

Figure 1   *Prior, likelihood and posterior distributions arising from GREAT trial of home thrombolysis.*

trial), the posterior probability that the reduction is at least 50% is only 5%, and a 95% interval runs from a 43% to 0% risk reduction.

The Subjective Interpretation of Probability

The normal use of probability describes long run frequency properties of repeated random events.

This is known as the *frequency* interpretation of probability, and so both Fisherian and Neyman–Pearson schools are often referred to as 'frequentist'. We have allowed probability to refer to generic uncertainty about any unknown quantity, and this is an application of the *subjectivist* interpretation of probability.

The Bayesian perspective thus extends the remit of standard statistical analysis, in that there is explicit concern for what it is reasonable for an observer to believe in the light of data. Thus the perspective of the *consumer* of the analysis is explicitly taken into account: for example, in a trial on a new drug being carried out by a pharmaceutical company, the viewpoints of the company, the regulatory authorities and the medical profession may be substantially different. The *subjective* nature of the analysis is therefore unapologetically emphasised, although it has been criticised elsewhere.[10] The prior distribution shown in Figure 1(a) was based on the subjective judgement of a senior cardiologist, informed by empirical evidence derived from one unpublished and two published trials.

Of course, conclusions strongly based on beliefs that cannot be supported by concrete evidence are unlikely to be widely regarded as convincing, and so it is important to attempt to find consensus on reasonable sources of external evidence. The assessment and use of prior beliefs is discussed further in pp. 280–3.

The Relation to the Use of Bayes' Theorem in Diagnostic Tests

If θ is something that is potentially observable, and $p(\theta)$ is available from known data, then the use of Bayes' theorem is uncontroversial. For example, it has long been established that sensitivity and specificity are insufficient characteristics to judge the result of a diagnostic test for an individual – the disease prevalence is also needed.

From the HTA perspective, the more interesting and controversial context is when the unknown θ is a quantity that is not potentially directly observable, such as the mean benefit of a new therapy in a defined group of patients. There have been many arguments[11–14] for the connection between the use of Bayes' theorem in diagnostic testing and in general clinical research, pointing out that just as the prevalence is required for the assessment of a diagnostic test, so the prior distribution on θ is required to supplement the usual information (*P*-values and confidence intervals) which summarises the likelihood. We need only think of the huge number of clinical trials that are carried out, with few clear successes, to realise that the 'prevalence' of truly effective treatments is low. Thus we should be cautious about accepting extreme results, such as observed in the GREAT trial, at face value.

The Prior Distribution

The next section provides a full discussion of the source and use of prior distributions, including elicitation from experts, the use of 'default'

priors to represent archetypal positions of ignorance, scepticism and enthusiasm and, when multiple related studies are being simultaneously analysed, the assumption of a common prior that may be 'estimated'.

Two important points should be emphasised immediately:

1 Despite the name 'prior' suggesting a temporal relationship, it is quite feasible that a prior distribution is decided *after* seeing the results of a study, since it is simply intended to summarise reasonable uncertainty given evidence external to the study in question.
2 There is no such thing as the 'correct' prior. Instead, researchers have suggested using a 'community' of prior distributions expressing a range of reasonable opinions.

Predictions

Suppose we wish to predict some future observations z, which depend on the unknown quantity θ through a distribution $p(z|\theta)$: for example, z may be the difference in outcomes to be observed on some future patients. Since our current uncertainty concerning θ is expressed by the posterior distribution $p(\theta|y)$, then we can integrate out the unknown θ from the product of $p(z|\theta)$ and $p(\theta|y)$ to obtain the *predictive* distribution $p(z|y)$ for the future observations z.

Such predictive distributions are useful in many contexts: Berry and Stangl[15] describe their use in design and power calculations, model checking, and in deciding whether to conduct a future trial. See pp. 284–6 and 288 for applications of predictions.

Decision-Making

There is a long history of attempts to apply the theory of optimal decision-making to medicine, in which (posterior) probabilities are combined with utilities, although the impact has been rather limited: Healy[16] gives a good tutorial introduction. Relevant applications within the HTA context include the explicit use of utility functions in the design and monitoring of clinical trials (see pp. 285–6 and 288 for further discussion and other examples).

Multiplicity

The context of clinical trials may present issues of 'multiple analyses of accumulating data, analyses of multiple endpoints, multiple subsets of patients, multiple treatment group contrasts and interpreting the results of multiple clinical trials'.[17] Observational data may feature multiple institutions, and meta-analysis involve synthesis of multiple studies. The general Bayesian approach to multiplicity involves specifying a common prior distribution for the substudies that expresses a belief in the expected 'similarity' of all the individual unknown quantities being estimated. This produces a degree of pooling, in which an individual study's results tend to be 'shrunk' towards the average result by an amount depending on the variability between studies and the precision of the individual study: relevant contexts include subset analysis, between-centre variability, and random-effects meta-analysis. This is discussed on pp. 283 and 286.

Computational Issues

The Bayesian approach applies probability theory to a model derived from substantive knowledge and can, in theory, deal with realistically complex situations. It has to be acknowledged, however, that the computations may be difficult, with the specific problem being to carry out the integrations necessary to obtain the posterior distributions of interest in situations where non-standard prior distributions are used, or where there are additional 'nuisance parameters' in the model. These problems in integration for many years restricted Bayesian applications to rather simple examples. However, there has recently been enormous progress in methods for Bayesian computation, generally exploiting modern computer power to carry out simulations known as Markov Chain Monte Carlo (MCMC) methods.[18]

Schools of Bayesians

It is important to emphasise that there is no such thing as *the* Bayesian approach, and that many ideological differences exist between the researchers whose work is discussed in this chapter. Four levels of Bayesian approach, of increasing 'purity', may be identified:

1 The *empirical* Bayes approach, in which a prior distribution is estimated from multiple experiments. Analyses and reporting are in frequentist terms.
2 The *reference* Bayes approach, in which a Bayesian interpretation is given to the conclusions expressed as posterior distributions, but an attempt is made to use 'objective' prior distributions.
3 The *proper* Bayes approach, in which informative prior distributions are used based on available evidence, but conclusions are summarised by posterior distributions without explicit incorporation of utility functions.

4 The *decision–theoretic* or 'full' Bayes approach, in which explicit utility functions are used to make decisions based on maximising expected utility.

Our focus in this chapter is on the third, proper, school of Bayesianism.

Further Reading

A wide-ranging introductory chapter by Berry and Stangl[15] in their textbook[19] covers a whole range of modelling issues, including elicitation, model choice, computation, prediction and decision-making. Non-technical tutorial articles include those by Lewis and Wears[20] and Lilford and Braunholtz.[21] Other authors emphasise different merits of Bayesian approaches in HTA: Eddy et al.[22] concentrate on the ability to deal with varieties of outcomes, designs and sources of bias, Breslow[23] stresses the flexibility with which multiple similar studies can be handled, Etzioni and Kadane[24] discuss general applications in the health sciences with an emphasis on decision-making, while Freedman[25] and Lilford and Braunholtz[21] concentrate on the ability to combine 'objective' evidence with clinical judgement.

There is a huge methodological statistical literature on general Bayesian methods, much of it quite mathematical. Cornfield[26] provides a theoretical justification of the Bayesian approaches, in terms of ideas such as *coherence*. A rather old article[27] is still one of the best introductions to the Bayesian philosophy. Good tutorial introductions are provided by Lindley[28] and Barnett,[29] while more recent books, in order of increasing technical difficulty, include those by Lee,[30] Gelman et al.,[31] Carlin and Louis,[32] and Bernardo and Smith.[33]

WHERE DOES THE PRIOR DISTRIBUTION COME FROM?

There is no denying that prior beliefs exist in medicine. For example, in the context of clinical trials, Peto and Baigent[34] state that 'it is generally unrealistic to hope for large treatment effects' but that 'it might be reasonable to hope that a new treatment for acute stroke or acute myocardial infarction could reduce recurrent stroke or death in hospital from 10% to 9% or 8%, but not to hope that it could halve in-hospital mortality'. However, turning informally expressed opinions into a mathematically expressible prior distribution is perhaps the most controversial aspect of Bayesian analysis. Four broad approaches are outlined below, ranging from the elicitation of subjective opinion to the use of statistical models to estimate the prior from data. Sensitivity analysis to alternative assumptions is considered vital, whatever the method used to construct the prior distribution.

From a mathematical and computational perspective, it is extremely convenient if the prior distribution is a member of a family of distributions that is *conjugate* to the form of the likelihood, in the sense that they 'fit together' to produce a posterior distribution that is in the same family as the prior distribution. For example, many likelihoods for treatment effects can be assumed to have an approximately normal shape,[35] and thus in these circumstances it will be convenient to use a normally shaped prior (the conjugate family), provided it approximately summarises the appropriate external evidence. Similarly, when the observed data are to be proportions (implying a binomial likelihood), the conjugate prior is a member of the 'beta' family of distributions which provide a flexible way of expressing beliefs about the magnitude of a true unknown frequency.

Modern computing power is, however, reducing the need for conjugacy, and in this section we shall concentrate on the source of the prior rather than its precise mathematical form.

Elicitation of Opinion

A true subjectivist Bayesian approach only requires a prior distribution that expresses the personal opinions of an individual but, if the health technology assessment is to be generally accepted by a wider community, it would appear to be essential that the prior distributions have some evidential or at least consensus support. In some circumstances there may, however, be little 'objective' evidence available and summaries of expert opinion may be indispensable.

There is a very large literature on eliciting subjective probability distributions from experts, with some good early references on statistical[36] and psychological aspects,[37] as well as on methods for pooling distributions obtained from multiple experts.[38] Chaloner[39] provides a thorough review of prior elicitation for clinical trials, including interviews with clinicians, postal questionnaires, and the use of an interactive computer program to draw a prior distribution. She concludes that fairly simple methods are adequate, using interactive feedback with a scripted interview, providing experts with a systematic literature review, using 2.5% and 97.5% percentiles, and using as many experts as possible. Berry and Stangl[15] discuss methods for eliciting conjugate priors and checking whether the assessments are consistent with each other.

Kadane and Wolfson[40] distinguish between *experiments to learn* for which only the prior of the experimenter needs to be considered, and *experiments to prove*, in which the priors (and utilities) of observers to be persuaded need to be considered. They discuss general methods of elicitation, and give an example applied to an observational study in healthcare.

The methods used in case studies can be divided into four main categories using increasingly formal methods:

1 *Informal discussion*: examples include Rosner and Berry,[41] who consider a trial of Taxol in metastatic breast cancer, in which a beta prior for the overall success rate was assessed using a mean 0.25 and 50% belief that the true success rate lay between 15% and 35%. Similarly, Lilford and Braunholtz[21] describe how priors were obtained from two doctors for the relative risk of venous thrombosis from oral contraceptives.

2 *Structured interviewing and formal pooling of opinion*: Freedman and Spiegelhalter[42] describe an interviewing technique in which a set of experts were individually interviewed and hand-drawn plots of their prior distributions elicited. Deliberate efforts were made to prevent the opinions being overconfident (too 'tight'). The distributions were converted to histograms and averaged to produce a composite prior. The approach was subsequently used in a bladder cancer trial and these priors used later in discussing initial and interim power of the study[43,44] – see p. 284.

3 *Structured questionnaires*: a technique in which a histogram is directly elicited via a questionnaire was used by Abrams et al.[45] for a trial of neutron therapy, and by Parmar et al.[46] to elicit prior distributions for the effect of a new radiotherapy regime (CHART). In this latter study the possible treatment effect was discretised into 5% bands, a distribution over these bands obtained from each of nine clinicians and an arithmetic mean taken.

4 *Computer-based elicitation*: Chaloner et al.[47] provide a detailed case study of the use of a rather complex computer program that interactively elicited distributions from five clinicians for a trial of prophylactic therapy in AIDS.

Summary of Evidence

If the results of previous similar studies are available it is clear that they may be used as the basis for a prior distribution. Three main approaches have been used:

1   *Use of a single previous trial result as a prior distribution*: Brown et al.[48] and Spiegelhalter et al.[35] both provide examples of prior distributions proportional to the likelihoods arising from a single pilot trial.
2   *Direct use of a meta-analysis of many previous studies*: Lau et al.[49] point out that cumulative meta-analysis can be given a Bayesian interpretation in which the prior for each trial is obtained from the meta-analysis of preceding studies, while Smith et al.[50] and Higgins and Whitehead[51] both use a meta-analysis of past meta-analyses as a basis for a prior distribution for the degree of heterogeneity in a current meta-analysis.
3   *Use of previous data in some discounted form*: Previous studies may not be directly related to the one in question, and we may wish to discount past evidence in some way. This approach has been most widely used in studies with non-concurrent controls (see p. 287, observational studies).

Default Priors

It would clearly be attractive to have prior distributions that could be taken 'off-the-shelf', rather than having to consider all available evidence external to the study in their construction. Four main suggestions can be identified:

1   *'Non-informative' priors*: There has been substantial research in the Bayesian literature into so-called *non-informative* or *reference* priors, which usually take the form of uniform distributions over the range of interest. Formally, a uniform distribution means the posterior distribution has the same shape as the likelihood function, which in turn means that the resulting Bayesian intervals and estimates will essentially match the traditional results, so that posterior tail areas will match one-sided *P*-values (ignoring any adjustment for sequential analysis).
    Results with such reference priors are generally quoted as one part of a Bayesian analyses. In particular, Burton[52] suggests that most doctors interpret frequentist confidence intervals as posterior distributions, and also that information prior to a study tends to be vague, and that therefore results from a study should be presented by performing a Bayesian analysis with a non-informative prior and quoting posterior probabilities for the parameter of interest being in various regions.

2   *'Sceptical' priors*: Informative priors that express scepticism about large treatment effects have been put forward both as a reasonable expression of doubt, and as a way of controlling early stopping of trials on the basis of fortuitously positive results. Mathematically speaking a sceptical prior about a treatment effect will have a mean of zero and some spread which determines the degree of scepticism. Fletcher et al.[53] use such a prior, while Spiegelhalter et al.[35] argue that a reasonable degree of scepticism may be equivalent to feeling that the alternative hypothesis is optimistic, formalised by a prior with only a small probability that the treatment effect is as large as the alternative hypothesis.
    This approach has been used in a number of case studies,[46,54] and has been suggested as a basis for monitoring trials[55] (see p. 285). A senior FDA biostatistician[56] has stated that he 'would like to see [sceptical priors] applied in more routine fashion to provide insight into our decision making'.
3   *'Enthusiastic' priors*: As a counter-balance to the pessimism expressed by the sceptical prior, Spiegelhalter et al.[35] suggest a prior centred on the alternative hypothesis and with a low chance (say 5%) that the true treatment benefit is negative. Use of such a prior has been reported in case studies[54,57] and as a basis for conservatism in the face of early negative results[55] (see p. 285).
4   *Priors with a point mass at zero ('lump-and-smear' priors)*: The traditional statistical approach expresses a qualitative distinction between the role of a null hypothesis, generally of no treatment effect, and alternative hypotheses. A prior distribution that retains this distinction would place a 'lump' of probability on the null hypothesis, and 'smear' the remaining probability over the whole range of alternatives. Cornfield repeatedly argued for this approach, which he termed the 'relative betting odds' on the null hypothesis,[58] both on a practical basis and as a rebuttal to the criticism of 'sampling to foregone conclusion' (see p. 285). It has been used in a cancer trial[59] and for sensitivity analysis in trial reporting[60] (see p. 286). Although such an analysis provides an explicit probability that the null hypothesis is true, and so appears to answer the question of interest, the prior might be somewhat more realistic were the lump to be placed on a small range of values representing the more plausible null hypothesis of 'no effective difference'.

Exchangeability and Hierarchical Models

The concept of exchangeability now needs to be introduced. Suppose we are interested in making inferences on many parameters $\theta_1, \ldots, \theta_k$ measured on k 'units' which may, for example, be subsets or clinics or trials. We can identify three different assumptions:

1 All the θs are identical, in which case all the data can be pooled and the individual units forgotten.
2 All the θs are entirely unrelated, in which case the results from each unit are analysed independently (for example using a fully specified prior distribution).
3 The θs are assumed to be 'similar' in the following sense. Suppose we were blinded as to which unit was which, and all we had was a label, say, A, B, C and so on. Then our prior opinion about any particular set of θs would not be affected by the labels, in that we have no reason to think specific units are systematically different. Such a set of θs are called 'exchangeable',[33] and this is mathematically equivalent to assuming they are drawn at random from some population distribution. Note that there does not need to be any actual sampling – perhaps these k units are the only ones that exist.

We emphasise that an assumption of exchangeability is a judgement based on our knowledge of the context, and if there are known reasons to suspect specific units are systematically different, then those reasons need to be modelled.

The Bayesian approach to multiplicity is thus to integrate all the units into a single model, in which it is assumed that $\theta_1, \ldots, \theta_k$ are drawn from some common prior distribution whose parameters are unknown: this is known as a hierarchical model. These unknown parameters may then be estimated directly from the data. Louis[61] reviews the area and provides a detailed case study, while other examples in clinical trials are described on p. 286.

A Guide to the Bayesian HTA Literature: Randomised Controlled Trials

General Arguments

Randomised controlled trials (RCTs) have provided fertile territory for arguments between alternative statistical philosophies. There are many specific issues in which a distinct Bayesian approach is identifiable, such as the ethics of randomisation, power calculations, monitoring, subset analysis, alternative designs and so on, and these are dealt with in separate sections below.

There are also a number of general discussion papers on the relevance of Bayesian methods to trials. These include general tutorial introductions at a non-technical[20] and slightly more technical level,[45] while Brophy and Joseph[62] explain the Bayesian approach by demonstrating its use in re-analysing data from the GUSTO trial of different thrombolytic regimes, using prior information from other studies. More detailed but non-mathematical discussions are given by Cornfield[58] and Kadane,[63] who particularly emphasises the internal consistency of the Bayesian approach, and welcomes the need for explicit prior distributions and loss function as producing scientific openness and honesty. Pocock and Hughes[64] again provide a non-mathematical discussion concentrating on estimation issues in trials, while Armitage[65] attempts a balanced view of the competing methodologies. Particular emphasis has been placed on the ability of Bayesian methods to take full advantage of the accumulating evidence provided by small trials.[66,67]

Somewhat more technical reviews are given by Spiegelhalter and colleagues.[35,68] Berry[69,70] has argued for a Bayesian decision-theoretic basis for clinical trial design, and this will be discussed further on p. 285.

Finally we refer to a special issue of *Statistics in Medicine* on 'Methodological and Ethical Issues in Clinical Trials', containing papers both for[68,69,71] and against[72] the Bayesian perspective, and featuring incisive discussion by Armitage, Cox and others.

Ethics and Randomisation

Is randomisation necessary?

Randomisation has two traditional justifications: it ensures that treatment groups are directly comparable (up to the play of chance), and it forms a physical basis for the probability distributions underlying the statistical procedures. Since Bayesian probability models are derived from subjective beliefs and do not require any underlying random mechanism, the latter requirement is irrelevant, and this has led some to question the need for randomisation at all, provided alternative methods of balancing groups can be established. For example, Urbach[71] argues that a 'Bayesian analysis of clinical trials affords a valid, intuitively plausible rationale for selective controls, and marks out a more limited role for randomisation than it is generally accorded', while Kadane[73] suggests updating clinician's priors and only assigning treatments that at least one clinician considers optimal. Papineau[74] refutes Urbach's position and claims that despite it not being essential for statistical inference, experimental randomisation forms a vital role in drawing causal conclusions. The relationship between randomisation and causal inferences is beyond the scope of this chapter, but in general the need for sound experimental design appears to dominate philosophical statistical issues.[75] In fact, Berry and Kadane[76] suggest that if there are several parties who make different decisions and observe different data, randomisation may be a strictly optimal procedure since it enables each observer to draw their own appropriate conclusions.

When is it ethical to randomise?

If we agree that randomisation is in theory useful, then the issue arises of when it is ethical to randomise. This is closely associated with the process of deciding when to stop a trial (discussed further on p. 285) and is often represented as a balance between individual and collective ethics.[77] It has been argued that a Bayesian model naturally formalises the individual ethical position,[78,79] in that it explicitly confronts the personal belief in the clinical superiority of one treatment.

Specification of Null Hypotheses

Attention in a trial usually focuses on the null hypothesis of treatment equivalence expressed by $\theta = 0$, but realistically this is often not the only hypothesis of interest. Increased costs, toxicity and so on may mean that a certain improvement would be necessary before considering the new treatment clinically superior, and we shall denote this value θ_{SUP}. Similarly, the new treatment might not actually be considered clinically inferior unless the true benefit were less than some threshold denoted θ_{INF}. The interval between θ_{INF} and θ_{SUP} has been termed the 'range of equivalence':[80] often θ_{INF} is taken to be 0.

This is not a specifically Bayesian idea,[65] and there are several published examples of the elicitation and use of such ranges of equivalence.[42,81]

Alternative Hypotheses, Power and Sample Size of Trials

Trials have traditionally been designed to have reasonable power, defined as the chance of correctly detecting an alternative hypothesis. Power

is generally set to 80% or 90%, and the alternative hypothesis may best be defined as being both 'realistic and important'. The requirement for the trial being designed to detect a plausible difference has naturally led to the use of prior distributions: either the prior mean could be the alternative hypothesis or the power for each value of θ could be averaged with respect to the prior distribution to obtain an 'expected' or 'average' power, which should be a more realistic assessment of the chance that the trial will yield a positive conclusion. It is natural to express a cautionary note issued on projecting from previous studies,[82] and possible techniques for discounting past studies is very relevant (see pp. 287–8).

The use of power calculations is so rooted into trial design that alternatives are rarely mentioned. However, it is natural within a Bayesian context to be less concerned with hypothesis testing and more focused on the eventual precision of the posterior distribution of the treatment effect. There is an extensive literature on non-power-based Bayesian sample size calculations which may be very relevant for trial design.[83,84]

Monitoring and Interim Analyses and Predictions

Introduction

Whether or not to stop a trial early is a complex ethical, financial, organisational and scientific issue, in which statistical analysis plays a considerable role.[77] Furthermore, the monitoring of sequential clinical trials can be considered the 'front line' between Bayesian and frequentist approaches, and the reasons for their divergence 'reach to the very foundations of the two paradigms'.[24]

Four main statistical approaches can be identified:

1 *Formal frequentist*: attempts to retain a fixed Type I error through tightly controlled stopping boundaries. Whitehead[3,72] is a major proponent, and Jennison and Turnbull[85] provide a detailed review.

2 *Informal non-Bayesian*: best exemplified in trials influenced by Richard Peto's group, in which protocols state[86] that the data monitoring committee should only alert the steering committee if there is '**both** (a) 'proof beyond reasonable doubt' that for all, or for some, types of patient one particular treatment is clearly indicated . . ., **and** (b) evidence that might reasonably be expected to influence the patient management of many clinicians who are already aware of the results of other main studies'.

3 *Informal Bayesian*: uses probabilities derived from a posterior distribution for monitoring, without formally pre-specifying a stopping criterion.

4 *Decision-theoretic Bayesian:* explicitly assesses the losses associated with consequences of stopping or continuing the study.

Here we briefly describe some of the huge literature on this subject.

Monitoring using the posterior distribution

Following the 'informal Bayesian' approach, it is natural to consider terminating a trial when one is confident that one treatment is better than the other, and this may be formalised by assessing the posterior probability that the treatment benefit θ lies above or below some boundary, such as the ends of the range of equivalence. It is generally recommended that a range of priors are considered, and possible applications have been reported in a variety of trials.[41,46,59,87–90] Fayers et al.[55] provide a tutorial on such an approach.

Monitoring using predictions

Investigators and funders are often concerned with the question: given the data so far, what is the chance of getting a 'significant' result? The traditional approach to this question is 'stochastic curtailment',[91] which calculates the conditional power of the study, given the data so far, for a range of alternative hypotheses.[85]

From a Bayesian perspective it is natural to average such conditional powers with respect to the current posterior distribution, just as the pre-trial power was averaged with respect to the prior to produce the average or expected power (see p. 284). This has been illustrated in a variety of contexts.[23,92–94] The technique has been used with results that currently show approximate equivalence to justify the 'futility' of continuing,[95] and may be particularly useful for data monitoring committees and funders[96] when accrual or event rates are lower than expected.

Monitoring using a formal loss function

The full Bayesian decision-theoretic approach requires the specification of losses associated with all combinations of possible true underlying states and all possible actions. The decision whether to terminate a trial is then, in theory, based on the whether termination has a lower expected loss than continuing, where the expectation is with respect to the current posterior distribution, and the consequences of continuing have to consider all possible future actions – the computationally intensive technique of 'dynamic programming' is required.

For example, Berry et al.[97] consider a trial of influenza vaccine for Navajo children, in which they attempt to model the consequences of continuing a trial for each successive month. The level of detail required for such an analysis has been criticised as being unrealistic,[23,35] but it has been argued that trade-offs between benefits for patients within and outside the trial should be explicitly confronted.[24]

The frequentist properties of Bayesian methods

Although the long-run sampling properties of Bayesian procedures should in theory be irrelevant, there have been many investigations of these properties.[41,98–100] In particular, Grossman et al.[101] show that a sceptical prior (p. 282), centred on zero and with precision equivalent to that arising from an 'imaginary' trial of around 26% of the planned sample size, gives rise to boundaries that have Type I error around 5% for five interim analyses, with good power and expected sample size. Thus an 'off-the-shelf' Bayesian procedure has been shown to have good frequentist properties.

One contentious issue is 'sampling to a foregone conclusion'.[102] This mathematical result proves that repeated calculation of posterior tail areas will, *even if the null hypothesis is true*, eventually lead a Bayesian procedure to reject that null hypothesis. This does not, at first, seem an attractive frequentist property of a Bayesian procedure. Nevertheless, Cornfield[103] argued strongly that you would only be concerned about this behaviour were you to entertain the possibility that the null hypothesis were precisely true, and if this is the case then you should be placing a lump of probability on it, as discussed on p. 282. He shows that if you assume such a lump, however small, then the problem disappears. Breslow[23] agrees with this solution, but Armitage retains his concern.[104]

The Role of 'Scepticism' in Confirmatory Studies

After a clinical trial has given a positive result for a new therapy, there remains the problem of whether a confirmatory study is needed. Fletcher et al.[53] argue that the first trial's results might be treated with scepticism, and Berry[105] points out that using a sceptical prior is a means of dealing with 'regression to the mean', in which extreme results tend to return to the average over time. Parmar et al.[106] consider two trials and show that, when using a reasonable sceptical prior, doubt can remain after both the first trial and the confirmatory trial about whether the new treatment provides a clinically important benefit.

Sensitivity Analysis, Robustness and Reporting

An integral part of any good statistical report is a sensitivity analysis of assumptions concerning the form of the model (the likelihood). Bayesian approaches have the additional concern of sensitivity to the prior distribution, both in view of its controversial nature and because it is by definition a subjective assumption that is open to valid disagreement. There is therefore a need to consider the impact of a 'community of priors'.[107]

A 'robust' Bayesian approach, in which an attempt is made to characterise the class of priors leading to a given decision, is illustrated by Hughes[108] and others.[109,110] There is limited experience of reporting such analyses in the medical literature, and it has been suggested that a separate 'interpretation' section is required to display how the data in a study would add to a range of currently held opinions.[35]

Subset and Multi-Centre Analysis

The discussion on multiplicity on pp. 277–80 has already described how multiple simultaneous inferences may be made by assuming a common prior distribution with unknown parameters, provided an assumption of exchangeability (the prior does not depend on units' identities) is appropriate. Within the context of clinical trials this has immediate relevance to the issue of estimating treatment effects in subgroups of patients.

Published applications are generally based on assigning a reference (uniform) prior on the overall treatment effect, and then assuming the subgroup-specific deviations from that overall effect have a common prior distribution with zero mean. This prior expresses scepticism about widely differing subgroup effects. Donner[111] sets out the basic ideas, and Simon and co-authors elaborate the techniques in several examples.[112,113] Explicit estimation of individual institutional effects[114,115] relates strongly to the methods used for institutional comparisons of patient outcomes (see p. 288).

Cost–Effectiveness of Carrying Out Trials: 'Payback Models'

'By explicitly taking into consideration the costs and benefits of a trial, Bayesian statistical methods permit estimation of the value to a health care organization conducting a randomised trial instead of continuing to treat patients in the absence of more information.'[116] Detsky[117] conducted an early attempt to model the impact of a trial in terms of future lives saved. In other examples,[116,118] sample-sizes are explicitly determined by a trade-off between the cost of the trial and the expected future benefit.

More generally, the role of decision analysis in health services research has been emphasised by Lilford and Royston.[119]

Data-Dependent Allocation

So far we have only covered standard randomisation designs, but a full decision-theoretic approach to trial design would consider data-dependent allocation so that, for example, in order to minimise the number of patients getting the inferior treatment, the proportion randomised to the apparently superior treatment could be increased as the trial proceeded. An extreme example is Zelen's 'play-the-winner' rule in which the next patient is given the currently superior treatment, and randomisation is dispensed with entirely.[120] Tamura et al.[121] report one of the few adaptive clinical trials to take place, in patients with depressive disorder. The review by Armitage[122] describes the practical problems in carrying out such trials.

Alternative Trial Designs

Equivalence Trials

There is a large statistical literature on trials designed to establish equivalence between therapies. From a Bayesian perspective the solution is straightforward: define a region of equivalence (see p. 284) and calculate the posterior probability that the treatment difference lies in this range – a threshold of 95% or 90% might be chosen to represent strong belief in equivalence. Several examples of this remarkably intuitive approach have been reported.[23,123–126]

Crossover and repeated N-of-1 trials

The Bayesian approach to crossover designs, in which each patient is given two or more treatments in an order selected at random, is fully reviewed by Grieve.[127] More recent references concentrate on Gibbs sampling approaches.[128,129] N-of-1 studies can be thought of as repeated crossover trials in which interest focusses on the response of an individual patient, and Zucker et al.[130] pool multiple N-of-1 studies using a hierarchical model.

Factorial designs

Factorial trials, in which multiple treatments are given simultaneously to patients in a structured design, can be seen as another example of multiplicity and hence a candidate for hierarchical models. Simon and Freedman[131] and Miller and Seaman[132] suggest suitable prior assumptions that avoid the need to decide whether interactions do or do not exist.

Other Aspects of Drug Development

Other aspects of drug development include:

1 *Pharmacokinetics*: The 'population' approach to pharmacokinetics is well established, and is essentially an empirical Bayes procedure. Proper Bayes analysis has been extensively reported by Wakefield and colleagues.[133,134]

2 *Phase 1 trials*: Phase 1 trials are conducted to determine that dosage of a new treatment which produces a risk of a toxic response which is deemed to be acceptable. The primary Bayesian contribution to the development of methodology for Phase 1 trials has been the Continual Reassessment Method developed by O'Quigley and colleagues,[135] and extended by Goodman et al.[136] amongst others. A prior for a parameter underlying a dose–toxicity curve is updated sequentially and used to find the current 'best' estimate of the dosage.

3 *Phase 2 trials*: Phase 2 clinical trials are carried out in order to discover whether a new treatment is promising enough to be submitted to a controlled Phase 3 trial, and often a number of doses might be compared. Bayesian work has focussed on monitoring and sample size determination. Monitoring on the basis of posterior probability of exceeding a desired threshold response rate has been recommended by Mehta and Cain,[137] while Heitjan[57] adapts the proposed use of sceptical and enthusiastic priors (see p. 285).

Thall and co-workers have also developed stopping boundaries for Phase 2 studies based on posterior probabilities of clinically important events,[138] although Stallard[139] has criticised this approach as being demonstrably suboptimal when evaluated using a full decision-theoretic model with a monetary loss function. Finally, Whitehead and colleagues[140,141] have taken a full decision-theoretic approach to allocating subjects between Phase 2 and Phase 3 studies.

A GUIDE TO THE BAYESIAN HTA LITERATURE: OBSERVATIONAL STUDIES

Since the probability models used in Bayesian analysis do not need to be based on actual randomisation, non-randomised studies can be analysed in exactly the same manner as randomised comparisons, perhaps with extra attention to adjusting for co-variates in an attempt to control for possible baseline differences in the treatment groups. The dangers of this approach have, of course, been well described in the medical literature,[142] but nevertheless there are circumstances where randomisation is either impossible or where there is substantial valuable information available in historical data. There is, of course, then a degree of subjective judgement about the comparability of groups, which fits well into the acknowledged judgement underlying all Bayesian reasoning.

The fullest Bayesian analysis of non-randomised data for HTA is probably the Confidence Profile Method of Eddy and colleagues,[143] but discussion of this technique is placed within evidence synthesis (p. 288). In this section we consider three aspects of non-randomised comparisons: direct analysis of epidemiological data including case-control studies; the use of historical controls; and comparisons of institutions on the basis of their outcomes.

Epidemiological Data

The results from an epidemiological study, whether of a cohort or case-control design, provide a likelihood which can be combined with prior information using standard Bayesian methods. Case-control designs have been considered in detail,[144,145] while Lilford and Braunholz's tutorial article is based on likelihoods arising from case-control studies.[21]

There is also a substantial literature on Bayesian methods for complex epidemiological modelling, particularly concerning problems with measurement error and spatial correlation.[146–148]

Using Historical Controls

A Bayesian basis for the use of historical controls in clinical trials, generally in addition to some contemporaneous controls, was first suggested by Pocock,[149] and has since been particularly developed within the field of carcinogenicity studies.[150] The crucial issue is the extent to which the historical information can be considered equivalent to contemporaneous data. Three broad approaches have been taken.

1   Assume the historical control groups are exchangeable with the current control group, and hence build or assume a hierarchical model for the response within each group.[151,152] This leads to a degree of pooling between the control groups, depending on their observed or assumed heterogeneity.
2   If there is only one historical group, then assume a parameter representing the probability that any past individual is exchangeable with current individuals, so discounting the contribution of past data to the likelihood, as used by Berry[15,153] in reanalysis of the ECMO study.
3   Assume that the parameter being estimated in historical data is some function of the parameter that is of interest, thus explicitly modelling potential biases, as in the Confidence Profile Method.[143]

Institutional Comparisons

A classic 'multiplicity' problem arises in the use of performance indicators to compare institutions with regard to their health outcomes or use of particular procedures. Analogously to subset estimation (p. 286), hierarchical models can be used to make inferences based on estimating a common prior or 'population' distribution.[154,155] An additional benefit of using Markov Chain Monte Carlo methods is the ability to derive uncertainty intervals around the rank order of each institution.[156]

A GUIDE TO THE BAYESIAN HTA LITERATURE: EVIDENCE SYNTHESIS AND POLICY-MAKING

Meta-analysis

Hedges[157] reviews Bayesian approaches to meta-analysis, which is similar to that assumed for random effects models, but requires that prior distributions are specified for the mean effect size and the between- and within-study variances. This leads to wider interval estimates. Several authors[158–160] have implemented a hierarchical model. Empirical Bayes approaches have received most attention in the literature until recently, largely because of computational difficulties in the use of fully Bayesian modelling.[161–163]

Cross-Design Synthesis

As noted when discussing observational studies, in some circumstances randomised evidence will be less than adequate due to economic, organisational or ethical considerations.[164] Considering all the available evidence, including that from non-randomised studies may then be necessary or advantageous. Cross-design synthesis, an approach for synthesising evidence from different sources, has been outlined[165] and subsequently applied to a data on breast cancer screening.[166,167] A Bayesian hierarchical model approach specifically allows for the quantitative within- and between-sources heterogeneity, and for a priori beliefs regarding qualitative differences between the various sources of evidence. It has yet to be established when such analyses are appropriate, as there is concern that including studies with poorer designs will weaken the analysis, though this issue is partially addressed by conducting sensitivity analyses under various assumptions.

Confidence Profile Method

This approach was developed by Eddy and colleagues and promulgated in a book with numerous worked examples and accompanying software,[143] as well as tutorial articles.[22,168] They use directed conditional independence graphs to represent the qualitative way in which multiple contributing sources of evidence relate to the quantity of interest, explicitly allowing the user to discount studies due to their potential internal bias or their limited generalisability. Their analysis is essentially Bayesian, although it is possible to avoid prior specification and use only the likelihoods. The necessity to make explicit subjective judgements, and the limited capacity and friendliness of the software, has perhaps limited the application of this technique.

Policy-Making

The use of Bayesian ideas in decision-making is a huge area of research and application, in which attention is more focussed on the utility of consequences rather than the use of Bayesian methods to revise beliefs.[169] This activity blends naturally into cost–effectiveness analysis which is outside the domain of this chapter, but nevertheless the subjective interpretation of probability is essential, since the expressions of uncertainty required for a decision analysis can rarely be based purely on empirical data.

The journal *Medical Decision Making* contains an extensive collection of policy analyses based on maximising expected utility, some of which particularly stress the importance of Bayesian considerations.[170]

IMPLICATIONS FOR FUTURE RESEARCH

The HTA field has been slow to adopt Bayesian methods, perhaps due to a reluctance to use prior opinions, unfamiliarity with the techniques, mathematical complexity, lack of software, or the innate conservatism of the medical establishment and regulatory authorities.

There are strong philosophical reasons for using Bayesian approaches in HTA, but the current literature emphasises the practical claims of being able to handle complex inter-related problems, as well as making explicit and accountable what is usually implicit and hidden, and so to clarify discussions and disagreements. The main advantage is that Bayesian analyses can tell us directly what we want to know: how should this piece of evidence change what we currently believe?

There are clearly a number of perceived problems with the Bayesian approach, largely concerning the source of the prior and the interpretations of the conclusions. There are also practical difficulties in implementation and software. It seems appropriate, therefore, that any serious introduction of Bayesian principles into HTA should be gradual and in parallel with traditional approaches, and in such a way as to facilitate examination of the sensitivity of results to prior distributions. This is emphasised in the international statistical guidelines for submissions to regulatory agencies, in which it is stated that 'the use of Bayesian and other approaches may be considered when the reasons for their use are clear and when the resulting conclusions are sufficiently robust'.[171]

Practical methodological developments to promote the appropriate introduction and extension of the use of Bayesian methods in HTA include:

(a) preparation of an extended set of case studies showing practical aspects of the Bayesian approach, in particular for prediction and handling multiple substudies, in which mathematical details are minimised, and
(b) development of standards for the performance and reporting of Bayesian analyses, the first steps towards which – the Bayes-Watch check-list – are reported in the full report of the project on which this chapter is based.[2]

REFERENCES

1. Spiegelhalter DJ, Myles JM, Jones DR, Abrams KR. An introduction to Bayesian methods in health technology assessment. *Br. Med. J.* 1999; **319**: 508–12.
2. Spiegelhalter DJ, Myles JM, Jones DR, Abrams KR. Bayesian methods in health technology assessment. *Health Technology Assessment* 2000, to appear.
3. Whitehead J. *The Design and Analysis of Sequential Clinical Trials*, 2nd edn. Chichester: J Wiley & Sons, 1997.
4. Senn S. *Statistical Issues in Drug Development.* Chichester: J. Wiley & Sons, 1997.
5. Rothman KJ. No adjustments are needed for multiple comparisons. *Epidemiology* 1990; **1**: 43–6.
6. Perneger TV. What's wrong with Bonferroni adjustments. *Br. Med. J.* 1998; **316**: 1236–8.
7. GREAT group. Feasibility, safety and efficacy of domiciliary thrombolysis by general practitioners: Grampian region early anisteplase trial. *Br. Med. J.* 1992; 305: 548–53.
8. Bayes T. An essay towards solving a problem in the doctrine of chances. *Phil. Trans. Roy. Soc.* 1763; **53**: 418.
9. Pocock SJ, Spiegelhalter DJ. Domiciliary thrombosis by general practitioners. *Br. Med. J.* 1992; **305**: 1015.
10. Cooper MW. Should physicians be Bayesian agents? *Theoret. Med.* 1992; **13**: 349–61.
11. Staquet MJ, Rozencweig M, Von Hoff DD, Muggia FM. The delta and epsilon errors in the assessment of cancer clinical trials. *Cancer Treatment Rep.* 1979; **63**: 1917–21.
12. Pocock S. *Clinical Trials: A Practical Approach.* Chichester: Wiley, 1983.
13. Diamond GA, Forrester JS. Clinical trials and statistical verdicts: probable grounds for appeal. *Ann. Intern. Med.* 1983; **98**: 385–94.
14. Browner WS, Newman TB. Are all significant p values created equal? The analogy between diagnostic tests and clinical research. *JAMA* 1987; **257**: 2459–63.
15. Berry DA, Stangl DK. Bayesian methods in health-related research. In: Berry DA, Stangl DK (eds). *Bayesian Biostatistics.* New York: Marcel Dekker, 1996, pp. 3–66.
16. Healy MJR. Probability and decisions. *Arch. Dis. Child.* 1994; **71**: 90–4.
17. Simon R. Problems of multiplicity in clinical trials. *J. Statist. Planning Inference* 1994; **42**: 209–21.
18. Gelman A, Rubin DB. Markov chain Monte Carlo methods in biostatistics. *Statist. Methods Med. Res.* 1996; **5**: 339–55.
19. Berry DA, Stangl DK (eds). *Bayesian Biostatistics.* New York: Marcel Dekker, 1996.
20. Lewis RJ, Wears RL. An introduction to the Bayesian analysis of clinical trials. *Ann. Emergency Med.* 1993; **22**: 1328–36.

21. Lilford RJ, Braunholtz D. For debate – the statistical basis of public policy – a paradigm shift is overdue. *Br. Med. J.* 1996; **313**: 603–7.

22. Eddy DM, Hasselblad V, Shachter R. A Bayesian method for synthesizing evidence: The confidence profile method. *Int. J. Technol. Assess. Health Care* 1990; **6**: 31–55.

23. Breslow N. Biostatistics and Bayes. *Statist. Sci.* 1990; **5**: 269–84.

24. Etzioni RD, Kadane JB. Bayesian statistical methods in public health and medicine. *Annu. Rev. Public Health* 1995; **16**: 23–41.

25. Freedman L. Bayesian statistical methods – a natural way to assess clinical evidence. *Br. Med. J.* 1996; **313**: 569–70.

26. Cornfield J. The Bayesian outlook and its applications. *Biometrics* 1969; **25**: 617–57.

27. Edwards WL, Lindman H, Savage LJ. Bayesian statistical inference for psychological research. *Psychol. Rev.* 1963; **70**: 193–242.

28. Lindley DV. *Making Decisions*, 2nd edn. Chichester: J. Wiley & Sons, 1985.

29. Barnett V. *Comparative Statistical Inference (Second Edition)*. Chichester: J. Wiley & Sons, 1982.

30. Lee PM. *Bayesian Statistics: an Introduction*. London: Edward Arnold, 1989.

31. Gelman A, Carlin J, Stern H, Rubin DB. *Bayesian Data Analysis*. New York: Chapman & Hall, 1995.

32. Carlin BP, Louis TA. *Bayes and Empirical Bayes Methods for Data Analysis*. London: Chapman & Hall, 1996.

33. Bernardo JM, Smith AFM. *Bayesian Theory*. Chichester: J. Wiley & Sons, 1994.

34. Peto R, Baigent C. Trials: the next 50 years. *Br. Med. J.* 1998; **317**: 1170–1.

35. Spiegelhalter DJ, Freedman LS, Parmar MKB. Bayesian approaches to randomized trials. *J. Roy. Statist. Soc. Series A – Statistics Society* 1994; **157**: 357–87.

36. Savage LJ. Elicitation of personal probabilities and expectations. *J. Am. Statist. Assoc.* 1971; **66**: 783–801.

37. Tversky A. Assessing uncertainty (with discussion). *J. Roy. Statist. Soc. B* 1974; **36**: 148–59.

38. Genest C, Zidek JV. Combining probability distributions: a critique and an annotated bibliography (with discussion). *Statist. Sci.* 1986; **1**: 114–48.

39. Chaloner K. Elicitation of prior distributions. In: Berry DA, Stangl DK (eds). *Bayesian Biostatistics*. New York: Marcel Dekker, 1996, pp. 141–56.

40. Kadane JB, Wolfson LJ. Priors for the design and analysis of clinical trials. In: Berry DA, Stangl DK (eds). *Bayesian Biostatistics*. New York: Marcel Dekker, 1996, pp. 157–84.

41. Rosner GL, Berry DA. A Bayesian group sequential design for a multiple arm randomized clinical trial. *Statist. Med.* 1995; **14**: 381–94.

42. Freedman LS, Spiegelhalter DJ. The assessment of subjective opinion and its use in relation to stopping rules for clinical trials. *The Statistician* 1983; **32**: 153–60.

43. Spiegelhalter DJ, Freedman LS. A predictive approach to selecting the size of a clinical trial, based on subjective clinical opinion. *Stat. Med.* 1986; **5**: 1–13.

44. Spiegelhalter DJ. Probabilistic prediction in patient management and clinical trials. *Stat. Med.* 1986; **5**: 421–33.

45. Abrams K, Ashby D, Errington D. Simple Bayesian analysis in clinical trials – a tutorial. *Controlled Clinical Trials* 1994; **15**: 349–59.

46. Parmar MKB, Spiegelhalter DJ, Freedman LS. The CHART trials: Bayesian design and monitoring in practice. *Stat. Med.* 1994; **13**: 1297–312.

47. Chaloner K, Church T, Louis TA, Matts JP. Graphical elicitation of a prior distribution for a clinical trial. *Statistician* 1993; **42**: 341–53.

48. Brown BW, Herson J, Atkinson EN, Rozell ME. Projection from previous studies – a Bayesian and frequentist compromise. *Controlled Clinical Trials* 1987; **8**: 29–44.

49. Lau J, Schmid CH, Chalmers TC. Cumulative meta-analysis of clinical trials builds evidence for exemplary medical care. *J. Clin. Epidemiol.* 1995; **48**: 45–57.

50. Smith TC, Spiegelhalter DJ, Parmar MKB. Bayesian meta-analysis of randomized trials using graphical models and BUGS. In: Berry DA, Stangl DK (eds). *Bayesian Biostatistics*. New York: Marcel Dekker, 1996, pp. 411–27.

51. Higgins JP, Whitehead A. Borrowing strength from external trials in a meta-analysis. *Stat. Med.* 1996; **15**: 2733–49.

52. Burton PR. Helping doctors to draw appropriate inferences from the analysis of medical studies. *Stat. Med.* 1994; **13**: 1699–713.

53. Fletcher A, Spiegelhalter D, Staessen J, Thijs L, Bulpitt C. Implications for trials in progress of publication of positive results. *Lancet*, 1993; **342**: 653–7.

54. Freedman LS, Spiegelhalter DJ, Parmar MKB. The what, why and how of Bayesian clinical trials monitoring. *Stat. Med.* 1994; **13**: 1371–83.

55. Fayers PM, Ashby D, Parmar MKB. Bayesian data monitoring in clinical trials. *Stat. Med.* 1997; **16**: 1413–30.

56. O'Neill RT. Conclusions: 2. *Stat. Med.* 1994; **13**: 1493–9.

57. Heitjan DF. Bayesian interim analysis of phase ii cancer clinical trials. *Stat. Med.* 1997; **16**: 1791–802.

58. Cornfield J. Recent methodological contributions to clinical trials. *Am. J. Epidemiol.* 1976; **104**: 408–21.

59. Freedman LS, Spiegelhalter DJ. Application of Bayesian statistics to decision making during a clinical trial. *Stat. Med.* 1992; **11**: 23–35.

60. Hughes MD. Reporting Bayesian analyses of clinical trials. *Stat. Med.* 1993; **12**: 1651–63.

61. Louis TA. Using empirical Bayes methods in biopharmaceutical research. *Stat. Med.* 1991; **10**: 811–29.

62. Brophy JM, Joseph L. Placing trials in context using Bayesian analysis – GUSTO revisited by Reverend Bayes. *JAMA* 1995; **273**: 871–5.

63. Kadane JB. Prime time for Bayes. *Controlled Clinical Trials* 1995; **16**: 313–18.

64. Pocock SJ, Hughes MD. Estimation issues in clinical trials and overviews. *Stat. Med.* 1990; **9**: 657–71.

65. Armitage PA. Inference and decision in clinical trials. *J. Clin. Epidemiol.* 1989; **42**: 293–9.

66. Lilford RJ, Thornton JG, Braunholtz D. Clinical trials and rare diseases – a way out of a conundrum. *Br. Med. J.* 1995; **311**: 1621–5.

67. Matthews JNS. Small clinical trials – are they all bad? *Stat. Med.* 1995; **14**: 115–26.

68. Spiegelhalter DJ, Freedman LS, Parmar MKB. Applying Bayesian ideas in drug development and clinical trials. *Stat. Med.* 1993; **12**: 1501–17.

69. Berry DA. A case for Bayesianism in clinical trials. *Stat. Med.* 1993; **12**: 1377–93.

70. Berry DA. Decision analysis and Bayesian methods in clinical trials. *Cancer Treatment Res.* 1995; **75**: 125–54.

71. Urbach P. The value of randomization and control in clinical trials. *Stat. Med.* 1993; **12**: 1421–31.

72. Whitehead J. The case for frequentism in clinical trials. *Stat. Med.* 1993; **12**: 1405–19.

73. Kadane JB. Progress toward a more ethical method for clinical trials. *J. Med. Philos.* 1986; **11**: 385–404.

74. Papineau D. The virtues of randomization. *Br. J. Philos. Sci.* 1994; **45**: 437–50.

75. Hutton JL. The ethics of randomised controlled trials: a matter of statistical belief? *Health Care Analysis* 1996; **4**: 95–102.

76. Berry SM, Kadane JB. Optimal Bayesian randomization. *J. Roy. Statist. Soc. Series B. Methodological* 1997; **59**: 813–19.

77. Pocock S. Statistical and ethical issues in monitoring clinical-trials. *Br. Med. J.* 1992; **305**: 235–40.

78. Lilford RJ, Jackson J. Equipoise and the ethics of randomization. *J. R. Soc. Med.* 1995; **88**: 552–9.

79. Palmer CR. Ethics and statistical methodology in clinical trials. *J. Medical Ethics* 1993; **19**: 219–22.

80. Freedman LS, Lowe D, Macaskill P. Stopping rules for clinical trials incorporating clinical opinion. *Biometrics* 1984; **40**: 575–86.

81. Fleming TR Watelet LF. Approaches to monitoring clinical trials. *J. Natl Cancer Inst.* 1989; **81**: 188–93.

82. Korn EL. Projection from previous studies. A caution [letter; comment]. *Controlled Clinical Trials* 1990; **11**: 67–9.

83. Hutton JL, Owens RG. Bayesian sample size calculations and prior beliefs about child sexual abuse. *Statistician* 1993; **42**: 399–404.

84. Adcock CJ. The Bayesian approach to determination of sample sizes – some comments on the paper by Joseph, Wolfson and Du Berger. *J. Roy. Statist. Soc. Series D* 1995; **44**: 155–61.

85. Jennison C, Turnbull BW. Statistical approaches to interim monitoring of medical trials: a review and commentary. *Statist. Sci.* 1990; **5**: 299–317.

86. Collins R, Peto R, Flather M, and ISIS-4 Collaborative Group. ISIS-4 – a randomized factorial trial assessing early oral captopril, oral mononitrate, and intravenous magnesium- sulfate in 58,050 patients with suspected acute myocardial infarction. *Lancet* 1995; **345**: 669–85.

87. Berry DA. Monitoring accumulating data in a clinical trial. *Biometrics* 1989; **45**: 1197–211.

88. Carlin BP, Chaloner K, Church T, Louis TA, Matts JP. Bayesian approaches for monitoring clinical trials with an application to toxoplasmic encephalitis prophylaxis. *Statistician* 1993; **42**: 355–67.

89. George SL, Li CC, Berry DA, Green MR. Stopping a clinical trial early – frequentist and Bayesian approaches applied to a CALGB trial in non-small-cell lung cancer. *Stat. Med.* 1994; **13**: 1313–27.

90. Dersimonian R. Meta-analysis in the design and monitoring of clinical trials. *Stat. Med.* 1996; **15**: 1237–48.

91. Halperin M, Lan KKG, Ware JH, Johnson NJ, DeMets DL. An aid to data monitoring in long-term clinical trials. *Controlled Clinical Trials* 1982; **3**: 311–23.

92. Spiegelhalter DJ, Freedman LS, Blackburn PR. Monitoring clinical trials: Conditional of predictive power? *Controlled Clinical Trials* 1986; **7**: 8–17.

93. Choi SC, Pepple PA. Monitoring clinical trials based on predictive probability of significance. *Biometrics* 1989; **45**: 317–23.

94. Quian J, Stangl DK, George S. A Weibull model for survival data: Using prediction to decide when to stop a clinical trial. In: Berry DA, Stangl DK (eds). *Bayesian Biostatistics.* New York: Marcel Dekker, 1996, Chapter 6.

95. Ware JH, Muller JE, Braunwald E. The futility index: an approach to the cost-effective termination of randomized clinical trials. *Am. J. Med.* 1985; **78**: 635–43.

96. Korn EL, Simon R. Data monitoring committees and problems of lower than expected accrual or event rates. *Controlled Clinical Trials* 1996; **17**: 526–35.

97. Berry DA, Wolff MC, Sack D. Decision making during a phase III randomized controlled trial. *Controlled Clinical Trials* 1994; **15**: 360–78.

98. Ho CH. Some frequentist properties of a Bayesian method in clinical trials. *Biometric. J.* 1991; **33**: 735–40.

99. Lewis RJ, Berry DA. Group sequential clinical trials – a classical evaluation of Bayesian decision-theoretic designs. *J. Am. Statist. Assoc.* 1994; **89**: 1528–34.

100. Lewis RJ. Bayesian hypothesis testing: Interim analysis of a clinical trial evaluating phenytoin for the prophylaxis of early post-traumatic seizures in children. In: Berry DA, Stangl DK (eds). *Bayesian Biostatistics*. New York: Marcel Dekker, 1996, pp. 279–96.

101. Grossman J, Parmar MKB, Spiegelhalter DJ, Freedman LS. A unified method for monitoring and analysing controlled trials. *Stat. Med.* 1994; **13**: 1815–26.

102. Armitage P, Mcpherson K, Rowe BC. Repeated significance tests on accumulating data. *J. Roy. Statist. Soc. A* 1969; **132**: 235–44.

103. Cornfield J. A Bayesian test of some classical hypotheses – with applications to sequential clinical trials. *J. Am. Statist. Assoc.* 1966; **61**: 577–94.

104. Armitage P. Discussion of Breslow (1990). *Statist. Sci.* 1990; **5**: 284–6.

105. Berry DA. When is a confirmatory randomized clinical trial needed? *J. Natl Cancer Inst.* 1996; **88**: 1606–7.

106. Parmar MKB, Ungerleider RS, Simon R. Assessing whether to perform a confirmatory randomized clinical trial. *J. Natl Cancer Inst.* 1996; **88**: 1645–51.

107. Kass RE, Greenhouse JB. Comments on 'Investigating Therapies of potentially great benefit: ECMO' by JH Ware. *Statist. Sci.* 1989; **4**: 310–17.

108. Hughes MD. Practical reporting of Bayesian analyses of clinical trials. *Drug Information J.* 1991; **25**: 381–93.

109. Greenhouse JB, Wasserman L. Robust Bayesian methods for monitoring clinical trials. *Stat. Med.* 1995; **14**: 1379–91.

110. Carlin BP, Sargent DJ. Robust Bayesian approaches for clinical trial monitoring. *Stat. Med.* 1996; **15**: 1093–106.

111. Donner A. A Bayesian approach to the interpretation of subgroup results in clinical trials. *J. Chron. Dis.* 1982; **35**: 429–35.

112. Simon R. Statistical tools for subset analysis in clinical trials. *Rec. Res. Cancer Res.* 1988; **111**: 55–66.

113. Simon R, Dixon DO, Friedlin B. Bayesian subset analysis of a clinical trial for the treatment of HIV infections. In: Berry DA, Stangl DK (eds). *Bayesian Biostatistics*. New York: Marcel Dekker, 1996, pp. 555–76.

114. Skene AM, Wakefield JC. Hierarchial models for multicentre binary response studies. *Stat. Med.* 1990; **9**: 919–29.

115. Stangl D. Hierarchical analysis of continuous-time survival models. In: Berry DA, Stangl DK (eds). *Bayesian Biostatistics*. New York: Marcel Dekker, 1996, pp. 429–50.

116. Hornberger J, Eghtesady P. The cost-benefit of a randomized trial to a health care organization. *Controlled Clinical Trials* 1998; **19**: 198–211.

117. Detsky AS. Using economic-analysis to determine the resource consequences of choices made in planning clinical-trials. *J. Chron. Dis.* 1985; **38**: 753–65.

118. Claxton K, Posnett J. An economic approach to clinical trial design and research priority-setting. *Health Economics* 1996; **5**: 513–24.

119. Lilford R, Royston G. Decision analysis in the selection, design and application of clinical and health services research. *J. Health Serv. Res. Policy* 1998; **3**: 159–66.

120. Zelen M. Play the winner rule and the controlled clinical trial. *J. Am. Statist. Assoc.* 1969; **64**: 131–46.

121. Tamura RN, Faries DE, Andersen JS, Heiligenstein JH. A case-study of an adaptive clinical trial in the treatment of out-patients with depressive disorder. *J. Am. Statist. Assoc.* 1994; **89**: 768–76.

122. Armitage P. The search for optimality in clinical trials. *Int. Statist. Rev.* 1985; **53**: 15–24.

123. Selwyn MR, Dempster AP, Hall NR. A Bayesian approach to bioequivalence for the 2×2 changeover design. *Biometrics* 1981; **37**: 11–21.

124. Racine A, Grieve AP, Fluhler H, Smith AFM. Bayesian methods in practice – experiences in the pharmaceutical industry. *Appl. Statist. J. Roy. Statist. Soc. Series C* 1986; **35**: 93–150.

125. Grieve AP. Evaluation of bioequivalence studies. *Eur. J. Clin. Pharmacol.* 1991; **40**: 201–2.

126. Baudoin C, O'Quigley J. Symmetrical intervals and confidence intervals. *Biometrical J.* 1994; **36**: 927–34.

127. Grieve AP. Bayesian analyses of two-treatment crossover studies. *Statist. Methods Med. Res.* 1994; **3**: 407–29.

128. Forster JJ. A Bayesian approach to the analysis of binary crossover data. *Statistician* 1994; **43**: 61–8.

129. Albert J, Chib S. Bayesian modelling of binary repeated measures data with application to crossover trials. In: Berry DA, Stangl DK (eds). *Bayesian Biostatistics*. New York: Marcel Dekker, 1996, pp. 577–600.

130. Zucker DR, Schmid CH, McIntosh MW, Agostino RB, Selker HP, Lau J. Combining single patient (n-of-1) trials to estimate population treatment effects and to evaluate individual patient responses to treatment. *J. Clin. Epidemiol.* 1997; **50**: 401–10.

131. Simon R, Freedman LS. Bayesian design and analysis of two × two factorial clinical trials. *Biometrics* 1997; **53**: 456–64.

132. Miller MA, Seaman JW. A Bayesian approach to assessing the superiority of a dose combination. *Biometrical J.* 1998; **40**: 43–55.

133. Racine-Poon A, Wakefield J. Bayesian analysis of population pharmacokinetic and instantaneous pharmacodynamic relationships. In: Berry DA, Stangl DK (eds). *Bayesian Biostatistics.* New York: Marcel Dekker, 1996, pp. 321–54.

134. Wakefield J, Bennett J. The Bayesian modeling of covariates for population pharmacokinetic models. *J. Am. Statist. Assoc.* 1996; **91**: 917–27.

135. O'Quigley J, Pepe M, Fisher L. Continual reassessment method – a practical design for phase I clinical trials in cancer. *Biometrics* 1990; **46**: 33–48.

136. Goodman SN, Zahurak ML, Piantadosi S. Some practical improvements in the continual reassessment method for phase I studies. *Stat. Med.* 1995; **14**: 1149–61.

137. Mehta CR, Cain KC. Charts for the early stopping of pilot studies. *J. Clin. Oncol.* 1984; **2**: 676–82.

138. Thall PF, Simon R. A Bayesian approach to establishing sample size and monitoring criteria for phase ii clinical trials. *Controlled Clinical Trials* 1994; **15**: 463–81.

139. Stallard N. Sample size determination for phase II clinical trials based on bayesian decision theory. *Biometrics* 1998; **54**: 279–94.

140. Whitehead J. Designing phase II studies in the context of a program of clinical research. *Biometrics* 1985; **41**: 373–83.

141. Brunier HC, Whitehead J. Sample sizes for phase II clinical trials derived from Bayesian decision theory. *Stat. Med.* 1994; **13**: 2493–502.

142. Byar DP, Simon RM, Friedewald WT, Schlesselman JJ, DeMets DL, Ellenberg JH, Gail MH, Ware JH. Randomized clinical trials. Perspective on some recent ideas. *N. Engl. J. Med.* 1976; **295**: 74–80.

143. Eddy DM, Hasselblad V, Shachter R. *Meta-Analysis by the Confidence Profile Method: the Statistical Synthesis of Evidence.* San Diego: Academic Press, 1992.

144. Zelen M, Parker RA. Case control studies and Bayesian inference. *Stat. Med.* 1986; **5**: 261–9.

145. Ashby D, Hutton J, McGee M. Simple Bayesian analyses for case-control studies in cancer epidemiology. *The Statistician* 1993; **42**: 385–97.

146. Richardson S, Gilks WR. A Bayesian approach to measurement error problems in epidemiology using conditional independence models. *Am. J. Epidemiol.* 1993; **138**: 430–42.

147. Bernardinelli L, Clayton D, Pascutto C, Montomoli C, Ghislandi M, Songini M. Bayesian analysis of space-time variation in disease risk. *Stat. Med.* 1995; **14**: 2433–43.

148. Ashby D, Hutton JL. Bayesian epidemiology. In: Berry DA, Stangl DK (eds). *Bayesian Biostatistics.* New York: Marcel Dekker, 1996, pp. 109–38.

149. Pocock S. The combination of randomised and historical controls in clinical trials. *J. Chron. Dis.* 1976; **29**: 175–88.

150. Ryan LM. Using historical controls in the analysis of developmental toxicity data. *Biometrics* 1993; **49**: 1126–35.

151. Tarone RE. The use of historical control information in testing for a trend in proportions. *Biometrics* 1982; **38**: 215–20.

152. Dempster AP, Selwyn MR, Weeks BJ. Combining historical and randomized controls for assessing trends in proportions. *J. Am. Statist. Assoc.* 1983; **78**: 221–7.

153. Berry DA, Hardwick J. Using historical controls in clinical trials: application to ECMO. In: Berger JO, Gupta S (eds). *Statistical Decision Theory and Related Topics V.* New York: Springer-Verlag, 1993, pp. 141–56.

154. Goldstein H, Spiegelhalter DJ. Statistical aspects of institutional performance: league tables and their limitations (with discussion). *J. Roy. Statist. Soc. A* 1996; **159**: 385–444.

155. Normand SL, Glickman ME, Gatsonis CA. Statistical methods for profiling providers of medical care: Issues and applications. *J. Am. Statist. Assoc.* 1997; **92**: 803–14.

156. Marshall EC, Spiegelhalter DJ. League tables of in-vitro fertilisation clinics: how confident can we be about the rankings? *Br. Med. J.* 1998; **317**: 1701–4.

157. Hedges LV. Bayesian meta-analysis. In: Everitt BS, Dunn G (eds). *Statistical Analysis of Medical Data: New Developments.* London: Arnold, 1998, pp. 251–76.

158. DuMouchel W, Berry DA. Bayesian meta-analysis. In: DuMouchel W, Berry DA (eds). *Statistical Methodology in the Pharmaceutical Sciences.* New York: Marcel Dekker, 1989, pp. 509–29.

159. Smith TC, Spiegelhalter DJ, Thomas A. Bayesian approaches to random-effects meta-analysis: a comparative study. *Stat. Med.* 1995; **14**: 2685–99.

160. Abrams K, Sansó. Approximate Bayesian inference for random effects meta-analysis. *Stat. Med.* 1998; **17**: 201–18.

161. Raudenbush SW, Bryk AS. Empirical Bayes meta-analysis. *J. Educational Statist.* 1985; **10**: 75–98.

162. Stijnen T, Van Houwelingen JC. Empirical Bayes methods in clinical trials meta-analysis. *Biometrical J.* 1990; **32**: 335–46.

163. Carlin JB. Meta-analysis for 2×2 tables – a Bayesian approach. *Stat. Med.* 1992; **11**: 141–58.

164. Black N. Why we need observational studies to evaluate the effectiveness of health care. *Br. Med. J.* 1996; **312**: 1215–18.

165. General Accounting Office. *Cross design synthesis: a new strategy for medical effectiveness research*. Washington, DC: General Accounting Office, 1992.

166. Abrams K, Jones DR. Meta-analysis and the synthesis of evidence. *IMA J. Mathematics Appl. Med. Biol.* 1995; **12**: 297–313.

167. Smith TC, Abrams KR, Jones DR. Using hierarchical models in generalised synthesis of evidence: an example based on studies of breast cancer screening. Technical Report 95-02, Department of Epidemiology and Public Health, University of Leicester, 1995.

168. Shachter R, Eddy DM, Hasselblad V. An influence diagram approach to medical technology assessment. In Oliver RM, Smith JQ (eds). *Influence Diagrams, Belief Nets and Decision Analysis*. Chichester: Wiley, 1990, pp. 321–50.

169. Weinstein MC, Fineberg HV. *Clinical Decision Analysis*. Philadelphia: W.B. Saunders, 1980.

170. Parmigiani G, Samsa GP, Ancukiewicz M, Lipscomb J, Hasselblad V, Matchar DB. Assessing uncertainty in cost-effectiveness analyses: application to a complex decision model. *Medical Decision Making* 1997; **17**: 390–401.

171. International Conference on Harmonisation. *Statistical Principles for Clinical Trials*, 1998. Available on http://www.ipfma.org/pdfifpma/ e9.pdf.

17

Methods for Evaluating Organisation- or Area-Based Health Interventions

MARTIN GULLIFORD, OBIOHA UKOUMUNNE,
SUSAN CHINN, JONATHAN STERNE,
PETER BURNEY and ALLAN DONNER

SUMMARY

In clinical research, intervention is usually at the level of the individual patient, but in health services research it is often at the level of the health service organisational unit or geographical or administrative area. Areas and organisations represent discrete clusters of individual patients or healthy subjects and evaluation may be difficult. This is because: (i) often only a few clusters may be included in a study; (ii) evaluation may be at the level of the individual subject whilst intervention is at the cluster level; and (iii) individual responses are often correlated within clusters. This chapter discusses the ways that these problems may be addressed in designing and analysing area- or organisation-based evaluations. It is important to include an adequate number of organisational clusters in each intervention group so that the effect of intervention may be distinguished from underlying variability between clusters. As with evaluation at the individual level, randomisation is the preferred method for allocating units to groups. Restricted randomisation is often advantageous in cluster randomised studies, because baseline imbalances may occur when the number of clusters is small. The pair matched design has specific limitations when compared to designs with replication within strata. When randomisation is not feasible, restricted allocation may help to reduce bias. In order to estimate the required number of individuals for a cluster based study, the results of a standard sample size calculation should be increased by the design effect or variance inflation factor. Including more clusters will enhance the generalisability of the results and allow more flexible approaches to analysis, and it is desirable to include at least ten clusters per group to permit analysis at the individual level. Three approaches to analysis are considered: (i) cluster level analysis in which the cluster means or proportions are employed as the observations; (ii) adjusted individual analysis using standard individual level tests after adjusting for the design effect; and (iii) regression methods for clustered data. The latter approach will often be preferred because adjustment for individual and cluster level confounders will increase precision in randomised studies and reduce bias in non-randomised designs. The recommendations of our review are summarised in the form of a checklist.

INTRODUCTION

In clinical epidemiology interventions are usually implemented at the level of the individual patient, and the accepted method of evaluation is the randomised controlled trial. In health services research, interventions are often implemented at the level of health service organisation or in geographical or administrative areas. Evaluation of organisation-based interventions presents a number of problems and the use of randomisation is currently neither well accepted nor widely practised. This chapter reviews the ways that the problems associated with organisation-based evaluation may be addressed; it is particularly concerned with quantitative studies that measure the effectiveness of organisational interventions by evaluating their outcomes.

PROBLEMS OF ORGANISATION-BASED EVALUATIONS

Hierarchical Structure of Data in Health Services Research

In clinical research, individual patient outcomes are usually considered as independent observations at a single level. Data from organisation-based evaluations often have a *hierarchical* structure. Observations may be made at two or more *levels*. Responses at lower levels are *nested* or *clustered* within higher levels, and individual outcomes are often correlated within *clusters*.

Clustering is an almost universal feature of social organisation. When considering community based health interventions, individual healthy subjects can be considered to be clustered within health authorities, towns, schools, workplaces or neighbourhoods. For healthcare interventions, individual patients can be considered to be clustered within general practices, hospital clinics or hospital wards. Sometimes there are several levels of clustering. For example, children are clustered within classes, which in turn are nested within schools, and schools within local authorities. Patients are clustered according to their general practitioner, general practitioners are nested within general practices, which in turn are nested within health authorities.

Three Problems

The hierarchical structure of data from organisation-based evaluations is associated with three problems:

1 It may be difficult to study an adequate number of organisational clusters.
2 The level of intervention (and unit of assignment) may differ from the level of evaluation.

3 Individual-level outcomes are often correlated within organisational clusters.

Including Adequate Numbers of Organisational Units

Organisation-based evaluations typically include only small numbers of organisational clusters. However, because differences between clusters must be taken into account in evaluating the effect of an intervention, the validity of the study will be more dependent on the number of clusters than on the number of individuals. One of the challenges presented by organisation-based evaluations is to include a sufficient number of organisational units in order to allow the study to give valid, generalisable results.

Distinction Between Cluster-Level and Individual-Level Evaluation

A key problem in organisation-based evaluation is that the level of measurement is often different from the level of intervention and unit of assignment. Organisation-level interventions are easier to evaluate when inferences from evaluation are intended at organisation level because the organisational clusters can then be considered as the units of analysis. For example, the consequences of different methods of funding primary care services might be evaluated according to whether certain types of practice had better facilities. However, organisation-level interventions are often designed to modify individual level outcomes. For example, a study might aim to determine whether setting up a general practice asthma clinic resulted in fewer symptoms and better respiratory outcomes in the practice's patients. In this instance intervention is at cluster – that is at practice – level, but inferences are intended at individual level.[1] This leads to the 'unit of analysis problem' where standard individual level analyses are performed inappropriately in an organisation-based evaluation. Whiting-O'Keefe et al. found that this type of error was present in 20 out of 28 healthcare evaluations which they studied.[2]

Correlation of Responses Within Organisations

Standard statistical methods are based on the assumption that individual responses are independent of one another. In the context of organisation-based evaluations, responses are rarely independent because areas and organisations tend to contain individuals who are more similar to each other than they are to individuals in other areas or organisations. In other words, because individual responses within an organisational cluster usually show some correlation, variation among individuals in different organisations may be greater than variation among individuals within the same organisation.[1-3] There are at least three reasons why this might be the case.[3-6] Firstly, subjects may select the organisational cluster to which they belong. For example, people with similar characteristics may tend to move into similar neighbourhoods. Patients may choose their doctor according to characteristics such as age, gender or ethnic group. Secondly, organisation level variables might influence all cluster members in a similar direction and each cluster will be subject to distinct influences. For example, patient outcomes may differ systematically among surgeons performing the same procedure.[7] Thirdly, individuals within clusters may interact, influence each other and tend to conform, as might happen in a school classroom or a psychotherapeutic group.

In general, because individual members of the same cluster are unlikely to be independent with respect to health outcomes,[8] standard statistical methods for calculating sample sizes, assessing power and analysing data are not appropriate for use in organisation-based evaluations. Use of standard methods may result in the required sample size being underestimated and standard methods of analysis will give confidence intervals that are too narrow and *P*-values that are too small.[9]

METHODS

The focus for this review included both randomised and non-randomised evaluations of existing services, but we did not include qualitative methods nor methods of health economic evaluation. The literature search was restricted to the English language. References were retrieved from personal collections, from hand-searches of relevant journals, from the electronic databases Medline, EMBASE and ERIC (Education Resources Information Centre). Limited searches were also made on the world wide web for literature and multilevel modelling software. Because the search process identified a very large number of citations, these were initially screened for relevance to the focus of the review. Relevant papers were retrieved, assessed against conventional epidemiological and statistical principles and qualitative judgements were made of their validity. We synthesised the

best evidence into a series of methodological recommendations.[10]

Two areas of study were particularly relevant to the present review. From the field of cardiovascular disease prevention, work on the design and analysis of community intervention trials had particular relevance to the design of intervention studies in health services research.[11] From the field of educational research, work on the analysis of hierarchical data in the assessment of school performance was particularly relevant to the evaluation of existing healthcare services.[12]

The review is divided into three sections. In the next section we review factors affecting the choice of study design. We then discuss sample size estimation for organisation-based evaluations. Finally, we review different approaches to analysis of data from organisation-based evaluation.

A CLASSIFICATION OF STUDY DESIGNS

Healthcare interventions may be evaluated either in the context of experimental studies, sometimes called intervention studies, or in the context of observational designs (Figure 1). The former should be used to evaluate new interventions and the latter are more appropriately used to evaluate the quality of existing services and to generate hypotheses for evaluation in randomised studies. In its epidemiological sense the term 'observational' refers to studies in which there is no intervention. In order to avoid confusion, it is important to make the distinction between *healthcare interventions* and *experimental interventions*. Observational studies of healthcare interventions do not incorporate experimental interventions initiated by the investigator.

Minimum Number of Clusters

Health services researchers are often asked to evaluate interventions implemented in single clusters. In the field of coronary heart disease prevention, the North Karelia project provides a well-known example.[13] This study, carried out in Finland, aimed to reduce coronary heart disease risk factors by a range of health promotion interventions carried out in a single intervention county in comparison with a single control county. This type of evaluation is sometimes strengthened by including more than one control cluster, as illustrated in a recent evaluation of a

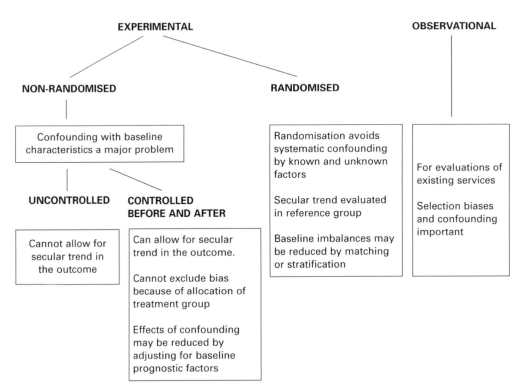

Figure 1   *A classification of study designs.*

regional trauma centre.[14] A few commentators have suggested that a one-to-one comparison of clusters can be rigorous enough to generalise the results, so long as the clusters are typical.[13,15] However, the validity of this type of design will always be questioned.

If only one cluster is allocated to each group the intervention effect cannot be separated from the natural variability among clusters.[16] In other words, it is impossible to say whether the difference between two clusters is the result of the intervention, or simply reflects the underlying variation among clusters. At least three or four clusters per group will be required to detect a significant intervention effect. Studies with as few as six clusters per group[17] have been used to demonstrate the effect of an intervention, but more clusters will often be needed – particularly when small intervention effects are of interest.

The evaluation of an intervention in one or a few clusters will provide a weak basis on which to generalise findings for policy formulation. Researchers need to advise health decision-makers and service providers that, although of local interest, evaluation of interventions implemented in one or two clusters is unlikely to yield decisive, generalisable results.

Observational Designs

Observational designs commonly used in health-care evaluation include cohort studies and single or repeated cross-sectional surveys. The usefulness of observational designs is limited by the problems of confounding and bias. However, Black[18] emphasised the continuing need for observational studies when randomisation is not possible. For the present review it is sufficient to note that it is essential that the design and analysis of observational studies should take into account the hierarchical structure of the data using the same principles that were developed for intervention studies and complex surveys.

Intervention Studies

In organisation-based intervention studies, *clusters of individuals* are allocated to *groups* which receive the same *intervention*. An *uncontrolled* study includes an intervention group, but no comparison or control group in which the intervention does not take place. Changes in the outcome may result from any of the factors which contribute to the secular trend and potential effects of intervention cannot be evaluated.

Table 1 *Summary of design recommendations for evaluation of organisation-based interventions*

Design	Recommendation	Example
Observational designs	Not recommended for evaluating effectiveness. May be appropriate for monitoring organisational performance.	Comparison of myocardial infarction mortality among hospitals[81]
Uncontrolled designs	Not recommended for evaluating effectiveness. May be appropriate for local audits.	Evaluation of a new way of organising a single anticoagulant clinic[91]
Quasi-experimental designs (controlled before and after)	Randomised designs to be preferred. Rejection of randomisation should be justified. Restricted allocation (matching or stratification) recommended.	Before and after evaluation of a regional trauma centre with two control regions[14]
Randomised designs	Recommended	Da Qing study of diabetes prevention in which 33 health clinics were randomised[92]
Restricted allocation	Recommended when the number of clusters is small, for stratifying variables that are known to be associated with the outcome. Matched pairs designs (in which there are two clusters per stratum) may be inefficient because of loss of degrees of freedom for analysis, unless there is a very strong association of the stratifying variable with the outcome. Valid estimates of between-cluster variation are less easy to obtain. Stratified designs do not share the limitations of the matched pairs design.	British Family Heart Study in which pairs of general practices were studied in 13 towns. One practice in each town was randomised to receive a nurse-led intervention to reduce cardiovascular risk factors in practice patients[29]
Cohort designs	More appropriate for short-term studies of individual outcomes. Bias likely to increase with duration of study.	Da Qing study[92] British Family Heart Study[29]
Cross-sectional designs	More appropriate for studies of community level health indicators. May be less susceptible to bias, but with lower power.	An HIV prevention programme was evaluated by means of repeat surveys of men patronising gay bars[28]

Uncontrolled studies are therefore not recommended for use in health technology assessment (see Figure 1 and Table 1).

Non-randomised *controlled* studies with *before- and after- evaluation* in both the intervention and control groups (sometimes known as '*quasi-experimental*' studies) can be used to separate the effects of intervention from secular trends. The major limitation of such studies is that baseline characteristics may differ between the intervention and control groups, thus confounding both the intervention effect and the secular trend. The effects of confounding can be reduced by using restricted forms of allocation, for example, by matching or stratifying clusters according to important prognostic factors before allocating them to intervention and control groups. Allowance can also be made for confounding at the time of analysis. Nevertheless, estimated effects of intervention may still be biased by unknown confounders or by residual confounding. For this reason random allocation of clusters is to be preferred in health technology assessment, and convincing justification should always be given for the use of non-randomised designs. A detailed discussion of non-randomised designs was provided in Cook and Campbell's book[19] and a range of examples are provided in our full report.[20]

In the simplest form of *randomised* design, all clusters are independently randomised to intervention or control groups. We noted earlier that organisation-based evaluations often include relatively small numbers of clusters. Whereas individually randomised trials often include sufficiently large numbers to preclude important imbalances between treatment and control groups, this is rarely the case for organisation-based evaluations. Simple randomisation is unlikely to produce groups that are balanced with respect to baseline prognostic variables and *restricted randomisation* may then be used to produce groups which are more balanced.[21]

Restricted Randomisation

The aim of restricted randomisation is to produce intervention and control groups that are more evenly balanced with respect to prognostic variables than if simple randomisation were used. Clusters are first divided into strata according to prognostic characteristics and then randomised within strata. This increases the statistical power, since estimates of the outcome are more precise.[1,3,11,22–24] Clusters should only be stratified on variables that are known to be highly correlated with the outcome of interest,[16,21–23,25] for example, baseline levels of the outcome variable.[26]

Restricted allocation may also reduce bias in quasi-experimental studies.[11,23] Murray recommended that non-random assignment of a small number of poorly matched or unmatched units to intervention groups is inadvisable and should be avoided.[27] Thus, some form of restricted allocation is mandatory for non-randomised intervention studies.

Paired Designs

The paired design is a special case of the stratified design in which there are only two clusters per stratum and one cluster is randomised to each group. In matched pairs designs, clusters are paired with respect to baseline characteristics that are associated with the outcome and randomly allocated within pairs to intervention and control groups. The matched pairs design has important limitations which should be recognised. Firstly, it may be difficult to find matching variables that can be used to create distinct pairs, particularly for a large number of clusters.[23,25] A second potential problem is that in the event that a particular cluster drops out of the study, the other cluster (and thus the entire stratum) must be eliminated, causing a reduction in study power. Such a problem was described in a recent community randomised trial of prevention of human immune deficiency virus (HIV) transmission.[28] Thirdly, because a paired analysis considers the differences between clusters within pairs, the power of the study will depend on the number of pairs rather than the number of clusters. This loss of degrees of freedom means that a matched analysis may be less powerful than an unmatched analysis when the number of pairs is small. For pairing to be successful the decrease in experimental error

needs to be sufficiently large to offset the reduction in degrees of freedom.[25] The power of a study will inevitably be reduced by matching on a variable that is unrelated to the outcome if a matched analysis is used. If the number of clusters is small, then an unmatched randomised design will usually be more efficient because of the loss of degrees of freedom associated with the matched analysis.[25] Diehr et al.[16] suggested that in studies with small numbers of clusters, if pre-intervention matching seems to be required at the outset, an unmatched analysis will usually be more powerful than a matched analysis. However, strong correlates of the outcome may make matching worthwhile for very small studies, as was described in a study of prevention of HIV transmission in Tanzania. In this study, intervention communities were pair matched with control communities according to baseline indicators of risk of transmission of HIV and other sexually transmitted diseases.[17]

Finally, Klar and Donner[23] cautioned that the matched pairs design may be less suitable for organisation-based evaluations because of the difficulty of separating the effect of intervention from between-cluster variation within pairs, and hence in estimating the value of the intracluster correlation. Thompson et al.[29] recently proposed that random effects meta-analysis can be applied to the analysis of paired cluster randomised designs. One variance component can be used to allow for both natural variation between clusters and variation in the intervention effect from stratum to stratum. Natural variation between clusters is not estimated explicitly, but is still allowed for in the analysis. This approach will be restricted to studies with the relatively large number of cluster pairs required to estimate variance components with reasonable precision.[30]

Stratified Designs

Under the stratified design, two or more clusters from each of several strata are allocated to each intervention group.[31] As for the matched pairs design, the clusters are grouped into strata according to one or more variables which are related to the outcome, but the stratified design differs qualitatively from the matched pairs design because there is *replication* of clusters within each intervention–stratum combination. It is therefore possible to obtain an estimate of between-cluster variation from a stratified organisation-based trial as the cluster effect can be separated from both the intervention effect and the stratum effect.

Using the completely randomised design as the benchmark in their simulations, Klar and Donner[23] found that compared to the matched pairs design there is little loss in power for stratified designs when strata are not related to outcome. Another advantage of the stratified design over the matched design is that for studies in which there are a large number of clusters it is easier to construct meaningful strata.[1,23] In the light of these advantages, Klar and Donner[23] suggest that the stratified design is under-utilised in comparison to the matched pairs design and should be considered more often. The stratified design requires at least some strata to have two or more clusters assigned to each intervention.

Design Issues for Follow-Up

Two designs can be used for sampling individuals from within clusters in organisation-based studies with follow-up. Under the *repeated cross-sectional* design a fresh sample of individuals is drawn from each of the clusters at each measurement occasion. Under the *cohort* design, data are collected from the same sample of individuals at each time point. When the ratio of sample size to population size is high, a cohort will be generated within the framework of a repeated cross-sectional design as individuals may be sampled repeatedly by chance.[21] The overlap of repeated cross-sectional samples may be engineered deliberately, and some community intervention studies have set out to achieve this mixed design.[21,32] If the main objective is to determine how an intervention changes the behaviour of individuals, then a cohort design should be used. Cohort studies provide the opportunity to link behavioural changes directly to individual level prognostic factors. When the main objective is to determine how an intervention affects a cluster-level index of health such as risk-factor prevalence, then a repeated cross-sectional design should be used as it will generate data which are representative of the study clusters throughout the study period. Cohorts are subject to ageing, migration, death, loss to follow-up and other factors which affect representativeness.[21,24,33] In choosing the most suitable design for follow-up, the aim of the intervention needs to be clearly defined so that the appropriate choice is made.

When cohort or repeated cross-sectional designs are considered equally appropriate and there are no biases, cohort designs will generally offer greater statistical power because measurements made on the same subject over time are often correlated and estimates of the intervention effect have a smaller variance than those calculated from repeated cross-sectional data.[21,24,33-35] The greater the correlation between measurements made on the same individual the more powerful the cohort design will be

in relation to the repeated cross-sectional one.[32,36-38] In deciding between the two designs, the relative costs should also be considered.[39]

SAMPLE SIZE REQUIREMENTS

When estimating the sample size it is important to take into account the planned method of analysis. If the intention is to analyse cluster-level outcomes, such as the proportion of general practices running a diabetic clinic, then a conventional sample size calculation may be performed to estimate the required number of clusters, using an estimate of the variance of the cluster-level outcome. If individual level analyses are to be performed, it will be necessary to allow for both within- and between-cluster variation by multiplying the sample size estimate obtained using standard formulae by an appropriate *variance inflation factor* or *design effect*.

Within-Cluster and Between-Cluster Variation

In studies at the individual level, variation is between individuals. In organisation-based studies, because of the correlation of individual level responses within clusters, there are two separate components of variation, within-cluster variation and between-cluster variation. Standard statistical methods for sample size estimation and analysis do not recognise these two components of variation in the outcome and cannot be applied directly to organisation-based studies with evaluation at the individual level. Standard sample size calculations, carried out using estimates of between-individual variation, will lead to sample size estimates that are too small. Appropriate methods for sample size calculation and analysis need to include estimates of within- and between-cluster variation.

Estimating within- and between-cluster components of variance

The overall variation in subject responses may be decomposed into its two constituent components, within-cluster and between-cluster variation, using analysis of variance. Variance components may be estimated using a one-way analysis of variance of the outcome with the clustering variable included as a random effect. The algebraic form of the appropriate model is

$$y_{ij} = \alpha + \beta_j + e_{ij} \qquad (1)$$

where y_{ij} is the response of the *i*th individual within the *j*th cluster, α is the mean of the responses, β_j is the random effect of the jth cluster, and e_{ij} is the random error component for the ith individual in the jth cluster. The β_j are independently and Normally distributed with zero mean and constant variance, σ_b^2. The e_{ij} are independently and Normally distributed with zero mean and constant variance σ_w^2. Estimates of the between- and within-cluster variance components are calculated from the analysis of variance table

$$\hat{\sigma}_b^2 = (MSB - MSW) / n_0 \qquad (2)$$

$$\hat{\sigma}_w^2 = MSW \qquad (3)$$

where MSB is the between-cluster mean square and MSW is the within-cluster mean square. n_0 is a measure of average cluster size which is appropriate when clusters are variable in size:[40]

$$n_0 = \frac{1}{J-1} \left[N - \frac{\sum n_j^2}{N} \right] \qquad (4)$$

where J is the number of clusters, N is the total number of individuals and n_j is the number of individuals in the jth cluster.

The analysis of variance approach can be extended to more complex designs which include other categorical and continuous variables that are important in the design of the study from which variance components have to be estimated. Thus, there may be two intervention groups, several strata, and several time points at which measurements are made. Further details are provided in standard texts.[41]

The intra-class correlation coefficient (ρ)

Within-cluster and between-cluster components of variance may be combined in a single statistical measure of between cluster variation, the intraclass correlation coefficient. The *intraclass correlation coefficient* (ρ) is defined as the proportion of the true total variation in the outcome that can be attributed to differences between the clusters. Algebraically ρ is given by:

$$\rho = \frac{\sigma_b^2}{\sigma_b^2 + \sigma_w^2}. \qquad (5)$$

Equations (2) and (3) can be substituted into Equation (5) and rearranged to show that the intra-class correlation[42] is given by:

$$\hat{\rho} = \frac{MSB - MSW}{MSB + (n_0 - 1)\,MSW}. \qquad (6)$$

If individuals within the same cluster are no more likely to have similar outcomes than individuals in different clusters then the intra-class correlation will be zero. Conversely, if all individuals in the same cluster are identical with

respect to the outcome, then the intra-class correlation is 1. In the context of organisation-based evaluations, the intra-class correlation coefficient will usually assume small positive values; negative values can usually be attributed to sampling error.

The analysis of variance model can also be used to calculate the intra-class correlation coefficient when the outcome is dichotomous. In this case, the resulting estimate is a version of the kappa coefficient, which itself is an intraclass correlation coefficient.[43,44]

The Design Effect

In order to take account of between cluster variation, standard sample size formulae applied at the individual level need to be increased by the *design effect*. The design effect (*Deff*) is defined as the ratio of the variance of the estimated outcome under the cluster sampling strategy (σ_c^2) to the variance that would be expected for a study of the same size using simple random sampling (σ_{srs}^2) and is given by:[45,46]

$$Deff = \frac{\sigma_c^2}{\sigma_{srs}^2}. \qquad (7)$$

The design effect has also been referred to as the variance inflation factor.[3,9] In evaluations of organisation-based interventions the design effect will usually be greater than unity because of between-cluster variation. An interpretation of design effect is the number of times more subjects an organisation-based evaluation should have compared with one in which individuals are randomised, in order to attain the same power.

It can be shown that the design effect is given approximately by

$$Deff = 1 + (n - 1)\rho \qquad (8)$$

where *Deff* is the design effect, n is the average cluster size (or number of individuals sampled per cluster), and ρ is the intraclass correlation coefficient of the outcome.[45,46] Thus, the standard sample size calculation should be multiplied by a factor lying between unity and the average cluster size. The design effect will tend to be large when the cluster size is large, even though ρ tends to be smaller for larger clusters.[47] The intra-class correlation coefficient is more generalisable than the design effect because it is independent of the number of individuals that are sampled from within each cluster, and can therefore be readily compared across studies of similar design and purpose. Estimates of ρ can then be used to calculate the design effect of proposed studies at the planning stage.

Total Number of Individuals

When the aim of the study is to estimate the difference between intervention group means, the standard normal deviate sample size formula for comparing two independent groups should be multiplied by the design effect.[48] The required number of individuals per group, N, is given by

$$N = \frac{2 M \sigma^2}{\delta^2} \quad x \, [1 + (n - 1)\rho] \qquad (9)$$

where n is the cluster size, ρ is the intra-class correlation coefficient, σ^2 is the variance of the outcome measure under simple random sampling, and the δ is the true difference between group means that can be detected. The value of M depends on the levels of power $(1 - \beta)$ and significance (α) and whether the test is to be one-sided or two-sided. Values for M are given in many texts, for example Ref. 49. When unequal cluster sizes are anticipated, Donner et al.[48] suggested the use of either the expected average cluster size, or more conservatively the expected maximum cluster size.

When the study will estimate the difference between group proportions, an adapted version of the standard sample size for comparing two proportions may be used.[8,48] The required number of individuals per group, N, is:

$$N = \frac{M \, [\pi_T (1 - \pi_T) + \pi_C (1 - \pi_C)]}{(\pi_T - \pi_C)^2} \\ x \, [1 + (n - 1)\rho] \qquad (10)$$

where N is the number of individuals per group, ρ is the intra-class correlation coefficient with respect to the binary trait, π_T is the expected event rate in the treatment group, π_C is the expected event rate in the control group and n is the cluster size. M has the values defined above. An equivalent method is given by Cornfield.[9] Sample size formulae appropriate for matched pairs and stratified designs are given by Hsieh,[50] Thompson et al.,[29] Shipley et al.[51] and Donner.[52]

Number of Clusters

In practice, when designing organisation-based evaluations the investigator often needs to estimate both the required total number of individuals and the required number of clusters. If the cluster size is predetermined, the required number of clusters can be estimated by dividing the total number of individuals required by the average cluster size. When it is feasible to sample individuals within clusters, the power of the study may be increased either by increasing the number of clusters or the number of individuals sampled within clusters. Examples of appropriate calculations were given by Thompson et al.[29] and Kerry and Bland.[53]

Increasing the number of clusters rather than the number of individuals within clusters has several advantages.[29] The results of the study will usually appear to be more generalisable if the intervention has been implemented in a number of different clusters. A larger number of clusters also allows more precise estimation of the intra-class correlation coefficient and more flexible approaches to analysis.[29] As a general rule, individual-level or multi-level approaches to analysis will require at least 20 clusters (at least 10 per group). Furthermore, there is a limit to the extent to which power may be increased solely by increasing the number of individuals within clusters because increasing the cluster size also increases the design effect.[29] The relative cost of increasing the number of clusters in the study, rather than the number of individuals within clusters, will be an important consideration when deciding on the final structure of the study.

Obtaining Estimates of the Intra-Class Correlation Coefficient

In order to carry out sample size calculations it is necessary to estimate the intra-class correlation coefficient from previous studies which are as similar as possible in terms of design to the one being planned. That is, studies that used similar clusters, contained similar types of individuals, and used the same outcome. We report a wide range of components of variance and intra-class correlations elsewhere.[20,54] Some examples are given in Table 2. Since the intra-class correlation coefficient will be known imprecisely, it is sensible to take this imprecision into account and carry out a sensitivity analysis on the estimated sample size.[55,56] If confidence limits of the intra-class correlation coefficient are available, these may be used to perform a sensitivity analysis.

Where possible, covariates other than design variables should be allowed for when estimating the intra-class correlation coefficient.[54,57–60] By controlling for covariates the size of ρ, the design effect and the required sample size can be reduced; cluster-level rather than individual-level covariates will usually be more important in this regard.[58,60] In order to translate this into a power advantage, the same covariates must also

Table 2   *Examples of intra-class correlation coefficients for design of area- or organisation-based interventions*

Cluster type	Variable	Source of data	Unit type	Average cluster size	Number of clusters	Intra-class correlation coefficient	Design effect
Health authority	Coronary heart disease mortality	Public Health Common Data Set 1995	Men < 65 years	198,419	105	0.0000283	6.62
Postcode sector	Systolic blood pressure	Health Survey for England 1994[93]	Adults > 15 years	17	711	0.0192	1.31
Household	Eats fruit at least once a day	Health Survey for England 1994[93]	Adults > 15 years	1.72	9053	0.328	1.24
Elderly care unit	Very satisfied with care	RCP Wound Care Audit[94]	Patient with wound	96.27	25	0.042	5.00
General practice	Has symptoms of asthma	Premaratne et al. 1997[95]	Patients registered with GPs	299.1	42	0.0096	3.86

be controlled for when evaluating the intervention effect of the study.

An example: sample size calculation allowing for clustering

To provide a numerical example we consider the planning of an audit of clinical care. Suppose an audit was to be carried out in the offices of single-handed general practitioners (GP) and at clinics held in primary care health centres (HC). We might propose to find out whether the proportion of all attenders who were taking anti-hypertensive treatment was the same in the two clinical settings.

Suppose it were assumed that about half (50%) of the health centre attenders and 40% of GP attenders were taking antihypertensive medication. How many subjects would be required to detect this difference? Using a standard sample size calculation with $\alpha = 0.05$ and power = 0.80, if 408 subjects from each setting were included in the study then there would be sufficient power to detect a difference in case-mix of this magnitude. However, because the subjects were to be sampled from a number of different clinics it would also be necessary to allow for between-cluster variation. We estimated that the average number sampled per clinic (in other words the cluster size) would be about 50. We did not know the intra-class correlation coefficient, so we carried out a sensitivity analysis using values of 0.01, 0.05 and 0.1. The results are shown in Table 3. After allowing for between-cluster variation, the sample size requirement was inflated to 608 if the ICC was 0.01 or 2,407 if the ICC was 0.1. Thus, 12 clinics per group would suffice if the ICC was 0.01, but 48 clinics per group would be needed if the ICC was as high as 0.1. If the number sampled per clinic could be increased to 100, then eight clinics would be required if the ICC was 0.01, but 44 clinics would be needed if the ICC was 0.1. In deciding on the final design of

Table 3   *Results of sample size calculation to detect a difference in proportions of 10%. Prevalence in control group = 50%, $\alpha = 0.05$, $1 - \beta = 0.8$*

	Number sampled per cluster = 50			Number sampled per cluster = 100		
Estimated ICC	Design effect	Individuals required per group	Clusters required per group	Design effect	Number required per group	Clusters required per group
0.0	1.00	408	8	1.00	408	4
0.01	1.49	608	12	1.99	812	8
0.05	3.45	1408	28	5.95	2428	24
0.1	5.9	2407	48	10.9	4447	44

the study it would be necessary to consider the feasibility and costs of increasing the number of clinics in the study rather than the number of individuals sampled per clinic.

METHODS OF ANALYSIS

Choice of Analytical Approach

When observations are made at the cluster-level, standard statistical methods may be used. For example, the effectiveness of smoking control policies might be evaluated using the proportion of smoke-free workplaces as an outcome. Standard statistical methods would not be appropriate for the analysis of individual-level outcomes, such as whether individuals gave up smoking, because the individual responses are likely to be correlated within organisational clusters such as workplaces.

There are three appropriate approaches to analysis of individual-level data:

1 Cluster-level analysis with the cluster means or proportions as the unit of analysis.
2 Individual level univariate analysis with standard errors adjusted for the design effect.
3 Regression analysis using methods for clustered data, allowing for both individual and cluster-level variation.

The choice of analytical approach may be restricted by the design of the study and by the number of clusters and individuals included in the sample. Univariate methods of analysis will not usually be appropriate for non-randomised studies because it will be necessary to allow for confounding by using multiple regression analysis. Analysis of data at the individual level, either by means of adjusted univariate tests or regression methods for clustered data, will require data from 20 to 25 clusters in order to allow the estimation of between-cluster variation with reasonable precision. When there are fewer than 10 clusters per group it may be more appropriate to analyse at the cluster level.

Cluster-Level Analysis

For cluster-level analyses, one or more summary measures of the response for all individuals in a cluster are derived; for example, the mean blood pressure for all patients or the proportion with hypertension. When cluster-level analyses are implemented, the unpaired t-test can be used with as few as three or four clusters per group but there should be sufficient individuals in each cluster to ensure the stability of the cluster specific estimates. Cluster-level analysis will

usually give similar results to adjusted individual analysis but may be less efficient if the precision of estimates can be increased by controlling for individual-level covariates. When cluster sizes are unequal, weighted versions of tests can be used.

Regression analyses may be carried out using the cluster-specific estimates as observations, but this approach is often limited by the small number of clusters. Cluster-level confounders may be included directly in these analyses. Individual-level confounders cannot be included directly, but cluster-specific estimates may be standardised for individual level characteristics such as age and sex.

Univariate Individual-Level Analyses Adjusted for the Design Effect

Univariate individual level analyses consider the outcome values for individual subjects as the observations. In order to allow for clustering of data, the design effect is incorporated into standard statistical formulae for hypothesis testing and confidence interval estimation. The univariate approach may often be less appropriate for non-randomised designs. The intra-class correlation coefficient may be estimated from the study data and about 20 clusters are required to calculate ρ with reasonable precision.[61]

The approach can be illustrated with reference to the estimation of a difference between two proportions. The standard error used to construct confidence intervals for the difference between proportions $\hat{P}_1 - \hat{P}_2$ can be adapted to give a method which is appropriately used when the groups include clusters of equal or varying size:

$$\hat{SE}(\hat{P}_1 - \hat{P}_2) = \left[\frac{Deff_1\hat{P}_1\hat{Q}_1}{N_1} + \frac{Deff_2\hat{P}_2\hat{Q}_2}{N_2}\right]^{1/2} \quad (11)$$

where $Deff_k$ is the variance correction factor, or design effect, for the kth group, $Q_k = 1 - P_k$, N_k is the number of individuals in the kth group. An equivalent approach may be used for continuous outcomes. Donner and Klar[1,62] provided details of adjusted individual level methods and illustrated them with an application to a binary outcome from a cluster randomised study.[61]

Adaptation of standard regression methods for individual-level analysis

It will often be necessary to use regression analysis, either to increase precision in randomised studies or to allow for confounding in non-randomised studies. It is not appropriate to carry out standard individual-level regression analyses with clustered data. As for the adjusted individual-level univariate tests, the variances of the regression coefficients need to be increased by the design effect. In the past, standard regression methods were adapted to account for clustering, either by including an indicator variable as a fixed effect for each cluster in individual-level analyses, or by aggregating data to the cluster-level, but both these approaches have well documented shortcomings.[65–67] An approach that is being used increasingly to adapt standard regression methods for clustering is the estimation of *robust standard errors* (or robust variance estimates). This approach allows the requirement that the observations be independent to be relaxed, and leads to corrected standard errors in the presence of clustering. Robust standard errors may be derived using the linear, logistic or other regression commands in the statistical package Stata.[68]

Regression Methods for Clustered Data

A number of approaches to the regression analysis of clustered data have been developed over the past few years, and these provide a useful alternative to cluster-level analysis and use of adjusted individual-level univariate tests. There are two common approaches to the regression analysis of clustered or multi-level data, random effects modelling and marginal modelling using Generalised Estimating Equations.

Random effects models

The random effects model is an extension of the generalised linear model which can be used to allow for the clustering of data within areas or organisations.[64,69–72] The term random effects modelling refers to the fact that the mean response is treated as varying randomly between clusters. Several other terms, for example, multi-level modelling[69] and hierarchical linear modelling[70] are commonly used and emphasise the multi-level, hierarchical nature of the data being analysed. A full discussion of random effects models is provided by Goldstein.[69]

Random effects models allow for the correlation of responses within organisations by explicitly modelling between-cluster variation. This approach also facilitates the inclusion in the analysis of cluster-level confounders in addition to individual-level confounders. With normally distributed outcomes, the form of a random effects model is:

$$y_{ij} = \alpha + \beta x_{ij} + u_j + e_{ij} \qquad (12)$$

where y_{ij} is the outcome response of the *i*th individual in the *j*th cluster, α is the constant or

intercept, β is the regression coefficient for covariate x, x_{ij} is the covariate value for the *i*th individual in the *j*th cluster, u_j is the random effect for the *j*th cluster and e_{ij} is the level one residual for the *i*th individual in the *j*th cluster. This model differs from the standard linear regression model by the incorporation of the random effect, u_j. This represents the amount by which the intercept for the *j*th cluster differs from the overall mean value α. Through u_j the dependence between observations within the same cluster is modelled explicitly. When there is no variation between clusters the random effects model is equivalent to standard regression analysis. Random effects models may be generalised to allow one or more regression coefficients to vary randomly between clusters. Random effects models may be estimated using the statistical packages SAS[73] and Stata.[68] In addition, there are a number of specialist packages available of which the most popular in the UK is MLn/MLwiN.[74] Random effects models can also be implemented in a Bayesian framework.[75]

The estimation of random effects models for non-normally distributed outcomes (for example, random effects logistic regression) presents considerable computational difficulties. Because full maximum-likelihood estimation procedures are not available, approximations (e.g. penalised quasi-likelihood[76]) are used. These may give rise to biased estimates and practical difficulties, for example, non-convergence. This is an area of active development.[77–79] For binary outcomes the method of Generalised Estimating Equations presents fewer difficulties (see below).

It is important to emphasise the substantial sample sizes that are required for random effects modelling. Duncan et al. suggest that a minimum of 25 individuals in each of 25 clusters may be required for analysis at a single level of clustering.[80] The requirement for a reasonably large number of clusters may often limit the application of random effects models to intervention studies in healthcare, but random effects modelling of observational data on health service performance will often be appropriate. For example, Leyland and Boddy[81] used this approach to study whether mortality of patients with myocardial infarction varied in different hospitals.

Generalised Estimating Equations (GEEs)

The method of generalised estimating equations is an alternative approach to the regression analysis of clustered data.[82–85] The method uses what is sometimes referred to as a population averaged or marginal modelling approach. Unlike the random effects model, the GEEs method does not model the within-cluster dependence explicitly. Instead, the GEEs method assumes a correlation matrix which describes the nature of the association within clusters and obtains estimates of standard errors which are corrected for clustering. Robust variance estimates which produce corrected standard errors even if the within cluster correlation structure has been specified incorrectly are generally used. The statistical packages Stata[68] and SAS[73] can be used to implement GEEs.

In the context of organisation-based evaluations the GEEs approach suffers from the disadvantages that it requires a large number of clusters,[84] it can only be used to model data with one level of clustering, and it is not possible to allow associations to vary between clusters. In spite of these disadvantages the GEEs approach is useful because correct standard errors and *P* values may be obtained without use of complex modelling of variance structures, as in random effects modelling. When the outcome is binary, GEEs may provide the most feasible approach to the regression analysis of data from organisation-based evaluations.

Applications of Multi-Level Analysis to Health Data

The practical application of multi-level analysis to the evaluation of healthcare is still at an early stage of development. Some applications up to 1996 were reviewed by Rice and Leyland,[64] and up to 1998 by Duncan et al.[80] For example, this approach may be applicable if cluster sampling is used to recruit individuals from different clinics.[86] In a study of neonatal mortality in relation to activity level in neonatal units, GEEs were used to adjust for the correlation of infant outcomes within hospitals.[87]

Duncan et al.[80] make the point that random effects models will be more useful than GEEs when the evaluator wants to distinguish the effects of the organisational or geographical context from the characteristics of individuals sampled within the organisation or area. This distinction is often important in observational evaluations of existing health services. For example, in comparing the performance of different institutions after allowing for differences in case mix,[81] or comparing healthcare processes and outcomes in different geographical areas.[80]

Goldstein and Speigelhalter[12] discussed some of the statistical issues in comparisons of institutional performance. They showed that it is important to carry out the correct hierarchical analysis in which individual responses are modelled as nested within hospitals or health authorities. This type of analysis in which organisational units are treated as random effects, leads to cluster-specific estimates which are shrunk towards the population mean with confidence intervals that are more appropriate when compared to a conventional fixed effects analysis. Over the past few years there has been increasing interest in monitoring the performance of health services by ranking organisational units into league tables. Goldstein and Speigelhalter[12] showed that regression methods for clustered data find a direct application in the analysis of this kind of data. In particular, an appropriate analysis can be used to generate confidence intervals for the rankings of organisational units as well as for the cluster-specific outcomes. The confidence intervals for ranks will often be very wide, and even when there are large differences in outcomes between units, ranks will often be imprecise and unstable indicators of performance.[88] Thus, league table rankings should not be used without additional information concerning their degree of imprecision.

An example: analysis allowing for clustering

To illustrate how an analysis might be performed in order to allow for clustering, we analysed data obtained from an audit of clinical care (Table 4). The aim of this analysis was to see whether there was a difference between the proportion of attenders who were receiving antihypertensive treatment at health centre clinics (HC) compared with attenders at single-handed general practitioners (GPs).

Initial inspection of the data showed that there were 26 clinics, including 18 health centres and eight single-handed GPs. The number of patients sampled per clinic was quite variable. The proportion of patients treated for hypertension seemed to be higher at the health centre clinics, but the health centre patients were older than those attending the GPs. The value for ρ estimated from the 26 clinics was 0.259, but it might not be justified to assume a common value for ρ at both types of clinic, since the estimated value for ρ in the HC clinics was 0.107 while for the GP clinics it was 0.013. However, the number of GP clinics was small and possibly not sufficient to obtain a stable estimate for ρ.

These observations suggest that certain approaches to analysis will be more appropriate than others. Because age is associated with both blood pressure and clinic type it will be necessary to carry out analyses which allow for differences in age among clinic types. Donner and Klar[61] pointed out that adjusted individual level

Table 4 *Data from clinical audit. Figures are frequencies (% of row total)*

Clinic type	Number of patients	On BP treatment	Mean age (years)	Women
HC	62	47 (76)	63	46 (74)
HC	51	44 (86)	62	34 (67)
HC	43	41 (95)	65	33 (77)
HC	43	32 (74)	64	27 (63)
HC	35	28 (80)	63	26 (74)
HC	21	9 (43)	69	7 (33)
HC	83	69 (83)	66	61 (73)
HC	68	24 (35)	56	43 (63)
HC	59	28 (47)	60	34 (58)
HC	74	39 (53)	59	45 (61)
HC	67	53 (79)	64	52 (78)
HC	44	27 (61)	59	28 (64)
HC	63	44 (70)	62	40 (63)
HC	76	39 (51)	63	49 (64)
HC	36	15 (42)	55	27 (75)
HC	66	41 (62)	60	42 (64)
HC	37	24 (65)	64	27 (73)
HC	47	32 (68)	57	42 (89)
GP	45	5 (11)	52	28 (62)
GP	43	6 (14)	52	29 (67)
GP	36	9 (25)	54	31 (86)
GP	89	14 (16)	46	69 (78)
GP	120	19 (16)	46	81 (68)
GP	21	8 (38)	53	13 (62)
GP	120	31 (26)	54	87 (73)
GP	84	19 (23)	47	49 (58)
HC subtotal	975	636 (65)	61	663 (68)
GP subtotal	558	111 (20)	49	387 (69)
Total	1533	747 (49)	57	1050 (68)

BP, blood pressure; HC, health centre; GP, general practitioner.

hypothesis tests which assume a common value for the design effect across groups will be less applicable to non-randomised data.

The results of several different methods of analysis are shown in Table 5. Initially, cluster-level analyses were performed using the cluster-specific proportions as observations. A non-parametric rank sum test shows a significant difference between the two clinical settings with an approximate z statistic of 3.95. The two-sample t-test gave a mean difference in the cluster-specific proportions of 0.439 (95% confidence interval (CI) 0.307 to 0.571). Analyses were also performed at the individual level. An analysis which made no allowance for the clustering of responses gave a difference between the two proportions of 0.453 with 95% CI from 0.409 to 0.498 and a z statistic of 17.1. However, a standard statistical analysis would be

incorrect because, as we noted above, between clinic variation is present. In order to construct CIs, the design effect should be incorporated into the formula for the standard error for the difference in two proportions as shown in Equation (11). The design effect for the health centre clinics is 6.66, and for the single-handed general practitioners is 1.90. The standard error of the difference in proportions was 0.0458. The difference was still 0.453, but the corrected CIs were from 0.363 to 0.543. This result showed that the difference between the two audits was estimated less precisely after allowing for between-clinic variation. The corresponding adjusted chi-squared test[61] yielded a χ^2 of 113.0 (df 1). Note however that this test assumes a common value for ρ.

An alternative approach to the analysis is to use logistic regression. A conventional logistic regression analysis showed that the relative odds of patients being on antihypertensive medication in the health centre clinics compared with the GP clinics were 7.56 (5.91 to 9.66). The z statistic obtained from this model was 16.1. This analysis was modified to allow for clustering within clinics by estimating robust standard errors giving the same odds ratio 7.56, but the 95% CIs were from 4.88 to 11.69 with a z statistic of 9.1. Analyses were adjusted for age and sex and the relative odds were reduced to 5.46 (CIs 3.66 to 8.15). The method of GEEs offered an alternative approach to regression analysis. This was carried out by specifying a logistic link function, an exchangeable correlation structure, and robust standard errors to allow for clustering within clinics. The analysis adjusted for age and sex gave an odds ratio of 5.06 (CIs 3.32 to 7.70) which was similar to the result obtained using logistic regression with robust standard errors, but this analysis adjusted the estimate for clustering as well as the standard error. We used the Stata software to perform both the logistic regression and GEEs analyses.[68]

A third approach to the analysis of these data is to use random effects logistic regression to model the variation in response at clinic level. We initially used a simplified model which assumed the same variation at level 2 (that is, clinic level) for both settings. The adjusted analysis gave a higher odds ratio (6.16) and slightly wider CIs (3.39 to 11.18), when compared to the logistic regression and GEE analyses. The level 2 variance on the log odds scale was 0.387 with a standard error of 0.139. We used MLn[89] to fit the random effects logistic regression models with second-order PQL estimation.

The incorrect individual level analyses with no adjustment for clustering gave narrower confidence intervals and larger z statistics than do

Table 5   *Results obtained using different methods of analysis to compare the proportion of attenders on antihypertensive treatment at health centre clinics and at single-handed general practitioners*

Method		Estimate (95% CI)	*z* statistic
		Difference	
Cluster-level analysis		(95% CI for difference)	
Rank sum test		–	3.95
Two-sample *t*-test		0.439 (0.307 to 0.571)	*t* = 6.85
Individual analysis – difference of proportions			
Standard univariate test		0.453 (0.409 to 0.498)	17.1
Univariate test adjusted for design effect		0.453 (0.363 to 0.543)	$\chi^2 = 113.0$ (df 1)*
		Odds ratio	
Univariate individual analysis – logistic regression methods		(95% CI for odds ratio)	
Standard logistic regression	– univariate	7.56 (5.91 to 9.66)	16.1
	– adjusted for age and sex	5.46 (4.22 to 7.08)	12.9
Logistic regression, robust standard errors	– univariate	7.56 (4.88 to 11.69)	9.1
	– adjusted for age and sex	5.46 (3.66 to 8.15)	8.3
Generalised estimating equations	– univariate	7.32 (4.62 to 11.57)	8.5
	– adjusted for age and sex	5.06 (3.32 to 7.70)	7.6
Random effects logistic regression	– univariate	8.47 (4.51 to 15.91)	6.6
	– adjusted for age and sex	6.16 (3.39 to 11.18)	6.0

* Refers to adjusted chi-squared test.[61]

Table 6   *Check-list for design and analysis of area- and organisation-based interventions*[90]

1. Recognise areas or organisational clusters as the units of intervention.
2. Justify allocation of entire clusters of individuals to groups.
3. Randomise clusters to intervention and control groups whenever possible, justify use of non-randomised designs.
4. Include a sufficient number of clusters. Studies in which there are less than four clusters per group are unlikely to yield conclusive results.
5. Multiply standard sample size formulae by the design effect in order to obtain the number of individuals required to give a study with the same power as one in which individuals are randomised. Estimates of the intra-class correlation coefficient should be obtained from earlier studies.
6. Consider stratification of clusters in order to reduce error in randomised studies and bias in quasi-experimental studies. Some stratification should usually be used unless the number of clusters is quite large. Researchers should be aware of the limitations of the matched pairs design (i.e. a design with only two clusters per stratum).
7. Choose between cohort and repeated cross-sectional sampling for studies that involve follow-up. The cohort design is more applicable to individual level outcomes, and may give more precise results, but is more susceptible to bias. The repeated cross-sectional design is more appropriate when outcomes will be aggregated to cluster-level, and is usually less powerful, but is less susceptible to bias.
8. Standard statistical methods, applied at the individual level, are not appropriate because individual values are correlated within clusters. Univariate analysis may be performed either using the cluster means or proportions as observations, or using individual-level tests in which the standard error is adjusted for the design effect. Where there are fewer than about 10 clusters per group, a cluster-level analysis may be more appropriate.
9. When individual- and/or cluster-level prognostic variables need to be allowed for, regression methods for clustered data are appropriate. Provided there are sufficient clusters, use of regression methods for clustered data may also provide a more flexible and efficient approach to univariate analysis.
10. Authors should publish estimates of components of variance and the intra-class correlation coefficient for the outcome of interest when reporting organisation level evaluations.

any of the methods which allow for clustering of responses. Carrying out a two-sample *t*-test using the cluster-specific proportions as observations provided the most accessible method of analysis and gave a valid result. However, as it was also necessary to adjust for individual level confounders, one of the regression methods for clustered data was to be preferred. Ordinary logistic regression with robust standard errors gave a similar result to that obtained using generalised estimating equations in these data. Logistic regression was more accessible, and was computationally less intensive with shorter analysis times, but the GEE approach adjusted both the estimate and the standard error for clustering and was to be preferred for this reason. Random effects logistic regression might have allowed additional modelling of the variance at cluster level which could have been useful if the analysis was to focus on the performance of particular primary care clinics.

CONCLUSIONS

The approach of clinical epidemiology emphasises the individual patient or healthy subject as the unit of investigation. Data from organisation- or area-based evaluations in health services research often have a hierarchical structure which should be explicitly recognised in designing and analysing studies. The particular need to include a sufficient number of organisational clusters in intervention and control groups, to randomise them, and to use statistical methods of analysis which are appropriate for clustered data should be emphasised. A check-list of items which we have reported previously[90] is shown in Table 6.

It is relevant to recognise possible reasons why evaluations may be designed using suboptimal methods. Firstly, health services researchers are often asked to evaluate interventions implemented in one or two clusters. Secondly, the resources required for evaluating interventions in large organisational clusters may be substantial, and this is likely to explain the tendency to study small numbers of clusters in primary research and to use routinely available data to study larger numbers of clusters. Finally, appropriate methods for the analysis of hierarchical data have only recently become widely available, and the extent to which they may be usefully applied in the practice of healthcare evaluation may not yet have been realised. Consideration of these constraints is as relevant for commissioners of research as for researchers. In spite of these constraints, there is a widening consensus that validity of health services research

studies will be enhanced by adopting approaches to study design and analysis that explicitly acknowledge the hierarchical structure of data from evaluations of health services.[2,3,12,20,64,80,90]

ACKNOWLEDGEMENTS

This work was funded by a contract from the UK National Health Service Health Technology Assessment Programme. The views expressed are those of the authors and do not necessarily reflect those of the NHS Research and Development Programme. The authors thank Dr D Mahabir for permission to present the audit data.

REFERENCES

1. Donner A, Klar N. Cluster randomization trials in epidemiology: theory and application. *J. Statistical Planning Inference* 1994; **42**: 37–56.
2. Whiting-O'Keefe QE, Henke C, Simborg DW. Choosing the Correct Unit of Analysis in Med Care Experiments. *Med Care* 1984; **22**: 1101–14.
3. Simpson JM, Klar N, Donner A. Accounting for cluster randomization: a review of primary prevention trials, 1990 through 1993. *Am. J. Public Health* 1995; **85**: 1378–83.
4. Dwyer JH, MacKinnon DP, Pentz MA, Flay BR, Hansen WB, Wang EY, Johnson CA. Estimating intervention effects in longitudinal studies. *Am. J. Epidemiol.* 1989; **130**: 781–95.
5. Williams PT, Fortmann SP, Farquhar JW, Varady A, Mellen S. A comparison of statistical methods for evaluating risk factor changes in community-based studies: an example from the Stanford Three-Community Study. *J. Chron. Dis.* 1981; **34**: 565–71.
6. Kelder SH, Jacobs DR, Jr., Jeffery RW, McGovern PG, Forster JL. The worksite component of variance: design effects and the Healthy Worker Project. *Health Education Res.* 1993; **8**: 555–66.
7. McArdle CS, Hole D. Impact of variability among surgeons on post-operative morbidity and mortality and ultimate survival. *Br. Med. J.* 1991; **302**: 1501–5.
8. Donner A. Approaches to sample size estimation in the design of clinical trials – a review. *Stat. Med.* 1984; **3**: 199–214.
9. Cornfield J. Randomization by group: a formal analysis. *Am. J. Epidemiol.* 1978; **108**: 100–2.
10. Slavin RE. Best-evidence synthesis: an intelligent alternative to meta-analysis. *J. Clin. Epidemiol.* 1995; **48**: 9–18.

11. Koepsell TD, Diehr PH, Cheadle A, Kristal A. Invited commentary: symposium on community intervention trials. *Am. J. Epidemiol.* 1995; **142**: 594–9.

12. Goldstein H, Spiegelhalter DJ. League Tables and Their Limitations: Statistical Issues in Comparisons of Institutional Performance. *J. Roy. Statist. Soc.*, A 1996; **159**: 385–443.

13. Puska P, Salonen JT, Tuomilehto J, Nissinen A, Kottke TE. Evaluating community-based preventive cardiovascular programs: problems and experiences from the North Karelia project. *J. Community Health* 1983; **9**: 49–64.

14. Nicholl J, Turner J. Effectiveness of a regional trauma system in reducing mortality from major trauma: before and after study. *Br. Med. J.* 1997; **315**: 1349–54.

15. Puska P, Holland WW, Detels R, Knox G (eds). *Oxford Textbook of Public Health. 12, Intervention and experimental studies.* Oxford: Oxford Medical Publications; 1991, pp. 177–87.

16. Diehr P, Martin DC, Koepsell T, Cheadle A. Breaking the matches in a paired *t*-test for community interventions when the number of pairs is small. *Stat. Med.* 1995; **14**: 1491–504.

17. Hayes R, Mosha F, Nicoll A, Grosskurth H, Newell J, Todd J, Killewo, J, Rugemalila J, Mabey D. A community trial of the impact of improved sexually transmitted disease treatment on the HIV epidemic in rural Tanzania: 1. *Design. AIDS* 1995; **9**: 919–26.

18. Black N. Why we need observational studies to evaluate the effectiveness of health care. *Br. Med. J.* 1996; **312**: 1215–18.

19. Cook TD, Campbell DT. *Quasi-experimentation. Design and analysis issues for field settings.* Chicago: Rand McNally College Publishing Company, 1979.

20. Ukoumunne OC, Gulliford MC, Chinn S, Sterne J, Burney PGJ. Methods for evaluating area-wide and organisation-based interventions in health and health care. *Health Technology Assessment* 1999; **3**(5).

21. Koepsell TD, Wagner EH, Cheadle AC, Patrick DL, Martin DC, Diehr PH, Perrin EB, Kristal AR, Allan-Andrilla CH, Dey LJ. Selected methodological issues in evaluating community-based health promotion and disease prevention programs. *Annu. Rev. Public Health* 1992; **13**: 31–57.

22. Freedman LS, Green SB, Byar DP. Assessing the gain in efficiency due to matching in a community intervention study. *Stat. Med.* 1990; **9**: 943–52.

23. Klar N, Donner A. The Merits of Matching: A Cautionary Tale. *Stat. Med.* 1997; **16**: 1573–64.

24. Green SB, Corle DK, Gail MH, Mark SD, Pee D, Freedman LS, Graubard, BI, Lynn WR. Interplay between design and analysis for behavioural intervention trials with community as the unit of randomization. *Am. J. Epidemiol.* 1995; **142**: 587–93.

25. Martin DC, Diehr P, Perrin EB, Koepsell TD. The effect of matching on the power of randomised community intervention studies. *Stat. Med.* 1993; **12**: 329–38.

26. Kirkwood BR, Morrow RH. Community-based intervention trials. *J. Biosocial Sci.* 1989; **10**: 79–86.

27. Murray DM. Design and analysis of community trials: lessons from the Minnesota Heart Health Program. *Am. J. Epidemiol.* 1995; **142**: 569–75.

28. Kelly JA, Murphy DA, Sikkema J, McAuliffe TL, Roffman RA, Solomon LJ, Winett RA, Kalichman SC, the Community HIV Prevention Research Collaborative. Randomised, controlled, community-level HIV prevention intervention for sexual-risk behaviour among homosexual men in US cities. *Lancet* 1997; **350**: 1500–5.

29. Thompson SG, Pyke SD, Hardy RJ. The design and analysis of paired cluster randomised trials: an application of meta-analysis techniques. *Stat. Med.* 1997; **16**: 2063–79.

30. Donner A, Hauck W. Estimation of a common odds ratio in case-control studies of familial aggregation. *Biometrics* 1988; **44**: 369–78.

31. Donner A, Donald A. Analysis of data arising from a stratified design with the cluster as unit of randomization. *Stat. Med.* 1987; **6**: 43–52.

32. Diehr P, Martin DC, Koepsell T, Cheadle A, Psaty BM, Wagner EH. Optimal survey design for community intervention evaluations: cohort or cross-sectional? *J. Clin. Epidemiol.* 1995; **48**: 1461–72.

33. Gail MH, Mark SD, Carroll RJ, Green SB, Pee D. On design considerations and randomization-based inference for community intervention trials. *Stat. Med.* 1996; **15**: 1069–92.

34. Gail MH, Byar DP, Pechacek TF, Corle DK. Aspects of statistical design for the Community Intervention Trial for Smoking Cessation (COMMIT). *Controlled Clinical Trials* 1992; **13**: 6–21.

35. Koepsell TD, Martin DC, Diehr PH, Psaty BM, Wagner EH, Perrin EB, Cheadle A. Data analysis and sample size issues in evaluations of community-based health promotion and disease prevention programs: a mixed-model analysis of variance approach. *J. Clin. Epidemiol.* 1991; **44**: 701–13.

36. Murray DM, Hannan PJ. Planning for the appropriate analysis in school-based drug-use prevention studies. *J. Consult. Clin. Psychol.* 1990; **58**: 458–68.

37. Donner A, Klar N. Statistical considerations in the design and analysis of community intervention trials. *J. Clin. Epidemiol.* 1996; **49**: 435–9.

38. Feldman HA, McKinlay SM. Cohort versus cross-sectional design in large field trials: precision, sample size, and a unifying model. *Stat. Med.* 1994; **13**: 61–78.

39. McKinlay SM. Cost-efficient designs of cluster unit trials. *Prevent. Med.* 1994; **23**: 606–11.

40. Armitage P, Berry G. *Statistical Methods in Medical Research*. 2nd edn. Oxford: Blackwell Science, 1987.

41. Snedecor GW, Cochran WG. *Statistical methods*. 6th edn. Ames, Iowa: Iowa State University Press, 1967.

42. Donner A. The analysis of intraclass correlation in multiple samples. *Ann. Hum. Genet.* 1985; **49**: 75–82.

43. Fleiss JL, Cohen J. The equivalence of weighted kappa and the intraclass correlation coefficient as measures of reliability. *Education Psychol. Measure* 1973; **33**: 613–19.

44. Fleiss JL. *Statistical methods for rates and proportions*. 2nd edn. Chichester: Wiley; 1981, pp. 211–36.

45. Moser CA, Kalton G. *Survey Methods in Social Investigation*. Aldershot: Dartmouth Publishing Company Limited, 1993, pp. 61–78.

46. Kish L. *Survey Sampling*. London: John Wiley & Sons, 1965, pp. 148–81.

47. Donner A. An empirical study of cluster randomization. *Int. J. Epidemiol.* 1982; **11**: 283–6.

48. Donner A, Birkett N, Buck C. Randomization by cluster. Sample size requirements and analysis. *Am. J. Epidemiol.* 1981; **114**: 906–14.

49. Pocock SJ. *Clinical trials. A practical approach*. Chichester: John Wiley & Sons, 1983.

50. Hsieh FY. Sample size formulae for intervention studies with the cluster as unit of randomization. *Stat. Med.* 1988; **7**: 1195–201.

51. Shipley MJ, Smith PG, Dramaix M. Calculation of power for matched pair studies when randomization is by group. *Int. J. Epidemiol.* 1989; **18**: 457–61.

52. Donner A. Sample size requirements for stratified cluster randomization designs. *Stat. Med.* 1992; **11**: 743–50.

53. Kerry SM, Bland JM. Sample size in cluster randomisation. *Br. Med. J.* 1998; **316**: 549.

54. Gulliford MC, Ukoumunne OC, Chinn S. Components of variance and intraclass correlations for the design of community-based surveys and intervention studies. Data from the Health Survey for England 1994. *Am. J. Epidemiol.* 1999; **149**: 876–83.

55. Mickey RM, Goodwin GD. The magnitude and variability of design effects for community intervention studies. *Am. J. Epidemiol.* 1993; **137**: 9–18.

56. Hannan PJ, Murray DM, Jacobs DR, Jr., McGovern PG. Parameters to aid in the design and analysis of community trials: intraclass correlations from the Minnesota Heart Program. *Epidemiology* 1994; **5**: 88–95.

57. Mickey RM, Goodwin GD, Costanza MC. Estimation of the design effect in community intervention studies. *Stat. Med.* 1991; **10**: 53–64.

58. Murray DM, Short B. Intraclass correlation among measures related to alcohol use by young adults: estimates, correlates and applications in intervention studies. *J. Studies Alcohol.* 1995; **56**: 681–94.

59. Siddiqui O, Hedeker D, Flay BR, Hu FB. Intraclass correlation estimates in a school-based smoking prevention study – outcome and mediating variables, by sex and ethnicity. *Am. J. Epidemiol.* 1996; **144**: 425–33.

60. Raudenbush SW. Statistical analysis and optimal design for cluster randomized trials. *Psychol. Methods* 1997; **3**: 173–85.

61. Donner A, Klar N. Methods for comparing event rates in intervention studies when the unit of allocation is a cluster. *Am. J. Epidemiol.* 1994; **140**: 279–89.

62. Donner A, Klar N. Confidence interval construction for effect measures arising from cluster randomization trials. *J. Clin. Epidemiol.* 1993; **46**: 123–31.

63. Aitkin M, Longford N. Statistical modelling issues in school effectiveness studies. *J. Roy. Statist. Soc. A* 1986; **149**: 1–43.

64. Rice N, Leyland A. Multilevel models: applications to health data. *J. Health Services Res. Policy* 1996; **1**: 154–64.

65. Zucker DM. An analysis of variance pitfall: The fixed effects analysis in a nested design. *Education Psychol. Measurement* 1990; **50**: 731–8.

66. Singer JD. An Intraclass Correlation Model for Analysing Multilevel Data. *J. Exp. Education* 1987; **55**: 219–28.

67. Brown RL, Baumann LJ, Cameron L. Single-level analysis of intervention studies with hierarchically structured data: a cautionary note. *Nursing Res.* 1996; **45**: 359–62.

68. Stata Corporation. *Stata statistical software. release 5*. College Station, Texas. Stata Press, 1997.

69. Goldstein H. *Multilevel Statistical Models*. London: Arnold, 1996.

70. Bryk AS, Raudenbush SW. *Hierarchical Linear Models*. London: Sage, 1992.

71. Longford NT. *Random Coefficient Models*. Oxford: Oxford University Press, 1995.

72. Arnold CL. An introduction to hierarchical linear models. *Measurement and Evaluation Counsel Develop.* 1992; **25**: 58–90.

73. SAS Institute Inc. *SAS/STAT User Guide. Version 6. Volume 2*. 4th edn. Cary, North Carolina: SAS Institute, 1990, pp. 1127–34.

74. Kreft IGG, de Leeuw J, van der Leeden R. Review of five multilevel analysis programs:

BMDP-5V, GENMOD, HLM, ML3, VARCL. *Am. Statist.* 1994; **48**: 324–35.

75. Speigelhalter DJ. Bayesian graphical modelling: a case study in monitoring health outcomes. *Appl. Statist.* 1998; **47**: 115–33.

76. Breslow E, Clayton DG. Approximate inference in generalized linear mixed models. *J. Am. Statist. Assoc.* 1993; **88**: 9–25.

77. Guo SW, Lin DY. Regression analysis of multivariate grouped survival data. *Biometrics* 1994; **50**: 632–9.

78. Hedeker D, Gibbons RD. A random-effects ordinal regression model for multilevel analysis. *Biometrics* 1994; **50**: 933–44.

79. Ten Have TR, Landis JR, Hartzel J. Population-averaged and cluster-specific models for clustered ordinal response data. *Stat. Med.* 1996; **15**: 2573–88.

80. Duncan C, Jones K, Moon G. Context, composition and heterogeneity: using multi-level models in health research. *Soc. Sci. Med.* 1998; **46**: 97–117.

81. Leyland AH, Boddy FA. League tables and acute myocardial infarction. *Lancet* 1998; **351**: 555–8.

82. Liang K, Zeger SL. Longitudinal data analysis using generalized linear models. *Biometrika* 1986; **73**: 13–22.

83. Zeger SL, Liang KY. Longitudinal data analysis for discrete and continuous outcomes. *Biometrics* 1986; **42**: 121–30.

84. Zeger SL, Liang KY, Albert PS. Models for longitudinal data: a generalized estimating equation approach. *Biometrics* 1988; **44**: 1049–60.

85. Diggle PJ, Liang KY, Zeger SL. *Analysis of Longitudinal Data.* Oxford: Oxford University Press, 1996.

86. Reid SE, Simpson JM, Britt HC. Pap smears in general practice: a secondary analysis of the Australian Morbidity and Treatment Survey 1990 to 1991. *Aust. N.Z. J. Public Health* 1997; **21**: 257–64.

87. Phibbs CS, Bronstein JM, Buxton E, Phibbs RH. The effects of patient volume and level of care at the hospital of birth on neonatal mortality. *JAMA* 1996; **276**: 1054–9.

88. Marshall EC, Speigelhalter DJ. Reliability of league tables of in vitro fertilisation clinics: retrospective analysis of live birth rates. *Br. Med. J.* 1998; **316**: 1701–5.

89. Paterson L. Woodhouse G. *Multilevel modelling applications. A guide for users of MLn.* London: Institute of Education, 1996.

90. Ukoumunne OC, Gulliford MC, Chinn S, Sterne J, Burney P, Donner A. Evaluation of health interventions at area and organisation level. In: Black N, Brazier J, Fitzpatrick R, Reeves B (eds). *Methods for Health Care Services Research.* London: BMJ Books, 1998.

91. Taylor FC, Ramsay ME, Renton A, Cohen H. Methods for managing the increased workload in anticoagulant clinics. *Br. Med. J.* 1996; **312**: 286.

92. Pan XR, Li GW, Hu YH et al. Effect of diet and exercise in preventing NIDDM in people with impaired glucose tolerance. The Da Qing IGT and Diabetes Study. *Diabetes Care* 1997; **20**: 537–44.

93. Colhoun H, Prescott-Clarke P. *Health survey for England 1994.* London: HMSO, 1996.

94. Royal College of Physicians Research Unit. *Older people's programme. National chronic wound audit.* London: Royal College of Physicians, 1997.

95. Premaratne UN, Sterne JAC, Webb J, et al. Clustered randomised trial of an intervention to improve the management of asthma: Greenwich asthma study. *Br. Med. J.* 1999; **318**: 1251–5.

18

Handling Uncertainty in Economic Evaluation

ANDREW H. BRIGGS and ALASTAIR M. GRAY

SUMMARY

The aim of this chapter is to present an overview of a structured review of the way in which uncertainty has been handled in economic evaluation, to examine data on the actual distributional form and variance of healthcare costs, and to devise guidelines to improve current practice.

A search of the literature was undertaken to identify published economic evaluations that reported results in terms of cost per life year or cost per quality-adjusted life year. Articles which met the search criteria were reviewed using a proforma designed to collect summary information on the disease area, type of intervention, nature of data, nature of results, study design and methods used to handle uncertainty in the study. These results were then entered as keywords onto a database, to allow interrogation and cross-referencing of the database by category.

Subsets of this data set were then employed to focus in on two specific areas of interest. Firstly, all studies reporting UK results were reviewed in detail and information on the baseline results, the methods underlying those results, the range of results representing uncertainty and the number of previously published results quoted in comparison were entered onto a relational database. By matching results by the methods employed using a retrospective application of a methodological 'reference case', a subset of results with improved comparability was identified and a rank ordering of these results was then attempted. Where a range of values accompanied the baseline results, the implications of

this uncertainty for the rank ordering was also examined.

Secondly, studies that reported patient-level cost data were reviewed in detail to consider how they had reported the distribution and variance of healthcare costs. In addition, five available datasets of patient-level cost data were examined in order to show how the healthcare costs in those data were distributed and to elucidate issues surrounding the analysis and presentation of healthcare cost differences.

Economists are not simply concerned with costs, but also with health outcomes, and the results of economic evaluation are usually presented in the form of a ratio. Where patient-level data are available, it is natural to represent uncertainty in point estimates by presenting confidence intervals. Ratio statistics pose particular problems for confidence interval estimation and recently proposed methods for estimating confidence intervals for cost–effectiveness ratios are reviewed.

A total of 492 articles to date have been found to match the search criteria and have been fully reviewed and entered onto the database. Analysis of the database shows that the vast majority of studies use one-way sensitivity analysis methods only. Of some concern is that almost 20% of studies did not attempt any analysis to examine uncertainty, although there is weak evidence to show that this situation has improved over time.

Of these 492 studies, 60 reported results for the UK. From these UK studies, 548 baseline cost–effectiveness results were extracted relating to 106 methodological scenarios. Application of a retrospective 'reference case' gave a single methodological scenario for each article with 333 associated baseline results. These results were converted to a common cost base year and rank ordered to give a comprehensive 'league table' of UK results. Of the 333 results, 61 had an associated full range of values to represent uncertainty. Alternative rankings based on the high or low values from this range showed that there could be considerable disruption to the rank order based on the baseline point estimates only.

The review of patient-level cost data showed that 53 of the 492 studies on the database had patient-level cost data, and that just 15 of these had reported some measure of cost variance. Only four studies had calculated 95% confidence intervals for cost. A review of five available cost data sets showed that cost data were not normally distributed, and in two cases showed substantial skewness.

The review of methods for calculating confidence intervals for cost–effectiveness ratios results in the recommendation that the parametric Fieller's method or non-parametric bootstrap approach be used. Cost–effectiveness acceptability curves are identified as a method of presenting uncertainty in studies that has several advantages over the presentation of confidence intervals.

INTRODUCTION

Health economics is a burgeoning discipline, particularly in the area of the economic evaluation of healthcare interventions. During the 1980s, much of the literature concerning economic analysis related to justifying the application of economic thinking to the healthcare sector. In the 1990s, with a much wider acceptance of the need to evaluate economically new and existing healthcare interventions, the focus has become more methodological – with much more attention being placed on the appropriate methods to employ when evaluating healthcare interventions. The most popular evaluative technique for economic evaluation is cost–effectiveness analysis,[1] and many cost–effectiveness studies present only point estimates of the value for money of particular healthcare interventions, although it is clear that there is often considerable uncertainty in the evaluative process.

The cost–effectiveness (CE) plane[2,3] is often employed to show how decisions can be related to both costs and effects. The CE plane (Figure 1) is divided into four quadrants indicating four possible situations in relation to the additional costs and additional health outcome effects of a

new therapy compared to the standard therapy. Where one therapy is simultaneously cheaper and more effective than the other (quadrants II and IV on the CE plane), it is clearly the treatment of choice and is said to dominate. However, where one intervention is both more effective and more costly (quadrants I and III), then the decision is no longer clear. Rather, a judgement must be made concerning whether the difference in costs resulting from a switch in therapy is justified by the difference in effectiveness that such a switch would bring about. If it is possible to define some maximum acceptable value for the incremental cost–effectiveness ratio (ICER), then this 'ceiling' value of the ratio can be used to judge whether the treatment in question is cost-effective. The ceiling value of the ICER can be represented by the (slope of the) dashed line on the CE plane of Figure 1. If the incremental costs and effects are plotted to the right of this line on the CE plane, then the treatment is considered cost-effective, while points to the left of this line represent cost-ineffective interventions.

Cost–effectiveness analysis is essentially a comparative methodology and, in the absence of a clearly defined ceiling ICER appropriate for decision-making, results have meaning primarily in terms of comparison to other reported cost–effectiveness results. In this review, we therefore concentrate on economic evaluations that report cost per life year or cost per quality-adjusted life year (QALY) results, since it is possible to compare these results across different disease/treatment areas. It is common for point estimates of cost–effectiveness to be grouped together and presented in rank order in so-called cost–effectiveness league tables. The implication of constructing such league tables is that those interventions with low cost per (QA)LY results should take precedence over interventions with higher cost per (QA)LY results.

The use of point estimates in constructing such tables raises problems. Consider Figure 2, where the point estimates for seven different healthcare interventions are plotted in increasing order of magnitude (this is adapted from Table II by Petrou and colleagues[4]). The 'I' bars on this figure represent the estimated range of uncertainty around the point estimates. It is immediately apparent that the range of uncertainty is so wide that it would be possible to rank these interventions in a completely different order than that obtained from the point estimates. Thus, if policy-makers are to be fully informed when making decisions based on the results of economic evaluations, it is imperative

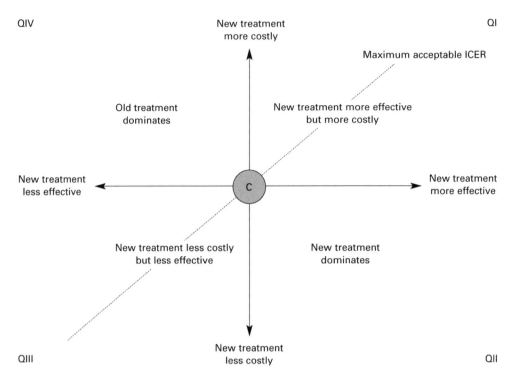

Figure 1   *The cost–effectiveness plane. ICER, incremental cost–effectiveness ratio.*

that analysts estimate and present the level of uncertainty inherent in their results.

Uncertainty in economic evaluation is pervasive, entering the evaluative process at every stage. It is useful to distinguish uncertainty related to the data requirements of a study (the resource use and health outcome consequences of a particular intervention and the data required to value those consequences) from uncertainty related to the process of evaluation. Uncertainty in the data requirements of a study arises through natural variation in populations, which means that estimates based on samples drawn from that population will always be associated with a level of uncertainty which is inversely related to sample size. Examples of uncertainty due to the evaluative process include: the need to extrapolate when conducting evaluations, for example from a clinical outcome measure (such as cholesterol lowering) to a health outcome measure (reduced morbidity and mortality due to heart disease); uncertainty related to generalising from the context of the study to other contexts and to different patient populations; and the uncertainty related to choice of analytical methods when conducting economic evaluation (e.g. whether to include indirect costs in the analysis).[5]

The standard method for handling uncertainty due to sampling variation is statistical analysis. Where patient specific resource use and health outcome data have been collected (for example, as part of a prospective clinical trial) in a so-called stochastic analysis,[6] then statistical techniques have been developed to calculate confidence intervals around point estimates of cost–effectiveness (although the methods required to estimate confidence limits around a ratio statistic are less straightforward than for many other statistics).

In practice, however, a relatively small proportion of all economic evaluations are conducted alongside clinical trials. Instead, data are synthesised from a number of different sources – including reviews of the literature, hospital records and even clinical judgement – in a deterministic analysis. Hence, standard statistical methods cannot be employed. Moreover, even where a stochastic analysis is possible, the remaining levels of uncertainty that are not related to sampling variation need exploration and quantification. To do this, a technique known as sensitivity analysis is used, which involves systematically examining the influence of the variables and assumptions employed in an evaluation for the estimated cost–effectiveness results.

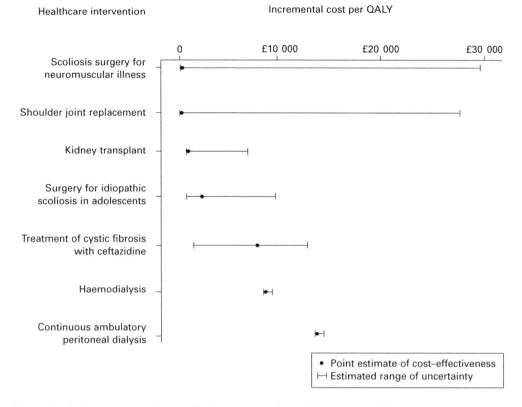

Figure 2 *Point estimates of cost–effectiveness together with estimates of the associated uncertainty. (Adapted from Table II of Petrou et al.[4])*

There are three main forms of sensitivity analysis.[7] A one-way sensitivity analysis examines the impact of each variable independently, while holding all other variable constant. By contrast, an extreme scenario analysis involves setting each variable to simultaneously take the most optimistic (pessimistic) value from the point of view of the intervention under evaluation in order to generate a best (worst) case scenario. In real life the components of an evaluation do not vary in isolation, nor are they perfectly correlated; hence a one-way sensitivity analysis might be expected to underestimate uncertainty, while an extreme scenario analysis might be expected to overestimate uncertainty. A third technique, known as probabilistic sensitivity analysis, involves allowing the variables in the analysis to vary simultaneously across a plausible range according to predefined distributions. Probabilistic analysis will normally produce a result lying between the ranges implied by one-way sensitivity analysis and extreme scenario analysis, and therefore may produce a more realistic interval.[8]

In the following sections, we report the results of a major review of the economic evaluation literature. The review is conducted at a number of levels of detail. The overall review process is described on pp. 318–22, including the search and identification methods used and the criteria for inclusion in the final sample. Descriptive statistics for the overall review are then presented, including the methods employed by analysts to quantify uncertainty in their study. The results of a detailed review of all studies reporting results for UK healthcare interventions is reported on pp. 322–7. This includes the development of a relational cost–effectiveness database with the ability to match study results by the underlying methods employed by analysts. A subset of studies for which patient level cost information are available is examined in detail on pp. 327–31 in order to see how healthcare cost data are reported. To aid the discussion, actual healthcare cost information from a number of available data sets is reported. The particular problem of calculating confidence intervals for cost–effectiveness ratios and reviews recently proposed methods for estimating confidence limits for cost–effectiveness ratios are examined on pp. 331–4. Finally, guidelines are proposed based on the findings of this review.

STRUCTURED REVIEW OF
COST–EFFECTIVENESS STUDIES

In this section, the selection and review of studies is described in detail. The aim was to identify and review as many published studies reporting results in terms of cost per (quality-adjusted) life year gained as possible. This form of study was chosen as it is the results of these studies that are commonly grouped together and reported in cost–effectiveness league tables.

Selection Process

Evidence that many literature reviews have in the past been unstructured, selective and subjective[9] has lent support to recent interest in systematic reviews of the medical literature, in particular the methods proposed by the Cochrane Collaboration.[10] Systematising the literature review process should reduce potential biases and improve the potential for other researchers to reproduce the results of the review.

In reviews of clinical evaluations, the well-documented existence of publication bias has led some researchers to devote substantial effort to searching the 'grey literature' in an attempt to identify all studies which have addressed the topic of interest. The existence or importance of publication bias in economic evaluations is less clear. Given the considerable resources required to search the grey literature, and given that published studies represent those results that are publicly available to policy- and decision-makers in the health service and to other analysts, the search strategy for this review was designed to identify only published economic evaluations. Due to the close association between systematicity and the 'Cochrane' style review process outlined above, we prefer to use the term 'structured review' to describe our review process.

The main focus of the search strategy was the electronic searching of available computerised databases. Three SilverPlatter™ databases – Medline, CINAHL and Econlit – and two BIDS (Bath Information Data Services) databases – EMBASE and the Social Science Citation Index – were searched. All identified studies then underwent an initial screen to eliminate clearly inappropriate studies.

Two other electronic databases were searched. Firstly, the database compiled by the Centre for Reviews and Dissemination (CRD) at York University; and secondly, the Office of Health Economics (OHE) and International Federation of Pharmaceutical Manufacturers' Associations

(IFPMA) Health Economic Evaluations Database (HEED), available on CD-ROM.

To supplement the electronic searching, where reviewed studies made comparisons with cost per life year figures obtained from other referenced published studies, these studies were obtained and, providing they met the criteria laid out above, then became part of the review sample. Additional articles were obtained from a published review of cost-utility studies.[11] Finally, an *ad hoc* group of studies of which we were aware and that met the criteria, but which had not been identified were included in the review sample. The overall identification process is illustrated in Figure 3. All identified studies were reviewed using a check-list of questions concerning the study, and the results were entered into a database, the full details of which can be found in the final report.[12] Selected results from the review database are presented below.

Results of the Review

In all, 492 studies published up to the end of 1996 were fully reviewed and entered onto the database, representing a substantial body of literature. As Figure 4 shows, the number of published studies has been growing exponentially. Figure 5 shows the relative shares of the published studies by area of the world. Of course, since only publications reported in the English language were reviewed, the relative shares of European and Rest of the World Studies are under-represented. However, it is clear that North American studies still dominate the English language literature, as was observed over 10 years ago.[13] Figure 6 summarises the study designs in the database, which will have an influence over the methods employed by analysts to quantify uncertainty. Of the 492 studies, 37 (7%) had conducted an economic analysis alongside a clinical trial and 10 (2%) had been conducted prospectively, but not in a trial situation. A secondary analysis of trial data had been conducted in 27 (5%) and a retrospective evaluation had taken place in 47 (9%) of studies. By far the majority of articles had presented a predominantly modelling based approach to their study, with data synthesised from a number of different sources. In 33% of articles, the authors had chosen to present their model in formal decision analytic type terms, with just over half employing a Markov model-type approach and the rest employing a standard decision tree approach.

A breakdown of methods employed by analysts to represent uncertainty in their results is presented in Figure 7. As the majority of

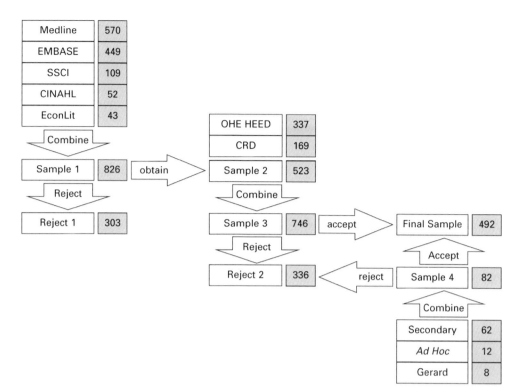

Figure 3   *Schematic diagram of the overall identification and review process.*

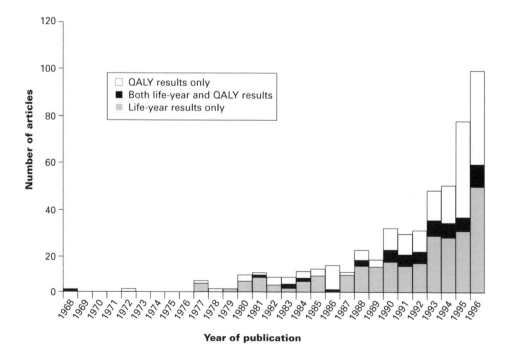

Figure 4   *Growth in the cost–utility analysis literature up to and including 1996.*

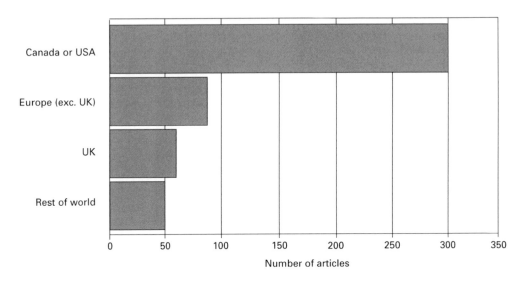

Figure 5   *Studies on the database by country to which the results are applicable.*

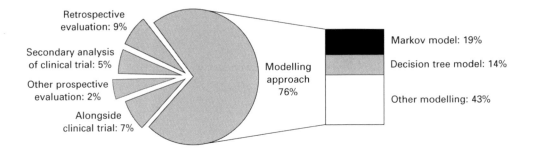

Figure 6   *Proportions of articles on the database by type of study.*

study designs were based on modelling-type approaches, it is not surprising that the majority of analyses used some form of sensitivity analysis, most commonly a simple one-way sensitivity analysis. Some form of statistical analysis was attempted in just 5% of studies, although this was rarely related to the cost–effectiveness ratio itself. Of some concern was that 17% of analysts failed to provide any attempt to quantify the inherent uncertainty in their results.

Discussion

Very few studies identified in our review are based on primary data collection, the majority relying instead on modelling techniques to synthesise data from a number of different sources. This pattern may change over the coming years with the increasing tendency to incorporate an economic component into clinical trials, and this

may produce more studies reporting standard statistical confidence intervals around cost–effectiveness ratios. Of the 24 studies on the database that incorporated some form of statistical analysis of uncertainty, only three attempted any kind of statistical analysis of the cost–effectiveness ratio itself. This may be due in part to the complexities of calculating confidence intervals for a ratio, a problem addressed in recent research – an overview of which is given on pp. 331–4.

It is worrying that 17% of studies do not attempt to quantify in any way the uncertainty in their analysis, especially given the proliferation of published reviews and guidelines for analysts, reviewers and editors in recent years which emphasise the importance of sound evaluative methods, including the use of sensitivity analysis. To examine whether there is any evidence that this situation has improved over time, Figure 8 shows the percentage of articles on the

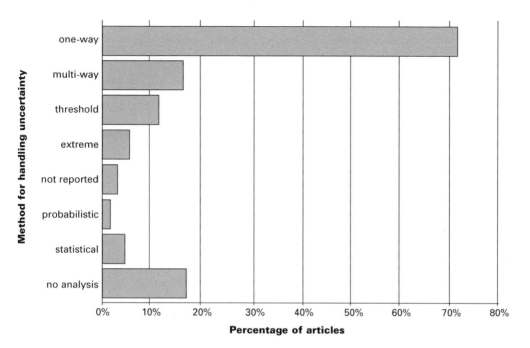

Figure 7   *How articles handled uncertainty in their results.*

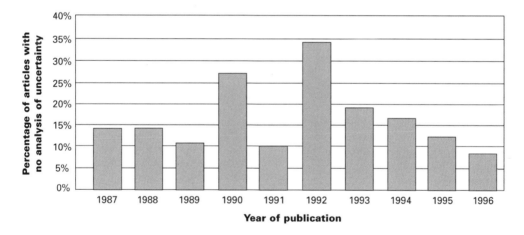

Figure 8   *Percentage of analysts failing to undertake any analysis of uncertainty by year of publication.*

database which failed to employ any methods for quantifying uncertainty, by year of publication over the past 10 years. Although no clear trend is discernible over the whole period, there would appear to be some improvement from 1992 onwards, giving grounds for optimism that methodological standards are improving. However, the reliance on simple one-way sensitivity analysis is less encouraging, as this method is likely to underestimate the level of uncertainty

compared to a statistical 95% confidence interval.[7] By contrast, extreme scenario analysis, which might be expected to overestimate such an interval and could therefore be seen as a more conservative approach, was only used by 6% of analysts. The methods of probabilistic sensitivity analysis may offer a compromise between these two methods,[8] but have so far been underutilised in the economic evaluation literature. A further concern is that the use of one-way sensitivity analysis often seemed less than comprehensive, with only select variables subjected to the analysis. We deal directly with this problem in the next section, as we consider the detailed review of all studies reporting cost–effectiveness results for the UK.

A DETAILED REVIEW OF UK COST–EFFECTIVENESS STUDIES

Performing a reliable economic evaluation is not a simple task. Firstly, the underlying methodological framework is still being debated among health economists. Secondly, there is often uncertainty surrounding data and assumptions, and a lack of consensus over how to handle this. Finally, there is subjectivity in presenting and interpreting results. What to one analyst is clearly 'a highly cost-effective use of resources' may to another analyst seem poor value for money.

The recent development of agreed guidelines for analysts, reviewers, editors and decision-makers should help to standardise methodologies and improve techniques for handling uncertainties over data and assumptions. Here we concentrate on the presentation and interpretation of results, and suggest an approach derived from a structured review of published UK cost–effectiveness studies identified from the overall database reported in the previous section.[a] A total of 60 studies[b] were identified that had presented cost per life-year or cost per QALY results in a UK context – the bibliographic references for these studies are listed in full in Appendix 3 of the full report.[12]

The Structured Review

Each of the 60 studies was reviewed with respect to: (i) the methods employed in the study; (ii) the baseline results reported; and (iii) the range of values reported to represent uncertainty. Additionally, any external cost–effectiveness results quoted by authors to compare with their own results was also recorded.

The first stage of the review process was to identify each 'methodological scenario' deployed by the analysts. For example, Field and colleagues,[14] in their evaluation of health promotion strategies in primary care presented results for two scenarios: firstly, where health outcomes generated by the programmes were discounted at the same rate as costs; and secondly, where those health outcomes were not discounted. In the second stage, the baseline results given by the analysts were then reviewed and attached to the appropriate scenario. It is

clear that many such baseline results can be presented for each scenario, relating to the disease in question, the type of intervention, and the clinical characteristics and age/sex distribution of the patient population. For example, Dusheiko and Roberts[15] evaluated interferon treatment for both hepatitis B and C; Daly and colleagues[16] presented baseline results for three different combinations of hormone replacement therapy for menopausal women; and Fenn and colleagues[17] presented baseline results for thrombolytic therapy by age and by sex subgroups of patients attending with symptoms of acute myocardial infarction. For the third stage, all ranges of values reported around each baseline result to represent uncertainty were recorded. For example, Freemantle and colleagues[18] reported that their baseline estimate of £51 717 per life-year saved by the use of selective serotonin re-uptake inhibitors for the prevention of suicide could vary from £31 000 to £155 000 per life-year saved when each parameter was varied separately across a plausible range of values (a so-called one-way sensitivity analysis), and from £19 000 to £173 000 per life-year saved when these parameters were varied simultaneously (a so-called multi-way analysis).

The final stage of the review was to record all references to other cost–effectiveness results made by analysts. The number of results quoted was recorded, along with the value of each result, the source, and the therapeutic area. As well as providing an opportunity to assess whether the external results chosen by analysts for comparison truly reflected the range of values found in the main review, this process provided a useful check on the identification process of the overall review – references not already on the database were obtained and reviewed.

Results from the Database

A summary of the entries on each level of the database is given in Table 1. A total of 60 studies which reported cost per (QA)LY results were identified and reviewed, and from these a total of 106 methodological scenarios, 548 baseline results, 209 ranges of values and 248 externally quoted ICERs were recorded. The mean, minimum and maximum values for each level in relation to the next level in the database hierarchy are also given. A range of values to represent uncertainty for at least one of the baseline results was recorded for 66% of studies, and 61% of studies quoted an external ICER for comparison with their own results.

Table 1   *Summary of the relational elements of the database*

	Articles	Methodological scenarios	Base-line results	Range of values	External ICERs
Total	60	106	548	209	268
Mean per article	N/A	1.77	9.13	3.48	4.47
Minimum	N/A	1	1	0	0
Maximum	N/A	6	82	42	21
Proportion (%)*	N/A	100	100	66	61

* Proportion of articles which report at least one of each element.
N/A, not available.

A major criticism of cost–effectiveness league tables is that they often contain results derived from studies using different methods.[19–21] In presenting results from our database we adopt an approach similar to the recent U.S. Panel on Cost–Effectiveness in Health and Medicine,[22] which recommended that all studies report a 'reference case analysis' using standard methods, in order to increase the comparability of studies. We defined a methodological 'reference case' with respect to the perspective of the analysis and the rate of discount, in which only costs to the health service are included and the Treasury recommended 6% rate of discount is applied to both costs and health outcomes.[c] We then selected one methodological scenario for each article that most closely reflected our 'reference case' and deviations from the reference case were recorded. In total, 333 baseline results were associated with these 60 scenarios and, 61 of the baseline cost–effectiveness results had a full range of values[d] to represent uncertainty. Almost half of the results were in cost per QALY terms and 55% were in cost per LY terms, with just 8% of baseline results presented both with and without quality of life adjustment.

The 333 baseline ICER results were inflated to represent a common base year (1996) using the combined Hospital and Community Health Services pay and price inflation index.[23] Where no cost base year was reported, we assumed this to be the article publication year minus two years. Once all results were in a common base, we rank ordered the results, employing the QALY result in preference to the life-year result when both were available. Figure 9 presents the minimum, maximum, mean and decile points from this rank ordering exercise. It is clear from the figure that the range of reported ICERs is huge (from £9 to £900 000 per (QA)LY) and that there is a pronounced skew to the results such that the median of £4961 is very much lower than the mean of £30 376.[e]

Extracts from the rank ordering of interventions are shown in Table 2. Results shown are the (closest) corresponding baseline to the

results shown in Figure 9. The rank ordering of the baseline results is shown adjacent to the article identifier (full bibliographic details are available in the full report). Any deviations from the reference case of appropriate methods are listed. Descriptions of the patient subgroup and the study comparator (against which incremental costs and health outcomes were judged) is also given. Of the 333 results, 61 had an associated full range of values to represent uncertainty. The full report presents alternative rankings based on the high or low values from this range, and showed that there could be considerable disruption to the rank order based on the baseline point estimates only.

Since 61% of articles quoted external UK ICERs from other studies for comparison with their own results, it was possible to compare the distribution of these external ICERs (similarly inflated to 1996 values) with the baseline results

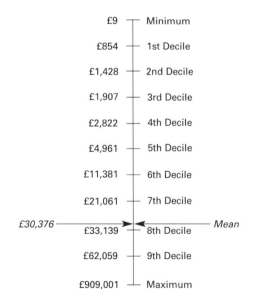

£9	Minimum
£854	1st Decile
£1,428	2nd Decile
£1,907	3rd Decile
£2,822	4th Decile
£4,961	5th Decile
£11,381	6th Decile
£21,061	7th Decile
£30,376 → ← Mean	
£33,139	8th Decile
£62,059	9th Decile
£909,001	Maximum

Figure 9   *Summary of the distribution of the rank-ordered ICERs.*

Table 2 *Extract from the 'league table' of analysed ICERs*

Article ID	Rank	Deviations from reference case	Intervention description	QALY?	ICER	Range?	Method 1 = one-way 2 = multi-way	No. of parameters	Low ICER	High ICER
Phillips 1993	1	No mention of discounting for health outcomes	Introduction of the 'Heartbeat Wales' no smoking programme compared to no programme	✗	£9	✓	2	2		£97
Russell 1990	33	No averted costs included/ Health outcomes discounted at 5%	Screening for abdominal aortic aneurysm and early repair compared to no screening for men aged 65 years	✓	£849	✗				
Parkin 1986	65	No averted costs/Health outcomes discounted at 5%/Inappropriate ICER	5-yearly screening programme for women aged 25 to 65 years compared to an opportunistic screening programme	✗	£1,428	✓	1	1	£886	
Haigh 1991	97	Costs and health outcomes discounted at 5%	Thrombolytic therapy administered between 7 and 24 hours of onset of symptoms suggesting acute myocardial infarction for patients aged between 55 and 64 years compared to no therapy	✓	£1,906	✗				
Hatziandreu 1994	129	Costs and health outcomes discounted at 5%	Selective serotonin reuptake inhibitors compared to tricyclics for preventing suicide in depressed female patients age 35 with two previous depressive episodes	✓	£2,820	✓	2	8	£1,073	£6,830
Akehurst 1994A	162	No averted costs included	Nicorette patch in addition to GP counselling to help smokers to quit	✗	£4,994	✗				
Pharoah 1996	194	Averted costs not included/ Costs and health outcomes discounted at 5%	Statin therapy compared to no statin therapy for males aged 55–64 with existing heart disease (MI) and cholesterol concentrations of 6.6–7.2 mmol L^{-1}	✗	£11,440	✗				

Drummond 1992	226	No averted costs included/ Costs and health outcomes discounted at 5%/Not clear whether appropriate incremental analysis was undertaken	ACE inhibitor therapy for male hypertensives (100 mmHg) aged 40 compared to no therapy	✓	£21,173	✓	1	2 £39,523
Anderson 1993	253	No averted costs included/ Health outcomes not discounted	Implantable cardioverter defibrillator (ICD) compared to no ICD for patients with cardiac fibrillation and with non-sustained ventricular tachycardia and inducible arrhythmia not suppressed by drugs	✗	£30,516	✗		
Field 1995	258	No averted costs included	Screening strategy for heart disease risk factors with appropriate treatment and cholesterol-lowering drugs for total cholesterol >7.5 mmol compared to screening with cholesterol lowering drugs for total cholesterol >8.5 mmol for reducing risk factors for heart disease in women	✗	£33,210	✗		
Richards 1996	290		Home parenteral nutrition compared to no feeding in patients with intestinal failure aged under 44 years	✓	£62,137	✓		
Anderson 1993	322	No averted costs included/ Health outcomes not discounted	Implantable cardioverter defibrillator (ICD) compared to no ICD for patients with cardiac fibrillation and inducible arrhythmia suppressed by drugs plus high ejection fraction	✗	£909,001	✗		

MI, myocardial infarction.

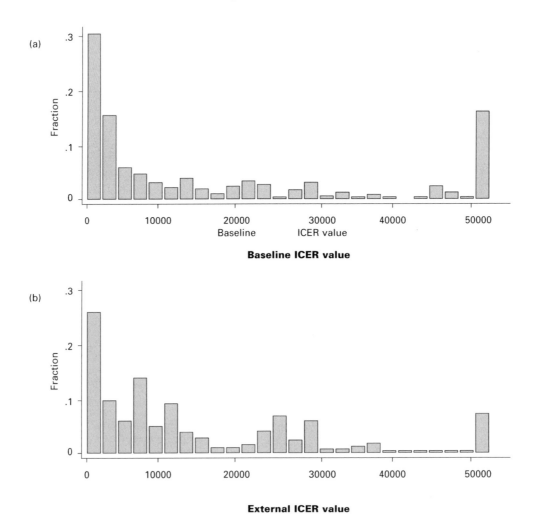

Figure 10 *Histogram of the distribution of (a) baseline ICERs from the database analysis and (b) external ICERs quoted in studies for comparison.*

from the rank ordering exercise. Histograms for these two distributions are presented in Figure 10, emphasising that the cost–effectiveness results chosen by analysts to compare with their own results tend to be higher than those recorded in our structured review of overall results.[f]

Discussion

Cost–effectiveness analysis is a comparative methodology, in which results have meaning primarily in relation to opportunity cost as measured by other cost–effectiveness results. It follows that the greater the number of results available for comparison, the more accurately can the relative cost–effectiveness of any particular study be judged. The 'league table' has

to date been a common way of making a comparison against other treatments routinely provided in the health service, i.e. other treatments which by inference society/healthcare providers are already revealing a willingness to provide at the calculated cost–effectiveness ratio. However, league tables – or other lists of external comparators – are seldom comprehensive. In our review, the 61% of studies which referred to external comparators quoted on average only six UK cost–effectiveness results. Thus, assessment of the relative cost–effectiveness of an intervention is generally made on the basis of very incomplete information. This is especially so when analysts are trying to get some grip on mean or median values – what is *routinely* provided and regarded as a currently acceptable norm across the health sector. This scope for subjective opinion and interpretation of cost–effectiveness results has been an important factor in the controversies over research sponsorship.[24]

Assessing the results of a cost–effectiveness analysis against a structured review, such as that reported here of all UK studies published up to 1996, should allow a better assessment of relative cost–effectiveness. For example, rather than vague and inevitably subjective comments that a particular result 'compares well with existing uses of healthcare resources', analysts (or the reader) could place results within a distribution – 'below the median figure for all published UK cost–effectiveness results', or 'within the first decile of published UK cost–effectiveness results'. Of course, it should be noted that our database – as with league tables – is based purely on published results, and does not imply that the interventions are necessarily in use. A published ICER should not be equated with a currently accepted use of healthcare resources. The acceptance of a more broadly based but methodologically similar set of comparisons across the full spectrum of health-related interventions, as proposed here, might encourage adherence to standards, and meanwhile should help to reduce the amount of subjectivity involved in interpreting results.

DISTRIBUTION AND VARIANCE OF COST DATA

With many more economic analyses being planned prospectively, analysts are increasingly in possession of patient-level data on the health-care costs of alternative interventions. A common belief is that such healthcare cost data are (positively) skewed rather than following a normal distribution, and concerns have been raised about what this may mean for standard statistical tests.[25] In this section we first examine how analysts reporting patient-level data on health-care costs have reported the distribution of that data. Secondly, we examine available healthcare cost data to see to what extent they are in fact skewed, and we discuss the implications that this may have for the statistical analysis of cost data.

Review of Studies Reporting Patient-Level Cost Data

From the full set of 492 studies identified in pp. 318–22, 26 studies were found which had collected patient specific resource/cost data as part of a randomised controlled trial (RCT), and a further 27 were identified which had collected patient-specific resource/cost data as part of a

non-RCT study. In total, therefore, 53 of the 492 studies in the database (11%) reported collecting patient-specific resource/cost data in a way that allowed some measure of variance to be reported.[g]

Details were extracted from this set of studies on the study design; whether or not patient-level data had been collected on resource use and on cost (and if so the sample size used); the size of the trial population from which any resource sample was drawn; the number of arms in a trial; the number of centres from which resource or cost data were collected; and the mean follow-up period. Also recorded was whether the study reported a resource use mean, variance or distributional form; the number of cost components reported, and for the control and intervention arm(s) the reported mean or median cost, the measures of cost variance reported, any mention of the distributional form of the cost data, any significance tests for cost differences.

Of the 53 studies, 17 reported some statistical measure of variance concerning use of resources, and 25 reported some statistical measure of variance concerning costs. Three studies mentioned the distributional form of resource use data (two normal, one positively skewed). In terms of the measures of cost variance reported, five articles gave a standard error, seven a standard deviation, four gave 95% confidence intervals, two gave an interquartile range, and 11 gave a range. In addition, one study reported an indeterminate measure – of the form 'mean ± x' – which was probably either a standard error or standard deviation, but could not be classified. In only four cases did articles report more than one measure of variance: standard deviation and range (two), standard error and interquartile range (one), standard error and range (one).

In the 26 RCT-related articles, 12 articles reported the value of the mean difference in costs between trial arms, and three of these articles reported some measure of variance in mean cost difference (95% confidence intervals). Eight articles either reported the *P*-value for a significance test of mean cost difference (four articles) or reported that the difference in mean costs was not statistically significant (four). In the 27 non-RCT-related articles, none reported a mean cost difference with associated variance between the patient groups or interventions being compared (one reported a mean cost difference with no measure of variance), and only one article reported a significance test for mean cost difference.

In summary, therefore, only a tiny fraction of the published cost–effectiveness results retrieved (15/492, or 3%) reported some conventional measure of variance (SD, SE, 95% CI) around the mean cost estimates they used to calculate cost–effectiveness ratios.

From the 15 articles identified above as reporting patient-specific mean cost data and conventional statistical measures of variance, a total of 32 mean cost figures with associated standard error, standard deviation or confidence interval were extracted (for example, a three-arm trial with data for each patient group gave three observations). The mean cost was 37 836 (in different denominations), the mean standard deviation was 40 150 and the corresponding mean of the coefficients of variation was 1.01. For the 28 out of 32 observations for which a sample size was reported, the mean sample size was 78 (SD 82, median 37, range 2 to 279).

Five Data Sets Describing Patient-Level Cost Data

In addition to the review described above, we obtained and analysed five healthcare cost data-sets to examine the variance and distributional form of the data, and to explore the potential to employ data transformation techniques when analysing and presenting the data. A description of each of the five data sets can be found in the full report. Briefly, each data set contained patient-level resource use data for a treatment and control arm of a clinical trial, and these resource data were weighted by unit cost information to give patient-level costs associated with the interventions under evaluation. Histograms for each arm of the five data sets is given in Figure 11. It is clear that these patient-level cost data do not seem to follow a normal distribution, with many showing evidence of substantial skewness.

In these circumstances, the median is often used as a measure of central tendency rather than the mean. However, although median cost provides useful descriptive information (particularly when presented alongside the mean), it is inappropriate to use median costs in a cost analysis, as we are interested both in the average per patient cost of a particular treatment and the total cost of care for a patient group. Multiplying the median cost by the number of patients treated will not give the total cost of treatment for that patient group. Since, ultimately, someone will have responsibility for a budget from which total costs of care will have to be met, the appropriate statistic for analysts in economic analyses (and decision-makers applying the results of such analyses) is the mean cost per patient. A further problem with median statistics is that convenient measures of dispersion, such as standard deviations or standard error do not exist as they do for the mean.

The non-normality of the data presented above may cause problems for parametric statistical tests for the equality of two means. The standard *t*-test is based on an assumption of normality of the underlying data and on the assumption that the two population variances are equal. Although the *t*-test is known to be *robust*, i.e. that moderate failure to meet the assumptions of normality and equal variance will not affect the results very much,[26] it is not clear just how great the departures from normality/equal variance must be before the *t*-test becomes inappropriate. It is clear from the *central limit theorem*, for example, that although the underlying data may not be normally distributed, the sampling distribution of the difference between two means, like the means themselves, will approximate the normal distribution for large sample sizes.[27] A useful result is that the skew coefficient of the population will be reduced by a factor of $\sqrt{n}$ in the sampling distribution of the mean of that population, where n is the sample size.[h] However, it is still not clear what value of skew in a sampling distribution is 'large enough' to cause concern, such that some of the large skewness observed in the five data sets described above may be problematic despite the sample sizes concerned. We therefore consider two alternatives to the standard parametric approach that might be employed for the analysis and presentation of the above data: the use of transformations to an alternative scale of measurement in order that the data more closely conform to the standard statistical assumptions; and the non-parametric approach of bootstrapping, which makes no assumptions concerning the distributional form of the underlying data.

Transformations

The transformation of data from one scale to another can be used to overcome problems associated with non-normality of data and unequal variance. Fortunately, transformations which normalise data will often also provide more equal variances.[28] In the final report we consider three of the most commonly used transformations: the (natural) log transformation; the square-root transformation; and the reciprocal transformation, and present the results from the five data sets on the transformed scales.

Although, in a statistical sense, transformed scales of measurement are no less appropriate for analysing differences between two arms of a study than the untransformed scale, transformation can lead to problems of interpretation for economic analyses. It is not clear what the magnitude of differences mean on the transformed scales; hence analysts are likely to want

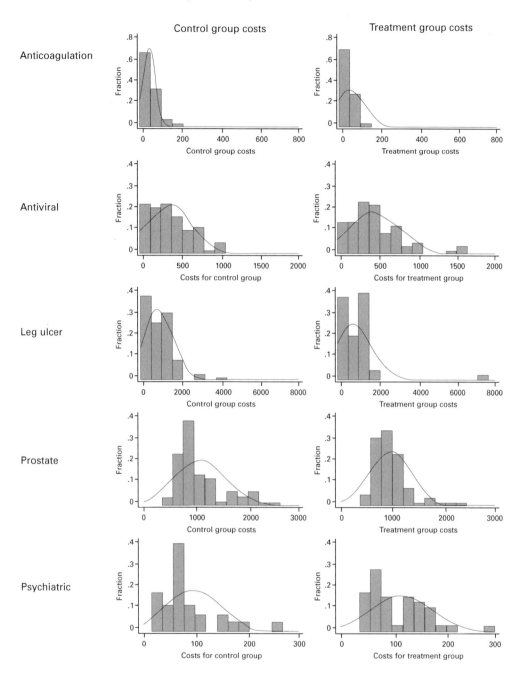

Figure 11   *Histograms showing the distribution of costs for the control and treatment arms for the five data sets. Overlaid are normal distributions with the same mean and variance as the data.*

to back-transform point estimates of central tendency and confidence limits from the transformed scale to the original scale. This is a simple process of using the inverse function for point estimates of the original cost data on the transformed scale.[29] Unfortunately, the cost *differences* observed following a square-root transformation or reciprocal transformation are not interpretable when back-transformed.[30] Cost differences under a log transformation do have an

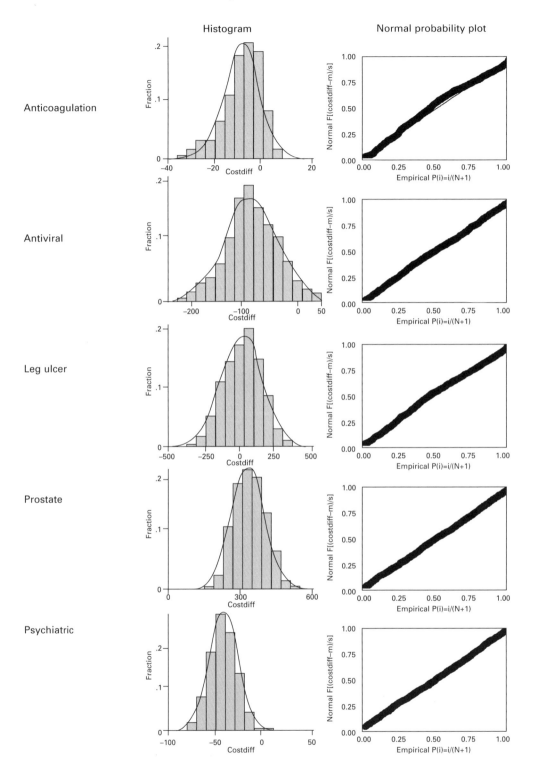

Figure 12   *Histograms of bootstrapped cost data with normal distributions overlaid and normal probability plots for the five data sets.*

interpretation when back-transformed since the difference of two log values is equal to the log of their ratio. The antilog transformation of a log value gives the geometric mean; hence the anti-log of the mean log difference gives the ratio of the geometric mean in the control group to the geometric mean in the treatment group. Similarly, the antilog transformation of the confidence limits for the difference in log values gives the confidence limits to this ratio of the geometric means in each group.[30] Hence, a significant result after back-transformation is indicated by a confidence interval that excludes unity (i.e. where the ratio of the geometric means is the same).

However, although *an* interpretation is possible after back-transforming results on a log-transformed scale, an *economic* interpretation is still problematic for two reasons. Firstly, the geometric mean is not the appropriate summary statistic for economic analyses, for the same reason the median was argued to be inappropriate above. Secondly, the back-transformation does not result in the original scale of measurement. If the aim is to combine information on cost with information on effect to produce a cost–effectiveness ratio, we need to express cost on the original scale (e.g. in pounds and pence).

Non-parametric bootstrapping[i]

The bootstrap approach is a non-parametric method that makes no distributional assumptions concerning the statistic in question. Instead, it employs the original data and computing power in a re-sampling exercise in order to give an empirical estimate of the sampling distribution of that statistic. Successive random samples of size n are then drawn from $\mathbf{x}$ *with replacement*[j] to give the bootstrap re-samples. The statistic of interest is then calculated for each of these re-samples, and these bootstrap replicates of the original statistic make up the empirical estimate of the statistic's sampling distribution.

The results of bootstrapping the sampling distribution of the cost differences between treatment and control arms of the five datasets are presented in Figure 12. What the bootstrap estimates of the sampling distributions show is the extent to which, in each case, the sample size of the study is sufficiently large that the assumption of a normal sampling distribution (from the central limit theorem) is justified. Where the sampling distribution approximates the normal distribution, we need not be too concerned about the violations of the assumptions underlying the *t*-test results reported above. It is clear that, for the antiviral example,

the prostate example and the psychiatric example, the bootstrap estimate of the sampling distribution closely approximates a normal distribution. Hence, for these studies we are unlikely to want to transform results onto an alternative scale, since we can be happy that the sample sizes are sufficient that the untransformed *t*-test results are robust.

By contrast, for the anticoagulation example and the leg ulcer example, the bootstrap results predict that some non-normality remains in the sampling distribution due to the relatively small sample sizes in relation to the extreme non-normality of the underlying data. In these examples, there may be a case for transforming the data to ensure that the assumptions underlying the *t*-test results are met. However, the bootstrap method can also be used to estimate confidence limits for the cost difference, which may be preferable to employing parametric techniques on a transformed scale. The most straightforward method of bootstrap confidence interval estimation is the percentile method, by choosing the 2.5th and 97.5th percentile values from the vector of cost differences to represent the 95% confidence interval limits. The bootstrap 95% percentile confidence interval for the anticoagulation data cost difference is −£21.91 to £8.03, while for the leg ulcer data, the 95% percentile confidence interval is −£258.36 to £242.96. These intervals are not symmetrically positioned around the point estimate of cost difference, reflecting the non-normality of the bootstrap estimate of the sampling distribution.

CONFIDENCE INTERVALS FOR COST–EFFECTIVENESS RATIOS

Analysts will increasingly be in possession of patient-level data on both cost and health outcome as more economic analyses are conducted alongside clinical trials. The overall review in pp. 318–22 found that just 24 studies had attempted any form of statistical analysis in looking at their data, and in only three cases was this analysis related to the ICER itself. Standard statistical methods of confidence interval estimation do not apply to the ICER since the variance of a ratio statistic is intractable. There has been much recent research into possible methods for estimating confidence intervals for the ICER stemming from a seminal paper by O'Brien and colleagues.[6] In this section, we offer an overview of this recent literature in order to elucidate the strengths and weaknesses of the alternative approaches. We also consider the use of an alternative approach to representing uncertainty in cost–effectiveness information and discuss the continuing role of sensitivity analysis for handling uncertainty not related to sampling variation.

Confidence Interval Estimation Methods

In recognition of the problem associated with standard statistical methods for estimating confidence limits for the ICER, a number of analysts have proposed alternative methods,

including methods based on confidence boxes,[6] confidence ellipses,[31] the Taylor series expansion,[6] Fieller's theorem[32,33] and non-parametric bootstrapping.[32,34,35] Each of the approaches outlined above are illustrated using patient-specific data[k] obtained from a clinical trial that compared a drug therapy treatment group with a placebo control group.[36] The representation of uncertainty based on each of the methods outlined above is shown in Figure 13 for the clinical trial data. The horizontal and vertical 'I' bars represent the 95% confidence intervals on incre-

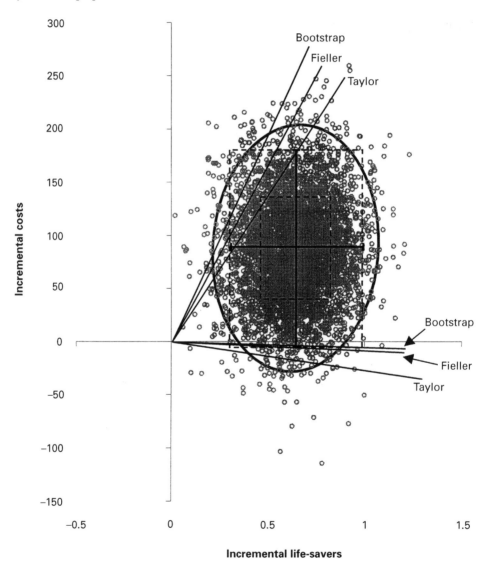

Figure 13   *Example of alternative confidence intervals using data from a clinical trial. (Rays from the origin represent the confidence intervals for Taylor, Fieller and bootstrap methods; rays representing confidence intervals for ellipse method and box methods are not shown in order to avoid cluttering the figure.)*

Table 3 *Comparing methods of confidence interval estimation: a numerical example*

Method	Lower limit	Upper limit	Interval length
Confidence box:			
Standard	−5.2	606.7	611.9
Revised	49.3	290.8	241.5
Taylor series	−21.89	295.94	317.83
Confidence ellipse	−48.7	523.4	572.1
Fieller's theorem	−8.3	380.6	388.9
Bootstrap percentile	−5.9	392.0	397.9

mental effects and cost separately, which intersect at the ICER point estimate of 137.18. The dashed box is the confidence box generated by these intervals. The ellipse shown joins points of equal probability (assuming a joint normal distribution) such that the ellipse covers 95% of the integrated probability. Also shown are 5000 bootstrap replications of the incremental effect and incremental cost pairs and the rays whose slopes correspond to the upper and lower 95% confidence limits of the ICER, as calculated by the Taylor, Fieller and bootstrap (percentile) methods. The confidence limits for each of the different methods, together with the interval length, are shown in Table 3. A full review and details for calculating these confidence limits can be found in the final report.

What is immediately apparent from this analysis is that the symmetrical nature of the Taylor series method gives a very different balance to the interval than the other methods. It is also interesting to observe that, in this example, the interval from the ellipse method is not internal to the interval from the box method, a result that contradicts recent representations in the literature.[8,37]

Figure 13 and Table 3 emphasise the differences in confidence intervals that can be obtained for the same data when employing different methods. However, it is not possible to judge which method is most appropriate on the basis of a single example. Recall that the definition of a 95% confidence interval is that the true population parameter will be included in the interval 95% of the time in repeated sampling. In order to estimate the accuracy of the intervals obtained by different methods, simulation experiments, where the true population ICER is defined, can be undertaken. Such experiments involve drawing samples of costs and effects from predefined distributions, calculating confidence intervals for the estimated ICER, and recording whether the true value is contained within the interval. This simulation is then repeated a large number of times and the proportion of times the true value of the ICER is contained within the interval is used to judge the coverage properties of the confidence interval calculation methods. The results of two such articles have shown that Fieller's method and bootstrap methods outperform the other methods.[38,39]

Given that the Monte Carlo evaluation studies show the bootstrap method to be a good overall method, the bootstrap can be used to show the inaccuracies of the inferior methods from Table 3 and Figure 13. For the Taylor series method, 6.8% of the bootstrap replications gave ICERs that were above the upper estimate of the confidence limit, while 1.5% were below the lower limit, suggesting an overall confidence interval of 91.7%. The ellipse method had an overall confidence interval of 98.4% (0.74% bootstrap replications below the lower limit and 0.84% above the upper limit), a greater overspecification than the standard box method at 96.9% (2.56% below and 0.56% above). The potential pit-falls of the revised box approach are plainly apparent (note that cost and effect differences in the numerical example used in Table 3 are almost independent), since the method gives just an 80% confidence interval: 12.6% of the bootstrap replications fell below the lower limit and 7.3% were above the upper limit.

Cost–Effectiveness Acceptability Curves

In the final report we identify a number of potential problems for confidence intervals as a method for representing uncertainty in the cost–effectiveness of healthcare interventions. These relate to the interpretation of negative ratios, the one-sided nature of the decision problem, uncertainty concerning the maximum acceptable or ceiling ICER appropriate for decision making, and the adherence to conventional levels of statistical significance.

Cost–effectiveness acceptability curves offer an alternative approach to presenting and thinking about uncertainty in cost–effectiveness analysis. Although originally proposed by van Hout and colleagues,[31] they have received comparatively little attention in the recent literature. If we define a ceiling cost–effectiveness ratio appropriate for decision-making, this can be represented on the cost–effectiveness (CE) plane (see Figure 1) as a ray passing through the origin, with slope equal to the ICER ceiling value. This divides the CE plane into two, and van Hout and colleagues refer to the area of the

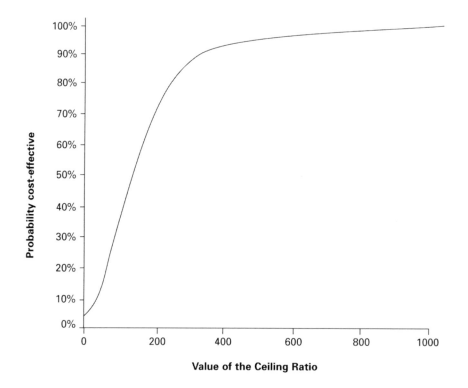

Figure 14   *The cost–effectiveness acceptability curve.*

CE plane lying to the right of the ceiling ratio as the acceptability surface. They advocate the construction of a cost–effectiveness acceptability curve on the basis of the probability an intervention is cost-effective in relation to all possible values of the ceiling ratio from 0 to ∞ (equivalent to rotating the ceiling ratio line on the CE plane from the horizontal through to the vertical).

The cost–effectiveness acceptability curve for the clinical trial data is shown in Figure 14. For all possible values of the ceiling ratio (x-axis), the probability that the intervention is cost-effective is shown (y-axis). Note that the point of inflexion on the cost–effectiveness acceptability curve occurs at the midpoint of the probability function and corresponds to the baseline cost–effectiveness data for the clinical trial data of 137.18. The point at which the curve crosses the vertical axis corresponds to the P-value associated with the incremental cost of the intervention, and the limit to which the curve is tending corresponds to the P-value associated with the incremental effect of the intervention.[1] Although cost–effectiveness acceptability curves are closely related to P-value functions, strictly their interpretation of showing the probability that an intervention is cost-effective given that

the data requires a Bayesian approach to statistical analysis.

This section has been concerned primarily with handling uncertainty in cost–effectiveness analysis arising from sampling variation. However, it is important to remember that sensitivity analysis methods have a continuing role alongside statistical methods for handling other important types of uncertainty in economic evaluation. A further advantage of cost–effectiveness acceptability curves is that a range of different curves arising from a number of sensitivity analyses may be easier to interpret than a corresponding number of confidence intervals.

GUIDELINES ARISING FROM THE REVIEW

In this concluding section we present the guidelines arising from the findings in our structured review. Full details and justification for these guidelines are given in the full report.

1   Analysts should aim to present results using a methodological reference case in order to increase the comparability of results between studies.

2 Analysts should be aware of the potential for the incremental cost–effectiveness ratio to vary at the margin.

3 Analysts should avoid selective comparison of their results with the results from other studies.

4 Analysts should ensure that they consider the potential implications of uncertainty for the results of their analysis.

5 Interval estimates should accompany each point estimate presented.

6 Where sensitivity analysis is employed to estimate an interval, analysts should be comprehensive in their inclusion of all variables in the analysis.

7 When reporting sensitivity analysis, analysts should be aware of the probabilistic nature of the reported range.

8 When reporting patient-level cost information, analysts should make more use of descriptive statistics.

9 Even when data are skewed, economic analyses should be based on means of distributions.

10 When reporting statistical tests of cost-differences, analysts should be aware that significance tests may be more powerful on a transformed scale, but that confidence limits should be reported on the original scale.

11 Where patient-level data on both cost and effect are available, the parametric approach based on Fieller's theorem or the non-parametric approach of bootstrapping should be employed to estimate a confidence interval for the cost–effectiveness ratio.

12 Sensitivity analysis has a continuing role in handling uncertainty not related to sampling variation.

13 Consideration should be given to using cost–effectiveness acceptability curves to present uncertainty in stochastic cost–effectiveness studies.

Acknowledgements

This report was funded by the NHS Executive through the National Co-ordinating Centre for Health Technology Assessment. A number of people have contributed directly to the production of this report. Professor Paul Fenn and Professor Alistair McGuire provided helpful comment on the design of the research, and Professor Fenn also made constructive comments on the review of methods for calculating confidence intervals. Dr David Smith and Sir David Cox provided statistical advice on the interpretation and use of transformations, and provided comments on the review of confidence interval methods reported. Simon Dixon of the Sheffield Health Economics Group provided the leg ulcer data used as one of the examples, and Professor Paul Fenn and colleagues provided access to their data for another of the examples. We are grateful also to the editors and anonymous referees of *Journal of Health Service Research & Policy* and *Health Economics* who provided feedback on articles to be published based on parts of this report. This feedback has contributed to the revision of this final report. The Institute of Health Sciences library staff provided help in obtaining many of the articles included in the review. Revision of the report and updating of the database to include the 1996 publication year was made possible through a joint MRC/Anglia and Oxford Region Special Training Fellowship held by A.B. Responsibility for the views expressed in this paper, and for all remaining errors, is our own.

Notes

a. Although we focus on UK studies, the general principles employed in this section are internationally applicable.

b. One of the specified criteria for inclusion on the overall database was that studies were published journal articles. We made two exceptions to this rule by including the Forrest Report[40] on breast cancer screening and the Standing Medical Advisory Committee report[41] on cholesterol testing. Both were felt to be high-quality reports that had been influential from a policy perspective without being published in a journal.

c. The UK Treasury has recently revised their recommendation concerning the rate of discount for health outcomes from 1.5 to 2%, while the recommended rate for costs stays at 6%. We adopt the previous recommendation here as that was applicable when the review was started, and when most analysts were conducting their studies.

d. We defined a 'full range' as being two-sided and excluded those results for which the sensitivity analysis range was 'one-sided' in either direction such that the baseline result was also a high or low value for the range.

e. The reported distribution of the ICER results and other statistics excluded 10 of the 333 baselines in which the intervention in question was dominated by the comparator.

f. Overall, external ICERs quoted by analysts tend to under-represent the low values and over-represent the mid-range values. However, analysts appear not to quote the very highest ICER results available.

g. A further 12 studies (three RCT, nine non-RCT) were identified which had collected patient-specific information in the course of the analysis, but analysed it in such a way (aggregating resource use in each arm of a trial, applying unit costs and then dividing by *n*, or variants of this approach) that it was not possible to calculate inter-patient cost variance.

h. This is a precise result, under standard parametric assumptions, that can be derived from the definition of the skew coefficient.

i. In the final report, we also consider other commonly used non-parametric rank order tests. However, we argue that these are not appropriate for cost analysis where difference in *mean* cost is the prime concern.

j. Of course, sampling from **x** without replacement *n* times, would simply yield **x** itself.

k. This is the same antiviral cost dataset from pp. 327–31, but this time we include an analysis of health outcome.

l. Note that due to the one-sided nature of the curve, the *P*-values associated with a two-sided hypothesis test would be twice the values from Figure 12.

References

1. Backhouse M, Backhouse RJ, Edey SA. Economic evaluation bibliography. *Health Economics* 1992; **1**(Suppl.): 1–235.

2. Anderson JP, Bush JW, Chen M, Dolenc D. Policy space areas and properties of benefit-cost/utility analysis. *JAMA* 1986; **255**: 794–5.

3. Black WC. The CE plane: A graphic representation of cost-effectiveness. *Med. Decis. Making.* 1990; **10**: 212–14.

4. Petrou S, Malek M, Davey PG. The reliability of cost–utility estimates in cost-per-QALY league tables. *PharmacoEconomics* 1993; **3**: 345–53.

5. Briggs AH, Sculpher MJ, Buxton MJ. Uncertainty in the economic evaluation of health care technologies: the role of sensitivity analysis. *Health Economics* 1994; **3**: 95–104.

6. O'Brien BJ, Drummond MF, Labelle RJ, Willan A. In search of power and significance: issues in the design and analysis of stochastic cost-effectiveness studies in health care. *Med. Care* 1994; **32**: 150–63.

7. Briggs AH. Handling uncertainty in the results of economic evaluation. *OHE Briefing Paper No. 32*, 1995.

8. Manning WG, Fryback DG, Weinstein MC. Reflecting uncertainty in cost–effectiveness analysis. In: Gold MR, Siegel JE, Russell LB, Weinstein MC (eds). *Cost-effectiveness in health and medicine*. New York: Oxford University Press, 1996.

9. Light RJ, Pillemer DB. *Summing up: the science of reviewing research*. Cambridge: Harvard University Press, 1984.

10. Chalmers I, Altman DG. *Systematic reviews*. London: BMJ, 1995.

11. Gerard K. Cost–utility in practice: a policy maker's guide to the state of the art. *Health Policy* 1992; **21**: 249–79.

12. Briggs AH, Gray AM. Handling uncertainty when performing economic evaluation of health care interventions: a structured review of published studies with special reference to the distributional form and variance of cost data. *Health Technology* 1999; **3**.

13. Blades CA, Culyer AJ, Walker A. Health service efficiency: appraising the appraisers – a critical review of economic appraisal in practice. *Soc. Sci. Med.* 1987; **25**: 461–72.

14. Field K, Thorogood M, Silagy C, Normand C, O'Neill C, Muir J. Strategies for reducing coronary risk factors in primary care: which is most cost effective? *Br. Med. J.* 1995; **310**: 1109–12.

15. Dusheiko GM, Roberts JA. Treatment of chronic type B and C hepatitis with interferon alfa: an economic appraisal [see comments]. *Hepatology* 1995; **22**: 1863–73.

16. Daly E, Roche M, Barlow D, Gray A, McPherson K, Vessey M. HRT: an analysis of benefits, risks and costs. *Br. Med. Bull.* 1992; **48**: 368–400.

17. Fenn P, Gray AM, McGuire A. The cost-effectiveness of thrombolytic therapy following acute myocardial infarction. *Br. J. Clin. Pract.* 1991; **45**: 181–4.

18. Freemantle N, House A, Song F, Mason JM, Sheldon TA. Prescribing selective serotonin re-uptake inhibitors as strategy for prevention of suicide. *Br. Med. J.* 1994; **309**: 249–53.

19. Gerard K, Mooney G. QALY league tables: handle with care. *Health Economics* 1993; **2**: 59–64.

20. Mason J, Drummond M, Torrance G. Some guidelines on the use of cost effectiveness league tables. *Br. Med. J.* 1993; **306**: 570–2.

21. Drummond M, Torrance G, Mason J. Cost-effectiveness league tables: more harm than good? *Soc. Sci. Med.* 1993; **37**: 33–40.

22. Gold MR, Siegel JE, Russell LB, et al. *Cost-effectiveness in health and medicine*. New York: Oxford University Press, 1996.

23. Department of Health. *Hospital and Community Health Services pay and price index*. London: Department of Health, 1996.

24. Hillman AL, Eisenberg JM, Pauly MV, Bloom BS, Glick H, Kinosian B, Schwartz JS. Avoiding bias in the conduct and reporting of cost-effectiveness research sponsored by pharmaceutical companies. *N. Engl. J. Med.* 1991; **324**: 1362–5.

25. Coyle D. Statistical analysis in pharmaco-economic studies. *PharmacoEconomics* 1996; **9**: 506–16.

26. Altman DG. *Practical statistics for medical research*. London: Chapman & Hall, 1991.

27. Armitage P, Berry G. *Statistical methods in medical research*. 3rd edn. Oxford: Blackwell Scientific Publications, 1994.

28. Bland JM, Altman DG. Transforming data. *Br. Med. J.* 1996; **312**: 770.

29. Bland JM, Altman DG. Transformations, means, and confidence intervals. *Br. Med. J.* 1996; **312**: 1079.

30. Bland JM, Altman DG. The use of transformation when comparing two means. *Br. Med. J.* 1996; **312**: 1153.

31. van Hout BA, Al MJ, Gordon GS, Rutten FF. Costs, effects and C/E-ratios alongside a clinical trial. *Health Economics* 1994; **3**: 309–19.

32. Chaudhary MA, Stearns SC. Estimating confidence intervals for cost-effectiveness ratios: An example from a randomized trial. *Statist. Med.* 1996; **15**: 1447–58.

33. Willan AR, O'Brien BJ. Confidence intervals for cost-effectiveness ratios: an application of Fieller's theorem. *Health Economics* 1996; **5**: 297–305.

34. Briggs AH, Wonderling DE, Mooney CZ. Pulling cost-effectiveness analysis up by its bootstraps: a non-parametric approach to confidence interval estimation. *Health Economics* 1997; **6**: 327–40.

35. Obenchain RL, Melfi CA, Croghan TW, Buesching DP. Bootstrap analyses of cost effectiveness in antidepressant pharmacotherapy. *PharmacoEconomics* 1997; **11**: 464–72.

36. Fenn P, McGuire A, Phillips V, Backhouse M, Jones D. The analysis of censored treatment cost data in economic evaluation. *Med. Care* 1995; **33**: 851–63.

37. Drummond MF, O'Brien B, Stoddart GL, Torrance G. *Methods for the economic evaluation of health care programmes*. 2nd edn. Oxford: Oxford University Press, 1997.

38. Polsky D, Glick HA, Willke R, Schulman K. Confidence intervals for cost-effectiveness ratios: a comparison of four methods. *Health Economics* 1997; **6**: 243–52.

39. Briggs AH, Mooney CZ, Wonderling DE. Constructing confidence intervals around cost-effectiveness ratios: an evaluation of parametric and non-parametric methods using Monte Carlo simulation. *Stat. Med.* 1999; **18**: 3245–62.

40. Forrest P. *Breast cancer screening*. London: HMSO, 1986.

41. Standing Medical Advisory Committee. *Blood cholesterol testing: the cost-effectiveness of opportunistic cholesterol testing*. Report by the Standing Medical Advisory Committee to the Secretary of State for Health, 1990.

19

A Review of the Use of the Main Quality of Life Measures, and Sample Size Determination for Quality of Life Measures, Particularly in Cancer Clinical Trials

MICHAEL J. CAMPBELL, STEVEN A. JULIOUS,
SARAH J. WALKER, STEVE L. GEORGE
and DAVID MACHIN

Summary

A literature search was carried out up to 1995 on the use of three quality of life (QoL) instruments used by the British Medical Research Council in designing trials for cancer clinical trials. These were the Hospital Anxiety and Depression Scale (HADS), the Rotterdam Symptom Checklist (RSCL) and the European Organisation for Research and Treatment in Cancer Questionnaire (EORTC QLQ-C30). These instruments are described in detail and their relative merits highlighted. The results showed a steady increase in the number of citations for each instrument. Two instruments, the HADS and the RSCL, were then examined using data from a clinical trial of 310 patients with small-cell lung cancer. An understanding of the QoL score distributions was achieved by investigating the raw scores of the HADS anxiety and RSCL psychological domains. The distribution of the raw HADS anxiety scores of patients at baseline was negatively skewed. The distribution of the raw RSCL psychological distress scores was positively skewed, with possibly three modes. The raw scores of neither questionnaire were Normally distributed, and there is no simple transformation that would make them Normal, because of the number of modes. Therefore, the usual mean and standard deviation are not adequate to summarise the distributions and non-parametric techniques which make no assumptions about the shape of the distribution that should be used for testing.

Methods for determining effect sizes and sample size calculations for data that are not Normally distributed were reviewed and applied to the cancer data sets. Different sample sizes were required depending on the outcome measure, and a small saving on the sample size was made when the ordinality of the outcome measure was taken into account. Finally, recommendations were made for further research.

Introduction

Towards the end of the 1940s the importance of measuring a person's quality of life (QoL) began to be realised, especially in the care of patients with cancer.[1] Methods for this evaluation were developed and began to be used in clinical trials and clinical practice. Currently, there are a large number of different QoL questionnaires, indices and scales being used and translated for many countries. However, many of these instruments are either based on somewhat general classifications of health, or are restricted to one physical illness. De Haes and Van Knippenberg[1] found that the philosophy and definition of QoL differed from one instrument to another, and that many of these instruments also had other methodological problems, particularly with respect to their reliability, validity and design.

The majority of early instruments for assessing QoL are:

(a) lengthy and complicated for both physicians and patients;
(b) difficult to score, often requiring trained personnel;
(c) restricted to physical function, with little regard to social and emotional issues;
(d) not validated or tested for reliability; and
(e) not able to differentiate between people with different levels of QoL.

WHY THIS ISSUE IS IMPORTANT

Quality of life is particularly important in palliative medicine because, for many cancers, little improvement in cure rates or survival times has been achieved in recent years.

Sample size issues are important for the planning of clinical trials. Studies that are either too small or too large may be judged unethical,[2] although there is some disagreement over this.[3] For example, a study that is too large could have demonstrated clinical improvement before the end of the trial had been reached, and so some patients may have been randomised to a treatment that could have been shown to be inferior. On the other hand, provided that it is not a life-or-death situation, large trials give the opportunity for examining a variety of end-points, and possibly subgroups of patients. A trial that is too small will have no power to demonstrate a meaningful effect, and so may be regarded as a waste of resources; moreover, patients are being put through the potential trauma of a trial for no tangible benefit. Inconclusive trials can also make the conduct of subsequent trials difficult if a marginal benefit that may have arisen by chance is shown. However, it could also be argued that any evidence is better than none, and provided that the results are reported they may be included in a formal synthesis by overview. The problem here is that it is difficult to publish inconclusive results, although matters are im-

proving with, for example large databases of therapeutic trials in the Cochrane Collaboration.

Increasingly, QoL is being chosen as a major end-point in clinical trials, and thus is one of the main determinants of the size of a sample. It is now recognised that QoL measures often have very skewed distributions and the usual sample size calculations are not valid.[4-6] Thus, we decided to review the distributional form of some commonly used QoL measures and methods used to determine sample sizes in clinical studies.

This chapter considers the following issues:

1 To discover which QoL measures are being used in cancer studies.
2 To obtain an understanding of the distribution of the score of three regularly used QoL instruments.
3 To provide guidelines for methods of sample size estimation for QoL data.

METHODS

Literature Search

The literature search was conducted using the EMBASE section contained within the Bath Information Data Services (BIDS) database. The most general strategy was used; search expressions being entered into the 'title, abstract or keywords' option. The keywords used were 'sample size', 'effect size', 'quality of life', 'sample size + quality of life' and 'cancer + clinical trial'. This led to a vast number of QoL instruments that were being used in all types of studies and populations. Because of the large number of QoL instruments initially found, it was decided that this project should concentrate on the three QoL questionnaires that have been used by the British Medical Research Council in their cancer clinical trials. These are the Hospital Anxiety and Depression Scale (HADS),[7] the Rotterdam Symptom Checklist (RSCL)[8] and the European Organisation for Research and Treatment in Cancer Questionnaire (EORTC QLQ-C30).[9]

Concentrating on these three instruments, a second and more precise search was carried out, seeking papers that cited the original paper describing the questionnaire. This has shown a steady increase in the number of cancer clinical trials using these three questionnaires as outcome measures. This can be seen in more detail in the results section within this chapter. Although the searches revealed an increase in the number of citations, and hence an apparent increase in usage of these three QoL questionnaires, it is not certain that the actual frequency of their usage has been determined. Certainly papers will not have been found due to the keywords not being in their title or abstract, or the authors not being cited. Other clinical trials may not have been published because they were conducted in the pharmaceutical industry, which frequently does not publish its results in peer-reviewed journals. More might have been missed due to the 'negative finding bias' of researchers and journals. Another factor which could not be measured is the possible lag effect in the use of QoL instruments. The measure being used is the number of published articles using QoL measures. However, the usage may be more widespread as it takes time to design, conduct, report and publish a clinical trial, resulting in a lag between the use of QoL measures and the article quoting them. If these factors remain constant, however, the apparent increase in use should reflect reality.

We have not investigated whether these questionnaires are being used by oncologists and physicians in clinical practice in the UK. In a recent paper[10] on QoL perspectives of 60 oncologists in America and Canada, only 7% stated that they formally both collected and used QoL information. An important question that needs to be answered is, 'How to really incorporate QoL issues into clinical practice?'

Data Sets

Five data sets were obtained from the Medical Research Council Cancer Trials Office in Cambridge. These studies have already been published.[11–13] One data set will be explored in detail here.[11] These data provide scores for different QoL dimensions and subgroups of lung cancer patients receiving either a standard or a new treatment. The QoL questionnaires were completed together at different times over 6 months. The sample size estimates from these data are not generalisable to other studies, unless the patients in these studies are sufficiently similar. However, the methods of calculation and the issues raised by the application of these methodologies are generalisable

Sample size calculations have been described in a number of recent papers and a book,[14–17] and one based on this work published recently.[6]

Background

Descriptions of the three QoL questionnaires under review are given below.

The Hospital Anxiety and Depression Scale (HADS)

This was developed by Zigmond et al.[7] in 1983. It was designed to measure two psychological dimensions of QoL, those of anxiety and depression, in patients who were physically ill, and therefore it excluded somatic symptoms that might be due to illness. It is a self-rating questionnaire which a patient completes in the waiting room before meeting a doctor in order to reflect how they have felt during the past week. The questionnaire has 14 items which split equally into the two subscales; each question has four possible responses with scoring levels of between 0 and 3. For this question, the responses are 'most of the time' (3), 'a lot of the time' (2), 'time to time' or 'occasionally' (1), and 'not at all' (0).

The total score for the seven questions in each of the two subscales lies therefore between 0 and 21. Patients can be categorised into one of three clinically predefined categories. A total score of 0–7 implies normality, 8–10 is borderline, and a score of 11–21 suggests that a patient has significant anxiety or depression.

The advantages of the HADS are that it is short, has a simple scoring system, is accepted by patients, is easy to understand, and is quick to complete and administer. Silverstone et al.[18] suggested that the HADS does not accurately diagnose the presence of major depressive disorders in either medical or psychiatric patients. Nonetheless, they concluded that the HADS should continue to be used as a clinical indicator of the possibility of a depressive disorder. Moorey et al.[19] have carried out factor analysis on the structure and stability of the HADS using principal-components analysis on the two subscales separately. Their results suggest that the items on the two subscales do separate the concepts of anxiety and depression extremely well, and they concluded that the HADS is a useful instrument for measuring these dimensions in cancer patients. They also felt that for patients with early stage cancer the repeated administration of its two subscales was justified, and provided the physician with practical facts concerning the patient's progress.

The Rotterdam Symptom Checklist (RSCL)

This was designed by De Haes et al.[8] in 1990, initially as an instrument to measure the symptoms reported by cancer patients participating in clinical research. It incorporates 38 items, each rated on a 4-point scale (between 0 and 3) and measures both physical and psychological dimensions. The psychological dimension contains eight questions, and hence has a total score ranging from 0 to 24. It has two clinically predefined categories where a total score of 0–10 is considered to be a Non-Case and a patient scoring 11–24 is considered a Case of being psychologically distressed. Conversely, the interpretation of the physical dimension (activities of daily living), which has seven questions with a total score ranging from 0 to 21, is reversed, with a higher score implying a better physical condition. The four possible responses and scores to each question are 'able' (3), 'with difficulty' (2), 'only with help' (1) and 'unable' (0).

The RSCL advantages are that it is clearly laid out, is easy to score, is readily administered by nurses, it takes 5–10 min to complete, and it can be divided into distinct subscales scores for the physical and psychological areas. This instrument was carefully designed from a pool of items based on existing questionnaires and involved check-lists from interviews with cancer patients. Patients indicate how much they have experienced particular symptoms over the past week. Maguire et al.[20] considered that the RSCL was a good, clear and simple questionnaire which has been validated against 'gold standard' interviews. They found it to have both high sensitivity and specificity in measuring the psychological dimensions. It has been employed successfully within busy clinics, and appears as effective for patients with both early or advanced cancer, and seems to measure the physical and social dimensions equally well. The reliability of the RSCL has again been assessed using principal component analyses, and details of the three studies used for this validation can be found in De Haes and Van Knippenberg.[1]

The European Organisation for Research and Treatment in Cancer Questionnaire (EORTC QLQ-C30)

This was designed by Aaronson et al.[9] in 1993, and is a 30-item core questionnaire containing multi- and single-item scales that reflect the multi-dimensionality of QoL. It contains five functional scales, three symptom scales, a global health QoL scale, and six individual items. The core QLQ-C30 questionnaire has a scale which is easy to score and is designed to evaluate several multi-dimensions of emotional, physical and social issues for heterogeneous groups of cancer patients. The responses for the physical items are 'yes or no' and for the symptom items categorical. An example of the social functioning dimension is 'Has your physical condition or medical treatment caused you financial difficulties?' These replies and their corresponding scores are 'very much' (4), 'quite a bit' (3), 'a little' (2) and 'not at all' (1).

In addition to the core, modules are used which relate to specific cancers, some of these are still in the development stage. The core also has 18 translations available at present, plus six pending translations and four English versions for English-speaking countries. Nine of these translations have a separate male and female version. Each is a patient self-rating questionnaire where the format changes according to the module being used. The core questionnaire is distributed at clinics by nurses and takes less than 10 min to complete. It is easy to score and produces both a total score and scores on each subscale. Whilst the scale has been carefully developed on the basis of existing instruments, its reliability and validity have still to be properly assessed, as the core has only been on release since 1993 and it still has to be checked against 'gold standard' interviews to see how it performs. Further details of the development of the EORTC QLQ-C30 and the EORTC studies that use it have been given recently.[27]

The relative merits of the three questionnaires are given in Table 1.

RESULTS OF LITERATURE REVIEW

In 1990, 27% of all deaths in England and Wales were due to cancer.[21] The numbers of cancer QoL clinical trial citations using just these three questionnaires as outcome measures per 1000 cancer deaths are displayed as rates and are presented in Table 2. This table gives an overall citation rate for all cancer types, and displays the rates for specific cancer QoL citations per 1000 specific cancer deaths.

The reason why the lung cancer rate is lower in comparison to the others, even though it is highly cited, is because of the large number of deaths from lung cancer. Conversely, the skin cancer rate appears high because of the low number of deaths: only about 2% of skin cancer patients actually die from skin cancer. Therefore, if one quoted the rates as QoL citations per 1000 cancer incident cases, the magnitude of these figures may alter.

Since the development of the HADS questionnaire in 1983 there has been a steady increase in citations both from generic and cancer trials, to total nearly 500. The frequency of citations is displayed in Figure 1 and indicates clearly an increase in popularity of the HADS in cancer clinical trials, whilst the cancer citations as a percentage of all HADS citations are shown

Table 1   *Questionnaire comparison*

	HADS	RSCL	EORTC
Year developed	1983	1990	1993
No. of questions	14	38	30
No. of dimensions	2	3	15
Scoring type	Categorical 0–3	Categorical 0–3	Categorical and Yes/No
Completion time (min)	5–10	5–10	Up to 10
Clinical categories	✓	✓	✓
Self-rating	✓	✓	✓
Generic	✓	x	x
Specific modules	x	x	✓
Translated	✓	✓	✓
Validated	✓	✓	x
Used as 'gold standard'	✓	✓	x
Psychological dimension	✓	✓	✓
Functional dimension	x	✓	✓
Social dimension	x	x	✓
Symptom dimension	x	✓	✓
Global QoL score	x	x	✓
Individual items	x	✓	✓

Table 2   *The rate of cancer QoL citations per 1000 cancer deaths*

Cancer	No. of deaths	No. of citations	Rate
All	76 000	233	3.07
Lung	39 000	21	0.54
Breast	15 000	49	3.27
Skin	500	4	8.00
Pancreas	6000	6	1.00

in Figure 2. On average, cancer studies form about 25% of all studies using the HADS, but the trend is no longer evident, suggesting that the use of the HADS in cancer studies reflects a general trend in the use of this questionnaire. A total of 121 HADS cancer trials were found using the BIDS citation search.

During the first 6 years following the HADS development (1984–1989), only trials from breast, lung and head and neck patients were published, with the majority of these citations just stating 'cancer' in the abstracts – 18 citations in all.

However, between 1990 and 1995 there has been a dramatic increase to 103 citations of QoL cancer trials, and also an increase in the types of cancer which now include melanoma, cervix, pancreatic, testicular, colorectal and leukaemia.

The RSCL questionnaire was developed in 1990, and its citations also indicate a steady increase in the 5-year period 1991–1995, giving a total of 63 citations (see Figure 3). The RSCL questionnaire has been used on a full range of

cancer patients since its development, including all those of the HADS questionnaire, plus gastric, prostate and mixed cancer trials.

It is too recent for the EORTC QLQ-C30 core questionnaire to have been widely cited since its development in 1993, but we identified a total of 52 citations in its first two years of use, see Figure 4. The EORTC QLQ-30 has been used in several types of cancer trials including bladder, penis, brain and oesophagus.

RESULTS FROM THE MRC QoL DATA SET

For the purpose of demonstrating the effect size, and hence the necessary sample size, the HADS and the RSCL questionnaires have been used. The data were from a previously published clinical trial run by the MRC which provided scores for the different QoL dimensions and subgroups of cancer patients receiving either a standard or new treatment. The standard consisted of a four-drug regime (etoposide, cyclophosphamide, methotrexate and vincristine), whilst the new, less-intensive treatment contained just two of these compounds (etoposide and vincristine).[11] The two treatment schedules were the same, comprising three cycles of chemotherapy at the same dosage. Each cycle was given on three consecutive days at 3-week intervals. Both questionnaires were completed together at different times over 6 months, survival permitting, by each of 310 patients with small-cell lung cancer and poor prognosis.

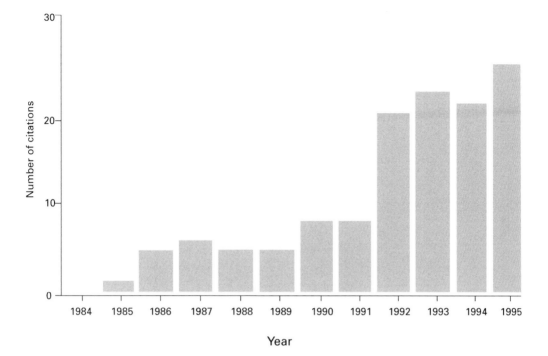

Figure 1 *Number of citations per year for the HADS questionnaire in cancer studies.*

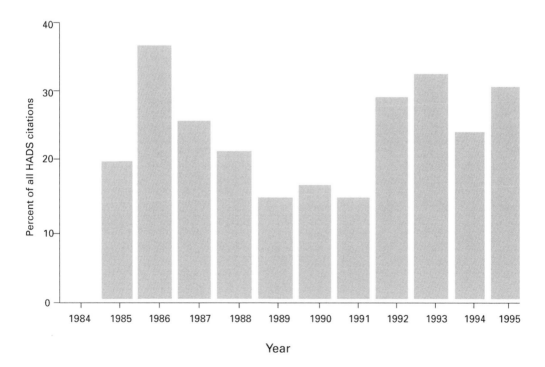

Figure 2 *Number of citations per year for the HADS questionnaire in cancer studies as a proportion of all HADS citations per year.*

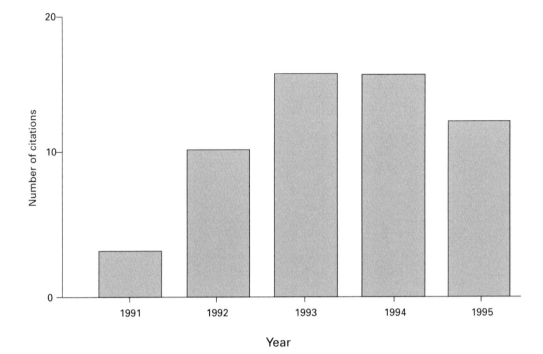

Figure 3   *Number of citations of the Rotterdam Symptom Checklist.*

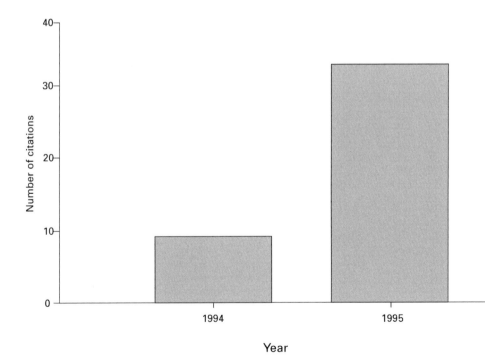

Figure 4   *Citations of the EORTC QLQ-C30.*

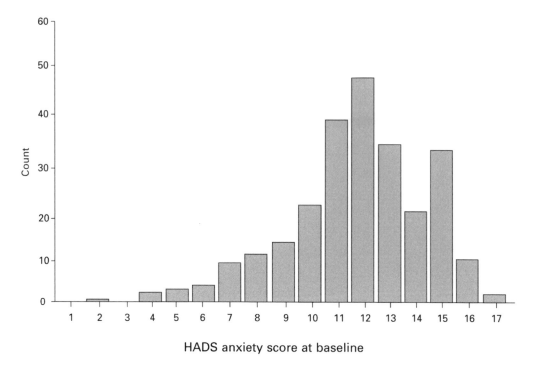

Figure 5   *Distribution of HADS anxiety scores at baseline (n = 310, 44 missing).*

QoL Score Distributions

An understanding of the QoL score distributions was achieved by investigating the raw scores of the HADS anxiety and RSCL psychological domains. The distribution of the raw HADS anxiety scores of the 310 lung cancer patients at baseline is shown in Figure 5, and is negatively skewed. The distribution of the raw RSCL psychological distress scores of the 310 lung cancer patients at baseline is shown in Figure 6; this is positively skewed, with possibly three modes.

It can be clearly seen from Figures 5 and 6 that the raw scores of neither questionnaire are Normally distributed, and that there is no simple transformation that will make them Normal, because of the number of modes. Therefore, the usual mean and standard deviation are not adequate to summarise the distributions, and non-parametric techniques – which make no assumptions about the shape of the distribution – should be used for testing.

Sample Size Methods

The main factor in determining sample size is the effect size. This is simply the size of the effect that is worth finding. It has been referred to as a 'clinically relevant' difference,[15,22] or perhaps more realistically as a 'cynically relevant difference'.[23] For a continuous outcome measure that is plausibly Normally distributed, the effect size is defined as the difference in means in the two treatment groups, that one would like to demonstrate. For a binary outcome, it is usually defined either as a difference in proportions, or more commonly as an odds ratio. If the proportion of patients achieving relief is p_1 in one group and p_2 in another, then the odds of achieving relief are $p_1/(1 - p_1)$ for the first group and $p_2/(1 - p_2)$ for the second group. The odds ratio is simply the ratio of these two odds, and can be applied to data where the outcome of interest has two or more categories.

In the two following equations, m is the number of patients required in each of two groups for a two-sided significance level α and power $1 - \beta$, where power is defined as the probability of rejecting the null hypothesis given that it is false. $Z_{1-\alpha/2}$ and $Z_{1-\beta}$ are the appropriate values from the standard Normal distribution for the $100(1 - \alpha/2)$ and $100(1 - \beta)$ percentiles respectively. Maximum power for a fixed number of patients is usually achieved by having an equal number of subjects in each group.

Parametric method[15]

The sample size required to compare two means μ_A and μ_B, assuming that the data have a

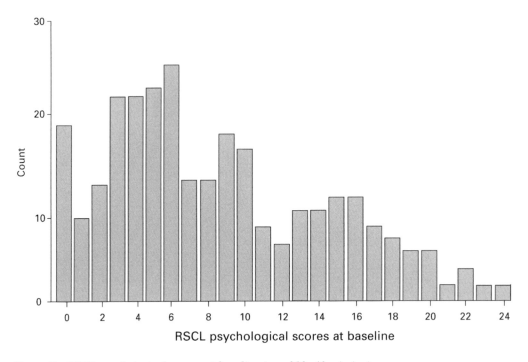

Figure 6 *RSCL psychological scores at baseline* (n = *310, 41 missing*).

Normal distribution, for a given effect size δ = $\mu_A - \mu_B$ is given in Equation (1).

$$m = \frac{2 * (Z_{1-\alpha/2} + Z_{1-\beta})^2}{d^2} + \frac{Z^2_{1-\alpha/2}}{2} \qquad (1)$$

Here, *m* is the total number needed in each group, *d* is the standardised difference, defined as δ/σ where σ is the population standard deviation of the measurements and δ, the effect size, is the minimum clinically significant difference. One important point to note is that the sample size is the same for +d and for −d; that is, whether the patients get better or get worse. One might expect that because of the central limit theorem for large samples, the assumption of Normality is reasonable. Thus for example with large samples a *z*-test gives a valid test, no matter what the distribution of the original data. However, the effect size is based on the standard *deviation*, which is a measure of individual variation. For a strongly skewed distribution, it matters whether one is trying to increase the score or decrease it.[5] Thus, with the HADS distribution in Figure 5, an intervention trying to *increase* the average score would require a different number of patients to one that tried to *decrease* it.

Non-parametric method[14,16]

Most QoL scales are ordinal; that is, the categories can be ordered, but numerical values should not be assigned to the scores (a value of 10 on the HADS does not mean that someone is twice as depressed as someone with a value of 5). The scores are often dichotomised, that is cut-offs are defined to make the scores binary (Case or Non-Case). However, dichotomising the data ignores valuable information on the ordering, and methods have been developed for sample sizes for ordered categorical (ordinal) data.[14] The minimum clinically significant effect is expressed as an odds ratio (OR). The advantage of the OR is that it can be estimated from a binary cut-off (for example borderline to case for the HADS) and then generalised from binary to ordered categorical variables. The sample size calculated stated in Equation (2), is based on the Mann–Whitney *U*-test, which allows for ties for ordered categorical data.

$$m = \frac{6\,(Z_{1-\alpha/2} + A_{1-\beta})^2 / (\log OR)^2}{\left[1 - \sum_{i=1}^{k} \bar{p}_i^3\right]} \qquad (2)$$

With this equation, *m* is the total number of patients required in each group, *OR* is the odds ratio of a subject being in a given category of less in one group compared to the other group, k is the number of categories and $\bar{p}_i$ is the mean proportion expected in category i, i.e. $\bar{p}_i = (p_{Ai} + p_{Bi})/2$ where p_{Ai} and p_{Bi} are the proportions expected in category i for the two groups A and B respectively. This equation is quite complicated to use, but rather than go through details here we refer the reader to two papers and a book that discuss its application in more detail.[6,15,16]

Equation (2) makes no assumptions about the distribution of data, but it does assume proportional odds, where the odds of being in a given category or less, in one treatment group are fixed relative to the odds of being in the same category or less in the other treatment group. Thus the *OR*s are identical for each pair of adjacent categories throughout the QoL scale. It is this assumption of a constant odds ratio (proportional odds) that allows one to generalise the *OR* calculated from a predetermined cut-off to the remaining categories of the scale.

The calculation is based on the proportions and cumulative distribution in each QoL category across dimensions. The application of the proportional odds in this formula assumes that when the distribution of the outcome for only one of the treatment arms is known, the expected cumulative proportions for the other arm can be obtained and from these the expected proportions derived for each pair of categories. Hence with prior knowledge of the distribution of just one treatment group, the *OR* and the sample size estimate can be calculated. This calculation gives different results for risks which are equal, but either represents an improvement (OR) or a deterioration (1/OR). This is sensible since it is harder to demonstrate an improvement than a deterioration in an outcome variable which takes

a limited number of values if the control group already has a high success rate.

Sample Size Comparison

The final outcome of the trial is summarised in Table 3 for the HADS and the RSCL, as a standardised difference in mean scores or as an odds ratio for either a Non-Case for the HADS and RSCL or for a borderline Case for the HADS alone. It can been seen that using either outcome the effect sizes are very small, and essentially there is little difference in the outcomes. However, for the HADS the assumption of a constant odds ratio would appear to be true. In Table 4 we ask the question 'Suppose we wished to design a new trial in similar patients as before, where the HADS anxiety dimension is to be the prime outcome. We assume the distribution of baselines was as in the earlier trial, and postulate as an effect size the observed effect in the earlier trial. What size sample would be required, with 80% power at 5% significance?' The effect sizes as measured by a difference in means or as an odds ratio both refer to the same data set, and so are attempting to summarise the same quantity, which is the difference in the distribution of the outcome measure under the two treatments. The sample size was estimated in three ways: (i) using Equation (1) and the difference in means; (ii) for the HADS dichotomising the data at two separate cut-off points and using the two separate ORs obtained in Equation (2) (a methodology often applied by researchers aware of the non-Normality of the data); and (iii) for the HADS taking the average of the two ORs and using all three categories again using Equation (2). For the RSCL there was only one score value for

Table 3   *Outcome of lung cancer trial*[10]

Standardised difference in means (HADS, anxiety) =		−0.0883
Odds ratios (HADS, anxiety) Non-Case (0–7) to Borderline (8–21)		0.92
Borderline (0–10) to Case (11–21)		0.93
Standardised difference in means (RSCL, anxiety =		0.0430
Odds ratios (RSCL, anxiety) Non-Case (0–10) to Case (11–24)		0.86

Table 4   *Sample size requirements for effect sizes from Table 3 (80% power and two-sided 5% significance level)*

Parametric (HADS)	2013
Binary (HADS) [Non-Case (0–7) – Borderline (8–21)]	9009
Binary (HADS) [Borderline (0–10) – Case (11–21)]	11 893
Ordinal (HADS)	8716
Parametric (RSCL)	8482
Binary RSCL [Non-Case (0–10) to Case (11–24)]	2760

separating Cases and Non-Cases, and so there is no way of extending the sample size calculations to ordinal data. The results are quite instructive. For the HADS, using a binary cut-off leads to a much higher sample size than that using the parametric methods. Methods for ordered categorical data result in a marginal saving of the sample size, compared with simple binary cut-offs. One might imagine that because the parametric method utilises much more information, the sample sizes would always be much smaller than for the binary method. However, for the RSCL this was not the case, with the parametric method requiring more subjects. This was because of the lack of Normality in the RSCL, so that the parametric assumptions are invalid.

From this exercise we learned that: (i) lack of Normality seriously affects the parametric method; (ii) a constant odds ratio model is reasonable for HADS for this data set; and (iii) different outcome measures (e.g. the HADS and the RSCL) have markedly different sample size requirements.

DISCUSSION AND CONCLUSIONS

The European Guidelines for the number of patients needed when conducting a clinical trial are given in a paper by Lewis et al.[24] The sample size should always be large enough to yield a reliable conclusion, and be the smallest necessary to reach this conclusion and the intended aim of the trial. If the sample size is too small, the usefulness of the results will be reduced because of the inadequate number of patients and clinically significant changes may be concealed. However, if the sample size is too large the trial will incur a waste of resources and patients may continue to receive a less effective or even dangerous treatment. These reasons to calculate an adequate sample size before conducting a clinical trial are well known.

Fayers and Machin[17] reported that it is also known that many randomised clinical trials with treatment comparisons are of an insignificant size to place weight behind the trial conclusions. Additionally, they recommend that one should calculate the sample size for a number of likely estimates of the effect size, to try and give an opinion as to whether the proposed trial is likely to be impractical.

It is evident that the methodology which assumes a symmetric Normal distribution for the QoL dimensions give symmetric sample sizes, as the parametric techniques for Normal data, shown in Equation (1), depend only on the absolute value of the difference regardless of the sign of the expected effect size. However, the non-parametric techniques, shown in Equation (2), for the QoL dimensions give markedly different sample sizes according to the direction of the expected effect size.

Our results have shown that many researchers quote means and standard deviations and imply a Normal distribution. We have demonstrated that this assumption in sample size calculations can lead to unrealistically sized studies, and we have highlighted the discrepancies between parametric and non-parametric techniques. We recommend that all researchers publish the distribution of the scores at baseline and at final outcome.

Our recommendations are to use the non-parametric formula, Equation (2), for the sample size estimations. This will allow health professionals involved in the care of cancer patients to develop interventions which maximise outcome in terms of both a patient's overall survival and their QoL.

INTERPRETATION OF TREATMENT EFFECTS

We have not been able to determine a clinically relevant treatment effect because we were dealing with retrospective data sets which show what *might* be achieved, but not what is *desirable* to achieve. It is important that a QoL measure can be responsive to change, and it is the change from baseline that is often the most important outcome. Guyatt et al.[25] discuss the interpretation of QoL scores. They suggest that even if the mean difference between a treatment and a control is appreciably less than the smallest change that is important, treatment may have an important impact on many patients. They suggest that the smallest change in a categorical variable that is important to a patient is 0.5 per question, with 1.0 being a moderate change and 1.5 being considered large. They describe a method by which these can be converted into a proportion of patients who benefit from a treatment, which can be compared to the number-needed-to-treat (NNT) provided with the usual clinical outcomes. We would not advise their method for the parallel group trial however, because it requires an assumption that responses within a patient are likely to be independent. Stockler et al.[26] looked at the responsiveness to change of the EORTC QLQ-C30[27] and compared it with a more specific instrument in prostate cancer. They concluded that the QLQ-C30 is responsive to changes in health-related quality of life, and suggest that the QLQ-30 is more responsive to global perceptions of health than the more specific questionnaire. However as Stucki et al.[28] point out, numerically equal gains in an ordinal score may differ in their meaning depending on the baseline health status. They recommend that the distribution of baseline health status measures and the distribution of responders by baseline status be reported in evaluative studies.

The sample size is most critically dependent on the estimation of the treatment effect size. If you halve the effect size, then you quadruple the sample size.[17] The effect size is commonly taken as a difference which is the minimum to be clinically meaningful, but its interpretation and specification are very subjective. The definition of a clinically significant difference is based on such things as experience of the QoL measure of interest and the population in which the QoL measure is being applied. This is not immediately straightforward, for different populations give different distributions for the QoL measures and different interpretations of what is a clinically significant effect size. However, there is at present limited experience of QoL measures in different populations, when compared to clinical end-points.

The specification of the treatment effect size is also important as one must also be able to put any results observed into a clinical context. A median reduction of 3 units must have a meaning regardless of statistical significance. If, using HADS as an example, a median reduction of 3 was observed, the interpretation of this reduction would have a different context if most subjects were classified as 'normal' in contrast to if most subjects were classified as 'depressed'. Patients who have higher scores on average have a higher potential for reduction.

Previously published work is an obvious source of information of what is a clinically significant treatment effect. However, one should not fall into the trap of simply setting the effect size to be what has been observed previously, without concurrent information as to whether it is meaningful to the patients.

One way of determining a clinically significant difference when there are no randomised trials available is through elicitation of possible differences using the opinion of individual clinicians with experience of the QoL measures.[29] Thus, one does not have a single estimate of an effect size, but a range or distribution of possible effects. This would lead to a range of possible sample sizes.

IMPLICATIONS FOR THE RESEARCHERS

It is now almost mandatory to include a sample size calculation in research protocols and to justify the size of clinical trials in papers. However, one of the most prevailing errors in clinical trials is a lack of justification of the sample size and one paper has concluded 'the reporting of statistical power and sample size needs to be improved'.[24] The identification of correct sample size estimates for use in clinical trials circumvents the unethical under- or over-recruitment of patients to a particular trial.

We have provided recommendations and produced a table which supplies evidence of the advantage of the non-parametric technique used for the sample size calculation with QoL outcomes. This will allow researchers to estimate more accurately sample sizes for future clinical trials involving these three commonly used QoL questionnaires as outcome measures in clinical trials and in clinical practice.

FURTHER RESEARCH

Five suggestions for further research are listed below:

1   To investigate patients' change in score over time. In particular, in many cancer patients, QoL scores may change quite rapidly, indicating a more restricted QoL and this is quickly followed by death. Research could be carried out to compare these scores with the scores of those who have survived, and then base the sample size estimate on the effect size over time. This might improve the sensitivity of QoL questionnaires to detect a significant treatment difference in longitudinal studies.

2   To quantify the effect of using covariates on sample size calculations. The consideration of covariates in calculating the clinically meaningful difference to be considered may be different in different subgroups of patients, and this will need to be corrected for in the sample size estimation.

3   The European Guidelines[24] state that the sample size should consider the possible number of patients that drop out of the trial, as it is the number of patients at the end of each trial which constitutes the sample size. Thus, further factors that need to be considered are the take-up rates (usually quite low) and drop-out rates (normally quite high) in a palliative care study. Rates for different types of patients and different scales could be provided from which inflation factors for the total sample size can be derived. Another area to consider is what is known as informative missing data. Data may be missing because, for example,

patients are too ill to complete the form and so simply treating these data as missing at random, and so ignoring patients with missing data, will give an unduly optimistic picture of the quality of life of a group. Similarly, patients who are immobile may simply ignore questions about pain on moving, so the fact that the response is missing is related to the condition of the patients and should not be ignored.

4 As previously stated, the frequency of use of these QoL instruments in clinical practice in the UK by specialist such as oncologists and physicians is unknown. Clinicians' perceptions of the usefulness of these instruments in making decisions about various treatment options for their patients could also be investigated.

5 To investigate the effect on sample size considerations in other therapeutic areas, the use of different instruments, and especially the SF-36 and EuroQoL (EQ-5D), should be undertaken.

References

1. De Haes JCJM, Van Knippenberg FCE. The quality of life of cancer patients – a review of the literature. *Soc. Sci. Med.* 1985; **20**: 809–17.

2. Altman DG. Statistics and ethics in medical research III – How large a sample? *Br. Med. J.* 1980; **281**: 1336–8.

3. Edwards SJL, Lilford RJ, Braunholtz D, Jackson J. Why 'underpowered' trials are not necessarily unethical. *Lancet* 1997; **350**: 804–7

4. Julious SA, George S, Campbell MJ. Sample size for studies using the short form 36 (SF36). *J. Epidemiol. Community Health* 1995; **49**: 642–4.

5. Campbell MJ, Julious SA, George SL. Estimating sample sizes for studies using the SF36 (reply to letter). *J. Epidemiol. Community Health* 1996; **50**: 473–4.

6. Julious SA, George S, Machin D, Stephen RJ. Sample sizes for randomised trials measuring quality of life in cancer patients. *Quality of Life Research* 1997; **6**: 109–17.

7. Zigmond AS, Snaith RP. The Hospital Anxiety and Depression Scale. *Acta Psychiatr. Scand.* 1983; **67**: 361–70.

8. De Haes JCJM, Van Knippenberg FCE, Neijt JP. Measuring psychological and physical distress in cancer patients – structure and application of the Rotterdam Symptom Checklist. *Br. J. Cancer* 1990; **62**: 1034–8.

9. Aaronson NK, Ahmedzai S, Bergman B, et al. The European Organisation for Research and Treatment of Cancer QLQ-C30: a quality of life instrument for use in international clinical trials in oncology. *J. Natl Cancer Inst.* 1993; **85**: 365–76.

10. Taylor KM, Macdonald KG, Bezjak A, Ng P, DePetrillo AD. Physicians' perspective on quality of life – An exploratory study of oncologists. *Quality of Life Research* 1996; **5**: 5–14.

11. Bleehen NM, Girling DJ, Hopwood P, Lallemand G, Machin D, Stephens RJ, Bailey AJ. Medical Research Council Lung Cancer Working Party: randomised trial of four-drug vs less intensive two-drug chemotherapy in the palliative treatment of patients with small-cell lung cancer (SCLC) and poor prognosis. *Br. J. Cancer* 1996; **73**: 406–13.

12. Bleehen NM, Bolger JJ, Girling DJ, Hasleton PS, Hopwood P, MacBeth FR, Machin D, Moghissi K, Saunders M, Stephens RJ, Thatcher N, White RJ. A Medical-Research Council (MRC) randomized trial of palliative radiotherapy with two fractions or a single fraction in patients with inoperable non-small-cell lung-cancer (NSCLC) and poor performance status. *Br. J. Cancer* 1992; **65**: 934–41.

13. Bleehan NM, Girling DJ, Machin D, et al. A randomized trial of three or six courses of etoposide, cyclophosphamide, methotrexate and vincristine or six courses of etoposide and ifosfamide in small-cell lung-cancer (SCLC) 2. Quality-of-life. *Br. J. Cancer* 1993; **68**: 1157–66.

14. Whitehead J. Sample size calculations for ordered categorical data. *Stat. Med.* 1993; **12**: 2257–73.

15. Machin D, Campbell MJ, Fayers P, Pinol A. *Statistical Tables for the Design of Clinical Studies*, 2nd edn. Oxford: Blackwell Science, 1997.

16. Campbell MJ, Julious SA, Altman DG. Estimating sample sizes for binary, ordered categorical, and continuous outcomes in two group comparisons. *Br. Med. J.* 1995; **311**: 1145–8.

17. Fayers PM, Machin D. Sample size – how many patients are necessary? *Br. J. Cancer* 1995; **72**: 1–9.

18. Silverstone PH. Poor efficacy of the Hospital Anxiety and Depression Scale in the diagnosis of major depressive disorder in both medical and psychiatric patients. *J. Psychosom. Res.* 1994; **38**: 441–50.

19. Moorey S, Greer S, Watson M, Gorman C, Rowden L, Tunmore R, Robertson B, Bliss J. The factor structure of factor stability of the hospital anxiety and depression scale in patients with cancer. *Br. J. Psychiatry* 1991; **158**: 255–9.

20. Maguire P, Selby P. Assessing quality of life in cancer patients. *Br. J. Cancer* 1989; **60**: 437–40.

21. Neal A, Hoskin P. *Clinical Oncology – A textbook for students*. Edward Arnold, 1994; 616–992.

22. Gardner MJ, Machin D, Campbell MJ. Use of checklists in assessing the statistical content of medical studies. *Br. Med. J.* 1986; **292**: 810–12.

23. Senn SJ. *Statistical Issues in Drug Development.* John Wiley & Sons, 1997.

24. Lewis JA, Jones DR, Rohmel J. Biostatistical methodology in clinical trials – a European guideline. *Stat. Med.* 1995; **14**: 1655–82.

25. Guyatt GH, Juniper EF, Walter SD, Griffith LE, Goldstein RS. Interpreting treatment effects in randomised trials. *Br. Med. J.* 1998; **316**: 690–3.

26. Stockler MR, Osoba D, Goodwin P, Corey P, Tannock IF. Responsiveness to change in health related quality of life in a randomised clinical trial: a comparison of the prostate cancer specific quality of life instrument (PROSQOL1) with analogous scales from the EORTC QLQ C30 and a trial specific module. *J. Clin. Epidemiol.* 1998: **51**: 137–45.

27. Kiebert GM, Curran D, Aaronson NK. Quality of life as an endpoint in EORTC clinical trials. *Stat. Med.* 1998; **17**: 561–70.

28. Stucki G, Daltroy L, Katz JN, Johannesson M, Liang MH. Interpretation of change scores in ordinal clinical scales and health status measures: the whole may not equal the sum of the parts. *J. Clin. Epidemiol.* 1996; **49**: 711–17.

29. Spiegelhalter DJ, Freedman LS, Parmar MK. Bayesian approaches to randomized trials. *J. Roy. Statist. Soc. A* 1994; **157**: 357–416.

20

Simultaneous Analysis of Quality of Life and Survival Data

LUCINDA J. BILLINGHAM, KEITH R. ABRAMS
and DAVID R. JONES

SUMMARY

The assessment of treatments for chronic diseases in clinical trials is often based on both length of survival and the quality of life experienced during that time. In longitudinal studies of quality of life where survival is also an end-point, patients are often severely ill, and it is a common occurrence for subjects to drop out of the study due to illness or death. This drop-out process may be related to the quality of life being experienced, rather than being at random. The missing quality of life data resulting from *informative drop-out* of this kind cannot be ignored in any analysis of the data since bias may result. Methods used to analyse longitudinal quality of life data must allow for informative drop-out.

Methods proposed for the analysis of quality of life and survival data in health technology assessment were identified from a search of the scientific and medical literature. They fall into three broad categories depending on whether the focus of the research is to compare treatments in terms of: (i) quality of life; (ii) survival; or (iii) both quality of life and survival simultaneously. Methods from the review were illustrated by application to a Cancer Research Campaign Phase III trial in lung cancer.

Methods that simultaneously analyse quality of life and survival data not only have the advantage of allowing for informative drop-out due to death, but also have the potential to be extended to allow for informative drop-out due to reasons other than death. These form the main body of literature for the review, and this chapter focuses on this area. Three different approaches to the simultaneous analysis of quality of life and survival data are examined. One approach is to combine quality and quantity of life into a single end-point and use *quality-adjusted survival analysis* methods to compare treatments. A second approach is to use *multi-state models* to model the movement of patients between various health states, defined by levels of quality of life and by death, and to explore how treatments differ in terms of these movements. Finally, a *simultaneous modelling* approach considers quality of life and survival as two simultaneous processes occurring in patients, and describes the data in terms of two inter-linked models.

In conclusion, the analysis of longitudinal quality of life data must consider the problem of informative drop-out. Methods that simultaneously analyse quality of life and survival data have the potential to deal with this problem. The choice of method in any application needs to consider the advantages and disadvantages of each method in conjunction with the question that the study is addressing.

BACKGROUND

Quality of life assessment has become an important issue in healthcare research and the study of new technologies, especially in many chronic diseases. Although length of survival is usually the standard end-point for assessing treatments in such clinical trials, informed clinical decisions generally require quantification and interpretation of quality of life measures, especially with respect to variation over time and the inter-relation with length of life. The role of quality of life will become even more prominent in the future as, for many diseases, especially cancer, improvements in survival due to treatment are either unlikely to be dramatic or likely to be made at the expense of quality of life.

There has been much research into the development of instruments with which to measure quality of life. This has resulted in a plethora of instruments[1] and in substantial amounts of quality of life data being gathered in trials. Consequently, methods that enable the effective and efficient analysis and interpretation of such data are needed. There are a number of previous reviews of the assessment and analysis of quality of life in clinical trials.[2–6]

In quality of life studies where survival is also an end-point, the patient population will not be stable over time. Patients are often severely ill, and subjects may have incomplete follow-up of quality of life for reasons related to disease or treatment, including death. This drop-out process may be related to the quality of life being experienced, rather than being at random, and is known as *informative drop-out*. In such situations, statistical analysis can be particularly problematic and this chapter reviews appropriate methods that yield unbiased and clinically relevant assessment of health technologies.

METHODS OF REVIEW

Literature Search

The scientific and medical literature were searched for relevant methodological articles. An article was defined as relevant if it included some sort of quality of life assessment over time, in circumstances where survival was also an issue, and it used either a known methodology of interest or a new and clearly detailed methodology.

Electronic searches were carried out systematically using the Science Citation Index, the Social Science Citation Index and the EMBASE database provided by BIDS (Bath Information and Data Service). Reference lists from articles defined as being relevant were 'exploded' such that they were checked to identify further relevant literature. Articles recommended by colleagues and from personal collections were also incorporated. These were supplemented by a hand-search of the journal *Quality of Life Research*.

The search produced 1127 references in total, of which 361 were considered to be relevant and were included in the review.[7] The literature search aimed to identify all methods proposed for the analysis of quality of life and survival data. It is not possible to determine if this aim has been achieved, but the broadness of the search strategy used, together with the method of exploding references, should have ensured a reasonably complete coverage of material in the field.

Illustrative Example: The MIC Study

The methods identified by the literature search are illustrated by application to data from a previously conducted study. The study is the second of two concurrent Phase III randomised trials of MIC (mitomycin, ifosfamide and cisplatin) chemotherapy in patients with non-small-cell lung cancer that were conducted at the Cancer Research Campaign Trials Unit at Birmingham University. The results from both trials are reported elsewhere,[8] and the worked examples here use just the quality of life and survival data from the second trial (MIC2), referred to here as the MIC study.

Patients in the MIC study were randomised to receive either standard palliative care (PAL), usually radiotherapy, or MIC chemotherapy to a maximum of four courses followed by palliative care (CT). The aim of the study was to compare treatments in terms of both length of survival and quality of life. The trial started in 1988 and closed in 1996, during which time 359 patients were randomised into the study. For practical reasons, quality of life was assessed in a subgroup of 109 patients from three centres, with 67 on the CT arm and 42 on the PAL arm. Quality of life was measured using a patient-completed questionnaire consisting essentially of 12 questions on various aspects of quality of life. Responses were measured on a four-level ordered categorical scale: 'none', 'a little', 'quite a bit' or 'very much'.

A single measure of quality of life is needed to illustrate the methods, and this may be as simple or as complex as required to reflect the quality of life of the patients. A malaise question, which asked if patients had been feeling 'generally ill', is chosen as the measure of quality of life to use in the analysis here. Due to the lack of data, the level of malaise, i.e. 'a little', 'quite a bit' or 'very much' has to be ignored, resulting in a binary quality of life outcome such that a patient either does or does not have malaise. Although this measure is very simplistic, it nonetheless illustrates the essentials of the methods and allows insight into the problems associated with the methods.

Quality of life was assessed only during the patient's treatment period. The study was designed such that patients on the CT arm completed five questionnaires at approximately 3-weekly intervals (one before each course of chemotherapy and one post treatment), whilst patients on the RT arm completed four questionnaires at approximately 3-weekly intervals. There was some variation in the timing, but 99% of questionnaires had been completed by 18 weeks and the 18-week period from entry to trial is defined as the analysis period for the study. Patients were severely ill and hence there were a considerable number of 'early' deaths and drop-outs from the quality of life study. Thirty-seven patients died within 18 weeks of entry to the trial, 29 of whom died before completing the full set of assessments. In total, 46 patients dropped out of the quality of life study. Ten of these drop-outs could be attributed directly to death in that they died within 3 weeks of the last completed assessment. The drop-out problem in the MIC study makes it a realistic example with which to illustrate methods for the assessment of quality of life and survival data.

Assumptions required for analysis of the MIC data

In the MIC study, the survival time within the 18-week analysis period for each patient was split into time with malaise and time without malaise according to the responses to the questionnaire at each quality of life assessment. Various assumptions are required to categorise patients into health states at all points of their survival time using the assessments made at discrete time points. If a patient's state of malaise changed between two assessments, then the change was assumed to happen at the mid-point between assessment dates and subjects were assumed to remain in a specified health state until a change occurred. The state of malaise that was reported at the last assessment was assumed to carry over until either death or 18 weeks, whichever came first. This may not be a reasonable assumption for patients who dropped out of the study, especially for those who dropped out early and then remained alive for the whole of the 18-week period. Sensitivity analysis should be used to examine the robustness of any conclusions with respect to the assumptions made.

METHODS FOR THE ANALYSIS OF QUALITY OF LIFE AND SURVIVAL DATA

Methods for analysing quality of life and survival data were found to fall into three broad categories according to the research question underlying the study, which in turn depends on the disease and treatments under investigation. The first category consists of methods where the primary aim of the study is to compare treatments in terms of quality of life whilst accounting for informative drop-out. The second consists of methods where the primary aim is to compare treatments in terms of survival whilst adjusting for the effects of quality of life. The third consists of methods for studies where quality of life and survival are both important end-points for assessing treatments, and the two end-points are to be analysed simultaneously.

If treatment comparison is primarily in terms of quality of life, then standard methods of longitudinal data analysis[9–11] can be applied. The application of such methods to quality of life data has been discussed,[12–17] but in situations where informative drop-out is present, they will give biased results since missing data are assumed to be missing at random. Missing data can be imputed using techniques such as 'last value carried forward',[18] but this could also result in bias. Modelling techniques that deal with informative drop-out have been developed.[19,20] The methods are not readily accessible to researchers and, with examples of their application to quality of life data being limited, further research into their application in this field is required.

If the aim of the analysis is to compare length of survival for different treatments then it may be necessary to incorporate changing quality of life values over time as a time-dependent co-variate. This may be done using standard survival analysis techniques such as Cox regression modelling.[21,22] If assessments of quality of life are infrequent, or data are missing for reasons other than death, then it may be difficult to adjust for changing quality of life with any degree of accuracy.

Methods that simultaneously analyse quality of life and survival data not only provide a means of comparing treatments in terms of the two end-points simultaneously, but also provide a means for overcoming problems of missing quality of life data, resulting from informative drop-out, when analysing either quality of life or survival as the primary end-point. For this reason, these methods are the focus of this chapter.

Three different approaches can be used to analyse quality of life and survival data simultaneously. The first approach considered is *quality-adjusted survival analysis* wherein treatments are compared in terms of a composite measure of quality and quantity of life, created by weighting periods of survival time according to the quality of life experienced. A second approach is to use *multi-state models* to describe the movement of patients between various health states, defined by levels of quality of life and death, and explore how treatments differ in terms of these transitions. Finally, a *simultaneous modelling* approach considers quality of life and survival as two simultaneous processes occurring in patients and describes the data in terms of two inter-linked models. These methods will be discussed, and the first two will be illustrated using data from the MIC study.

Quality-Adjusted Survival Analysis

Quality-adjusted survival analysis is based on the concept of QALYs (quality-adjusted life years)[23] where quality and quantity of survival are combined into a composite measure. In the general QALY model, survival time is split into periods spent in different health states where different quality of life is experienced. QALYs are calculated by summing these times with weights attached to each time period reflecting the quality of life experienced. The weights range from 0 to 1, with 0 representing quality of life equivalent to death and 1 representing perfect health. Negative weights can be used if the quality of life is thought to be worse than death. These weights are intended to reflect the relative desirability of the state and are sometimes referred to as 'health state utilities'.[24]

Special restricted forms of QALYs are TWiST (Time Without Symptoms or Toxicity)[25,26] and Q-TWiST (Quality-adjusted TWiST).[27,28] For TWiST, all periods of survival time with symptoms of disease or toxicity resulting from treatment are given a weight of 0, whilst all other time periods are given a weight of 1, so that as the term suggests, TWiST counts only time without symptoms or toxicity. The Q-TWiST end-point is a more general form of TWiST. It

was originally developed for a breast cancer application,[27] but has since been modified where necessary for use with other diseases such as rectal cancer[29] and AIDS.[30] With Q-TWiST, periods of survival time spent with symptoms of disease and toxicity resulting from treatment are each given weights between 0 and 1, rather than being ignored as they are in TWiST.

There are two main approaches to quality-adjusted survival analysis, depending on the level of aggregation of the quality of life and survival data. The subject-based approach combines quality of life and survival at the patient level, thus creating a single end-point for each subject on which to compare treatments, whilst the population-based approach aggregates quality of life and survival at a (predefined) group level. Both approaches will be discussed and illustrated using data from the MIC study.

Subject-based approach illustrated with data from the MIC study

QALWs (quality-adjusted life weeks) were calculated for each subject in the MIC study by allocating a weight of 1 to the time spent with no malaise, and a weight of 0.8 to the time spent with malaise to reflect the reduced quality of life during this time. The choice of weights was arbitrary and was made purely to illustrate the method. Table 1 gives an example of the calculations for a particular individual who survived for 16.85 weeks and whose quality-adjusted survival time was calculated as 16.21 weeks by down-weighting the 3.21 weeks spent with malaise by a factor of 0.8. The health states in the MIC study did not conform to the strict definition of TWiST or Q-TWiST, since at no time during the 18-week analysis period were the patients free of symptoms or toxicity, but a TWiST-type end-point was calculated by giving a weight of 1 to times with no malaise and a weight of 0 to times with malaise. For the example given in Table 1, time periods spent with no malaise were summed to give 13.64 weeks, and this forms the TWiST end-point for that subject.

So far, follow-up has only been discussed in terms of the study of quality of life over time, but it is now necessary to consider follow-up in

Table 1 *Example of QALY calculations in the MIC study*

Patient no.	Health state	Weeks	QALW	TWiST
93	No malaise	5.57	5.57	5.57
	Malaise	3.21	$0.8 \times 3.21 = 2.57$	0
	No malaise	8.07	8.07	8.07
		16.85	16.21	13.64

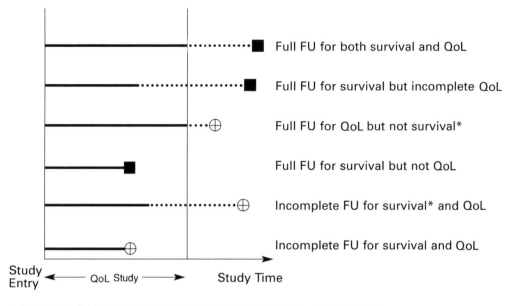

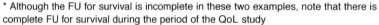

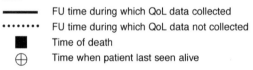

* Although the FU for survival is incomplete in these two examples, note that there is complete FU for survival during the period of the QoL study

KEY

———	FU time during which QoL data collected
·········	FU time during which QoL data not collected
■	Time of death
⊕	Time when patient last seen alive

Figure 1   *Examples of differing follow-up (FU) in studies of quality of life (QoL) and survival.*

terms of the study of survival time. It should be noted that the follow-up in terms of these two end-points could be different (see Figure 1). In studies of survival time, subjects may either be lost-to-follow-up during the course of the study, or may be followed-up for the period of the study, but not die. For these patients, although the actual survival time is not known, the data provide a lower bound for the value. These are known as *censored survival times* and standard survival analysis techniques are specifically designed to account for any censored data. The methods, however, are only valid if the mechanism that causes the individual's survival time to be censored is unrelated to the actual unobserved survival time. When the censoring mechanism is not independent of survival time, *informative censoring* occurs and standard methods for survival analysis are invalid.[22] It should be noted that informative censoring is a different concept to the previously discussed concept of informative drop-out (see Background), which

relates to completeness of follow-up in terms of quality of life data.

In calculating QALYs for each subject, there may be individuals who have censored survival times and therefore the number of QALYs for these individuals will also be censored. It therefore seems appropriate to apply standard survival analysis techniques to this quality-adjusted survival time, as for a standard survival end-point. This approach, however, may be invalid and give biased results because the censoring mechanism is related to the QALY end-point, resulting in informative censoring.[23] For example, if two patients both have the same censored survival time (say 2 years) and one patient spends their survival time in poor quality of life (valued at say 0.5), whilst the other has good quality of life (valued at say 1), then the QALY time for the first individual will be censored earlier (i.e. 1 year) than the second individual (2 years), purely because of their quality of life. One method for overcoming this problem is to restrict the analysis to a time period for which all patients have an *observed* survival time. Then, as there are no censored survival times, informative censoring will not be a problem and standard survival techniques can be used. If there are a number of survival times censored at an early time point, then this approach may not be practical. An alternative population-based approach such as partitioned survival analysis,[23] which will be discussed later, may be used to overcome the problem.

In the MIC study, because the analysis was restricted to 18 weeks from study entry and all patients have complete follow-up during that time in terms of survival, there was no problem of informative censoring, and standard survival analysis techniques could be used.

Before presenting quality-adjusted survival times, the results of analysing the standard survival end-point should be noted. A standard analysis of the survival of patients in the MIC quality of life study within 18 weeks of trial entry showed that chemotherapy increased the length of survival compared to standard palliative care. The Kaplan–Meier survival curves for the two treatment groups are shown in Figure 2. The areas under the curves give the mean survival time accumulated over the 18 weeks, which was 16.2 weeks (standard error 0.48) for CT and 14.4 weeks (standard error 0.74) for PAL. A log-rank test showed this difference in

18-week survival to be statistically significant ($\chi^2 = 8.07$, $P = 0.005$).

Kaplan–Meier survival curves using the QALW end-point rather than survival are shown in Figure 3. At any time point the curves represent the proportion of patients having at least that quality-adjusted survival time. It should be noted that the steps do not represent deaths as they do with normal survival curves, but rather termination of a patient's QALW at that point. As the number of QALWs increases, so the proportion having at least that value decreases. The curves for the different treatments are similar, with the PAL curve decreasing more rapidly than that for CT. The areas under the curves give the mean quality-adjusted life weeks accumulated over 18 weeks which was 14.4 weeks (standard error 0.46) for CT and 13.0 weeks (standard error 0.70) for PAL, indicating better quality-adjusted survival with chemotherapy. A log-rank test showed no statistically significant difference between treatment arms ($\chi^2 = 1.33$, $P = 0.25$). Thus, although treatments differed in terms of survival within 18 weeks, they were not found to differ significantly in terms of quality-adjusted survival. This conclusion is based on weighting periods of malaise with the value of 0.8, and sensitivity analysis should be used to establish the robustness of conclusions to the choice of weights used to calculate the QALW end-point for each subject.

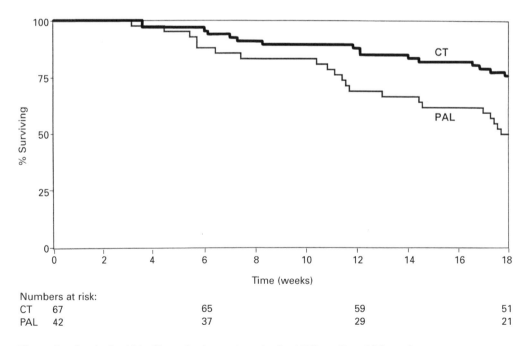

Figure 2 *Survival within 18 weeks for patients in the MIC quality of life study.*

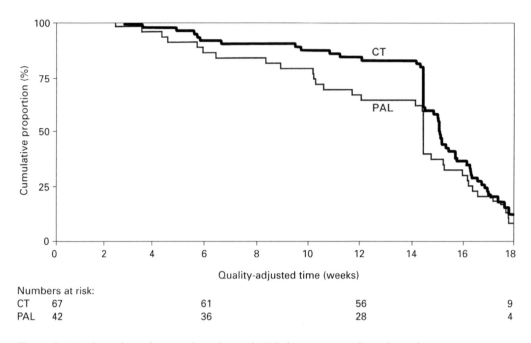

Figure 3   *Quality-adjusted survival analysis of MIC data using quality-adjusted life weeks (QALWs).*

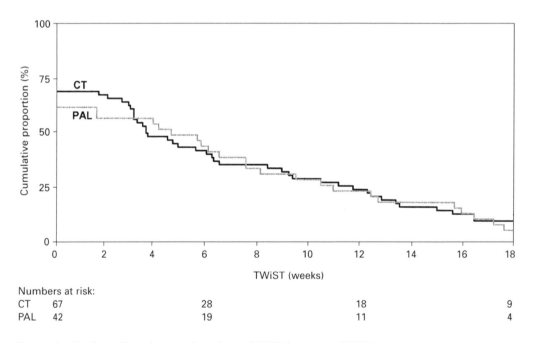

Figure 4   *Quality-adjusted survival analysis of MIC data using TWiST.*

Kaplan–Meier survival curves for each treatment group using the TWiST end-point are shown in Figure 4. The low starting point of the curves represents the proportion of patients whose whole survival time during the 18-week period was with malaise and hence have a TWiST of 0. The curves show no difference between treatments. The areas under the curves gives the mean TWiST accumulated over 18 weeks which was 6.6 weeks (standard error

0.81) for chemotherapy and 6.5 weeks (standard error 1.06) for palliative treatment. A log-rank test showed no statistically significant difference ($\chi^2 = 0.04$, $P = 0.85$).

The treatments significantly differ in terms of survival, but not in terms of quality-adjusted survival, possibly because the extra survival time obtained under chemotherapy is generally spent in poor quality of life. The extra variability in the quality-adjusted survival data may also have some impact in changing the significance of the results.

Partitioned survival analysis illustrated with data from the MIC study

It has already been noted that standard survival analysis of a QALY end-point, calculated for each individual, may lead to a problem of informative censoring. Population-based approaches, which combine quality of life and survival data at the population level rather than at the subject level, can overcome the problem of informative censoring. This is because survival analysis is carried out on *unweighted* survival times and the quality of life adjustments are applied at a later stage to summary measures of survival time. Various population-based approaches have been discussed,[29,31] but *partitioned survival analysis*[23,28] is the most widely used. In this approach, the time spent in each of a finite number of progressive health states is calculated as a mean for a group rather than on a patient-by-patient basis. A weighted sum of these mean times estimates the quality-adjusted survival time for the group. The method was devised and is generally used for a Q-TWiST end-point with three progressive health states: time spent with toxicity (TOX); TWiST; and time following relapse of disease (REL). Quality of life data do not generally create such health states, but the methodology may still be applicable by defining health states based on the quality of life outcomes. This approach is illustrated by application to the MIC data.

The first step in the method is to define a set of progressive health states that the patient passes through during their survival time. This is not always straightforward or possible. In the MIC data, patients appear to fluctuate from one state to another in no obvious pattern, and it is difficult to define progressive health states that are clinically meaningful. For illustrative purposes we chose a set of four progressive health states: a good state (*GOOD1*) followed by a poor state (*POOR1*) followed by a second good state (*GOOD2*) and a further poor state (*POOR2*). Good and poor health states were defined as time without and with malaise respectively, as determined from the quality of

life assessments. Time spent in the health states (t_i where i is a health state) were combined using a QALY model as defined in Equation (1) where both good states were allocated weights of 1. The two poor states were allocated different weights, u_1 and u_2 ($0 \leq u_1 \leq 1$, $0 \leq u_2 \leq 1$), on the assumption that the quality of life differs depending on whether it is the first or second time in that state.

$$QALW = t_{GOOD1} + u_1 t_{POOR1} + t_{GOOD2} + u_2 t_{POOR2} \quad (1)$$

The partitioned survival curves for the chemotherapy treatment group are shown in Figure 5(a). The curves are standard Kaplan–Meier survival curves with not only time to death represented, but also time to exiting each of the progressive health states. This partitions the area under the overall survival curve into areas representing time spent in each state. The area between curves is calculated and represents the mean time spent in the health states, restricted to the 18-week analysis period. These values can be put into the model as specified in Equation (1) to give the restricted mean quality-adjusted survival time for the chemotherapy treatment group as specified in Equation (2). The process is repeated for the palliative group to give Equation (3).

$$QALW_{CT} = 3.37 + 8.10u_1 + 3.16 + 1.66u_2 \quad (2)$$

$$QALW_{PAL} = 4.22 + 7.96u_1 + 2.15 + 0.19u_2 \quad (3)$$

At this point of the analysis there are two main options. If some knowledge exists regarding the values that u_1 and u_2 should take, then those values could be used to calculate the restricted mean quality-adjusted survival time for each treatment group; otherwise a special form of sensitivity analysis called a *threshold utility analysis* may be carried out.

In a threshold utility analysis, all possible pairs of values for the weights are considered, and values that give no difference between treatments in terms of restricted mean quality-adjusted survival time are determined. Weights, u_1 and u_2, can take any value between 0 and 1. The shaded area in Figure 6 shows all possible pairs of values that u_1 and u_2 can take, known as the *threshold utility plane*. The line in Figure 6, known as the *threshold line*, represents pairs of values for which the restricted mean quality-adjusted survival times in the two treatment groups are equal. This is calculated by putting $QALW_{CT}$, as specified in Equation (2), equal to $QALW_{PAL}$, as specified in Equation (3). The area above the line represents pairs of values for which quality-adjusted survival time is greater for CT than PAL, and below the line where quality-adjusted survival time is less for CT

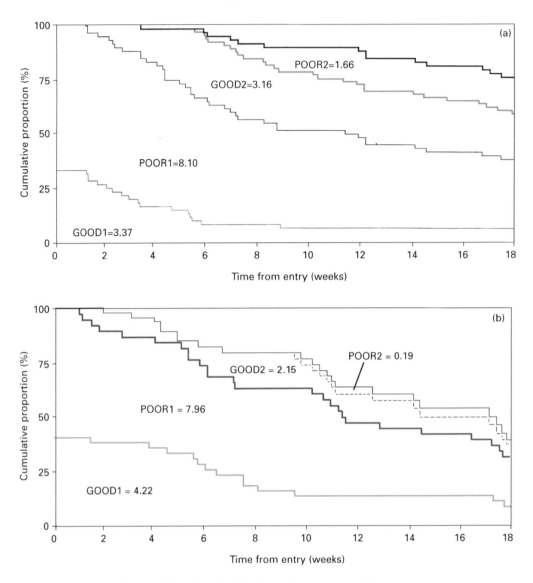

Figure 5   *Partitioned survival analysis for (a) chemotherapy arm and (b) palliative arm of the MIC study.*

compared to PAL. Figure 6 shows that all possible pairs of values of u_1 and u_2 fall above the line, so that whatever values of u_1 and u_2 are used in the model, the amount of quality-adjusted survival time will be greater under chemotherapy than under palliative treatment in this example.

Critical appraisal of quality-adjusted survival analysis

Quality-adjusted survival analysis provides a relatively straightforward approach for the simultaneous analysis of quality of life and survival data. It can be used with any quality of life instrument, providing it is possible to define meaningful health states from it. In some situations, it may be desirable to carry out separate analyses for each dimension in a multi-dimensional instrument.

The subject-based approach may suffer from the problem of informative censoring. This may be overcome by either restricting the analysis to an upper time limit, which may occur automatically anyway if the quality of life data collection is restricted to a limited time period, or using a population-based approach such as partitioned survival analysis.

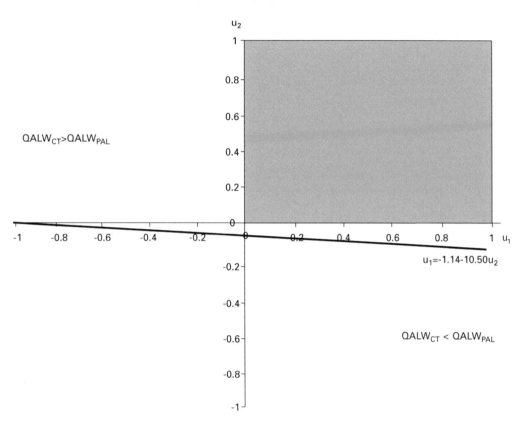

Figure 6   *Threshold utility analysis for the MIC study.*

Partitioned survival analysis may be problematic if the progressive health states required for the analysis are difficult to define, as in the MIC study. It also has the potential disadvantage of needing to be restricted to an upper time limit, although methods to investigate the effect of imposing an upper time limit can be applied.[23,32] Further, calculation of confidence intervals for the restricted mean quality-adjusted survival times requires use of the bootstrap method,[33] which may not be readily accessible to researchers. The method can incorporate co-variates[34] and in general, some of the limitations of quality-adjusted survival analysis may be overcome by using a parametric approach to the method.[35]

Quality-adjusted survival analysis overcomes the problem of missing quality of life data due to drop-out because of death, but it does not deal with other disease- or treatment-related reasons for drop-out. Values for the missing data can be imputed, or it may be possible to incorporate the time spent as a drop-out into the model with an appropriate weighting to reflect quality of life. Alternatively, methods that explicitly model the drop-out process, such as multi-state survival analysis or simultaneous modelling should be considered (see next sections).

Multi-state Survival Analysis

Multi-state models in survival analysis have been applied in a variety of clinical settings,[36–40] but have not been widely used for quality of life data. They provide a means for analysing quality of life and survival data simultaneously and allow for the dynamic nature of quality of life data.

The multi-state model is defined by a finite number of health states, including death, together with the possible transitions between them. The health states are described in terms of the nature and levels of quality of life experienced by patients during the study, and should be defined such that the number of patients passing from one state to another is sufficient for adequate modelling of the data.

The simplest multi-state model is the 'three-state illness–death model' which consists of two transient alive states, *alive and well* and *alive and ill*, and one absorbing death state. This type

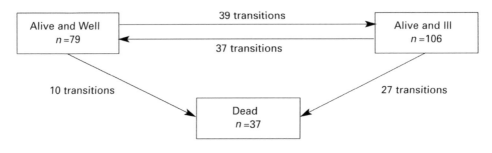

n = number of occasions when patients are in a health state and at risk of transition to another
(this may consist on no occasions for some patients and multiple occasions for others).

Figure 7   *Multi-state model for the MIC study.*

of model was used for the MIC study (see Figure 7) with patients categorised as being in an *alive and well* state if they had no malaise and in an *alive and ill* state if they had malaise at any level. Patients can move between the alive states any number of times during their follow-up until they finally move to the absorbing state of death. As one would expect, the 37 deaths that occurred within the 18-week analysis period came mostly from the *alive and ill* state.

The movement between health states is described by transition rates. A transition rate is the instantaneous potential of transition at any point in time, and is equivalent to the standard hazard rate function for a survival time distribution. The transition rates in a multi-state model can be represented by Cox regression models,[41] and are modelled using the transition times for patients. If exact transition times are not available then they need to be estimated for this type of analysis.

The transition rate from state i to state j at time t, $\lambda_{ij}(t)$, can be modelled using a Cox regression model as follows:

$$\lambda_{ij}(t) = \lambda_{0ij}(t) \exp(\underline{\beta}_{ij}^T \underline{x}_{ij}) \qquad (4)$$

where $\lambda_{0ij}(t)$ is a baseline transition rate for the transition from i to j, $\underline{x}_{ij}$ is a vector of covariates specific to that transition and $\underline{\beta}_{ij}$ is a vector of unknown regression coefficients.

In modelling the transition rate from state i to state j, simplifying assumptions that may be made include: (i) a Markov process; or (ii) a semi-Markov process. In a Markov process the transition rate from state i to state j is dependent only upon the present state occupied; in a semi-Markov process the transition rate is also dependent upon the *duration* of time in the present state.

The transition rates can either be modelled semi-parametrically using a Cox regression model, where the underlying baseline transition rate is left unspecified, or parametrically by

assuming the transition times follow a specific distribution with a parametric form for the baseline transition rate. The most commonly used distributions are the exponential and the Weibull distributions, the exponential simply being a special form of Weibull distribution. If an exponential is assumed, then the underlying baseline transition rate is taken as constant; otherwise for a Weibull distribution the underlying baseline transition rate is allowed to change over time.

Modelling transition rates in the MIC study

To model the transition rates in the three-state illness–death model for the MIC study (see Figure 7), exact times of transition from one state to another within the 18-week analysis period were needed for each patient. The exact dates of transition to death were known, but dates of transition between alive states had to be estimated. Estimation was based on the same assumptions that were used in the quality-adjusted survival analysis, in particular that health state changes occur midway between assessments (see previous section on Assumptions required for analysis of the MIC data).

The illustrative results presented here (see Figure 8) relate to a semi-parametric model with an underlying semi-Markov process. Other models are presented in the full project report.[7] The PHREG procedure in SAS[42] was used to analyse the data. Figure 8 shows, for each transition, the ratio of the transition rate for CT compared to the transition rate for PAL. Transition ratios greater than 1 indicate that the transition rate on CT is greater than that on PAL. The point estimates suggest that the hazard of moving between the 'alive' states is greater on CT compared to PAL, whilst the hazard of death from either of the 'alive' states is reduced with CT compared to PAL. This suggests that chemotherapy leads to greater

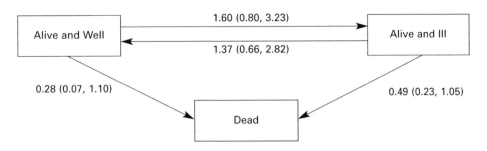

Figure 8 *Transition ratios (and 95% confidence intervals) for the MIC study assuming semi-Markov, semi-parametric models for each transition rate.*

fluctuations in quality of life whilst alive, but reduces the hazard of death. However, the 95% confidence intervals for the transition ratios (shown in brackets) are wide.

Multi-state survival analysis allows the effect of treatments on different health state transitions to be explored. If a single overall statement of the superior treatment is required explicitly then some sort of trade-off between these results would be needed.

Critical appraisal of multi-state survival analysis

Multi-state survival analysis provides a flexible approach for the simultaneous assessment of quality of life and survival data, and a greater biological insight may be gained, though the method can be problematic.

As with quality-adjusted survival analysis, the method – in theory – can be used with any quality of life instrument, providing they can be used to define meaningful health states. For multi-dimensional instruments, separate analyses may be desirable. Defining health states using quality of life data is subjective, and the effects of using different definitions should be considered as part of a sensitivity analysis. Definitions will differ depending on the quality of life variable to be used, the number of health states to be included, and the cut-off values used to discriminate between health states.

Another difficulty with the method is the need for exact dates of transition between health states. These can be estimated and the accuracy is determined by the frequency of the quality of life assessments. Alternative methods that do not require exact transition dates are available,[43] but these methods require specialised software that is not readily accessible to researchers.

One of the main advantages of the method is that provides a means of dealing with the problem of informative drop-out. The inclusion of death as a health state in the model deals with drop-out due to death and it may be possible to

deal with drop-out for other reasons by including a 'drop-out' health state. This approach allows the drop-out process to be explored.

Simultaneous Modelling

Simultaneous modelling is a developing area of methodology that currently has not been applied in a quality of life context, but potentially could provide a powerful approach to analysing quality of life and survival data. The change in quality of life over time and the time to death can be considered as two simultaneous processes occurring in patients, and can be modelled as such. Models are set up for each process, and Gibbs sampling may be used to fit the models simultaneously in a single analysis.[44,45]

Simultaneous modelling allows survival data to be incorporated into the model for quality of life data, thus adjusting for informative missing data caused by drop-out due to death. At the same time, the modelling of survival data with quality of life as a time-dependent co-variate is enhanced since co-variate values are estimated from the model for quality of life data over time fitted to all subjects. The approach can be generalised to model the drop-out process rather than the survival process and in this way overcome the problem of informative drop-out for reasons other than death.[46] It may be possible to extend the method to include models of a hierarchical nature that would account for the multi-dimensionality of quality of life data.

Study Design

The method of analysis needs to be decided upon at the design stage of a study so that appropriate quality of life data can be collected. The following issues should be considered.

1   Most methods of analysis are based on a single measure of quality of life. Using a multi-dimensional instrument will result in multiple measures of quality of life each potentially requiring a separate analysis. Selecting instruments that produce a global quality of life score or identifying specific dimensions at the design stage for hypothesis testing from a multi-dimensional instrument will reduce problems of multiple testing.
2   Quality of life assessments should be frequent enough to ensure accurate estimation of dates of health state transitions.
3   Assessments of quality of life should be planned such as to minimise non-compliance and thus reduce the problem of missing data.
4   Recording the reason for drop-out during data collection will maximise insight into the drop-out process and enable modelling of separate drop-out processes where necessary.
5   The number of subjects required for a study will depend on the method of analysis. Multi-state survival analysis, for example, needs a relatively large overall sample size, so that there are sufficient subjects in each transition for adequate modelling of the data.

Choosing the Appropriate Method

The choice of method should be based on the research question that the study aims to answer. The advantages and disadvantages of each method[7] should be considered carefully together with the relevance and interpretability of the results to clinicians and patients.

Methods used to analyse longitudinal quality of life data must consider the problem of informative drop-out.

Reporting the Analysis

Methods used should be reported clearly, with details of definitions and assumptions used in the analysis.

Sensitivity analysis should be carried out to assess the robustness of conclusions to any critical assumptions made in the analysis.

SUGGESTIONS FOR FUTURE RESEARCH

Further experience in the application of quality-adjusted survival analysis techniques specifically to quality of life data, rather than clinical data, is needed to enable a proper evaluation of such methods in this field.

Further research is needed to develop multi-state models, simultaneous modelling methods and hierarchical models in their practical application to quality of life and survival data, using both classical and Bayesian approaches. Consideration should be given to how methods could deal with the multivariate nature of the quality of life end-point.

A full review of available software for methods that simultaneously assess quality of life and survival data is needed to highlight areas requiring further development.

ACKNOWLEDGEMENTS

This research was funded under a National Health Service Health Technology Assessment Methodology Programme grant. We thank the Cancer Research Campaign Trials Unit at Birmingham University for supporting the secondment of Lucinda Billingham to Leicester University for the duration of the project. We are grateful to Dr Michael Cullen, Consultant and Honorary Reader in Medical Oncology at the Queen Elizabeth Hospital in Birmingham, for allowing us to use the MIC data as the illustrative example in this chapter. Finally, we would like to thank the editors for their useful comments.

REFERENCES

1. Bowling A. *Measuring health: a review of quality of life measurement scales.* Open University Press, 1991.
2. Cox DR, Fitzpatrick R, Fletcher AE, Gore SM, Spiegelhalter DJ, Jones DR. Quality-of-life assessment: can we keep it simple? *J. Roy. Statist. Soc. A* 1992; **155**: 353–93.
3. Hopwood P, Stephens RJ, Machin D. Approaches to the analysis of quality of life data: experiences gained from a Medical Research Council Lung Cancer Working Party palliative chemotherapy trial. *Quality of Life Research* 1994; **3**: 339–52.
4. Fletcher A, Gore SM, Jones DR, Fitzpatrick R, Spiegelhalter DJ, Cox DR. Quality of life measures in health care. II: Design, analysis and interpretation. *Br. Med. J.* 1992; **305**: 1145–8.
5. Schumacher M, Olschewski M, Schulgen G. Assessment of quality-of-life in clinical trials. *Stat. Med.* 1991; **10**: 1915–30.
6. Olschewski M, Schumacher M. Statistical analysis of quality of life data in cancer clinical trials. *Stat. Med.* 1990; **9**: 749–63.

7. Billingham LJ, Abrams KR, Jones DR. Methods for the analysis of quality of life and survival data in health technology assessment. *Health Technology Assessment* 1999; **3**(10).

8. Cullen MH, Billingham LJ, Woodroffe CM, et al. Mitomycin, ifosfamide and cisplatin in unresectable non-small cell lung cancer: effects on survival and quality of life. *J. Clin. Oncol.* 1999; **17**: 3188–94.

9. Matthews JNS, Altman DG, Campbell MJ, Royston P. Analysis of serial measurements in medical research. *Br. Med. J.* 1990; **300**: 230–5.

10. Diggle PJ, Liang K, Zeger SL. *Analysis of longitudinal data.* Oxford: Clarendon Press, 1994.

11. Goldstein H. *Multilevel statistical models.* 2nd edn. London: Edward Arnold, 1995.

12. Korn EL. On estimating the distribution function for quality of life in cancer clinical trials. *Biometrika* 1993; **80**: 535–42.

13. Hollen PJ, Gralla RJ, Cox C, Eberly SW, Kris MG. A dilemma in analysis: issues in the serial measurement of quality of life in patients with advanced lung cancer. *Lung Cancer* 1997; **18**: 119–36.

14. Zwinderman AH. Statistical analysis of longitudinal quality of life data with missing measurements. *Quality of Life Research* 1992; **1**: 219–24.

15. Beacon HJ, Thompson S. Multi-level models for repeated measurement data: application to quality of life data in clinical trials. *Stat. Med.* 1996; **15**: 2717–32.

16. Beacon HJ. *The statistical analysis of self assessed quality of life data in cancer clinical trials.* PhD Thesis. London: London School of Hygiene and Tropical Medicine, University of London, 1996.

17. Zwinderman AH. The measurement of change of quality of life in clinical trials. *Stat. Med.* 1990; **9**: 931–42.

18. Little RJA, Rubin DB. *Statistical analysis with missing data.* John Wiley & Sons, 1987.

19. Little RJA. Modelling the drop-out mechanism in repeated measures studies. *J. Am. Statist. Assoc.* 1995; **90**: 1112–21.

20. De Stavola BL, Christensen E. Multilevel models for longitudinal variables prognostic for survival. *Lifetime Data Analysis* 1996; **2**: 329–47.

21. Cox DR. Regression models and life tables. *J. Roy. Statist. Soc. B* 1972; **34**: 187–220.

22. Collett D. *Modelling survival data in medical research.* London: Chapman & Hall, 1994.

23. Glasziou PP, Simes RJ, Gelber RD. Quality adjusted survival analysis. *Stat. Med.* 1990; **9**: 1259–76.

24. Torrance GW. Utility approach to measuring health-related quality of life. *J. Chron. Dis.* 1987; **40**: 593–600.

25. Gelber RD, Gelman RS, Goldhirsch A. A quality-of-life-oriented endpoint for comparing therapies. *Biometrics* 1989; **45**: 781–95.

26. Gelber RD, Goldhirsch A. A new endpoint for the assessment of adjuvant therapy in postmenopausal women with operable breast cancer. *J. Clin. Oncol.* 1986; **4**: 1772–9.

27. Goldhirsch A, Gelber RD, Simes RJ, Glasziou P, Coates AS. Costs and benefits of adjuvant therapy in breast cancer: a quality-adjusted survival analysis. *J. Clin. Oncol.* 1989; **7**: 36–44.

28. Gelber RD, Cole BF, Gelber S, Goldhirsch A. Comparing treatments using quality-adjusted survival: the Q-TWiST method. *Am. Statistician* 1995; **49**: 161–9.

29. Gelber RD, Goldhirsch A, Cole BF, Weiand HS, Schroeder G, Krook JE. A quality-adjusted time without symptoms or toxicity (Q-TWiST) analysis of adjuvant radiation therapy and chemotherapy for resectable rectal cancer. *J. Natl Cancer Inst.* 1996; **88**: 1039–45.

30. Gelber RD, Lenderking WR, Cotton DJ, Cole BF, Fischl MA, Goldhirsch A, Testa MA. Quality-of-life evaluation in a clinical trial of zidovudine therapy in patients with mildly symptomatic HIV infection. *Ann. Intern. Med.* 1992; **116**: 961–6.

31. Hwang JS, Tsauo JY, Wang JD. Estimation of expected quality adjusted survival by cross-sectional survey. *Stat. Med.* 1996; **15**: 93–102.

32. Gelber RD, Goldhirsch A, Cole BF. Parametric extrapolation of survival estimates with applications to quality of life evaluation of treatments. *Controlled Clinical Trials* 1993; **14**: 485–99.

33. Hinkley DV. Bootstrap methods. *J. Roy. Statist. Soc. B* 1988; **50**: 321–37.

34. Cole BF, Gelber RD, Goldhirsch A. Cox regression models for quality adjusted survival analysis. *Stat. Med.* 1993; **12**: 975–87.

35. Cole BF, Gelber RD, Anderson KM. Parametric approaches to quality-adjusted survival analysis. *Biometrics* 1994; **50**: 621–31.

36. Kay R. Multistate survival analysis: an application in breast cancer. *Methods Inf. Med.* 1984; **23**: 157–62.

37. Hansen BE, Thorogood J, Hermans J, Ploeg RJ, van Bockel JH, van Houwelingen JC. Multistate modeling of liver transplantation data. *Stat. Med.* 1994; **13**: 2517–29.

38. Andersen PK. Multistate models in survival analysis: a study of nephropathy and mortality in diabetes. *Stat. Med.* 1988; **7**: 661–70.

39. Marshall G, Jones RH. Multistate models and diabetic retinopathy. *Stat. Med.* 1995; **14**: 1975–83.

40. Gentleman RC, Lawless JF, Lindsey JC, Yan P. Multistate Markov models for analyzing incomplete disease history data with illustrations for HIV disease. *Stat. Med.* 1994; **13**: 805–21.

41. Kay R. The analysis of transition times in multistate stochastic processes using proportional

hazard regression models. *Communications in Statistics – Theory and Methodology* 1982; **11**: 1743–56.

42. SAS Institute Inc. SAS technical report P–229, SAS/STAT software: changes and enhancements; Release 6.07. Cary, NC: SAS Institute Inc., 1992.

43. Kay R. A Markov model for analysing cancer markers and disease states in survival studies. *Biometrics* 1986; **42**: 855–65.

44. Faucett CL, Thomas DC. Simultaneously modelling censored survival data and repeatedly measured covariates: a Gibbs sampling approach. *Stat. Med.* 1996; **15**: 1663–85.

45. Berzuini C. Medical monitoring. In: Gilks WR, Richardson S, Spiegelhalter DJ (eds). *Markov Chain Monte Carlo in practice*. London: Chapman & Hall, 1995; Chapter 18.

46. Lindsey JK. Modelling longitudinal measurement dropouts as a survival process with time-varying covariates. Technical Report, Limburgs Universitair Centrum, Belgium, 1997.

Part V
CONSENSUS, REVIEWS AND META-ANALYSIS

INTRODUCTION by ANDREW STEVENS and KEITH R. ABRAMS

The research evidence both informing health technology assessment (HTA), and consequent on it, can be seen as being at three distances from the end user. Distance 1, primary research (well-designed randomised trials and observational studies) form a core means of providing data for HTA. Primary data collection has been dealt with extensively elsewhere in this book. However, at the heart of HTA is the logic of the need for systematic reviews, i.e. distance 2. The case for systematic reviews has been established beyond all reasonable doubt over the past decade.[1,2] Indeed, Chapters 21–23 in this section all amply illustrate that we have moved well past exhortations for systematicity in reviewing, to the scientific requirements of ensuring that systematicity is guaranteed. All three of these chapters explore methodological frontiers in systematic reviews. Distance 3 (closest to the end user) includes guidelines, syntheses of the evidence on multiple interventions and structured reviews aimed at end users. This group of 'products' has partly been necessitated by the increasing rigour used to synthesise evidence within systematic reviews. The scientific synthesis of evidence has the tendency both to narrow the topics and to increase the 'weight' of reviews, making them difficult to access in day-to-day planning, either at the clinical or at the health authority/insurance planning level. It is, however, also recognised that the primary

data needed for synthesised evidence will not always be present. Chapter 24, on consensus as a basis for guidelines, reflects both of these points.

It is worth rehearsing some of the key features of the systematic review revolution that have generated their wide usage and continuing methodological interest. First, systematic reviewing means *systematicity* of search. Precise rules for how far to search to produce a systematic review have not been universally agreed. The elements of searching can include not just the use of the many electronic databases (e.g. the Cochrane Library, Medline, CINAHL, Psychlit, Science Citation Index), but also hand-searching the relevant journals and identifying unpublished literature and conference proceedings.[3] The principle underlying the systematicity of searching is the avoidance of bias. The absence of a systematic search can be a sign of a review setting out to prove a point, rather than to appraise the evidence – a common feature of traditional reviews and editorials. Even when reviews have an unbiased intent, a systematic and comprehensive search is necessary because of the bias that can arise when studies with positive or dramatic findings are more likely to be published than those with negative or unexciting results. This 'publication bias' may be more of a problem with smaller studies. In Chapter 21, Song and colleagues analyse these issues and review a variety of methods for detecting and adjusting for publication bias in systematic reviews, which they suggest should be used critically in *any* systematic review or meta-analysis. They also stress that sensitivity analyses should cover both the effect of including or excluding unpublished studies and the choice of methods for assessing or adjusting for publication bias. They further conclude that the prospective registration of all research studies is probably the only way in which the effect of publication bias may be eliminated. In the meantime, further empirical research is required in order to assess the extent to which such bias affects current healthcare decision making.

A second feature of systematic reviewing is the *grading of the evidence*. The evidence for effectiveness or otherwise of healthcare has traditionally come from a variety of levels of evidence. Systematic reviews explicitly judge the quality of the evidence, and draw on the highest quality of evidence wherever practicable. A number of hierarchies of evidence are in common use for this purpose. All are very similar, rating randomised controlled trials (RCTs) highest, and evidence based on un-researched consensus lowest. A typical scale would run, therefore, from: (i) multiple RCTs, preferably large ones, suitably meta-analysed; (ii) at least one properly designed RCT of appropriate size; (iii) well controlled trials without randomisation; (iv) well-designed cohort or case control studies; (v) multiple time series or dramatic results from uncontrolled experiments; (vi) opinions of respected authorities based on clinical evidence, descriptive studies or expert committee; to (vii) small uncontrolled case series and samples. Notwithstanding this well accepted hierarchy,[4] it does not necessarily follow that moderate studies at one level are better than good studies at another level.

Therefore a third element of systematic reviews is the *critical appraisal* of the evidence – both of the studies collecting the primary data, and of the reviews. Critical appraisal is not new: it has long been of concern to journal editors (who receive, appraise and publish or reject) and to researchers (who find, appraise and synthesise). But it has now become a core skill for those planning to use evidence to support healthcare decisions – that is all those concerned with HTA. The underlying principles of critical appraisal concern the validity and applicability of the research discernible in published papers. Numerous check-lists have been developed to inform critical appraisal for primary research and review articles.[5] Typically, in the case of a review, the questions concern whether the review addresses a clearly focused issue, whether the search was appropriate,

whether the search was sensitive and specific, whether there was a quality assessment of the included studies, and whether the combination of the studies was undertaken reasonably. In Chapter 23, Moher and colleagues take such considerations further, questioning the quality assessments of RCTs included in meta-analyses. In other words, they probe at the sharp end of reviews, and demonstrate that in any meta-analysis, exploration of the sensitivity of the overall results to the quality of included studies is of paramount importance. However, they conclude that in the assessment of study quality, and its integration within a meta-analysis, both further empirical and methodological research is required.

A fourth component of systematic reviewing is that of *integrating the evidence*. Integrating evidence from different sources is essential, in reviews not just of trials and observational studies but also of cost–effectiveness analyses and qualitative research. The combining of evidence from multiple different studies is arguably at its most straightforward when the studies are all high-quality RCTs. Here, the synthesis can use meta-analysis in which the results of trials are quantitatively re-analysed collectively, ideally using original patient data. In Chapter 22, Sutton and colleagues demonstrate that this is far from straightforward in their exploration of the different statistical techniques which can be brought to bear on meta-analytic modelling. They use a running theme of the integration of studies on cholesterol reduction comparing a range of interventions, including drug, diet and surgery, to improve outcomes in terms of all-cause mortality. Whilst they review many of the fundamental meta-analytic methods, they also consider the use of more recently developed techniques such as meta-regression, Bayesian methods and methods for the synthesis of evidence when it arises from a variety of sources. They conclude that although the use of methods such as meta-regression may be useful in examining potential sources of between-study heterogeneity, the sensitivity of the overall results and conclusions to the choice of the specific meta-analytic methods used should also be *routinely* investigated.

Finally, the key feature of the systematic review revolution, if not of systematic reviews themselves, is the *interpretation and delivery* of the evidence. The scale and complexity of the evidence base of healthcare is at the same time vast and occasionally sparse. It needs to be interpreted and delivered to the user in a meaningful and valued form – irrespective of the fullness of the evidence for a particular element of healthcare. A number of initiatives has evolved to meet the need for interpretation and delivery, including tertiary reviews of disease-wide topics, guidelines, new information facilities, and dissemination initiatives. Guidelines are often at the heart of such initiatives. The construction and implementation of guidelines is a wide topic, beyond the scope of this book (but see Nuffield Institute of Health, 1994).[6] But as the need for clear guidance will often run ahead of systematic review evidence, a particularly important frontier, greatly at risk of abuse, is the construction of guidelines from consensus. In Chapter 24, Black and colleagues discuss consensus development methods and their use in creating clinical guidelines. What they have to say has a bearing on consensus methods for any purpose. In theory, consensus could be one of the means of synthesis and systematic reviews. As the authors note, consensus development is intended to make the best use of available information, although unlike synthesis of primary data, that can sometimes just be the collective wisdom of the participants. For that reason consensus development methods involve planning, individual judgement and group interaction. Not only do Black and colleagues analyse the literature on consensus, but they also perform the useful service of imposing scientific methods and rigorous thinking, even where data paucity can turn observers towards nihilism. Given the importance of sound judgement and precision in healthcare, and given the breadth of the technology frontier with which evidence based healthcare has to cope, it is important that they not do

so. Indeed the over-arching conclusion of the chapters in this section is that researchers must be aware that not only should the robustness of results and conclusions they draw to the empirical evidence used be assessed, but so too must their choice of methods.

REFERENCES

1. Mulrow CD. The medical review article: state of the science. *Ann. Int. Med.* 1987; **104**: 485–8.
2. Chalmers I, Altman D. *Systematic Reviews.* London: BMJ Publishing, 1995.
3. NHS Centre for Reviews and Dissemination. *Undertaking Systematic Reviews of Research On Effectiveness.* York: University of York, 1996.
4. Woolf SH, Battista RN, Anderson GM, Logan AG, Wang E and the Canadian Task Force on the Periodic Health Examination. Assessing the clinical effectiveness of preventive manoeuvres: analytic principles and systematic methods in reviewing evidence and developing clinical practice recommendations. *J. Clin. Epidemiol.* 1990; **43**: 891–905.
5. Critical Appraisal Study Programme. *Orientation Guide.* Oxford: Institute of Health Sciences, 1996.
6. NHS Centre for Reviews and Dissemination. Implementing Clinical Practice Guidelines: can guidelines be used to improve clinical practice? *Effective Health Care* 1992; **1**: 1–12.

21

Publication and Related Biases

FUJIAN SONG, ALISON EASTWOOD,
SIMON GILBODY, LELIA DULEY and ALEX SUTTON

SUMMARY

The available evidence demonstrates that research with significant results or favourable results is more likely to be published than that with non-significant or unfavourable results, although the extent and direction of such selective publication is uncertain, and may vary greatly depending on the circumstances. Investigators, journal editors, peer-reviewers and research sponsors may all be responsible for the existence of publication bias. Methods available to detect or adjust for publication bias in systematic reviews are by nature indirect and exploratory. Results from a sample of systematic reviews revealed that potential publication bias has been ignored in many published systematic reviews. It is concluded that all funded or approved studies should be prospectively registered. Further research about publication bias should be an integral part of research that explores alternatives to the conventional methods for generating, disseminating, preserving and utilising scientific research findings.

INTRODUCTION

In the face of a rapidly expanding volume of medical research, literature review is becoming increasingly important to summarise research evidence for clinical and health policy decision-making.[1] In contrast to traditional narrative review that has been criticised for being subjective, scientifically unsound, and inefficient,[2] systematic review could produce more reliable results by systematically locating, appraising and synthesising research evidence.[3]

However, if the published studies comprise a biased sample of all studies that have been conducted, the results of a literature review will be misleading.[4] For example, the efficacy of a treatment will be over-estimated if studies with positive results are more likely to be published than those with negative results. Although bias in published literature may imperil the validity of both traditional narrative review and systematic review, the problem of selective publication of studies has been highlighted only recently in medical research, coincided with an increasing use of meta-analysis and systematic review.[5]

Publication bias can be narrowly defined as 'the tendency on the parts of investigators, reviewers, and editors to submit or accept manuscripts for publication based on the direction or strength of the study findings'.[6] Chalmers and colleagues[7] considered publication bias more broadly to have three stages: (i) pre-publication bias in the performance of research; (ii) publication bias; and (iii) post-publication bias in interpretations and reviews of published studies. In this chapter, publication and related biases include bias due to selective publication and other biases due to the time, type, and language of publication, selective reporting of outcomes measured, duplicate publications, and selective citation of references.

This chapter presents the major results of a systematic review of studies that have examined methodological issues or provided empirical evidence concerning publication and related biases.[8] After a brief description of the methods used in this review, empirical evidence of publication and related biases are summarised and the potential sources of publication bias are discussed. Then, the methods for dealing with publication and related biases, classified according to the stage of a literature review, are described and their usefulness and weakness are discussed. The results of a survey of published systematic reviews are also presented to provide further evidence of publication bias, and to illustrate the methods used for dealing with publication bias. Finally, we summarise and discuss the major findings of this review and make recommendations for future research.

METHODS

The following databases were searched to identify relevant literature concerning empirical evidence and methodological issues pertaining to publication and related biases: the Cochrane Review Methodology Database, Medline, EMBASE, BIDS, Library and Information Science Abstracts, Psyclit, Sociofile, Eric, Dissertation Abstracts, MathSci, British Education Index, SIGLE, and ASSIA. The reference lists in identified articles were checked, and authors of some articles contacted to identify further studies.

It is difficult to define a clear and narrow criterion for including studies in this review because of the broad nature of related issues and the great diversity of relevant studies. Therefore, all studies relevant to publication-related biases were included, although studies may be excluded if the issue of publication bias is only mentioned but is not a major topic. The search results from the electronic databases were independently checked by two reviewers to identify all relevant studies and any difference was solved by discussion.

A survey of published systematic reviews was also undertaken, to identify further evidence of publication bias, and to illustrate what methods are currently used for detecting and reducing publication bias. A sample of systematic reviews was selected from the Database of Abstracts of Reviews of Effectiveness (DARE) produced by the NHS Centre for Reviews and Dissemination at the University of York. These published reviews were independently assessed by two reviewers using a data-extraction sheet to collect the following information: type of review (narrative or meta-analysis); whether the issue of publication bias was considered; whether unpublished studies or those published in non-English languages were searched for and included; any evidence on the existence, extent and consequence of publication bias; and the methods used for dealing with publication bias.

EVIDENCE OF PUBLICATION AND RELATED BIASES

The existence of publication bias was first suspected from the observation that a large proportion of published studies had rejected the 'null hypothesis'. In 1959, Sterling found that the results of 97% of studies published in four major psychology journals were statistically significant, concluding that studies with non-significant results might be under-represented.[9] In 1995, the same author concluded that practices leading to publication bias had not changed over a period of 30 years.[10]

An early example of the identification of publication bias in medical research is that by Chalmers and colleagues[11] who in 1965 attempted to explain the variability in reported rates of deaths due to serum hepatitis. They concluded that there was a tendency for clinicians or editors to publish unusual findings. It was suggested that small studies with unusually high or low fatality rates might have a greater chance to be reported than those with 'more average or mundane fatality rates'.

During the 1980s and 1990s, more evidence about the existence of publication bias has been provided by surveying authors, comparing published with unpublished studies, and following-up cohorts of registered studies.

Survey of Authors

According to a survey of 48 authors of articles submitted to the journal of *Personality and Social Psychology* in 1973, the probability of submitting for publication was 0.59 for studies with significant result and only 0.06 for studies with non-significant result.[12] A survey of 1000 members of the American Psychological Association found that studies with 'neutral or negative' findings were less likely to be submitted or accepted for publication.[13] Dickersin et al.[14] observed that the proportion of trials in which the new treatment was superior to the control therapy was 55% in 767 published studies compared to only 14% in 178 unpublished studies. In another survey, the rate of publication was 73% for 30 studies with significant results and 54% for 26 studies with non-significant findings.[15]

Published versus Registered Trials in a Meta-Analysis

The most direct and convincing evidence of the existence of publication bias comes from the comparison between unpublished and published results. In a meta-analysis that compared combination chemotherapy versus initial alkylating agent in advanced ovarian cancer, Simes found that overall survival was significantly higher in the combination chemotherapy group than in the initial alkylating agent group when the published trials were combined.[16] However, this survival advantage for combination chemotherapy was not found when all registered trials (both published and unpublished) were combined.

Follow-up of Cohorts of Registered Studies

The existence of publication bias has been consistently confirmed by studies which have followed-up cohorts of studies approved by research ethics committee or cohorts of trials registered by the research sponsors (Figure 1).[17–20] By pooling results from these cohort studies, the rate of publication of studies with significant results was significantly higher than those with non-significant results (overall odds ratio 2.54, 95% confidence interval (CI): 1.44 to 4.47).[21] The publication bias in favour of studies with significant results was confirmed in these studies by multivariate analysis adjusting for other factors such as study design, sample size and funding sources.

Studies with significant results were also more likely to generate multiple publications and more likely to be published in journals with a high citation impact factor when compared to studies with non-significant results.[17] It may be interesting to note that studies with a non-significant trend were less likely to be published than studies with no difference.[17,20]

Stern and Simes observed that clinical trials with statistically significant results were published much earlier than those with non-significant results (median 4.7 years versus 8.0 years).[20] This finding was confirmed using a cohort of randomised controlled trials on AIDS, in which it was found that the median time from starting enrollment to publication was 4.3 years for positive trials and 6.5 years for negative trials.[22] In a study of publication bias among studies examining the effects of passive smoking, it was found that the median time to publication was 5 years (95% CI: 4 to 7) for statistically non-significant studies and 3 years (95% CI: 3 to 5) for statistically significant studies ($P = 0.004$).[23]

Other Publication-Related Biases

The accessibility of research results is dependent not only on whether and when a study is published, but also on its format of publication. For example, research results published only in reports, working papers, theses or abstracts, often have limited dissemination, and may be termed as 'grey literature'.[24] Other biases that are publication related include language bias, outcome reporting bias, duplicate bias and citation bias. The available evidence about these biases are discussed below.

Grey literature bias

In 1964, Smart randomly selected 37 Ph.D. theses from *Dissertation Abstracts in Psychology* and found that theses with positive results were more likely to be published than those with negative results.[25] In the fields of psychological and educational research, several authors observed a tendency that the average effects estimated from journal articles were greater than the corresponding effects from theses and dissertations.[26–28]

A large number of study results are initially presented as abstracts at various scientific meeting or journals. Two studies found that submitted abstracts reporting positive results were more likely to be accepted for presentation than those reporting negative results.[29,30] On average, about half of abstracts were published in full after more than 12 months.[31] The association between significant results and full publication of abstracts have been observed in two studies[31,32] but not in others.[33–35]

Language and country bias

The effect of language bias was investigated by including 19 studies that had been originally excluded for linguistic reasons from 13 meta-analyses.[36] By doing this, one statistically non-significant result in a meta-analysis became statistically significant. By comparing 40 pairs of trials conducted by German-speaking investigators, it was found that authors were more likely to publish trials in an English-language journal if the results were statistically significant.[37] When 180 Scandinavian referees were asked to review two fictitious manuscripts in English or in the national language, the English version was on average given a higher quality score than the national-language version of the same manuscript.[38]

Ottenbacher observed that the estimated effect of spinal manipulation therapy was larger in studies reported in English-language journals published outside the United States than similar studies in journals published in the United States.[39] In a survey of Medline abstracts of trials evaluating acupuncture or other interventions, the proportion of studies with a positive

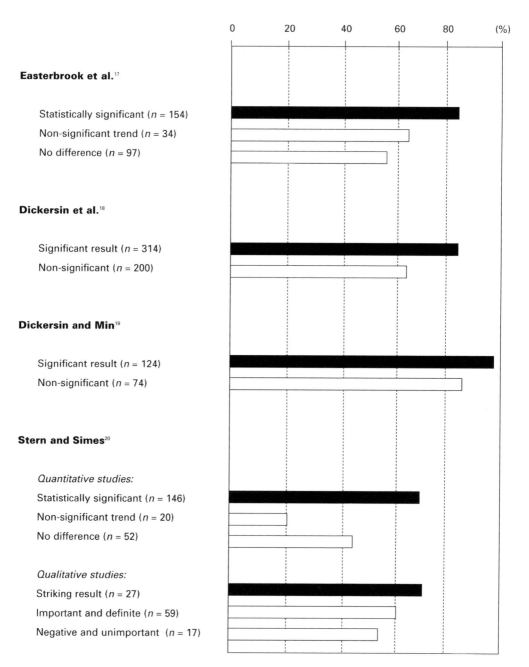

Figure 1   *Publication rate (%) and study results in registered studies.*

result was much higher for trials originating from China, Taiwan, Japan and Hong Kong than trials conducted in western countries such as USA, Sweden, UK, Denmark, Germany and Canada.[40] It was suggested that publication bias is a possible explanation for the unusually high proportions of positive results observed for some countries.

Outcome reporting bias

Outcome reporting bias happens when trials with multiple outcome measures report only those which are significant. In 45 clinical trials published in three general medical journals the median number of end-points was six per trial.[41] Tannock found that more than half of the implied statistical comparisons had not been reported in 32 oncology trials.[42] In addition, the methods of reporting and the completeness of information may influence the interpretation of study findings.[43–45]

Duplicate (multiple) publication

In a meta-analysis of ondansetron on postoperative emesis, Tramer et al.[46] found that efficacy was over-estimated when duplicate publications were included as compared with when they were excluded. This bias is often difficult to detect; for example, in a review of risperidone, it was found that identifying duplicate publications of the multicentre trials was far from obvious, because of the chronology of publications, changing authorship, lack of transparency in reporting, and the frequent citation of abstracts and unpublished reports.[47]

Citation (reference) bias

Citation bias may occur at the post-publication stage.[7] For example, supportive trials were found to be cited almost six times more often than non-supportive trials of cholesterol-lowering interventions.[48] By examining quotations in three influential reviews on diet–heart issues, it was found that only one of six relevant randomised trials with a negative result was cited, and this was only in one of the three reviews.[49] Conversely, the three reviews respectively cited two, four and six non-randomised trials with a positive result. However, in reviews of the clinical effectiveness of pneumococcal vaccine, non-supportive trials were more likely to be cited than supportive trials.[50] This may be because the reviews tended to cite more recently published trials in which outcomes were more frequently found to be non-supportive.

Koren and Klein compared newspaper coverage of one positive study and one negative study on radiation as a risk for cancer which were published in the same issue of *JAMA* in 1991.[51] Nine of the 19 newspaper reports covered only the positive study. In 10 other reports that covered both positive and negative studies, the average number of words was 354 for the positive study, and 192 for the negative study.

CONSEQUENCES OF PUBLICATION BIAS

Although the existence of publication bias is well demonstrated, there is limited empirical evidence about the consequences of publication bias. In the perinatal research, a study observed that routine hospitalisation was associated with more unwanted outcomes in women with un-

complicated twin pregnancies, but the findings remained unpublished for 7 years.[52] Chalmers pointed out that 'at the very least, this delay led to continued inappropriate deployment of limited resources; at worst, it may have resulted in the continued use of a harmful policy'.[52]

In 1980, a trial tested lorcainide in patients with acute and recovery myocardial infarction, and observed more deaths in the treatment group than in the placebo group (9/48 versus 1/47).[53] The trial results were not published because the development of lorcainide was stopped for 'commercial reasons'. About a decade later, an increased mortality was observed amongst patients treated with encainide and flecainide in two trials.[54,55] Encainide, flecainide and lorcainide all belong to a class of 1C anti-arrhythmic agents. If the results of the early trial in 1980 has been published, the mortality of patients included in the later two trials might have been avoided or reduced.

Based on the results of a meta-analysis of several small trials, intravenous magnesium was recommended as a treatment for acute myocardial infarction.[56] However, a subsequent large trial (ISIS-4) showed that the rate of death was higher in patients receiving intravenous magnesium than those receiving standard treatment (7.64% versus 7.24%, $P = 0.07$).[57] Publication bias has been identified as a possible explanation for the discrepant results from the meta-analysis and the following large trial.[58] The number of hospital admissions due to acute myocardial infarction was 116 635 in 1993–94 in England.[59] If all these patients had received intravenous magnesium, there would have been 466 more deaths than without using such therapy.

WHO IS RESPONSIBLE FOR PUBLICATION BIAS?

Publication bias may be introduced intentionally or unintentionally, consciously or unconsciously because of varying motivations or biased standards used to judge research evidence.[60] Investigators, journal editors, journal peer reviewers and research sponsors may all be responsible for the existence of publication bias, though the extent of such responsibility may be different in different circumstances.

Investigators and Authors Investigators may get inappropriate recommendations not to publish studies with non-significant results. For example, it has been suggested that non-significant research 'clutters up the journals and does more harm than good to the author's reputation in the minds of the discerning'.[61] Available evidence indicates that investigators are the main source of publication bias, for not writing up or submitting studies.[18,19] The most frequent reason given for failing to write up the study was the presence of a null result.[17,20] Studies with positive results were often submitted for publication more rapidly after completion than were negative studies.[22]

Chalmers and colleagues[7] observed that author's speciality was significantly associated with the enthusiasm for the procedure reviewed in an article. For example, 21 of the 29 radiotherapists were enthusiastic for radiotherapy after radical mastectomy when stage is not distinguished, compared with only five of 34 authors with other specialities. In a systematic review of the risks of stroke and death due to endarterectomy for symptomatic carotid stenosis, it was observed that the risk of stroke or death was highest in studies in which patients were assessed by a neurologist after surgery (7.7%) and lowest in studies with a single author affiliated with a department of surgery (2.3%).[62] It is possible that surgeons were less likely to report the results if the operative risk of stroke and death was high.

Editorial Policy of Journals

Although editorial rejection was not a frequent reason given by investigators for studies remaining unpublished,[17,18] it cannot be ruled out that authors do not submit studies with negative results because of anticipated rejection according to journals' instructions to authors and their own experience. In a survey of 80 authors of articles published in psychology or education journals in 1988, 61% of the 68 respondents agreed that if the research result is not statistically significant, there is little chance of the manuscript being published.[63] Weber et al.[34] found that anticipated rejection was given as a reason for failure to submit a manuscript by 20% of 179 authors. In another study, 17 of 45 submitted trials were rejected by at least one journal, and at least four negative trials with over 300 patients each were rejected two or three times, while no positive trial was multiply rejected.[22]

'Originality' is one of the most important criteria upon which journals decide whether a submitted paper will be accepted.[64] For example, according to the *Lancet*'s instruction to authors, articles published 'are selected, from among a huge number of submissions, if they are likely to contribute to a change in clinical practice or in thinking about a disease'.[65] Lack

of originality accounted for 14% of all reasons given for rejection of manuscripts in 1989 by the *American Journal of Surgery*.[66] Confirmatory trials, either positive or negative, have a low chance of being accepted.[67] A journal on diabetes clearly stated that 'mere confirmation of known facts will be accepted only in exceptional cases; the same applies to reports of experiments and observations having no positive outcome'.[68] *The New England Journal of Medicine* would normally reject epidemiological studies with a relative risk smaller than three.[69] Not surprisingly, editors will publish negative studies that may have a potential to change current practice by showing that a widely used intervention is ineffective.[70]

Peer Reviewing

Journal peer review has been defined as 'the assessment by experts (peers) of material submitted for publication in scientific and technical periodicals'.[71] The degree to which peer review contributes to publication bias was investigated by Mahoney, who examined the recommendations of 75 journal referees about a fictitious manuscript with identical experimental procedures but different results.[72] It was found that referees were biased against the manuscript which reported results contrary to their own perspectives. In another study, it was also found that referees' judgements on a fictitious research report was associated with their own preconceptions and experience.[73] However, Abbot and Ernst[74] did not find peer reviewing bias against positive or negative outcome in complementary medicine.

Research Funding Bodies and Commercial Interests

According to a telephone survey of 306 companies in the United States in 1994, 82% of companies interviewed asked investigators at universities 'to keep the results of research secret beyond the time needed to file a patent'.[75] Many clinical trials submitted by drug companies to licensing authorities have never been published.[76–78] Commercial interests and intellectual property are often the main reasons for the non-publication of clinical studies funded by drug companies.[79–81] Abraham and Lewis[80] argued that 'the present European medicines licensing system is biased in favour of commercial interests at the expense of medical science, public health, and the adequate provision of information for doctors and patients'.

Drug companies may be particularly unwilling to publish sponsored trials with unfavourable results.[82] Rennie describes two cases in which pharmaceutical companies attempted to suppress the publication of the negative results of research which they sponsored.[83] Other available evidence also indicates the selective publication of research results in favour of the interests of research sponsors.[84–90]

Companies may also try to prevent the publication of studies conducted by others when the findings of the studies will undermine their commercial interests. For example, a pharmaceutical company attempted to prevent the publication of a systematic review that would have negative economic impact on statins (cholesterol-lowering drugs).[91] In another case, a company that produces hormone bovine somatotropin blocked the publication of a meta-analysis with unsupportive results by using its legal rights over the raw data.[92]

METHODS FOR DEALING WITH PUBLICATION BIAS

Many methods have been suggested for preventing or testing publication bias. In this review the available methods are discussed according to the stage of a literature review: to prevent publication bias before a literature review (for example, prospective registration of trials); to detect publication bias during a literature review (for example, locating unpublished studies, fail-safe N or the file drawer method, funnel plot, modelling); or to minimise the impact of publication bias after a literature review (for example, confirmatory large-scale trials, up-dating the systematic review).

Prospective Registration of Trials and Freedom of Information

There is little disagreement that prospective registration of all trials at their inception is the best solution to eliminating publication bias.[93] If not all trials can be registered, a prospective registration of some trials may provide an unbiased sample of all studies that have been conducted.[4] There will be no publication bias in systematic reviews that are based only on prospectively registered trials; however, it has been argued that the assessment even in this case may be biased in favour of the priors in a Bayesian analysis, as the incomplete use of empirical evidence may add illegitimate weight to the priors based on subjective judgement.[94]

Easterbrook identified 24 registries of clinical trials after a survey of 62 organisations and 51

investigators in 13 countries in 1989.[95] Since then, more registries of clinical trials have been established.[96–100] Recently, prospective meta-analyses have been planned or conducted.[101,102] It should be stressed that trial registries often include published, unpublished or on-going trials and published trials may be retrospectively included in many trial registries.

It has been suggested that research ethics committees (or the Institutional Review Board in the United States) may play an important role in eliminating publication bias by requiring registration of trials at inception and requiring a commitment to disseminate research results as a condition of approval.[103,104] In Spain, a register of clinical trials has been established as a consequence of the law – a Royal Decree of 1978 and a Ministerial Order of 1982.[105] In the United States, the Food and Drug Administration (FDA) Modernization Act of 1997 includes a section which calls for the establishment of a federally funded database containing information on both government-funded and privately funded clinical trials of drugs designed to treat serious or life-threatening conditions.[106]

Recently the practice of incomplete release of information about licensed drugs in Europe for reasons of commercial interests and intellectual property has been challenged.[79–81,107,108] Abraham and Lewis[80] suggested that 'the secrecy and confidentiality of EU medicines regulation is not essential for a viable pharmaceutical industry', considering that European pharmaceutical companies often obtain data on competitors' products by using the US Freedom of Information Act. They also reported that the majority of industrialists and regulators interviewed (74%) in principle did not oppose greater public access to information.[80] There are some 'encouraging signs' within the pharmaceutical industry to improve public access to the findings of clinical studies that the industry sponsored.[81]

Changes in publication process and journals

It has been suggested that journals could reduce publication bias by accepting manuscripts for publication based mainly on the research protocol.[109] To motivate investigators to register their trials, it was also suggests that prospective registration should be a requirement laid down by journal editors and registering agencies.[110] By disclosing 'conflict of interest' or 'competing interests', potential bias due to sources of research funding may be revealed.[111]

Recently, over 100 medical journals around the world have invited readers to send in information on unpublished trials in a so-called 'trial amnesty',[112,113] and by the end of 1998, this trial amnesty has registered 150 trials.[98] Since the beginning of 1997, a general medical journal, *The Lancet*, has been assessing and registering selected protocols of randomised trials, and providing a commitment to publish the main clinical findings of the study.[65] However, there is little hope that conventional paper journals can solve the problem of publication bias because of space limitation and the requirement of newsworthy articles for maintaining or increasing the journals' circulation level.

Fox considered that medical journals have two basic functions: as a medical recorder, and as a medical newspaper.[114] The function of medical recorder is important for communication between investigators for the advancement of medical knowledge, while the function of medical newspaper is to disseminate information relevant to medical practice. Both of these two basic functions may benefit from the development of modern computer and Internet technology.[115]

Publication bias may be reduced by introducing new peer-reviewed electronic journals without space limitation, in which papers should be accepted based only on the research methodology or validity criteria, and not on the results.[52,116–118] Because the originality is no longer a requirement, these types of electronic journals will encourage the submission of trials with negative or non-striking results, and trials that simply replicate previous trials. Such journals would be mainly used as medical recorders and therefore would be most useful for investigators and people who conduct systematic reviews.

Systematic Review

For many types of publication-related biases (such as grey literature bias, language bias, citation bias and duplication bias), a systematic approach to searching, assessing and summarising published or unpublished studies is crucial. Conducting a thorough literature search when carrying out systematic reviews may reduce the risk of missing studies that are published in low-circulation journals or in the grey literature.

The risk of potential publication bias may be estimated according to its association with some study characteristics, such as observational studies or small sample size. In meta-analysis, larger studies are normally given greater weight than smaller studies. This procedure will have an advantage in reducing the impact of publication bias since less weight is given to smaller studies that are associated with a greater risk of publication bias. In addition, systematic reviews

can be up-dated in order to reduce the consequence of delayed publication of trials with unfavourable results. The methods that may be used in systematic reviews to deal with the problem of publication bias are discussed below.

Locating unpublished trials

Only limited success has been reported in identifying unpublished studies by sending questionnaires to investigators, organisation or research sponsors.[14,119] In a systematic review of near patient testing, no unpublished data were obtained by sending questionnaires to 194 academics and 152 commercial companies.[120] Because the quality of unpublished trials may be different from that of published trials, there is disagreement about whether unpublished studies should be included in meta-analyses.[70,121,122]

It has been suggested that the use of unpublished data can not necessarily reduce the bias in meta-analysis, particularly if the unpublished data are provided by interested sources such as pharmaceutical companies.[123]

Estimating the number of unpublished studies

Rosenthal's fail-safe N method (or the file–drawer method) is a statistical method to estimate the number of unpublished studies required, with zero treatment effect on average, to overturn a significant result in a meta-analysis.[124] If the number of unpublished studies required to overturn the statistically significant result is large, and therefore unlikely to exist, the risk of publication bias is considered to be low and thus the results obtained from published studies are deemed to be reliable.

The plausible number of unpublished studies may be hundreds in some areas or only a few in others. Therefore, the estimated fail-safe N should be considered in proportion to the number of published studies (K). Rosenthal suggested that the fail-safe N may be considered as being unlikely if it is greater than a tolerance level of '$5K + 10$'.[124]

A meta-analysis of risperidone versus typical neuroleptics in the treatment of schizophrenia shows that risperidone is associated with statistically significantly more patients who had clinically improved (odds ratio 0.75; 95% CI: 0.61 to 0.92) (Figure 2).[125] By applying Rosenthal's method, at least 23 unpublished studies with zero treatment effect on average are required in this meta-analysis to change the statistically significant result into a statistically non-significant result. Although the fail-safe N is two times greater than the published studies, it is less

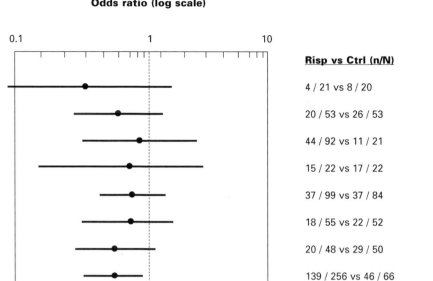

Figure 2 *Meta-analysis of risperidone for schizophrenia: number of patients classified as clinically not improved with risperidone (Risp) versus typical neuroleptic medication (Ctrl).*[125]

than 60 (that is, $5 \times 10 + 10$), a tolerance level suggested by Rosenthal.

Two problems with the fail-safe N method have been identified.[126] Firstly, the method over-emphasises the importance of statistical significance. Secondly, it may be misleading when the unpublished studies have an average effect that is in the opposite direction to the observed meta-analysis. If the unpublished studies reported contrary results compared to those in the published studies, the number of unpublished studies required to overturn a significant result would be smaller than that estimated assuming an average effect of zero in unpublished studies.

The fail-safe N estimated by using Rosenthal's method is not necessarily related to the actual number of unpublished studies. Using the *P*-values reported in the published studies, Gleser and Olkin proposed two general models for estimating the number (and its lower confidence

bound) of unpublished studies.[127] The models are based on the following three basic assumptions: (i) all studies, published and unpublished, are mutually statistically independent; (ii) the *P*-value in each study is based on a continuous test statistic; and (iii) the null hypothesis is true. Because these methods are based on the assumption that the null hypothesis is true, they cannot be used to estimate the effects of publication bias on effect size.

Funnel plot

Because of larger random error, the results from smaller studies will be more widely spread around the average effect. A plot of sample size versus treatment effect from individual studies in a meta-analysis should be shaped like a funnel if there is no publication bias.[2] If the chance of publication is greater for trials with statistically significant results, the shape of the funnel plot may become skewed.

Light and Pillemer described two ways in which the shape of the funnel plot can be modified when studies with statistically significant results are more likely to be published.[2] Firstly, assume that the true treatment effect is zero. Then the results of small studies can only be statistically significant when they are far away from zero, either positive or negative. If studies with significant results are published and studies with results around zero are not published, there will be an empty area around zero in the funnel plot. In this case, the funnel plot may not be obviously skewed but would have a hollow area inside. These polarised results (significant negative or positive results) may cause many debates; however, the overall estimate obtained by combining all studies is unlikely to be biased.

When the true treatment effect is small but not zero, small studies reporting a small effect size will not be statistically significant and therefore less likely to be published, while small studies reporting a large effect size may be statistically significant and more likely to be published. Consequently there will be a lack of small studies with small effect in the funnel plot, and the funnel plot will be skewed with a larger effect among smaller studies and a smaller effect among larger studies. This will result in an over-estimation of the treatment effect in a meta-analysis.

In a funnel plot, the treatment effects from individual studies are often plotted against their standard errors (or the inverse of the standard error) instead of the corresponding sample sizes (Figure 3). Use of standard errors may have some advantages because the statistical significance is determined not only by the sample size but also by the level of variation in the outcome measured, or the number of events in the case of categorical data. However, the visual impression of a funnel plot may change by plotting treatment effects against standard errors instead of against the inverse of standard errors.[128]

There are some limitations in the use of funnel plot to detect publication bias. For a funnel plot to be useful, there needs to be a range of studies with varying sizes. The funnel

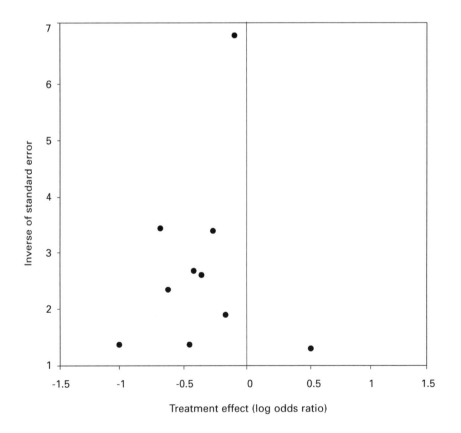

Figure 3   *Funnel plot of log odds ratio against inverse of standard error. Meta-analysis of risperidone versus typical neuroleptics for schizophrenia.*

plot is an informal method for assessing the potential publication bias subjectively, and different people may interpret the same plot differently. It should be stressed that a skewed funnel plot may be caused by factors other than publication bias. Other possible sources of asymmetry in funnel plots include different intensity of intervention, differences in underlying risk, poor methodological design of small studies, inadequate analysis, fraud, choice of effect measure, and chance.[129]

Rank correlation test

Begg and Mazumdar suggested that a rank correlation test can be used to examine the association between effect estimates and their variances, as a complementary method to the funnel plot.[130] The rank correlation test is a distribution-free method which involves no modelling assumptions. However, it suffers from a lack of power and so the possibility of publication bias cannot be ruled out when the test is non-significant.

According to simulated results, the power of the rank correlation test is related to several factors: the number of component studies in the meta-analysis; the underlying effect size parameter; the range of variances across studies; the strength of the selection function; and the presence of one-sided or two-sided selection pressures.[130] The test is fairly powerful for large meta-analyses with 75 component studies, but has only moderate power for meta-analyses with 25 component studies. In the meta-analysis of risperidone for schizophrenia,[125] the rank correlation test did not find an association between the estimated treatment effects and their variances (Spearman's rho correlation coefficient 0.018; $P = 0.96$).

Linear regression approach

Egger and colleagues[129] suggested a method to test the asymmetry of a funnel plot, based on a regression analysis of Galbraith's radial plot.[131] The standard normal deviate, defined as the log odds ratio divided by its standard error, is regressed against the estimate's precision (i.e. the inverse of the standard error). In this linear regression analysis, the intercept is used to measure asymmetry; a negative intercept indicates that smaller studies are associated with bigger treatment effects.

By applying this method, significant asymmetry was observed in 38% of 37 meta-analyses published in a selection of journals, and in 13% of 38 Cochrane reviews.[129] Egger et al. also identified four meta-analyses in which discordant funnel plots showed that the treatment effect was larger in meta-analyses than in the corresponding large trials. Using Egger et al.'s method, significant asymmetry was found in three of these four meta-analyses; however, when the rank correlation test was used, only one of the four meta-analyses showed significant asymmetry. Thus the linear regression method[129] appears to be more sensitive than the rank correlation test.[130]

The results of applying this method to the meta-analysis of risperidone for schizophrenia are shown in Figure 4. Because the intercept of the weighted regression is significantly less than zero, it indicates that the small studies are associated with a larger treatment effect.

In the original Galbraith radial plot, the slope of the line indicates the size and direction of effect; a greater gradient of the slope indicates a greater difference in the treatment effect.[131] However, for testing the asymmetry of a funnel plot, the gradient of the slope will become closer to zero or positive when the estimated effect is greater in smaller studies. The operating characteristics of this method need to be evaluated thoroughly by more analytic work, or computer simulations.[132]

Trim and fill method

The trim and fill method is a simple rank-based data augmentation technique to formalise the use of the funnel plot.[128] This recently developed method can be used to estimate the number of missing studies and, more importantly, to provide an estimate of the treatment effect by adjusting for potential publication bias in a meta-analysis. Briefly, the asymmetric outlying part of the funnel is firstly 'trimmed off' after estimating how many studies are in the asymmetric part. The symmetric remainder is then used to estimate the 'true' centre of the funnel. Finally, the 'true' mean and its variance are estimated based on the 'filled' funnel plot in which the trimmed studies and their missing 'counterparts' symmetric about the centre are replaced. In simulation studies, it was found that the method estimated the point estimate of the overall effect size approximately correctly and the coverage of the confidence interval is substantially improved, as compared to ignoring publication bias.[128]

Applying the Trim and Fill method to meta-analysis of risperidone for schizophrenia (see Figure 3) suggests that the original funnel plot would need three trials to fill on the right side. After filling with the assumed missing trials, the adjusted odds ratio (0.82, 95% CI: 0.68 to 1.01) become non-significant compared to that based on the published trials (0.75, 95% CI: 0.61 to

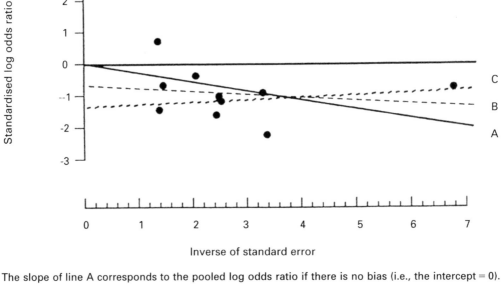

The slope of line A corresponds to the pooled log odds ratio if there is no bias (i.e., the intercept = 0). The line B is an unweighted regression in which the intercept is negative but not statistically significant (intercept = −0.704, P = 0.223). The line C is a weighted (by the inverse of variance) regression in which the intercept is significantly less than zero (intercept = −1.392, P = 0.016), therefore it indicates the existence of bias in favour of small trials.

Figure 4   *Linear regression method to test asymmetry of funnel plot: meta-analysis of risperidone for schizophrenia as an example.*

0.92). The advantage of risperidone versus conventional neuroleptics in clinical improvement for schizophrenia becomes smaller and no longer statistically significant after adjusting potential publication bias.

More sophisticated modelling methods

The impact of missing studies may also be assessed by using more sophisticated methods. Several selection modelling methods have been developed to investigate/adjust the results of a meta-analysis in the presence of publication bias. Many of these methods are related and based on weighted distribution theory derived from both classical[133–137] and Bayesian[138,139] perspectives, although other methods do exist.[140]

There are two aspects to the selection models which use weighted distribution theory: an effect size model which specifies what the distribution of the effect size estimate would be if there were no selection, and the selection model which specifies how this effect size distribution is modified by the selection process.[141] In some methods the nature of the selection process is pre-defined by the researcher, while in others it is dictated by the available data.

Unfortunately, the complexity of these methods means that they have largely been used only by statistical modelling experts. Hence, although applications of their use do exist,[139,142] they are limited in number and no comprehensive comparison of the methods has ever been carried out. For this reason, many feel they are still in the experimental stage of development, despite being considered for well over a decade.[143] Development of user-friendly software is required to bring the methods into more mainstream use. They have the potential to be a valuable tool for assessing the robustness of a meta-analyses results to publication bias; if not to adjust the pooled estimate *per se.*[143]

Confirmatory Large-Scale Trials

For the purpose of avoiding moderate biases and moderate random errors in assessing or refuting moderate benefits, a large number of patients in randomised controlled trials are required.[144] Large-scale trials are generally believed to be less vulnerable to publication bias; this is the fundamental assumption of many methods for detecting publication bias. Though the results of meta-analyses often agree with those of large trials, important discrepancies have been observed.[145–147] When the existence of publication bias is likely and the consequences of such bias are clinically important, a confirmatory, multi-centre large-scale trial may be conducted to provide more convincing evidence.

SURVEY OF PUBLISHED SYSTEMATIC REVIEWS

At the end of August 1998, 193 systematic reviews published in 1996 were included in the Database of Abstracts of Reviews of Effectiveness (DARE) at the NHS Centre for Reviews and Dissemination, University of York. These reviews have been selected to examine the issues and methods relevant to publication bias. Among the 193 systematic reviews, the majority (83%) evaluated the effectiveness of health interventions; 8% focused on adverse-effects of interventions; and 9% evaluated diagnostic technologies. In total, 131 of these reviews were meta-analyses in which the results of primary studies are combined quantitatively, while 62 were narrative systematic reviews in which quantitative pooling was not employed.

Searching for unpublished studies was reported more often in meta-analyses than in narrative systematic reviews (32% versus 16%). The methods used were mainly to write to investigators/authors, research organisations and pharmaceutical companies. Meeting proceedings were often searched to identify unpublished abstracts. By checking the reference lists of all 193 reviews, it was found that conference abstracts were included in some reviews in which unpublished studies were not explicitly searched for. In total, 35% of meta-analyses and 31% of narrative systematic reviews explicitly searched for, or included, unpublished studies. Seventeen meta-analyses explicitly excluded unpublished studies or abstracts because they were not peer-reviewed and were therefore considered to be unreliable.

Non-English language literature were searched for or included in 30% of the systematic reviews. However, language restrictions may still exist in some reviews that included non-English language literature. For example, the reviews were often limited to literature in major European languages, or English plus the reviewers' native languages.

The problem of potential publication bias was discussed or mentioned more frequently in the meta-analyses than in the narrative systematic reviews (46% versus 11%). Methods of testing publication bias were used in 27 of the 131 meta-analyses and in only one of the 62 narrative systematic reviews. The most commonly used methods were fail-safe N (in 14 reviews) and funnel plot-related methods (in 11 reviews). Other methods used included large-scale trials, sensitivity analysis, and comparing published with unpublished studies.

DISCUSSION

The existence of publication bias is demonstrated by showing an association between the chance or manner of publication and the strength or direction of study findings. It is therefore important to define what we mean by two basic concepts: publication and study findings.

The formats of publication include full publication in journals, presentation at scientific conferences, reports, book chapters, discussion papers, dissertations or theses. The studies presented at scientific meetings are often not considered to be published, and there are disagreements about how reliable they are. For example, 17 of the 133 meta-analyses surveyed in this review explicitly excluded abstracts because they were not peer-reviewed.

Study findings are commonly classified as being statistically significant or statistically non-significant. Sometimes, study results are classified as being negative versus positive,[22,40,148,149] supportive versus unsupportive,[50,90] or striking versus unimportant.[20] The classification of study findings are often dependent upon subjective judgement, and may therefore be unreliable.

In addition to the difficulties in defining publication and classifying outcomes, studies of publication bias themselves may be as vulnerable as other studies to selective publication of significant or striking findings.[4] Therefore, the available evidence about publication bias should be interpreted with caution.

The empirical evidence demonstrates that studies with significant results or favourable results are more likely to be published or cited than those with non-significant or unfavourable results. The extent and direction of such selective publication is still uncertain, and may vary greatly depending on the circumstances. In addition, there is little empirical evidence about the impact of publication and related biases on health policy, clinical decision-making and outcome of patient management.

Because of the lack of empirical evidence about the impact of publication bias, there is disagreement on the actual importance of publication bias in the evaluation of healthcare interventions. Some have argued that the potential consequences of publication bias are serious,[4,52,150] whilst others argue that positive studies are more important than negative studies and selective publication of positive studies is not a clinical problem.[151-153] At the very least, it is arguable that under-reporting research is scientific misconduct that may cause inappropriate patient care, and also it is unethical to mistreat the trust of patients involved and waste resources invested.[6,52]

Practitioners and researchers may have developed some immunity to publication bias, by waiting for confirmatory studies about a claimed advancement before changing their practice. This skepticism about new developments may reduce the impact of publication bias. However, the corollary of this is that the introduction of a new cost-effective technology may be unnecessarily delayed.

It seems that the most common reason for publication bias is that investigators fail to write-up or submit studies with non-significant results. Investigators may lose interest in non-significant results, or be motivated not to publish results that are unfavourable to their own interest. However, it is possible that investigators would not submit studies with non-significant results mainly because of anticipated rejection by journals. Paper-based journals often select manuscripts that are original with an important impact on practice. The potential role of research sponsors needs to be emphasised, because evidence has shown that studies with favourable results to funding body's interest are more likely to be disseminated.

Risk Factors for Publication Bias

Studies with small sample sizes tend to produce results with great variation and therefore give people a great range of results to select for publication. Simulations have demonstrated that small sample size is associated with a great extent of publication bias when only studies with significant results are published.[133,154] In practice, a small study with a non-significant result may be readily abandoned without trying to publish because it is easy and cheap to carry out in terms of time, staff and other resources invested. In addition, small trials may often be poorly designed and conducted. Therefore, the risk of publication bias will be great if many small trials have been conducted.[143]

The simulation results also indicated that the extent of bias, by selecting only the significant results to publish, is greater when the true effect is small or moderate than when the true effect is zero or large.[154] A small or moderate effect (or weak association) may be considered as a risk factor for publication bias. This risk factor may exist in most cases because clinical trials are mainly designed to assess healthcare interventions with small or moderate (but clinically important) effects.

The interest of investigators and funding bodies may be associated with publication bias. Therefore, the risk of bias may be great if all trials are funded by a single body with explicit or implicit reasons for favouring a particular finding. Conversely, when similar results are obtained from trials funded by different bodies with conflicting interests, the risk of bias due to funding bodies may not be important.

The design quality of studies may be associated with the risk of publication bias. Non-randomised studies, single-centre studies, Phase I and II trials might be more susceptible to publication bias than randomised studies, multi-centre studies and Phase III trials.[155,156] Risk factors for publication bias were assessed, but not consistently identified, across several cohort studies of publication bias.[17-20] Irwig and colleagues[157] suggested that publication bias is more of a problem for diagnostic tests than for randomised trials because 'many studies of test accuracy may use data collected primarily as part of clinical care, there may be no clear record of attempted evaluations'.

Implications for Decision-Makers and Researchers

The potential problem of publication and other selection biases should be taken into consideration by all who are involved in evidence based decision making. For research funding bodies and research ethics committees, all funded or approved studies should be prospectively registered and such registrations should be accessible to the public. The dissemination of research results should be considered as an integral part of research.

In all systematic reviews, a thorough literature search is crucial to identify all relevant studies, published or not. Whenever possible, registers of clinical trials should be used in a systematic review to identify relevant studies, and identified trials should be classified according to whether they are prospectively or retrospectively registered. The search of electronic databases alone is seldom sufficient and should be supplemented by checking references of relevant studies and contacting experts or organisations.[120]

Because even a thorough literature search cannot eliminate publication bias, the risk of publication bias should be assessed and, when estimated, should be incorporated into the review's conclusions and recommendations in systematic reviews. The risk of publication bias can be assessed, for example, according to the sample sizes of studies, the potential number of studies that may have been conducted, research sponsors, time of publication of studies, and heterogeneity across studies. Although it is still controversial, systematic reviews should not systematically exclude unpublished studies or abstracts presented at scientific meetings. The quality of unpublished studies or abstracts should be assessed using the same criteria for assessing published studies. Sensitivity analysis could be used in systematic reviews to compare the results with and without data from unpublished studies.

Some methods are available in systematic reviews to deal with publication bias, such as the fail-safe N method, funnel plot, rank correlation method, linear regression method, trim-and-fill method, and some complex modelling methods. Rosenthal's fail-safe N and funnel plot-related statistical methods are the most commonly used. These methods are mainly useful to detect publication bias, although some methods (such as trim-and-fill method) could provide an estimate by adjusting for the detected bias. It should be stressed that all these methods are by nature indirect and exploratory, because the true extent of publication bias is generally unknown.

There are some methodological difficulties in using the available methods to test and adjust for publication bias in meta-analyses. In most cases, it is impossible to separate the influence of factors other than publication bias on the observed association between the estimated effects and sample sizes across studies. The appropriateness of many methods is based on some strict assumptions that can be difficult to justify in the real practice. For these reasons, it seems reasonable to argue that these methods 'are not very good remedies for publication bias'.[6] The attempt at identifying or adjusting for publication bias in a systematic review should be mainly used for the purpose of sensitivity analyses, and the results should be interpreted with great caution.

Large-scale confirmatory trials become necessary after a systematic review has reported a clinically significant finding, but publication bias cannot be safely excluded as an alternative explanation. As compared with a universal register of all trials, large confirmatory trials are more selective about the research areas and objectives, but more flexible at the same time to minimise the impact of other biases, for example, biases related to study design, selection of control, participants and setting.

Recommendations for Future Research

Further research is needed to provide more reliable empirical evidence about publication and related biases. Especially, there is a lack of reliable evidence about the impact of publication bias on health decision-making and outcomes of patient management.

In the foreseeable future, many systematic reviews may still have to depend upon studies identified retrospectively from the published literature. The available methods for detecting or adjusting for publication bias should be evaluated and measures taken to make the more complex methods easier to use. Further research is also needed to develop new methods that are sensitive and easy to use for detecting or adjusting for publication bias in systematic reviews. In addition, there is a lack of methods that can be used to detect publication bias in narrative systematic reviews.

It is most important for future research to identify the cost-effective and feasible methods for preventing publication bias. Further research is needed to answer questions about how to establish and maintain prospective registration of clinical trials and observational studies; how to make all research findings accessible to the public; and how the developments in computer science and information technology can be used to solve the problem of publication bias. The problem of publication bias is unlikely to be solved by the conventional paper-based medical journals because of their intrinsic limitations. Further research about publication bias should be an integral part of research that explores alternatives to the conventional methods for generating, disseminating, preserving and utilising scientific research findings.

ACKNOWLEDGEMENTS

This work was supported by the NHS R&D Health Technology Assessment Programme. The authors would like to thank Kathleen Wright for assisting with the search and location of the literature; Sue Duval at University of Colorado Health Sciences Center for help in using the trim-and-fill method. We also thank Iain Chalmers, Trevor Sheldon, Jos Kleijnen, Andrew Stevens, and Keith Abrams for commenting on the early manuscript.

REFERENCES

1. Mulrow CD. Rationale for systematic reviews. *Br. Med. J.* 1994; **309**: 597–9.

2. Light RJ, Pillemer DB. *Summing up: the science of reviewing research.* Cambridge, Massachusetts, and London: Harvard University Press 1984.

3. Chalmers I, Altman DG. *Systematic Reviews.* London: BMJ Publishing Group 1995.

4. Begg CB, Berlin JA. Publication bias: a problem in interpreting medical data. *J. Roy. Statist. Soc. A.* 1988; **151**: 419–63.

5. Song F, Gilbody S. Increase in studies of publication bias coincided with increasing use of meta-analysis [letter]. *Br. Med. J.* 1998; **316**: 471.

6. Dickersin K. The existence of publication bias and risk factors for its occurrence. *JAMA* 1990; **263**: 1385–9.

7. Chalmers TC, Frank CS, Reitman D. Minimizing the three stages of publication bias. *JAMA* 1990; **263**: 1392–5.

8. Song F, Eastwood A, Gilbody S, Duley L, Sutton A. Publication and related biases in health techology assessment. *Health Technology Assessment* 2000; **4**(10).

9. Sterling TD. Publication decisions and their possible effects on inferences drawn tests of significance – or vice versa. *Am. Statist. Assoc. J.* 1959; **54**: 30–4.

10. Sterling TD, Rosenbaum WL, Weinkam JJ. Publication decisions revisited – the effect of the outcome of statistical tests on the decision to publish and vice-versa. *American Statistician* 1995; **49**: 108–12.

11. Chalmers TC, Grady GF. A note on fatality in serum hepatitis. *Gastroenterology* 1965; **49**: 22–6.

12. Greenwald AG. Consequences of prejudice against the null hypothesis. *Psychol. Bull.* 1975; **82**: 1–20.

13. Coursol A, Wagner EE. Effect of positive findings on submission and acceptance rates: a note on meta-analysis bias. *Professional Psychology* 1986; **17**: 136–7.

14. Dickersin K, Chan S, Chalmers TC, Sacks HS, Smith H, Jr. Publication bias and clinical trials. *Controlled Clinical Trials* 1987; **8**: 343–53.

15. Sommer B. The file drawer effect and publication rates in menstrual cycle research. *Psychol. Women Q.* 1987; **11**: 233–42.

16. Simes RJ. Publication bias: the case for an international registry of clinical trials. *J. Clin. Oncol.* 1986; **4**: 1529–41.

17. Easterbrook PJ, Berlin JA, Gopalan R, Matthews DR. Publication bias in clinical research. *Lancet* 1991; **337**: 867–72.

18. Dickersin K, Min YI, Meinert CL. Factors influencing publication of research results. Follow up of applications submitted to two institutional review boards. *JAMA* 1992; **267**: 374–8.

19. Dickersin K, Min. YI. NIH clinical trials and publication bias. *Online J. Curr. Clin. Trials* 1993; **Doc. No. 50**.

20. Stern JM, Simes RJ. Publication bias: evidence of delayed publication in a cohort study of clinical research projects. *Br. Med. J.* 1997; **315**: 640–5.

21. Dickersin K. How important is publication bias? A synthesis of available data. *Aids Education and Prevention* 1997; **9**: 15–21.

22. Ioannidis J. Effect of the statistical significance of results on the time to completion and publication of randomized efficacy trials. *JAMA* 1998; **279**: 281–6.

23. Misakian AL, Bero LA. Publication bias and research on passive smoking. Comparison of published and unpublished studies. *JAMA* 1998; **280**: 250–3.

24. Auger CP. *Information sources in grey literature*, 4th edn. London, Melbourne, Munich, New Providence, N.J: Bowker-Saur, 1998.

25. Smart RG. The importance of negative results in psychological research. *Can. Psychol.* 1964; **5**: 225–32.

26. Smith ML. Publication bias and meta-analysis. *Eval. Educ.* 1980; **4**: 22–4.

27. Glass GV, McGaw B, Smith ML. *Meta-analysis in social research.* London: Sage Publications, 1981.

28. White KR. The relation between socioeconomic status and academic achievement. *Psychological Bulletin* 1982; **91**: 461–81.

29. Koren G, Graham K, Shear H, Einarson T. Bias against the null hypothesis: the reproductive hazards of cocaine. *Lancet* 1989; **2**: 1440–2.

30. Callaham ML, Wears RL, Weber EJ, Barton C, Young G. Positive-outcome bias and other limitations in the outcome of research abstracts submitted to a scientific meeting. *JAMA* 1998; **280**: 254–7.

31. Scherer RW, Dickersin K, Langenberg P. Full publication of results initially presented in abstracts. A meta-analysis. *JAMA* 1994; **272**: 158–62.

32. DeBellefeuille C, Morrison CA, Tannock IF. The fate of abstracts submitted to a cancer meeting: factors which influence presentation and subsequent publication. *Ann. Oncol.* 1992; **3**: 187–91.

33. Chalmers I, Adams M, Dickersin K, et al. A cohort study of summary reports of controlled trials. *JAMA* 1990; **263**: 1401–5.

34. Weber EJ, Callaham ML, Wears RL, Barton C, Young G. Unpublished research from a medical specialty meeting. Why investigators fail to publish. *JAMA* 1998; **280**: 257–9.

35. Cheng K, Preston C, Ashby D, OHea U, Smyth R. Time to publication as full reports of abstracts of randomized controlled trials in cystic fibrosis. *Pediatr. Pulmonol.* 1998; **26**: 101–5.

36. Gregoire G, Derderian F, Lorier JL. Selecting the language of the publications included in a meta-analysis: is there a tower of babel bias? *J. Clin. Epidemiol.* 1995; **48**: 159–63.

37. Egger M, Zellweger-Zahner T, Schneider M, Junker C, Lengeler C, Antes G. Language bias in randomised controlled trials published in English and German. *Lancet* 1997; **350**: 326–9.

38. Nylenna M, Riis P, Karlsson Y. Multiple blinded reviews of the same two manuscripts. Effects of referee characteristics and publication language. *JAMA* 1994; **272**: 149–51.

39. Ottenbacher K, Difabio RP. Efficacy of spinal manipulation/mobilization therapy. A meta-analysis. *Spine* 1985; **10**: 833–7.

40. Vickers A, Goyal N, Harland R, Rees R. Do certain countries produce only positive results? A systematic review of controlled trials. *Controlled Clinical Trials* 1998; **19**: 159–66.

41. Pocock SJ, Hughes MD, Lee RJ. Statistical problems in the reporting of clinical trials. A survey of three medical journals. *N. Engl. J. Med.* 1987; **317**: 426–32.

42. Tannock IF. False-positive results in clinical trials: multiple significance tests and the problem of unreported comparisons. *J. Natl Cancer Inst.* 1996; **88**: 206–7.

43. Forrow L, Taylor WC, Arnold RM. Absolutely relative: how research results are summarized can affect treatment decisions. *Am. J. Med.* 1992; **92**: 121–4.

44. Naylor CD, Chen E, Strauss B. Measured enthusiasm: does the method of reporting trial results alter perceptions of therapeutic effectiveness? *Ann. Intern. Med.* 1992; **117**: 916–21.

45. Bobbio M, Demichelis B, Giustetto G. Completeness of reporting trial results: effect on physicians' willingness to prescribe. *Lancet* 1994; **343**: 1209–11.

46. Tramer MR, Reynolds DJM, Moore RA, McQuay HJ. Impact of covert duplicate publication on meta-analysis: a case study. *Br. Med. J.* 1997; **315**: 635–40.

47. Huston P, Moher D. Redundancy, disaggregation, and the integrity of medical research. *Lancet* 1996; **347**: 1024–6.

48. Ravnskov U. Cholesterol lowering trials in coronary heart disease: frequency of citation and outcome. *Br. Med. J.* 1992; **305**: 15–19.

49. Ravnskov U. Quotation bias in reviews of the diet-heart idea. *J. Clin. Epidemiol.* 1995; **48**: 713–19.

50. Hutchison BG, Oxman AD, Lloyd S. Comprehensiveness and bias in reporting clinical trials. Study of reviews of pneumococcal vaccine effectiveness. *Can. Fam. Physician* 1995; **41**: 1356–60.

51. Koren G, Klein N. Bias against negative studies in newspaper reports of medical research. *JAMA* 1991; **266**: 1824–6.

52. Chalmers I. Under-reporting research is scientific misconduct. *JAMA* 1990; **263**: 1405–8.

53. Cowley AJ, Skene A, Stainer K, Hampton JR. The effect of lorcainide on arrhythmias and survival in patients with acute myocardial infarction – an example of publication bias. *Int. J. Cardiol.* 1993; **40**: 161–6.

54. The Cardiac Arrhythmia Suppression Trial (CAST) Investigators. Preliminary report: effect of encainide and flecainide on mortality in a randomised trial of arrhythmia suppression after myocardial infarction. *N. Engl. J. Med.* 1989; **321**: 406–12.

55. The Cardiac Arrhythmia Suppression Trial II Investigators. Effect of the antiarrhythmic agent moricisine on survival after myocardial infarction. *N. Engl. J. Med.* 1992; **327**: 227–33.

56. Yusuf S, Koon T, Woods K. Intravenous magnesium in acute myocardial infarction: an effective, safe, simple, and inexpensive intervention. *Circulation* 1993; **87**: 2043–6.

57. ISIS–4 Collaborative Group. ISIS–4: a randomised factorial trial assessing early oral captopril, oral mononitrate, and intravenous magnesium sulphate in 58050 patients with acute myocardial infarction. *Lancet* 1995; **345**: 669–85.

58. Egger M, Davey-Smith G. Misleading meta-analysis: lessons from 'an effective, safe, simple' intervention that wasn't. *Br. Med. J.* 1995; **310**: 752–4.

59. The Government Statistical Service. *Hospital episode statistics. Volume 1. Finished consultant episodes by diagnosis, operation and specialty. England: financial year 1993–94.* London: Crown Copyright, 1995.

60. MacCoun R. Biases in the interpretation and use of research results. *Annu. Rev. Psychol.* 1998; **49**: 259–87.

61. Beveridge WIB. *The art of scientific investigation.* London: Mercury Books, 1961.

62. Rothwell PM, Slattery J, Warlow CP. A systematic review of the risks of stroke and death due to endarterectomy for symptomatic carotid stenosis. *Stroke* 1996; **27**: 260–5.

63. Kupfersmid J, Fiala M. A survey of attitudes and behaviors of authors who publish in psychology and education journals [comments]. *Am. Psychol.* 1991; **46**: 249–50.

64. Kassirer JP, Campion EW. Peer review: crude and understudied, but indispensable. *JAMA* 1994; **272**: 96–7.

65. The Lancet. http://www.thelancet.com.

66. Abby M, Massey MD, Galandiuk S, Polk HC. Peer review is an effective screening process to evaluate medical manuscripts. *JAMA* 1994; **272**: 105–7.

67. Zelen M. Guidelines for publishing papers on cancer clinical trials: responsibilities of editors and authors. *J. Clin. Oncol.* 1983; **1**: 164–9.

68. Editor. Manuscript guideline. *Diabetologia* 1984; **25**: 4A.

69. Taubes G. Epidemiology faces its limits. *Science* 1995; **269**: 164–9.

70. Angell M. Negative studies. *N. Engl. J. Med.* 1989; **321**: 464–6.

71. Bailar JC, Patterson K. Journal peer review: the need for a research agenda. *N. Engl. J. Med.* 1985; **312**: 654–7.

72. Mahoney MJ. Publication prejudices: an experimental study of confirmatory bias in the peer review system. *Cognitive Ther. Res.* 1977; **1**: 161–75.

73. Ernst E, Resch KL. Reviewer bias – a blinded experimental study. *J. Lab. Clin. Med.* 1994; **124**: 178–82.

74. Abbot NC, Ernst E. Publication bias: direction of outcome less important than scientific quality. *Perfusion* 1998; **11**: 182–4.

75. Blumenthal D, Causino N, Campbell E, Seashore K. Relationships between academic institutions and industry in the life sciences – an industry survey. *N. Engl. J. Med.* 1996; **334**: 368–73.

76. Hemminki E. Study of information submitted by drug companies to licensing authorities. *Br. Med. J.* 1980; **280**: 833–6.

77. Bardy AH. Report Bias in Drug Research. *Therapie* 1996; **51**: 382–3.

78. Bardy A. Bias in reporting clinical trials. *Br. J. Clin. Pharmacol.* 1998; **46**: 147–50.

79. Dent THS, Hawke S. Too soon to market: doctors and patients need more information before drugs enter routine use. *Br. Med. J.* 1997; **315**: 1248–9.

80. Abraham J, Lewis G. Secrecy and transparency of medicines licensing in the EU. *Lancet* 1998; **352**: 480–2.

81. Roberts I, Li-Wan-Po A, Chalmers I. Intellectual property, drug licensing, freedom of information, and public health. *Lancet* 1998; **352**: 726–9.

82. Lauritsen K, Kavelund T, Larsen LS, Rask-Madsen J. Withholding unfavourable results in drug company sponsored clinical trials. *Lancet* 1987; **i**: 1091.

83. Rennie D. Thyroid storm. *JAMA* 1997; **277**: 1238–43.

84. Kotelchuk D. Asbestos research: winning the battle but losing the war. *Health/PAC Bulletin* 1974; **61**: 1–27.

85. Davidson RA. Source of funding and outcome of clinical trials. *J. Gen. Intern. Med.* 1986; **1**: 155–8.

86. Rochon PA, Gurwitz JH, Simms RW, Fortin PR, et al. A study of manufacturer-supported trials of nonsteroidal anti-inflammatory drugs in the treatment of arthritis. *Arch. Intern. Med.* 1994; **154**: 157–63.

87. Bero LA, Galbraith A, Rennie D. Sponsored symposia on environmental tobacco-smoke. *JAMA* 1994; **271**: 612–17.

88. Barnes DE, Bero LA. Industry-funded research and conflict of interest: an analysis of research sponsored by the tobacco industry through the center for indoor air research. *J. Health Polit. Policy Law* 1996; **21**: 515–42.

89. Cho MK, Bero LA. The quality of drug studies published in symposium proceeding. *Ann. Intern. Med.* 1996; **124**: 485–9.

90. Stelfox HT, Chua G, O'Rourke K, Detsky AS. Conflict of interest in the debate over calcium-channel antagonists. *N. Engl. J. Med.* 1998; **338**: 101–6.

91. CCOHTA. *Canadian Coordinating Office For Health Technology Assessment: Annual Report 1997–1998.* Ottawa, 1998.

92. Millstone E, Brunner E, White I. Plagiarism or protecting public health. *Nature* 1994; **371**: 647–8.

93. Simes RJ. Confronting publication bias: a cohort design for meta analysis. *Stat. Med.* 1987; **6**: 11–29.

94. Kleijnen J, Knipschild P. Review Articles and Publication Bias. *Arzneim. Forsch./Drug Res.* 1992; **42**: 587–91.

95. Easterbrook PJ. Directory of registries of clinical trials. *Stat. Med.* 1992; **11**: 345–423.

96. Silagy CA. Developing a register of randomised controlled trials in primary care. *Br. Med. J.* 1993; **306**: 897–900.

97. Robertson SE, Mayans MV, Horsfall S, et al. The WHO Global Programme for Vaccines and Immunization Vaccine Trial Registry. *Bull. World Health Org.* 1997; **75**: 295–305.

98. Cochrane Controlled Trials Register. In: *The Cochrane Library (Issue 1).* Oxford: Update Software, 1999.

99. *The National Research Register.* The NHS R&D Information Systems Strategy. Leeds, 1998.

100. The Current Science Group. Current Controlled Trials. *http://www.controlled-trials.com.*

101. Downs JR, Gotto A, Clearfield M, Gordon D, Manolio T, Goldbourt U, et al. Protocol for a prospective collaborative overview of all current and planned randomized trials of cholesterol treatment regimens. *Am. J. Cardiol.* 1995; **75**: 1130–4.

102. Simes RJ. Prospective metaanalysis of cholesterol-lowering studies – the prospective pravastatin pooling (Ppp) project and the Cholesterol Treatment Trialists (Ctt) Collaboration. *Am. J. Cardiol.* 1995; **76**: C122–6.

103. Meinert CL. Toward prospective registration of clinical trials. *Controlled Clinical Trials* 1988; **9**: 1–5.

104. Savulescu J, Chalmers I, Blunt J. Are Research Ethics Committees behaving unethically? Some

suggestions for improving performance and accountability. *Br. Med. J.* 1996; **313**: 1390–3.

105. Dickersin K, Garcia Lopez F. Regulatory process effects clinical trial registration in Spain. *Controlled Clinical Trials* 1992; **13**: 507–12.

106. Chollar S. A registry for clinical trials [news]. *Ann. Intern. Med.* 1998; **128**: 701–2.

107. Freedom of information, when it suits (editorial). *Lancet* 1998; **352**: 665.

108. Bardy AH. Freedom of information. *Lancet* 1998; **352**: 229.

109. Newcombe RG. Discussion of the paper by Begg and Berlin: Publication bias: a problem in interpreting medical data. *J. Roy. Statist. Soc. A* 1988; **151**: 448–9.

110. Julian D. Meta-analysis and the meta-epidemiology of clinical research. Registration of trials should be required by editors and registering agencies [letter]. *Br. Med. J.* 1998; **316**: 311.

111. Smith R. Beyond conflict of interest: transparency is the key. *Br. Med. J.* 1998; **317**: 291–2.

112. Smith R, Roberts I. An amnesty for unpublished trials: send us details on any unreported trials. *Br. Med. J.* 1997; **315**: 622.

113. Horton R. Medical Editors Trial Amnesty. *Lancet* 1997; **350**: 756.

114. Fox T. *Crisis in communication: the functions and future of medical journals.* London: The Athlone Press, 1965.

115. Huth EJ. Electronic publishing in the health sciences. *Bull. PAHO* 1995; **29**: 81–7.

116. Berlin JA. Will publication bias vanish in the age of online journals? [editorial]. *Online J. Curr. Clin. Trials* 1992; **Jul 8; Doc. No. 12**.

117. Song F, Eastwood A, Gilbody S, Duley L. The role of electronic journals in reducing publication bias. *Med. Inform.* 1999; **24**: 223–9.

118. Chalmers I, Altman DG. How can medical journals help prevent poor medical research? Some opportunities presented by electronic publishing. *Lancet* 1998; **353**: 490–3.

119. Hetherington J, Dickersin K, Chalmers I, Meinert CL. Retrospective and prospective identification of unpublished controlled trials: lessons from a survey of obstetricians and pediatricians. *Pediatrics* 1989; **84**: 374–80.

120. McManus R, Wilson S, Delaney B, et al. Review of the usefulness of contacting other experts when conducting a literature search for systematic reviews. *Br. Med. J.* 1998; **317**: 1562–3.

121. Chalmers TC, Levin H, Sacks HS, Reitman D, Berrier J, Nagalingam R. Meta-analysis of clinical trials as a scientific discipline. I: control of bias and comparison with large co-operative trials. *Stat. Med.* 1987; **6**: 315–25.

122. Cook DJ, Guyatt GH, Ryan G, Clifton J, Buckingham L, Willan A, et al. Should unpublished data be included in meta analyses? Current convictions and controversies. *JAMA* 1993; **269**: 2749–53.

123. Davey-Smith G, Egger M. Meta-analysis: unresolved issues and future developments. *Br. Med. J.* 1998; **316**: 221–5.

124. Rosenthal R. The 'file drawer problem' and tolerance for null results. *Psychol. Bull.* 1979; **86**: 638–41.

125. Kennedy E, Song F, Hunter R, Gilbody S. Risperidone versus 'conventional' antipsychotic medication for schizophrenia. In: *The Cochrane Library (Issue 3).* Oxford: Update Software, 1998.

126. Evans S. Statistician's comments on: 'Fail safe N' is a useful mathematical measure of the stability of results [letter]. *Br. Med. J.* 1996; **312**: 125.

127. Gleser LJ, Olkin I. Models for estimating the number of unpublished studies. *Stat. Med.* 1996; **15**: 2493–507.

128. Duval S, Tweedie R. Trim and fill: a simple funnel plot based method of adjusting for publication bias in meta-analysis. *Am. Statist. Assoc. J.* (in press).

129. Egger M, Davey-Smith G, Schneider M, Minder C. Bias in meta-analysis detected by a simple, graphical test. *Br. Med. J.* 1997; **315**: 629–34.

130. Begg CB, Mazumdar M. Operating characteristics of a rank correlation test for publication bias. *Biometrics* 1994; **50**: 1088–101.

131. Galbraith RF. A note on graphical presentation of estimated odds ratios from several clinical trials. *Stat. Med.* 1988; **7**: 889–94.

132. Naylor CD. Meta-analysis and the meta-epidemiology of clinical research: meta-analysis is an important contribution to research and practice but it's not a panacea. *Br. Med. J.* 1997; **315**: 617–19.

133. Hedges LV. Estimation of effect size under nonrandom sampling: the effects of censoring studies yielding statistically insignificant mean differences. *J. Education. Stat.* 1984; **9**: 61–85.

134. Iyengar S, Greenhouse JB. Selection models and the file drawer problem. *Stat. Sci.* 1988; **3**: 109–35.

135. Hedges LV. Modelling publication selection effects in meta-analysis. *Stat. Sci.* 1992; **7**: 246–55.

136. Dear HBG, Begg CB. An approach for assessing publication bias prior to performing a meta-analysis. *Stat. Sci.* 1992; **7**: 237–45.

137. Vevea JL, Hedges LV. A general linear model for estimating effect size in the presence of publication bias. *Psychometrika* 1995; **60**: 419–35.

138. Cleary RJ, Casella G. An application of Gibbs sampling to estimation in meta-analysis: accounting for publication bias. *J. Education. Behav. Stat.* 1997; **22**: 141–54.

139. Givens GH, Smith DD, Tweedie RL. Publication bias in meta-analysis: a Bayesian data-augmentation approach to account for issues exemplified in the passive smoking debate. *Stat. Sci.* 1997; **12**: 221–50.

140. Copas J. What works? selectivity models and meta-analysis. *J. Roy. Statist. Soc. A* 1998; **162**: 95–109.

141. Hedges LV, Vevea JL. Estimating effect size under publication bias: Small sample properties and robustness of a random effects selection model. *J. Education. Behav. Statist.* 1996; **21**: 299–332.

142. Linde K, Clausius N, Ramirez G, et al. Are the clinical effects of homoeopathy placebo effects? A meta-analysis of placebo-controlled trials. *Lancet* 1997; **350**: 834–43.

143. Begg CB. Publication bias. In: Cooper H, Hedge LV (eds). *The Handbook of Research Synthesis.* New York: Russell Sage Foundation, 1994.

144. Peto R, Collins R, Gray R. Large-scale randomized evidence: large, simple trials and overviews of trials. *J. Clin. Epidemiol.* 1995; **48**: 23–40.

145. Villar J, Carroli G, Belizan JM. Predictive ability of meta-analyses of randomised controlled. *Lancet* 1995; **345**: 772–6.

146. Cappelleri JC, Ioannidis JPA, Schmid CH, Ferranti SDd, Aubert M, Chalmers TC, et al. Large trials vs meta-analysis of smaller trials. How do their results compare? *JAMA* 1996; **276**: 1332–8.

147. LeLorier J, Gregoire G, Benhaddad A, Lapierre J, Derderian F. Discrepancies between meta-analyses and subsequent large randomized, controlled trials. *N. Engl. J. Med.* 1997; **337**: 536–42.

148. Moher D, Dulberg CS, Wells GA. Statistical power, sample size, and their reporting in randomized controlled trials. *JAMA* 1994; **272**: 122–4.

149. Moscati R, Jehle D, Ellis D, Fiorello A, Landi M. Positive-outcome bias: comparison of emergency medicine and general medicine literatures. *Acad. Emerg. Med.* 1994; **1**: 267–71.

150. Moher D. Publication bias (letter). *Lancet* 1993; **342**: 1116.

151. Bailar JC. Discussion of the paper by Begg and Berlin: Publication bias: a problem in interpreting medical data. *J. Roy. Statist. Soc. A* 1988; **151**: 451.

152. Simon R. Discussion of the paper by Begg and Berlin: Publication bias: a problem in interpreting medical data. *J. Roy. Statist. Soc. A* 1988; **151**: 459–60.

153. de-Melker HE, Rosendaal FR, Vandenbroucke JP. Is publication bias a medical problem? [letter]. *Lancet* 1993; **342**: 621.

154. Lane DM, Dunlap WP. Estimating effect size: bias resulting from the significance criterion in editorial decisions. *Br. J. Math. Statist. Psychol.* 1978; **31**: 107–12.

155. Berlin JA, Begg CB, Louis TA. An assessment of publication bias using a sample of published clinical trials. *J. Am. Stat. Assoc.* 1989; **84**: 381–92.

156. Begg CB, Berlin JA. Publication bias and dissemination of clinical research. *J. Natl Cancer Inst.* 1989; **81**: 107–15.

157. Irwig L, Macaskill P, Glasziou P, Fahey M. Meta-analytic methods for diagnostic test accuracy. *J. Clin. Epidemiol.* 1995; **48**: 119–30.

22

Meta-Analysis in Health Technology Assessment

ALEXANDER J. SUTTON, DAVID R. JONES,
KEITH R. ABRAMS, TREVOR A. SHELDON
and FUJIAN SONG

SUMMARY

Use of systematic review and meta-analytic methods in health technology assessment (HTA) and related areas is now common. This chapter focuses on the quantitative pooling, or meta-analytical aspects of the systematic review process. Methods for combining binary, continuous and ordinal outcome data are discussed. Fixed effects, random effects and Bayesian modelling have all been advocated for meta-analysis. All are described, and the results from their corresponding analyses compared. Next, methods to include covariates, which could potentially explain between-study heterogeneity, are outlined. A practical example using binary outcomes is presented for all these methods. Brief consideration is given to new and other developments. These include methods for the review of disparate sources of data, including that from routine databases and audit data, which may be relevant when assessing HTA interventions, as well as that from RCTs.

CONTEXT

Systematic reviews and meta-analytic methods are now commonly used approaches to the assessment of health technology and related areas, and increasing adoption of such techniques is likely, partly in response to the empha-

sis on 'evidence based' approaches to medicine and healthcare and the explosion of publications beyond the capacity of all except specialist researchers. If combination of results from a set of studies investigating a common intervention is appropriate, synthesis of their results may yield a more precise estimate of the treatment or policy benefit and perhaps also reduce the bias associated with specific individual studies.[1] Combining several sources of evidence may also increase the generalisability of the results, and allow a full exploration of the effects in subgroups. More importantly, adopting the rigorous methods required to carry out a systematic review can highlight deficiencies in the existing literature, such as the existence of low quality of the primary studies. It can also draw attention to methodological differences between studies, for example, variation on the way an intervention is administered, or differences in the demographic characteristics of the study populations. Finally, rigorously performed systematic reviews can also inform future research priorities.

Coupled with this increase in the application of systematic reviews and/or meta-analyses has been the development of meta-analytic methods. This chapter is the result of an extensive review of this accelerating literature,[2] which had the purpose of identifying the different methodological and statistical methods which have been proposed. For this review we identified approximately 1000 potentially relevant references, a number of them from disciplines other than health research, such as education, psychology and sociology. A description of the review methods, including Medline and EMBASE search strategies used, is reported elsewhere,[2] and is available via the internet at

http://www.prw.le.ac.uk/epidemio/personal/kra1/ srotos.html.

It is beyond the possibilities of a single chapter to discuss and illustrate, in depth, all the

---

Guidelines for good systematic review/meta-analytic practice:

1 **Prior to commencing a review:** Specification in a protocol of the objectives, hypotheses (in both biological and healthcare terms), scope, and methods of the systematic review, before the study is undertaken.

2 **Data collection:** Compilation of as comprehensive a set of reports as possible of relevant primary studies, having searched for all potentially relevant data, clearly documenting all search methods and sources.

3 **Study quality assessment:** Assessment of the methodological quality of the set of studies (the method being based on the extent to which susceptibility to bias is minimised – and the specific system used reported). Any selection of studies on quality or other criteria should be based on clearly stated a priori specifications. The reproducibility of the procedures in stages 2 and 3 should also be assessed.

4 **Data identification:** Identification of a common set of definitions of outcome, explanatory and confounding variables, which are, as far as possible, compatible with those in each of the primary studies.

5 **Data extraction:** Extraction of estimates of outcome measures and of study and subject characteristics in a standardised way from primary study documentation, with due checks on extractor bias. Procedures should be explicit, unbiased and reproducible.

6 **Meta-analysis:** Perform, where warranted by the scope and characteristics of the data compiled, quantitative synthesis of primary study results (meta-analysis) using appropriate methods and models (clearly stated), in order to explore and allow for all important sources of variation (e.g. differences in study quality, participants, in the dose, duration, or nature of the intervention, or in the definitions and measurement of outcomes). This will often involve the use of mixed/hierarchical models, including fixed covariates to explain some elements of between-study variation, in combination with random effects terms.

7 **Qualitative summary:** Performance of a narrative or qualitative summary, where data are too sparse, or of too low quality, or too heterogeneous to proceed with a statistical aggregation (meta-analysis). In such cases, the process of conduct and reporting should still be rigorous and explicit.

8 **Sensitivity analysis:** Exploration of the robustness of the results of the systematic review to the choices and assumptions made in all of the above stages. In particular, the following should be explained or explored:
    (a) the impact of study quality/inclusion criteria
    (b) the likelihood and possible impact of publication bias
    (c) the implications of the effect of different model selection strategies, and exploration of a
        reasonable range of values for missing data from studies with uncertain results

9 **Reporting the results:** Clear presentation of key aspects of all of the above stages in the study report, in order to enable critical appraisal and replication of the systematic review. These should include a table of key elements of each primary study. Graphical displays can also assist interpretation and should be included where appropriate. Confidence intervals around pooled point estimates should be reported.

10 **Assessment and recommendations of review:** Appraisal of methodological limitations of both the primary studies and the systematic review. Any clinical or policy recommendations should be practical and explicit, and make clear the research evidence on which they are based. Proposal of a future research agenda should include clinical and methodological requirements as appropriate.

Figure 1 *Recommendations for meta-analytical practice.*

stages of carrying out a systematic review. The whole process is however, outlined here in a set of guidelines (Figure 1). For the most part these follow standard and widely agreed guidelines published previously.[3-5] The reader is recommended to consult these[3,4] for detailed descriptions of the procedural stages required in carrying out a high-quality systematic review. After a brief description of the project methods, it is meta-analytic methods (or quantitative synthesis – described in point 6 of the recommendations in Figure 1) on which we focus our attention for the remainder of this chapter. The review identified a considerable body of work on this topic, with increasingly sophisticated methods being developed over time. This is an area where previous guidelines have been less detailed. In addition to development of general methods, much research has been carried out which focuses on meta-analysis of specific outcome measures and data types, as well as other problems researchers face at the meta-analytic stage of a systematic review.

EXAMPLE: EFFECT ON MORTALITY OF LOWERING SERUM CHOLESTEROL LEVELS

A meta-analysis of cholesterol-lowering trials is used to illustrate the methods throughout the chapter. Since 1962 a series of randomised controlled trials (RCTs) have investigated the effect of lowering cholesterol levels on the risk from all-cause mortality, as well as specific causes. Our example draws on a data set consisting of 34 RCTs, originally analysed by Smith et al.[6] (see this paper for a listing of these trials; numbering in this chapter corresponds to theirs, although knowledge of this is not necessary). It should be noted that since this review was completed, further relevant trials have been carried out. It therefore should be stressed that the analyses presented are to *illustrate* the various methods discussed, and are in no way meant to provide a definitive analysis. The binary outcome used in the primary studies is total mortality.

AN INTRODUCTION TO META-ANALYTIC METHODS INCORPORATING FIXED EFFECTS MODELS

This section considers methods for combining binary outcome measures, which are probably the most common type of outcome used when assessing medical interventions. However, continuous and ordinal outcomes are also used;

these are mentioned briefly below, and further details given in Sutton et al.[2] Here, a practical approach is adopted throughout, with algebra and formulae kept to a minimum (though references are given to where technical details can be obtained). Fortunately, software is becoming available to implement all the methods described below, much of it freely available. A detailed review of this topic has been published elsewhere,[7] and software is available via the internet at *http://www.prw.le.ac.uk/epidemio/personal/kra1/srotos.html*; the reader is referred to these for details of practical implementation.

All the methods described below focus on pooling treatment estimates from different studies. This yields an overall pooled estimate of treatment effect, together with a confidence interval. Methods which only tally the numbers of studies showing beneficial and harmful effects, known as vote-counting, and ones which pool the *P*-values of significance tests from each study also exist.[8] Neither of these methods produces an overall pooled estimate and, due to this and other drawbacks, are not recommended for routine use and are not considered further here.

Binary Outcomes

When outcome data are binary in form, several different measures of treatment effect may be used (and are used in varying degrees of popularity); these are described briefly below. Firstly, it is convenient to arrange the data from each trial into the form of tables, like the one illustrated below in Table 1.

For example, cholesterol trial 16 (see the first line of Table 2) takes values: $a = 174$; $b = 250$; $c = 178$; and $d = 244$.

The odds ratio

The odds ratio can then be calculated by the formula $\frac{ad}{bc}$. This measure gives a relative measure of risk in the form of the ratio of the odds of an event in the two groups.[9] An odds ratio of less than 1, when comparing a new treatment to the control, would indicate an improvement on the new treatment; while a ratio greater than 1 would imply that the new treatment was less effective than any treatment received by the control group.

Table 1 *Outcome data from a single study*

	Failure/death	Success/alive
New treatment	a	b
Control	c	d

For the purposes of combining it is common – and recommended – to work in terms of the log odds ratios to provide a measure which is approximately normally distributed.[10] The estimate and corresponding confidence interval obtained can then be converted back onto an odds ratio scale by taking anti-logarithms. The (large sample) variance (a measure of the precision) of the natural log of the odds ratio is given by:

$$v_{Ln(OR)} = \frac{1}{a} + \frac{1}{b} + \frac{1}{c} + \frac{1}{d}. \qquad (1)$$

Other measures of effect based on binary outcome data

In addition to the odds ratio, other measures of comparative effect can be calculated from binary outcome data. The relative risk – defined as the probability of an event in the treatment group divided by the probability of an event in the control group – is one such alternative. Another is the risk difference – the difference between the probabilities of an event in the two groups. The reciprocal of the risk difference is often called the number needed to treat,[11] as it can be interpreted as the number of patients that need to be treated using the experimental treatment rather than the placebo/old treatment in order to prevent one additional adverse event. Less commonly used are the relative risk reduction (1 minus the relative risk), and the Phi coefficient, which can be used when a measure of the correlation (rather than difference) is required between two dichotomous variables.[12]

Which scale to use?

When deciding on the choice of measure to summarise studies, two opposing considerations are present: (i) whether it is statistically convenient to work with; and (ii) whether it conveys the necessary clinically useful information.[13] The number needed to treat is a measure that is being used increasingly when reporting the results of clinical trials. The motivation for its use is that it is more useful than the odds ratio and the relative risk for clinical decision-making.[11] However, its role as a measure of comparative treatment effects is limited.[14] Detailed discussions of the relative merits of using the other scales have been reported.[10,13] Historically, the odds ratio is most commonly reported for RCTs, while relative risks are often used for reporting observational studies. One should be aware that while analyses using different scales will often come to the same conclusion, in some instances considerably different results will be obtained.[15]

A simple fixed effects approach to meta-analysis: the inverse variance method

A simple model for pooling estimates from individual studies, often called the inverse variance-weighted method, can be calculated for all measurement scales and data types using the same general formula presented below. The method was first described by Birge[16] and Cochran[17] in the 1930s. The model assumes that all population effect sizes are equal, that is to say, the studies are all estimating one single true value underlying all the study results, hence the name fixed effects model. A mean effect size is calculated, giving each study estimate a weight directly proportional to its precision (i.e. inversely proportional to their variance).

More formally, for $i = 1, \ldots, k$ independent studies to be combined; let T_i be the observed effect size. A general formula for the weighted average effect size ($\bar{T}$) for these studies is thus:

$$\bar{T} = \frac{\sum\limits_{i=1}^{k} w_i T_i}{\sum\limits_{i=1}^{k} w_i}, \qquad (2)$$

where the optimal weights are inversely proportional to the variance in each study,[18] i.e.

$$w_i = \frac{1}{v_i}. \qquad (3)$$

The explicit variance formulae depends on the effect measure being combined. The formula for the variance of an odds ratio is given above; an exhaustive list of variance formulae for other measures has been reported elsewhere.[10,19] Approximate 95% confidence intervals can then be calculated for this pooled estimate:[12]

$$\bar{T} - 1.96 \times \sqrt{\frac{1}{\sum\limits_{i=1}^{k} w_i}} \leq \theta \leq \bar{T} + 1.96 \times \sqrt{\frac{1}{\sum\limits_{i=1}^{k} w_i}}, \quad (4)$$

where θ is the true treatment effect. On the mathematical level, this is essentially all that is required to synthesise study treatment effects at a basic level, though other 'real world' issues need considering, outlined later and in the guidelines. For a fuller coverage of this method see Fleiss,[12] or Shadish et al.[18]

Pooling the cholesterol data using the inverse-variance weighted method

For this illustrative analysis, only a subset of the 34 RCTs will be used. The subset of trials chosen consists of those in which patients were largely without pre-existing cardiovascular disease, so that cholesterol lowering was implemented predominantly as a primary intervention (identification (id.) numbers 16, 20, 24, 28, 29, 30 and 31). For clarity, data from these seven trials is reproduced in Table 2.

The odds ratio (OR) for each study is calculated (e.g. study id. 16: $OR = (174 \times 244)/(250 \times 178) = 0.954$). As previously mentioned, it is advisable to log transform the data before combining (e.g., id. 16: $LOR = -0.051$). The variance of LOR is calculated (e.g., id. 16: $Var(LOR) = 1/250 + 1/174 + 1/244 + 1/178 = 0.0195$). Confidence intervals for LOR can be constructed (e.g., id. 16: $-0.051 \pm 1.96 \sqrt{0.0195} = [-0.31$ to $0.22]$), and transforming back to the odds ratio scale (e.g., id. 16: $[e^{(-0.31)}$ to $e^{(0.22)}] = [0.73$ to $1.25]$).

The eighth column of Table 2 displays the point estimates along with their 95% CI for all seven studies. It can be seen from Table 2 that three of the point estimates are below one, indicating a reduced risk for people on the treatment (cholesterol-reducing) and four are above one indicating an increased risk for the treatment. However, with the exception of that for study 31, every confidence interval includes one. From this, we conclude that no significant treatment effect was detected when considering each study separately. The 95% CI of study 31 spans 1.07 to 1.59, indicating evidence of a statistically significant increased risk for the patients in the treatment arm. By combining these studies it is hoped that an estimate which is more generalisable than any of the individual study results (not least because studies using different populations are being combined), and more precise (through reducing the effect of sampling variations in estimates based on smaller numbers) can be produced.

The weighting given to each study (w_i) needs to be calculated; using the inverse variance-weighted method, this is simply equal to 1/Var(LOR) (e.g., for study 16: $w_i = 1/0.0195 = 51.38$). Column 11 of Table 2 shows the values for the rest of the studies.

Combining the results using formula, [Equation (2)], gives a point estimate of the log odds ratio: $LOR =$

$$\frac{[(51.38 \times -0.05) + \ldots + (98.489 \times 0.27)]}{(51.38 + \ldots + 98.48)}$$

$= 0.085$. An estimate of its variance is given by the reciprocal of the sum of the weights (i.e. $1/\sum_{i=1}^{k} w_i$); hence the standard error (square root of the variance) is given by: $SE(LOR) = \sqrt{1/(51.38 + \ldots + 98.48)} = 0.054$. Calculating

a 95% confidence interval for this pooled estimate using Equation (4), and converting back to the odds ratio scale gives: $OR = 1.09$ (0.98 to 1.21).

The results of this analysis are displayed graphically in Figure 2. This is a very common way of displaying the results of a meta-analysis, sometimes known as a forest plot. Each study's point estimate, together with its 95% CI, is displayed. The size of the box representing each point estimate is inversely proportional to the variance of the study, and hence proportional to the weight of that study in the analysis. Below the estimates of each study is the pooled estimate together with its 95% confidence interval. Results using two other methods are also displayed in this figure. These are described later.

The combined odds ratio is slightly greater than 1. However, because its corresponding confidence interval includes one, a conclusion that no evidence of a treatment effect exists is drawn from the combined results of the seven studies. The confidence interval around this estimate is narrow due to the large numbers of patients/events combined, and only just crosses unity. From this illustrative analysis, the possibility that cholesterol-lowering treatment may actually be harmful as a primary intervention cannot be ruled out.

Other fixed effect methods for combining odds ratios

Other fixed effect methods, specific to combining odds ratios, have been proposed. Under most conditions the estimates obtained from each method should be very similar to one another, but there are circumstances where they differ markedly.

A common alternative to the above is the Mantel–Haenszel method;[20] the use of which for meta-analysis has been described previously.[12] A variance estimate of the treatment effect calculated in this manner has been derived.[21,22] Using the Mantel–Haenszel estimate, a study with zero total events is completely excluded from the analysis if no continuity correction is used. This is unappealing, as a trial with zero events from 200 subjects would then be equally non-informative as a trial with no events but only 20 subjects. To get round this problem it has been recommended[23] that a continuity correction (adding 0.5 to each cell) should be used for sparse data. Another common method, first described by Peto et al.,[24] and more thoroughly by Yusuf et al.,[25] can be regarded as a modification of the Mantel–Haenszel method. An advantage it has over the latter method is that it can be used, without any corrections, if there are zeros

Table 2   Results of the seven primary studies investigating the effect of cholesterol lowering on mortality

Study id. number	No of subjects in treatment arm (nt)	No of subjects in control arm (nc)	No of deaths in treatment arm (dt) = a	No of deaths in the control arm (dc) = c	No still alive in treatment arm (nt − dt) = b	No still alive in the control arm (nc − dc) = d	Estimate of odds ratio (a × d)/(b × c) = OR [95% CI]	Log odds ratio (LOR) = ln(OR)	var(LOR) = 1/a + 1/b + 1/c + 1/d	w = 1/var(LOR)
16	424	422	174	178	250	244	0.95 [0.73, 1.25]	−0.051	0.0195	51.38
20	1149	1129	37	48	1112	1081	0.75 [0.48, 1.16]	−0.288	0.0497	20.13
24	4541	4516	269	248	4272	4268	1.08 [0.91, 1.29]	0.077	0.0082	121.68
28	1906	1900	68	71	1838	1829	0.95 [0.68, 1.34]	−0.051	0.0300	33.47
29	2051	2030	44	43	2007	1987	1.01 [0.66, 1.55]	0.010	0.0465	21.28
30	6582	1663	33	3	6549	1660	2.79 [0.85, 9.10]	1.026	0.3644	2.74
31	5331	5296	236	181	5095	5115	1.31 [1.07, 1.59]	0.270	0.0102	98.48

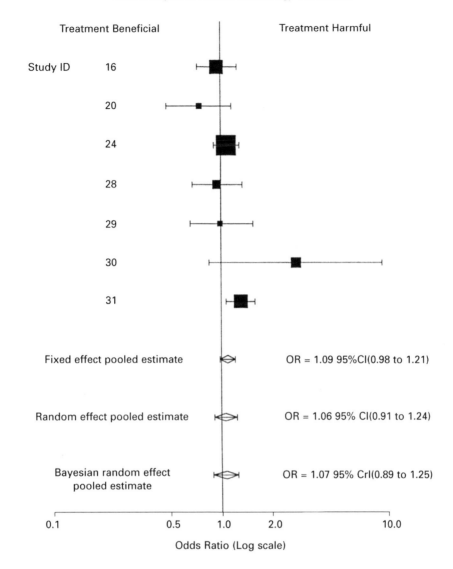

Figure 2 *Forest plot of RCTs of cholesterol lowering: results of meta-analysis using fixed effects, random effects and Bayesian models.*

present in cells for any of the studies. Combining the cholesterol studies using these two methods produces virtually the same results as the inverse variance-weighted method.

Having a number of different approaches to combine odds ratios at the researchers disposal, it would be desirable to have guidelines indicating when particular methods are most appropriate. The Peto method has come under strong criticism as it has been demonstrated that it is capable of producing seriously biased odds ratios and corresponding standard errors when there is severe imbalance in the numbers in the two groups being compared,[26] or when the estimated odds ratio is far from unity.[12] Conditions

have been described previously[27] for which the inverse-weighted and the Mantel–Haenszel methods are to be preferred respectively. If the number of studies to be combined is small, but the within-study sample sizes per study are large, the inverse-weighted method should be used. If one has many studies to combine, but the within-study sample size in each study is small, the Mantel–Haenszel method is preferred. Comparisons between the various methods have been carried out.[26] Other maximum likelihood and exact methods which are available[28–30] are only worth considering if cells from several studies have less than five observations, due to the much increased computation involved.

Combining Outcomes Measured on a Continuous Scale

Many of the continuous scales used to measure outcomes in the medical literature such as lung function, pulse rate, weight and blood pressure have the commonality that they are measured on a positive scale. For this reason it is possible – and common practice – to use a logarithmic transformation, after which the data are usually assumed to be normally distributed (a condition which is required for statistical inferences).[30] Usually, the value of interest is the difference in effect size between the treatment and control groups. If it can be assumed that all the studies estimate the same parameter, and that the estimates of continuous outcome measures are approximately normal, then the inverse variance-weighted method can be used directly, combining the data in their original metric. If different studies measured their outcomes on different scales then synthesis is still possible, but the data must first be standardised. This can be achieved by dividing the difference of interest by an estimate of its standard deviation; possible estimates of this standard deviation are discussed by Hedges and Olkin.[8] However, it should be noted that by doing this the resulting estimate may be difficult to interpret clinically. If the data are censored in any way, as is often the case for survival data, then special methods are needed.[2,31–33]

Combining Outcomes Measured on Ordinal Scales

If the outcome of interest is measured on a categorical scale and ordered in terms of desirability, then one can consider the data as ordinal, e.g. gastrointestinal damage is often measured by the number of lesions.[34] Two situations exist when combining ordinal data from different studies: (i) when the response variable (the outcome of interest) is the same in each study; and (ii) when different response variables are used in the studies. A unified framework has been described that can incorporate both possibilities.[35]

Assessing Heterogeneity

Using a fixed effects model to combine treatment estimates assumes no heterogeneity between the results of the studies; that is to say, the studies are all estimating a single 'true' value underlying all the study results. Hence, all observed variation in the treatment effects between the studies is considered due to sampling error

alone. Clearly, in many instances this may not seem realistic, possibly due to qualitative differences between the studies, e.g. differences in the way an intervention is administered, or differences between study populations. However, the decision will not always be clear-cut, and for this reason a formal test of heterogeneity is used as a guide to when the use of a fixed effect model is appropriate.

Test for Heterogeneity

The test devised by Cochran,[36] which is widely used, is given below (5). It tests the assumption that all the studies are estimating a single underlying effect size, and hence that the variation observed between study results is due to chance alone. The test involves calculating

$$Q = \sum_{i=1}^{k} w_i (T_i - \overline{T})^2, \qquad (5)$$

where k is the number of studies being combined, T_i is the treatment effect estimate in the ith study, and $\overline{T}$ is the inverse variance-weighted estimator of treatment effect (as calculated above), and w_i is the weight of that study (usually the inverse of the ith sampling variance) in the meta-analysis.

Q is approximately distributed χ^2 on $k - 1$ degrees of freedom under the null hypothesis, which is to say, when heterogeneity is not present. Hence, if the value for Q exceeds the upper-tail critical value of chi-square distribution with $k - 1$ degrees of freedom, the observed variance in study effect sizes is significantly greater than that expected by chance if all studies are estimating a common population effect size. Thus, one concludes that an assumption of homogeneity is not appropriate.

Choosing an appropriate critical value for this test is made difficult because of its low statistical power.[37] This means heterogeneity may indeed be present even if the Q statistic is not statistically significant. As a consequence, using a cut-off significance level of 0.10, rather than the usual 0.05, has been recommended.[38] This has become a customary practice in meta-analysis. The potential presence of publication biases (see later and Chapter 21) makes the interpretation of heterogeneity tests more complex.[39]

In addition to the formal test, several plots have been advocated to assist the exploration of heterogeneity in meta-analysis; these include a radial plot,[40] L'Abbé plot,[41,42] and a plot of normalized (z) scores[43] as well as the forest plot.

Due to the limitations of the test, and because it is unrealistic for there to be no between study heterogeneity (all studies vary in at least some respects), it has been suggested that rather than testing for heterogeneity, quantifying estimates of the between-study variability and incorporating these into the model is a more sensible approach.[44] In this way, some of the heterogeneity between studies is accounted for when inferences about the intervention effect are being made. This is addressed below using random effects models.

Cholesterol data example

Applying the test to the seven primary cholesterol studies produces a value of 10.1854 for Q. This is compared to a chi-squared statistic on six ($n - 1$ studies) degrees of freedom, giving a P-value of 0.117. In this case $P > 0.1$, and is therefore non-significant, but the result is marginal. It is clearly possible that study results may vary by a greater amount than chance alone would permit, and hence it is wise to consider using a method that would take this extra variation into account. These are described below.

RANDOM EFFECTS MODELS

Random effects models can be used when the assumption that all the studies are estimating the same underlying effect size is violated, and heterogeneity is present. Many meta-analysts regard the random effects model as always more appropriate than the fixed effects model for combining studies, regardless of the result of the test for heterogeneity.[45]

This model takes into account an extra variation component implied by assuming that the studies are estimating different (underlying) effect sizes. In addition, the variation caused by sampling error described in the fixed effects model is still present. These underlying effects are assumed to vary at random; to make modelling possible, they are assumed to vary according to a given distribution (usually the Normal).[46] This assumption has caused much dispute, since

each study is regarded as coming from a population of similar studies, a concept some people feel is unrealistic, though random effects models have a long history in other fields of application.

Hence, the total variation of the estimated effect size can be broken down into two components:

$$\begin{matrix} \text{Variance of} \\ \text{estimated} \\ \text{effects} \end{matrix} = \begin{matrix} \text{Between-study} \\ \text{random effects} \\ \text{variance} \end{matrix} + \begin{matrix} \text{Within-study} \\ \text{estimation} \\ \text{variance} \end{matrix}$$

If the random effects variance were zero, the above model would reduce exactly to the fixed effects model. Details of estimation of the underlying mean effects size and variance components parameters is omitted, but have been described clearly elsewhere.[18,46] Computer code is recommended for their practical implementation.[7] Random effects models can also be derived using Bayesian methods, an approach which is described later in this chapter.

Pooling the Cholesterol Data Example Using a Random Effects Model

The same studies used previously are combined below using a random effects model. Table 3 shows the weightings given to each study in the fixed and random effects models.

It is instructive to examine how these relative weightings differ between models. Using the random effects model, the larger studies have been down-weighted while the relative weighting of the smaller studies is increased. This trend generally holds true as the within-study weights are 'diluted' by the inclusion of the between study term.

Using the random effects model produces a pooled point estimate odds ratio of 1.06, and associated 95% confidence interval (0.91 to 1.24). The model estimates τ^2, the between-study variance, at 0.014.

A plot of the pooled results is included in Figure 2. This result can be compared with those obtained from fitting a fixed effects model.

Table 3   *Weighting of studies used in the random and fixed effects models*

Study id.	T_i	$\ln(T_i)$	w_i (% of total) (fixed effect)	w_i^* (% of total) (random effect)
16	0.95	−0.051	51.37 (14.7)	28.20 (17.3)
20	0.75	−0.288	20.13 (5.8)	15.23 (9.3)
24	1.08	0.077	121.68 (38.9)	41.29 (25.3)
28	0.95	−0.051	33.47 (9.6)	21.80 (13.4)
29	1.01	0.010	21.28 (6.1)	15.87 (9.7)
30	2.79	1.026	2.74 (0.8)	2.62 (1.6)
31	1.31	0.270	98.48 (28.2)	38.23 (23.4)

There, the point estimate was 1.09, slightly higher than that of the random effects model above (1.06). Comparing confidence intervals, using a fixed effects model gives 0.98 to 1.21, whilst using a random effects model gave 0.91 to 1.24. The random effects derived interval is thus wider, incorporating both higher and lower values than that of the corresponding fixed effects one. This will generally hold true; the random effects confidence interval will be wider, reflecting the inclusion of between study heterogeneity. Although the overall conclusion is similar to that given earlier by the fixed effects model – the treatment effect is non-significant – the result is more conservative.

Extensions to the Random Effects Model

One drawback of this model is that the sampling variance is assumed to be known, although in reality it is estimated from the data,[46] which means that the uncertainty associated with this estimation is not taken into account. Two recent advances have attempted to address this problem,[47,48] both of which produce confidence intervals which are wider than those by the traditional model described above, when the number of studies being combined is small. A further extension of the random effects model is a likelihood approach which avoids the use of approximating Normal distributions, and can be used when the assumptions of normality are violated.[49]

Debate over Choice Between Fixed Versus Random Effects Models

The argument over which model is theoretically superior has been running for many years, with many comments scattered throughout the literature. Random effects models have been criticised on grounds that unrealistic/unjustified distributional assumptions have to be made.[50] However, it has also been argued that they are consistent with the aims of generalisation of results of the meta-analysis.[51] A further consideration is that random effects models are more sensitive to publication bias.[52] Thus, neither fixed nor random effect analyses can be considered ideal.[45] As the next section discusses, it is better to explain the underlying causes of heterogeneity, if possible.

META-REGRESSION AND MIXED MODELS

Random effects models *account* for heterogeneity between studies, while meta-regression provides the researcher with a tool for exploring, and ultimately *explaining*, heterogeneity between studies by including study level covariates in the analysis. Investigating why study results vary systematically can lead to discovery of associations between study or patient characteristics and the outcome measure, not possible in the analysis of single studies (not least due to lack of power). This in turn can lead to clinically important findings and may eventually assist in individualising treatment regimes.[53] Covariates may characterise study design features, e.g. the dose level of a treatment, or may represent the mean of characteristics of patients, e.g. patient age in the study.

These modelling techniques can be used for the synthesis of randomised clinical trials or observational studies (for examples of its use, see Dickersin and Berlin[54]). In both cases, dose–response modelling is possible.[55,56] Modelling of effects of the underlying risk of patients is also feasible, but specialist methods are required,[57–60] due to the underlying problem of regression to the mean.[61] If regression to the mean is not accounted for properly, it will cause an exaggerated relationship between baseline risk and the outcome to be observed.

It should be stressed, however, that this type of analysis should be treated as exploratory, as associations between characteristics and the outcome can occur purely by chance, or may be due to the presence of confounding factors. Regression analysis of this type is also susceptible to ecological bias, which occurs if the relation between study means and outcomes do not correspond to the relations between individuals values and individuals outcomes.[62] Regression-type models are most useful when the number of studies is large, and cannot be sensibly attempted when very small numbers of studies are being combined.[51] A further restriction is that the data on covariates required may be limited in study reports.

Two main types of regression model are possible: one an extension of the fixed effects model, commonly known as a meta-regression model; and the other an extension of the random effects model, called a mixed model (because it includes both fixed and random terms). The meta-regression model is most appropriate when all variation (above that explainable by sampling error) between study outcomes can be considered accountable by the covariates included. A mixed model is appropriate when the predictive covariates only explain part of the variation/heterogeneity, as the random effect term can account for the remainder. However, in parallel to earlier argument concerning fixed and random effects models, it has been suggested that one should always include a random effects term as there will always be some degree of unexplainable heterogeneity.[63]

Several authors have put forward extensions/alternatives to the basic model.[64,65] Further extensions of mixed models are discussed in the Generalized Synthesis of Evidence (p. 403) and Bayesian (p. 402) methods sections below.

Fixed Effects Regression Model

A general meta-regression model, which can include continuous and discrete predictor variables, is clearly explained by Hedges et al.,[66] and is briefly summarised below. Taking the fixed effects model as a starting point; suppose now, that there are p known covariates $X_1, \ldots, X_p$ which are believed to be related to the effects via a linear model. Let $x_{i1}, \ldots, x_{ip}$ be the values of the covariates $X_1, \ldots, X_p$ for the ith study and $\beta_0, \beta_1, \ldots, \beta_p$ be the unknown regression coefficients, to be estimated, indicating the relationship between its associated covariate and the outcome. Then the $\beta_0 + \beta_1 x_{i1} + \ldots + \beta_p x_{ip}$ estimates the mean effect in the ith study.

The coefficients in the model are calculated via weighted least squares algorithms; any standard statistical package that performs weighted (multiple) regression can be used.[7]

When binary outcomes are being combined, a possible alternative to the above is to use logistic regression. This allows the outcome variables to be modelled directly (on the odds ratio scale), and removes the need for the normality assumption (see Sutton et al.[7] and Thompson[45] for details).

Cholesterol data example

Returning to the cholesterol-lowering trials, one covariate that the dataset includes is absolute cholesterol reduction. This is a measure of the difference in cholesterol reduction, on average, between the two arms in the RCTs. It seems reasonable to speculate that the trials in which a greater degree of lowering occurred may have achieved a more favourable treatment effect and hence produced a lower odds ratio estimate. This can be investigated using regression methods. The analysis is restricted to those nine trials in which diet was the main intervention (i.e. not the same ones as used before), and the relevant data are provided in Table 4. A fixed effects regression model, including absolute cholesterol reduction as a single covariate yielded the following model: $\ln(OR) = 0.034 - 0.208 \times$ (absolute cholesterol reduction). The standard error terms for the constant and cholesterol reduction coefficients are 0.26 and 0.36 respectively. The

Table 4 *Data used in the regression and mixed modelling examples*

Study id. number	Log odds ratio (LOR)	variance of LOR	Cholesterol reduction (mmol/l)
1	−0.71	0.073	0.4
7	−0.38	0.059	1.1
8	−0.13	0.124	0.6
9	−0.003	0.023	0.3
16	−0.23	0.049	0.9
17	−0.03	0.090	1.0
21	0.42	0.076	0.3
22	1.13	0.845	0.6
24	0.12	0.035	0.7

cholesterol reduction coefficient is negative, suggesting that trials in which cholesterol was lowered by greater amounts showed larger treatment benefits. However, the improvement in the model by including such a term is far from statistically significant ($P = 0.59$), and certainly further research would be needed to confirm such a result. (Thompson,[45] analysing a different set of cholesterol trials, and using a different outcome, did establish a significant relationship.) The trials, together with the fitted line, are displayed in Figure 3, where the size of the circular plotting symbol is proportional to the size of the trial.

Mixed Models (Random-Effects Regression)

A full description of mixed models for meta-analysis follows a logical extension of the regression model given above, and has been given elsewhere.[51,63] Their implementation is slightly more complex, but appropriate software is available.[7]

Cholesterol data example

The analysis carried out in the previous section using a fixed effects meta-regression model, may be repeated, this time using a mixed model. The model fitted is: $\ln(OR) = 0.081 - 0.239 \times$ (absolute cholesterol reduction), which has coefficients that are only marginally different from those of the previous model. The standard error terms for the constant and cholesterol reduction coefficients are 0.27 and 0.38 respectively, which are marginally larger than before due to the incorporation of a between-study variance term (estimate $= 0.052$). Again, the co-

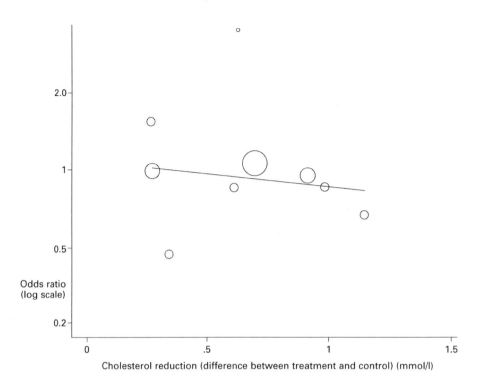

Figure 3 *Regression plot of cholesterol-lowering trials using diet: log odds ratio against absolute reduction in cholesterol (between arms), together with regression line.*

efficient for cholesterol reduction is not statistically significant.

BAYESIAN METHODS IN META-ANALYSIS

Over the past few years, Bayesian methods have become more frequently used in a number of areas of healthcare research, including meta-analysis.[67–69] Though much of this increase in their use has been directly as a result of advances in computational methods, it has also been partly due to their more appealing nature, and also specifically the fact that they overcome some of the difficulties encountered by other methods traditionally used. Philosophical and practical issues regarding their application in a number of areas in HTA are discussed in Chapter 16.

Many of the authors who have considered a Bayesian approach to meta-analysis have implemented a hierarchical model, frequently also making an assumption of Normality at one or more levels of the hierarchy.[70–75] For an up-to-date review and exposition of the Bayesian approach to meta-analysis, see Hedges et al.[76] In other areas of statistical science such Bayesian

hierarchical models have been used for some considerable time.[77,78] Whilst the underlying structure of such models is similar to that assumed for the random effects model described previously, the Bayesian formulation requires that prior distributions are specified for the mean effect size, and the between- and within-study variances. In estimating the parameters of such models a distinction should be drawn between *empirical* and *fully* Bayesian methods: a fully Bayesian approach specifies the prior distributions completely, whereas empirical Bayesian methods estimate such prior distributions from the data.[79] In a meta-analysis setting, empirical Bayes approaches have received much attention in the literature, as until recently the use of a fully Bayesian approach has been hampered by computational difficulties.[80–86]

Choice of Prior Distributions

When adopting a fully Bayesian approach considerable flexibility exists as to the specification of the prior distributions for the mean effect and the between- and within-study variances, though this is a non-trivial task, and the specific choice of prior distributions has recently received considerable attention.[87,88]

Having specified the prior distributions in terms of the relevant model parameters, estimation can then proceed using one of a number of computational approaches. However, the assumption of Normality that is frequently made – combined with the fact that there are often a reasonable number of studies in any specific meta-analysis – make such models particularly suited to Markov Chain Monte Carlo (MCMC) methods.[89] In particular, Gibbs sampling has been increasingly used in applied Bayesian analyses within a healthcare research setting[68,89,90] and a specific package BUGS[91] has been developed to facilitate its implementation.

Cholesterol data example

A fully Bayesian analysis is carried out on the cholesterol data in Table 2. Gibbs sampling, implemented via BUGS, was used for the analysis. Details of how this is done have been given elsewhere.[74] The posterior mean for the odds ratio was estimated to be 1.07 with an associated 95% *Credibility Interval* (a Bayesian measure of uncertainty similar to a Classical confidence interval) from 0.89 to 1.25. This is plotted at the bottom of Figure 2. Similarly, the posterior mean for the between-study variance was estimated to be 0.0241 with an associated 95% Credibility Interval from 0.0007 to 0.1352. The overall estimate of the odds ratio can be seen to be very similar to that obtained using the Classical random effects model previously, but the 95% Credibility Interval is slightly wider, reflecting the fact that uncertainty regarding the between-study variance has now been accounted for.

GENERALISED SYNTHESIS OF EVIDENCE

Generalised synthesis of evidence is the term given to combination of evidence on efficacy or effectiveness of a particular technology derived from a number of sources, not necessarily sharing common biases and designs. Although RCTs may be considered the 'gold standard' approach to assess the efficacy of an intervention, in some circumstances in health technology assessment, randomised evidence will be less than adequate due to economic, organisational or ethical considerations.[92] In these situations, considering all the available evidence, including that from non-randomised studies (such as case-control, cohort and database or audit data) may be beneficial. In addition, while RCTs may provide a robust estimate of the efficacy of an intervention, assessment of other types of data, derived from

more general populations, may indicate better its likely effectiveness in practice.

In 1992, the Program Evaluation and Methodology Division of the U.S. General Accounting Office (GAO)[93] reported an approach for synthesising evidence from different sources. They called this new method cross-design synthesis, though they cite the confidence profile method of Eddy et al.[94] as an influence. Their idea was to create methodology for a new form of meta-analysis that aims to capture the strengths of multiple-study designs (and the evidence they include) whilst minimising their weaknesses.

Operational methodology, in the spirit of that laid out by the GAO, has been developed by Smith et al.[87] This combines studies with disparate designs into a single synthesis, using a Bayesian hierarchical model approach. The hierarchical nature of the model specifically allows for the quantitative within- and between-sources heterogeneity, whilst the Bayesian approach can accommodate a priori beliefs regarding qualitative differences between the various sources of evidence. Prior distributions may represent subjective beliefs elicited from experts, or they might represent other data based evidence, which though pertinent to the issue in question is not of a form that can be directly incorporated, such as data from animal experiments.[95] This model can be viewed as an extension of the standard random effects model[46] described above, but with an extra level of variation to allow for variability in effect sizes, and different weightings, between different sources.

It has yet to be established when such analyses are appropriate, as there is concern that including studies with poorer designs will weaken the analysis, though this issue is partially addressed by conducting sensitivity analyses under various assumptions. However, the issue of quality assessment across studies of different designs needs addressing.

OTHER ISSUES IN META-ANALYSIS

Meta-Analysis of Observational and/or Epidemiological Studies

Many of the methods described above can be used to combine evidence from observational studies, but there may be problems additional to those encountered with RCTs.[43,96] A set of guidelines for the meta-analysis of environmental health data has been compiled,[97] much of which is applicable to observational studies in other areas.

Individual Patient Data

An alternative approach to combining aggregated study results is to gather individual patient data from the study investigators, and to carry out a meta-analysis at the patient level. Advantages of this approach include the ability to: (i) carry out detailed data checking; (ii) ensure the appropriateness of the analyses; (iii) update follow-up information; and (iv) carry out a survival-type analysis. Also, regression using patient level (as opposed to study level) covariates is possible.[98] These advantages come with the penalty that individual patient data meta-analyses are very time-consuming and costly.[99] It has yet to be established in which situations the extra effort is worthwhile.

Cumulative Meta-Analysis

Cumulative meta-analysis has been described as the process of performing a new meta-analysis every time a new trial relevant to a particular context is published.[100] Hence, it can be used to update meta-analyses and offers the care-giver and the healthcare consumer with answers regarding the effectiveness of a certain intervention at the earliest possible date.[101] Additionally, sequential combination of studies in chronological order, or ordered by some other factor, enables any trends present to be assessed.[102]

Economic Evaluation

Economic evaluations through meta-analysis are sometimes referred to as 'secondary economic evaluations', evaluations which use available data either alongside a review and meta-analysis of clinical trials, or as a summary of self-standing evaluations.[103] Despite the number of studies available, the process of reviewing and summing up economic evidence is relatively under-developed, and there are often problems due to substantial methodological variations between economic evaluations which on the surface appear similar.

Study Quality

It is common and desirable to assess the quality of the primary studies eligible for inclusion in the review. Exclusion of poor-quality studies, or at least a downweighting of them in a formal pooled analysis, may appear sensible, but no consensus has been reached as to the best way to proceed.

Publication and Related Biases

Publication biases exist because research yielding statistically significant, interesting, or 'welcome' results is more likely to be submitted, published or published quickly,[104] and published in English.[105] A commonly used method for detecting its presence is a plot of precision (such as the inverse of the effect size standard error or sample size) versus effect size; if no bias is present this plot should be shaped like a funnel, and hence is often referred to as a funnel plot.[106] If publication bias is present, the plot will typically be skewed, with a lack of small 'negative' studies. Recently, more formal statistical tests for its presence have been derived.[107,108] Methods also exist for adjusting the analysis when publication bias is suspected[109–111] but are still under development. The problem of publication bias is considered in more detail in Chapter 21.

Missing Data

Publication bias could be considered as data missing at the study level; less attention has been given to data missing from individual trials, such as relevant covariates. Although general methods such as imputation of unknown data do exist in other areas,[112] many of them have not been applied in a meta-analysis setting. There is clearly a need for the further development of appropriate methods in this area, particularly as the use of meta-regression increases.

Further Developments/Extensions to Meta-Analysis Methods

Although other methods for meta-analysis exist, these are mentioned only briefly here due to space limitations; further details can be found elsewhere.[2] Meta-analysis methods have been developed for the combination of specific types of data, such as time to event/survival,[31–33] and for data assessing the accuracy of diagnostic tests.[113] Extended methods are needed when multiple outcomes are being considered simultaneously in a single model.[114] Methods have also been developed which allow the meta-analysis of surrogate markers.[115,116] Some general approaches to meta-analysis are also being developed, e.g. prospective meta-analysis, where a meta-analysis is planned prior to the studies being carried out. This has the advantages that publication biases are minimised and a complete, pooled database is obtained with more consistent quality data across sites.[117]

DISCUSSION AND CONCLUSIONS

Systematic review methods including quantitative combination of study results are already common in health technology assessments (HTA) contexts, and are likely to become more common – perhaps almost universal – as moves towards evidence-based medicine and healthcare strengthen. This chapter describes the more basic and common methods of meta-analysis that may be employed, considers problems likely to be encountered in applications of meta-analysis in HTA, and briefly introduces other more complex or powerful approaches already established or under development. Some of these may prove especially valuable in HTA contexts.

REFERENCES

1. Sacks HS, Berrier J, Reitman D, Ancona-Berk VA, Chalmers TC. Meta-analysis of randomized controlled trials. *N. Engl. J. Med.* 1987; **316**: 450–5.

2. Sutton AJ, Abrams KR, Jones DR, Sheldon TA, Song F. Systematic reviews of trials and other studies. *Health Technology Assessment* 1998; 2(19).

3. Deeks J, Glanville J, Sheldon T. Undertaking systematic reviews of research on effectiveness: CRD guidelines for those carrying out or commissioning reviews. York: CRD 1996, Report #4.

4. Oxman AD. *The Cochrane Collaboration handbook: preparing and maintaining systematic reviews.* Oxford: Cochrane Collaboration, 1996.

5. Cook DJ, Sackett DL, Spitzer WO. Methodologic guidelines for systematic reviews of randomized control trials in health care from the Potsdam Consultation on Meta-Analysis. *J. Clin. Epidemiol.* 1995; **48**: 167–71.

6. Smith GD, Song F, Sheldon TA, Song FJ. Cholesterol lowering and mortality: The importance of considering initial level of risk. *Br. Med. J.* 1993; **306**: 1367–73.

7. Sutton AJ, Lambert PC, Hellmich M, Abrams KR, Jones DR. Meta-analysis in practice: a critical review of available software. In: Berry DA, Strangl DK (eds). *Meta-analysis in medicine and health policy.* New York: Marcel Dekker, 2000.

8. Hedges LV, Olkin I. *Statistical Methods for meta-analysis.* London: Academic Press, 1985.

9. Meinert CL. *Clinical trials dictionary: Terminology and usage recommendations.* Baltimore, Maryland: The Johns Hopkins Center for Clinical Trials, 1996.

10. Fleiss JL. Cooper H, Hedges LV (eds). *The handbook of research synthesis.* Chapter 17, Measures of effect size for categorical data. New York: Russell Sage Foundation, 1994, pp. 245–60.

11. Cook RJ, Sackett DL. The number needed to treat: a clinically useful measure of treatment effect. *Br. Med. J.* 1995; **310**: 452–4.

12. Fleiss JL. The statistical basis of meta-analysis. *Stat. Methods. Med. Res.* 1993; **2**: 121–45.

13. Sinclair JC, Bracken MB. Clinically useful measures of effect in binary analyses of randomized trials. *J. Clin. Epidemiol.* 1994; **47**: 881–9.

14. Dowie J. The number needed to treat and the 'adjusted NNT' in health care decision making. Presented at the conference 'From Research Evidence to Recommendations Exploring the Methods'; Harrogate 17–18 February 1997 (unpublished).

15. Deeks JJ, Altman DG, Dooley G, Sackett DLS. Choosing an appropriate dichotomous effect measure for meta-analysis: empirical evidence of the appropriateness of the odds ratio and relative risk. *Controlled Clinical Trials* 1997; **18**: 84s–85s.

16. Birge RT. The calculation of errors by the method of least squares. *Physiol. Rev.* 1932; **16**: 1–32.

17. Cochran WG. Problems arising in the analysis of a series of similar experiments. *J. Roy. Statist. Soc.* 1937; **4** (Suppl.): 102–18.

18. Shadish WR, Haddock CK. Cooper H, Hedges LV (eds). *The handbook of research synthesis.* Chapter 18, Combining estimates of effect size. New York: Russell Sage Foundation, 1994, pp. 261–84.

19. Rosenthal R. Cooper H, Hedges LV (eds). *The handbook of research synthesis.* Chapter 16, Parametric measures of effect size. New York: Russell Sage Foundation, 1994, pp. 231–44.

20. Mantel N, Haenszel W. Statistical aspects of the analysis of data from retrospective studies of disease. *J. Natl Cancer Inst.* 1959; **22**: 719–48.

21. Robins J, Breslow N, Greenland S. Estimators of the Mantel-Haenszel variance consistent in both sparse data and large-strata limiting models. *Biometrics* 1986; **42**: 311–23.

22. Robins J, Greenland S, Breslow NE. A general estimator for the variance of the Mantel-Haenszel odds ratio. *Am. J. Epidemiol.* 1986; **124**: 719–23.

23. Sankey SS, Weissfeld LA, Fine MJ, Kapoor W. An assessment of the use of the continuity correction for sparse data in meta-analysis. *Communications in Statistics-Simulation and Computation* 1996; **25**: 1031–56.

24. Peto R, Pike MC, Armitage P, Breslow NE, Cox DR, Howard SV, Mantel N, McPherson K, Peto J, Smith PG. Design and analysis of randomized clinical trials requiring prolonged observation of

each patient. II: Analysis and examples. *Br. J. Cancer* 1977; **35**: 1–39.

25. Yusuf S, Peto R, Lewis J, et al. Beta blockade during and after myocardial infarction: an overview of the randomised trials. *Prog. Cardiovasc. Dis.* 1985; **27**: 335–71.

26. Greenland S, Salvan A. Bias in the one-step method for pooling study results. *Stat. Med.* 1990; **9**: 247–52.

27. Fleiss JL. *Statistical methods for rates and proportions*. 2nd edn. New York: Wiley; 1981.

28. Emerson JD. Combining estimates of the odds ratio: the state of the art. *Stat. Methods Med. Res.* 1994; **3**: 157–78.

29. Hauck WW. A comparative study of conditional maximum likelihood estimation of a common odds ratio. *Biometrics* 1984; **40**: 1117–23.

30. Hasselblad VIC, McCrory DC. Meta-analytic tools for medical decision making: A practical guide. *Medical Decision Making* 1995; **15**: 81–96.

31. Dear KBG. Iterative generalized least squares for meta-analysis of survival data at multiple times. *Biometrics* 1994; **50**: 989–1002.

32. Hunink MGM, Wong JB. Meta-analysis of failure-time data with adjustment for covariates. *Medical Decision Making* 1994; **14**: 59–70.

33. Messori A, Rampazzo R. Metaanalysis of clinical-trials based on censored end-points – simplified theory and implementation of the statistical algorithms on a microcomputer. *Computer Methods and Programs in Biomedicine* 1993; **40**: 261–7.

34. Whitehead A, Jones NMB. A meta-analysis of clinical trials involving different classifications of response into ordered categories. *Stat. Med.* 1994; **13**: 2503–15.

35. Whitehead A, Whitehead J. A general parametric approach to the meta-analysis of randomised clinical trials. *Stat. Med.* 1991; **10**: 1665–77.

36. Cochran WG. The combination of estimates from different experiments. *Biometrics* 1954; **10**: 101–29.

37. Thompson SG, Pocock SJ. Can meta-analyses be trusted? *Lancet* 1991; **338**: 1127–30.

38. Fleiss JL. Analysis of data from multiclinic trials. *Controlled Clinical Trials* 1986; **7**: 267–75.

39. Matt GE, Cook TD. Cooper H, Hedges LV (eds). The handbook of research synthesis. Chapter 31, Threats to the validity of research synthesis. New York: Russell Sage Foundation, 1994, pp. 503–20.

40. Galbraith RF. A note on graphical presentation of estimated odds ratios from several clinical trials. *Stat. Med.* 1988; **7**: 889–94.

41. L'Abbé KA, Detsky AS, O'Rourke K. Meta-analysis in clinical research. *Ann. Intern. Med.* 1987; **107**: 224–33.

42. Sharp SJ, Thompson SG, Altman DG. The relation between treatment benefit and underlying risk in meta-analysis. *Br. Med. J.* 1996; **313**: 735–8.

43. Greenland S. Quantitative methods in the review of epidemiological literature. *Epidemiol. Rev.* 1987; **9**: 1–30.

44. National Research Council. *Combining Information: Statistical Issues and Opportunities for Research*. Washington, D.C. National Academy Press, 1992.

45. Thompson SG. Controversies in meta-analysis: the case of the trials of serum cholesterol reduction. *Stat. Methods Med. Res.* 1993; **2**: 173–92.

46. DerSimonian R, Laird N. Meta-analysis in clinical trials. *Controlled Clinical Trials* 1986; **7**: 177–88.

47. Hardy RJ, Thompson SG. A likelihood approach to meta-analysis with random effects. *Stat. Med.* 1996; **15**: 619–29.

48. Biggerstaff BJ, Tweedie RL. Incorporating variability in estimates of heterogeneity in the random effects model in meta-analysis. *Stat. Med.* 1997; **16**: 753–68.

49. Van Houwelingen HC, Zwinderman KH, Stijnen T. A bivariate approach to meta-analysis. *Stat. Med.* 1993; **12**: 2273–84.

50. Peto R. Why do we need systematic overviews of randomised trials? *Stat. Med.* 1987; **6**: 233–40.

51. Raudenbush SW. Cooper H, Hedges LV (eds). *The handbook of research synthesis*. Chapter 20, Random effects models. New York: Russell Sage Foundation, 1994, pp. 301–22.

52. Greenland S. Invited commentary: a critical look at some popular meta-analytic methods. *Am. J. Epidemiol.* 1994; **140**: 290–6.

53. Gelber RD, Goldhirsch A. The evaluation of subsets in meta-analysis. *Stat. Med.* 1987; **6**: 371–88.

54. Dickersin K, Berlin JA. Meta-analysis: state-of-the-science. *Epidemiol. Rev.* 1992; **14**: 154–76.

55. Tweedie RL, Mengersen KL. Meta-analytic approaches to dose-response relationships, with application in studies of lung cancer and exposure to environmental tobacco smoke. *Stat. Med.* 1995; **14**: 545–69.

56. Berlin JA, Longnecker MP, Greenland S. Meta-analysis of epidemiologic dose-response data. *Epidemiology* 1993; **4**: 218–28.

57. Thompson SG, Smith TC, Sharp SJ. Investigation underlying risk as a source of heterogeneity in meta-analysis. *Stat. Med.* 1997; **16**: 2741–58.

58. McIntosh MW. The population risk as an explanatory variable in research synthesis of clinical trials. *Stat. Med.* 1996; **15**: 1713–28.

59. Cook RJ, Walter SD. A logistic model for trend in $2 \times 2 \times$ kappa tables with applications to meta-analyses. *Biometrics* 1997; **53**: 352–7.

60. Walter SD. Variation in baseline risk as an explanation of heterogeneity in meta-analysis. *Stat. Med.* 1997; **16**: 2883–900.

61. Senn S. Importance of trends in the interpretation of an overall odds ratio in the meta-analysis of clinical trials. *Stat. Med.* 1994; **13**: 293–6.

62. Lau J, Ioannidis JP, Schmid CH. Summing up evidence: one answer is not always enough. *Lancet* 1998; **351**: 123–7.

63. Thompson SG, Sharp SJ. Explaining heterogeneity in meta-analysis: a comparison of methods. *Stat. Med.* 2000; **18**: 2693–708.

64. Berkey CS, Hoaglin DC, Mosteller F, Colditz GA. A random-effects regression model for meta-analysis. *Stat. Med.* 1995; **14**: 395–411.

65. Stram DO. Meta-analysis of published data using a linear mixed-effects model. *Biometrics* 1996; **52**: 536–44.

66. Hedges LV. Cooper H, Hedges LV (eds). *The handbook of research synthesis*. Chapter 19, Fixed effects models. New York: Russell Sage Foundation; 1994, pp. 285–300.

67. Breslow NE. Biostatisticians and Bayes (with discussion). *Statist. Sci.* 1990; **5**: 269–98.

68. Gilks WR, Clayton DG, Spiegelhalter D, Best NG, McNeil AJ, Sharples LD, Kirby AJ. Modelling complexity: applications of Gibbs sampling in medicine. *J. Roy. Statist. Soc. B* 1993; **55**: 39–52.

69. Berry DA, Stangl DK. *Bayesian Biostatistics*. New York: Marcel Dekker, 1996.

70. DuMouchel W, Berry DA (eds). *Statistical Methodology in the Pharmaceutical Sciences*. New York: Marcel Dekker, 1989, pp. 509–29.

71. DuMouchel WH, Harris JE. Bayes methods for combining the results of cancer studies in humans and other species (with comment). *J. Am. Statist. Assoc.* 1983; **78**: 293–308.

72. DuMouchel, W. Hierarchical Bayes linear models for meta-analysis. Research Triangle Park, NC: National Institute of Statistical Sciences, 1994; 27.

73. Abrams KR, Sanso B. Approximate Bayesian inference in random effects meta-analysis. *Stat. Med.* 1998; **17**: 201–18.

74. Smith TC, Spiegelhalter DJ, Thomas A. Bayesian approaches to random-effects meta-analysis: a comparative study. *Stat. Med.* 1995; **14**: 2685–99.

75. Skene AM, Wakefield JC. Hierarchical models for multicentre binary response studies. *Stat. Med.* 1990; **9**: 919–29.

76. Hedges LV. Everitt BS, Dunn G (eds). *Statistical analysis of medical data. New developments*. London: Arnold, 1998.

77. Box GEP; Tiao GC. *Bayesian inference in statistical analysis*. Massachusetts: Addison-Wesley; 1973.

78. Raiffa H, Schlaifer R. *Applied statistical decision theory*. Boston: Harvard Business School; 1961.

79. Louis TA. Estimating a population of parameter values using Bayes and empirical Bayes methods. *J. Am. Statist. Assoc.* 1984; **79**: 393–8.

80. Raudenbush SW, Bryk AS. Empirical Bayes meta-analysis. *J. Educ. Statist.* 1985; **10**: 75–98.

81. Zhou XH. Empirical Bayes combination of estimated areas under ROC curves using estimating equations. *Medical Decision Making* 1996; **16**: 24–8.

82. van Houwelingen HC, Stijnen T. Monotone empirical Bayes estimators based on more informative samples. *J. Am. Statist. Assoc.* 1993; **88**: 1438–43.

83. Waclawiw MA, Liang KY. Empirical Bayes estimation and inference for the random effects model with binary response. *Stat. Med.* 1994; **13**: 541–51.

84. Morris CN. Hierarchical models for combining information and for meta-analysis. *Bayesian Statistics* 1992; **4**: 321–44.

85. Stijnen T, Van Houwelingen JC. Empirical Bayes methods in clinical trials meta-analysis. *Biometrical J.* 1990; **32**: 335–46.

86. Carlin JB. Meta-analysis for 2×2 tables: a Bayesian approach. *Stat. Med.* 1992; **11**: 141–58.

87. Smith TC, Abrams KR, Jones DR. Using hierarchical models in generalised synthesis of evidence: an example based on studies of breast cancer screening. Department of Epidemiology and Public Health Technical Report 95-02. University of Leicester, 1995.

88. Smith TC, Abrams KR, Jones DR. Assessment of prior distributions and model parameterisation in hierarchical models for the generalised synthesis of evidence. Department of Epidemiology and Public Health Technical Report 96-01. University of Leicester, 1996.

89. Gilks WR, Richardson S, Spiegelhalter DJ. *Markov Chain Monte Carlo in practice*. London: Chapman & Hall, 1996.

90. Best NG, Spiegelhalter DJ, Thomas A, Brayne CEG. Bayesian analysis of realistically complex models. *J. Roy. Statist. Soc. A* 1996; **159**: 323–42.

91. Gilks WR, Thomas A, Spiegelhalter DJ. A language and program for complex Bayesian models. *The Statistician* 1994; **43**: 169–78.

92. Black N. Why we need observational studies to evaluate the effectiveness of health care. *Br. Med. J.* 1996; **312**: 1215–18.

93. General Accounting Office. *Cross design synthesis: a new strategy for medical effectiveness research*. Washington, DC. General Accounting Office, 1992.

94. Eddy DM, Hasselblad V, Shachter R. *Meta-analysis by the Confidence Profile Method*. San Diego: Academic Press, 1992.

95. Abrams KR, Hellmich M, Jones DR. Bayesian approach to health care evidence. Department of Epidemiology and Public Health Technical Report 97–01. University of Leicester, 1997.

96. Spitzer WO. Meta-meta-analysis: unanswered questions about aggregating data. *J. Clin. Epidemiol.* 1991; **44**: 103–7.

97. Blair A, Burg J, Foran J, et al. Guidelines for application of meta-analysis in environmental epidemiology. ISLI Risk Science Institute. *Regul. Toxicol. Pharmacol.* 1995: 189–97.

98. Boissel JP, Blanchard J, Panak E, Peyrieux JC, Sacks H. Considerations for the meta-analysis of randomized clinical trials: summary of a panel discussion. *Controlled Clinical Trials* 1989; **10**: 254–81.

99. Stewart LA, Clarke MJ. Practical methodology of meta-analyses (overviews) using updated individual patient data. Cochrane Working Group. *Stat. Med.* 1995; **14**: 2057–79.

100. Whiting GW, Lau J, Kupelnick B, Chalmers TC. Trends in inflammatory bowel disease therapy: a meta-analytic approach. *Can. J. Gastroenterol.* 1995; **9**: 405–11.

101. Antman EM, Lau J, Kupelnick B, Mosteller F, Chalmers TC. A comparison of results of meta-analyses of randomized control trials and recommendations of clinical experts: Treatments for myocardial infarction. *JAMA* 1992; **268**: 240–8.

102. Lau J, Schmid CH, Chalmers TC. Cumulative meta-analysis of clinical trials: builds evidence for exemplary medical care. *J. Clin. Epidemiol.* 1995; **48**: 45–57.

103. Jefferson T, DeMicheli V, Mugford M. *Elementary economic evaluation in health care. 8. Current issues*. London: BMJ Publishing Group, 1996.

104. Easterbrook PJ, Berlin JA, Gopalan R, Matthews DR. Publication bias in clinical research. *Lancet* 1991; **337**: 867–72.

105. Moher D, Fortin P, Jadad AR, Juni P, Klassen T, Le Lorier J, Liberati A, Linde K, Penna A. Completeness of reporting of trials published in languages other than English: implications for conduct and reporting of systematic reviews. *Lancet* 1996; **347**: 363–6.

106. Begg CB. Cooper H, Hedges LV (eds). *The handbook of research synthesis*. Chapter 25, Publication bias. New York: Russell Sage Foundation, 1994, pp. 399–409.

107. Begg CB, Mazumdar M. Operating characteristics of a rank correlation test for publication bias. *Biometrics* 1994; **50**: 1088–101.

108. Egger M, Smith GD, Schneider M, Minder C. Bias in meta-analysis detected by a simple, graphical test. *Br. Med. J.* 1997; **315**: 629–34.

109. Iyengar S, Greenhouse JB. Selection models and the file drawer problem. *Statist. Sci.* 1988; **3**: 109–35.

110. Dear KBG, Begg CB. An approach for assessing publication bias prior to performing a meta-analysis. *Statist. Sci.* 1992; **7**: 237–45.

111. Vevea JL, Hedges LV. A general linear model for estimating effect size in the presence of publication bias. *Psychometrika* 1995; **60**: 419–35.

112. Little RJA, Rubin DB. *Statistical analysis with missing data*. New York: Wiley, 1987.

113. Irwig L, Tosteson AN, Gatsonis C, Lau J, Colditz G, Chalmers TC, Mosteller F. Guidelines for meta-analyses evaluating diagnostic tests. *Ann. Intern. Med.* 1994; **120**: 667–76.

114. Berkey CS, Anderson JJ, Hoaglin DC. Multiple-outcome meta-analysis of clinical trials. *Stat. Med.* 1996; **15**: 537–57.

115. Daniels MJ, Hughes MD. Meta-analysis for the evaluation of potential surrogate markers. *Stat. Med.* 1997; **16**: 1965–82.

116. Tori V, Simon R, Russek-Cohen E, Midthune D, Friedman M. Statistical model to determine the relationship of response and survival in patients with advanced ovarian cancer treated with chemotherapy. *J. Natl Cancer Inst.* 1992; **84**: 407–14.

117. Margitic SE, Morgan TM, Sager MA, Furberg CD. Lessons learned from a prospective meta-analysis. *J. Am. Geriatr. Soc.* 1995; **43**: 435–9.

23

Assessing the Quality of Reports of Randomised Trials Included in Meta-Analyses: Attitudes, Practice, Evidence and Guides

DAVID MOHER, TERRY P. KLASSEN,
ALISON L. JONES, BA' PHAM, DEBORAH J. COOK,
ALEJANDRO R. JADAD, PETER TUGWELL
and MICHAEL MOHER

SUMMARY

Only limited information exists regarding the views of a broad spectrum of health service professionals involved in the conduct of meta-analyses, regarding quality assessment. Similarly, the extent to which meta-analysts assess trial quality, and how they incorporate a measure of its effect into the quantitative data synthesis, is limited. Although there is increasing evidence regarding the effects that low-quality trials have on the results of meta-analyses, few data exist to suggest whether any one method of quality assessment provides a more biased estimate than any other. Bringing this information together as the basis for practical guides is also lacking; this chapter attempts to provide answers to some of these issues.

Attitudes regarding quality assessment were examined by surveying a broad spectrum of meta-analysts, methodologists and editors of biomedical journals. The current practice of quality assessment, by meta-analysts, was evaluated by reviewing reports of meta-analysis of randomised trials. Logistic regression models were used to examine the effects of quality assessment on

the results of meta-analyses. Once these studies were completed, along with supplemental literature, guides were formulated.

The overwhelming majority of meta-analysts, methodologists and editors reported that assessment of the quality of randomised trials included in a meta-analysis was important. Most respondents believed that guidelines for assessing the quality of such trials included in a meta-analysis would increase the rigour and reporting of published meta-analyses. Most respondents also believed that such guidelines would make interpretation of meta-analysis easier for clinicians. Trial quality was assessed in about one-half of the reviewed meta-analyses. Of these, only one-quarter took such assessments into account during data analyses. Trials with a low-quality score, compared to a high-quality one, resulted in a significant increase in the benefits of interventions. The use of quality scores as a quality weight also identified exaggerated effect estimates.

It is recommended that the quality of reports of randomised trials, included in meta-analyses, should be assessed. Items used for such assessment should be included based on the existing empirical evidence available that they can influence treatment effects. Using a validated scale and component approach appears to be complementary. Quality assessments should be incorporated into meta-analyses through sensitivity analyses. Alternatively, the quality weighting method is showing promise as a valid option for incorporation of quality into overall treatment effect.

INTRODUCTION

Meta-analyses pool individual studies – either observational or randomised controlled trials (RCTs) – to provide an overall estimate of the effect of the treatment under consideration, and are a key component of evidence based healthcare. Today, the RCT is considered the most reliable method of assessing the efficacy of healthcare interventions.[1] However, poorly conducted RCTs may yield misleading results, and hence it is important for those involved in healthcare to be able to assess the reliability of the research evidence that is available.

Quality is a construct (a concept) that has been defined in a variety of ways. In this chapter, our focus is on internal validity and quality is defined[2] as 'the confidence that the trials design, conduct, analysis, and presentation has minimised or avoided biases in its intervention comparisons'. As a meta-analysis is conducted retrospectively, it is undoubtedly susceptible to certain sources of bias. The need to assess quality stems mainly from a desire to estimate the effects of such bias on the results of a randomised trial. Meta-analyses of RCTs have always included studies of variable methodological quality, and differences in quality between randomised trials may indicate that some are more biased than others. It seems only sensible that meta-analysts and others will want to account for such differences to ensure that their findings are valid.

The assessment of the quality of individual randomised trials included in meta-analyses has been viewed with some controversy,[3–5] yet only limited data exist to inform these views. At a fundamental level, we know little about the views of a broad spectrum of health service professionals involved in the conduct of meta-analyses, regarding quality assessment. Albeit several aspects of trial quality have been shown empirically to be important – including the adequacy of reporting the randomisation strategy, allocation concealment, and double-blinding procedures as well as the handling of drop-outs and withdrawals – the extent to which meta-analysts assess trial quality and how they incorporate a measure of its effect into the quantitative data synthesis is limited. Although there is

increasing evidence[6] regarding the effects that low-quality trials have on the results of meta-analyses, few data exists to suggest whether any one method of quality assessment provides a more biased estimate than any other. More broadly, little attention has been given to synthesising the available evidence to help develop practical guides to facilitate issues regarding quality assessment in the conduct and reporting of meta-analyses.

The importance of assessing trial quality and its use in analysis is something that many meta-analysts have not consistently taken into account until recently. There is an on-going movement towards developing methodologies to help reduce or avoid bias in the conduct and reporting of meta-analysis. Three approaches to assessing the quality of reports of RCT have been developed: (i) component assessment (items such as randomisation and blinding); (ii) checklists; and (iii) scales. However, there are still no set rules or regulations regarding the quality assessment of trials. Hence, the objectives of this chapter are to examine this issue and to provide empirically based recommendations on how to conduct meta-analyses with respect to quality assessment.

METHODS

To complete the research reported here, we first created a database of 491 meta-analyses of RCTs using the refined strategy reported in Table 1. Meta-analyses were included in the study if they included only randomised trials, and if they were published in the Cochrane Library or in paper-based journals indexed by Medline. For the latter, they had to be coded by indexers as meta-analyses, or described by the authors as systematic reviews, meta-analyses, integrative research reviews, overviews, quantitative syntheses, pooling or combining studies.

In a review of 36 Cochrane reviews, compared to 39 paper based ones, published in 1995, we found that Cochrane reviews included a description of the inclusion and exclusion criteria, assessed trial quality, were more frequently updated, and did not have language restrictions.[7] Such evidence suggests that the quality of reports of Cochrane reviews are superior (in some aspects) to paper ones, and since we are interested in producing systematic reviews with the least amount of bias, our results section includes a comparison of these two categories of meta-analyses.

In order to develop guidelines regarding quality assessment in the conduct and reporting of

Table 1 *Search strategy to identify systematic reviews and meta-analyses*

Set	Search terms
001	meta-analysis.pt,sh.
002	(meta-anal: or metaanal:).tw.
003	(quantitativ: review: or quantitativ: overview:).tw.
004	(systematic: review: or systematic: overview:).tw.
005	(methodologic: review: or methodologic: overview:).tw.
006	(integrative research review: or research integration:).tw.
007	review.pt,sh. or review:.tw. or overview:.tw.
008	quantitativ: synthes:.tw.
009	1 or 2 or 3 or 4 or 5 or 6 or 8
010	(medline or medlars).tw,sh. or embase.tw.
011	(scisearch or psychinfo or psycinfo).tw.
012	(psychlit or psyclit).tw.
013	(hand search: or manual search:).tw.
014	(electronic database: or bibliographic database:).tw.
015	(pooling or pooled analys: or mantel haenszel).tw.
016	(peto or der simonian or dersimonian or fixed effect:).tw.
017	10 or 11 or 12 or 13 or 14 or 15 or 16
018	7 and 17
019	9 or 18

Table 2 *Analysis procedures for each of the three studies in the methods section*

Study	Analysis
1 Assessing attitudes regarding quality assessment	• Pearson chi-squared for across-group comparisons • Separate comparison of editors versus reviewers and methodologists to see differences • Qualitative analysis of commentary (reviewed in duplicate)
2 Current practice of quality assessment	• Descriptive statistics for eight questions by source (MAPJ + CDSR) and for all 240 meta-analysis • Differences between MAPJ + CDSR compared using chi-squared and Fisher's exact test
3 Effects of quality assessment on the results of meta-analysis	• Paired *t*-test for mean differences in quality scores (masked versus unmasked) • Chi-squared + logistic regression for differences between masked + unmasked in proportion with adequately reported components • Reliability checked via replication of point estimate and 95% CI • Logistic regression models to examine impact of quality assessment • Quality scores incorporated into analysis as threshold a quality weight or individual component (e.g. double-blinding) • Sensitivity analysis for relationship between a component assessment of quality compared to a scale • Results reported as ROR and OR[14] • Mean residual deviance of fitted models reflects degree of heterogeneity between trials (adjusted for independent factors) • *F*-test for effects of heterogeneity ($P < 0.05$)

meta-analysis, three studies were conducted. One was a survey of reviewers, methodologists and editors designed to appraise attitudes regarding quality assessment. The second looked at the current practice of quality assessment of meta-analysis, and the third dealt with the effects of quality assessment on the results of meta-analysis. Each study is described here, and the details of the analysis can be found in Table 2.

Assessing Attitudes Regarding Quality Assessment

Sampling frame

To generate respondents for our questionnaire, we randomly sampled 240 (48.9%) of these 491 articles. We identified three sets of respondents; the first being the corresponding author of each meta-analysis in our sample (i.e. the systematic reviewers), the second set of respondents were the corresponding authors of the methodology articles included in our sample (the methodologists), and the third group were editors of the journals in which the meta-analyses were published (the editors).

Instrument development, format and administration

From our database, our personal files and through two focus groups of five clinical epidemiologists each, we generated candidate items for a questionnaire used as an instrument to appraise attitudes regarding quality assessment. To ensure clarity and to remove redundant or illogical items, we pre-tested this instrument by eliciting feedback from five methodologists. We mailed the modified questionnaire to all potential respondents.

We asked respondents a set of questions to elicit their views on the assessment and reporting of the quality of randomised trials included in meta-analyses. For the purposes of this survey, we asked respondents to consider trial quality in reference to whether the design, conduct and analysis are undertaken in such as way as to minimise bias. We also provided space for

commentary. We surveyed 155 meta-analysts, 74 methodologists and 107 editors of biomedical journals.

Current Practice of Quality Assessment by Meta-Analysts

We obtained hard copies of 240 published reports of meta-analysis of randomised trials [204 meta-analyses of paper journals (MAPJ) and 36 Cochrane Database of Systematic Reviews (CDSR)] and deleted all information related to the identity and affiliation of the authors, and the date of publication. We also deleted the name of the journal. Using the masked copies of the meta-analyses, we extracted information from each report using eight questions that addressed aspects directly related to quality assessments (Box 1). Information regarding journal, number of authors, language and year of publication of each meta-analysis was also extracted.

Effects of Quality Assessment on the Results of Meta-Analyses

We selected 11 meta-analyses involving 22 independent outcomes (due to non-overlapping trials) from which 127 randomised trials were identified and retrieved. Masked and unmasked quality assessments were completed using a validated scale[8] and individual components known to affect estimates of intervention effectiveness.[6] The scale consists of three items pertaining to descriptions of randomisation, masking, and drop-outs and withdrawals in the report of a randomised trial. The scoring ranges from 0 to 5, with higher scores indicating superior

---

Box 1   *Questions on quality assessment used to extract information from the meta-analyses*

1 **Were the trials subjected to any quality assessment?**
   (yes, no or cannot tell)

2 **If yes, what method of quality assessment did the author(s) report using?** (this included components, check-lists, scales, 'other methods' and 'not reported')

3 **Was the reproducibility of the quality assessments assessed?** (yes, no or cannot tell)

4 **If the author(s) reported assessing quality using a component approach, which one did they use?** (six options were given including 'other')

5 **If the author(s) reported assessing quality using a check-list, which one did they use?** (10 options were given, including 'other')

6 **If the author(s) reported assessing quality using a scale, which one did they use?** (22 options were given, including 'other'). The options were selected from a previous article[23]

7 **Were the quality scores incorporated into the quantitative analysis?** (yes, no or cannot tell/not reported)

8 **How were the quality scores incorporated into the quantitative analysis?** (weights, thresholds, input sequence for cumulative meta-analysis, or as a visual plot)

reporting. The individual components assess the adequacy of reporting of allocation concealment and are described in detail elsewhere.[6]

In addition to the quality assessment of each randomised trial the following data were also extracted: the number of events and patients in the control group, and the number of events and patients in the experimental group. The data were extracted independently by two people (A.L.J. and D.M.) and consensus was achieved for any discrepancies before data entry.

RESULTS: WHAT THE OPINION LEADERS FEEL SHOULD BE THE 'RULES'

Assessing Attitudes Regarding Quality Assessment

The response rates were 78% for meta-analysts, 74% for methodologists, and 60% for editors. The overwhelming majority of meta-analysts, methodologists and editors reported that assessment of the quality of randomised trials included in a meta-analysis was very or somewhat important (97%, 94% and 100%, respectively). We asked all respondents to consider how, in their role (or potential role) as editors of biomedical journals, they would deal with an otherwise rigorous meta-analysis in which the quality of randomised trials had not been assessed. Overall, 66% said they would be unenthusiastic about publishing it unless the quality of the trials was assessed, 5% were indifferent, and 28% said they would be willing to publish an otherwise rigorous meta-analysis if the trial quality was not assessed. Reviewers, methodologists and editors had different views ($P = 0.04$), editors being less enthusiastic about publishing a meta-analysis in which quality had not been assessed.

In considering ways in which the quality of randomised trials included in a meta-analysis should be assessed, use of a series of items as in a check-list was recommended by 45% of reviewers, 57% of methodologists and 62% of editors. Assessment of a series of items that would generate an overall summary score, i.e. a scale, was recommended by 28%, 30% and 38% of the respondents, respectively. Qualitative analysis yielded recommendations that a modest number of criteria be used by meta-analysts to assess and report trial quality.

Reliance solely on universal criteria was considered inappropriate, and specific items tailored to the question under investigation were thought to be important. For example, when evaluating trials comparing drug treatment versus sclerotherapy for bleeding oesophageal varices, traditional blinding of patients and care-givers is

impossible and may not be a reasonable quality assessment item; however, evaluation of re-bleeding events using explicit, a priori criteria by an adjudication committee blinded to treatment may minimise the chance of a biased outcome assessment, and could be a more discriminating quality assessment item.

Respondents also reported that quality assessment should ideally be based on empirical evidence of bias, i.e. that the essential features of study design that minimise bias should be represented. If quality assessment is a vague part of the analysis process this is likely to lead to a variety of problems.[2] For example, the *conduct* and *reporting* of trial quality assessment in meta-analyses may be conflated in instruments such as the 100-point scale[9] for 'quality rating of randomised trials'. This tool combines items about reporting style (e.g. inclusion of trial commencement and cessation dates), sample size, unrelated to study quality or systematic error (e.g. whether or not investigators included a power analysis), and features designed to minimise systematic error (e.g. treatment allocation, blinding, and losses to follow-up).

The majority of respondents believed that the methods used to develop a quality check-list or scale were somewhat or very important (92%, 94% and 95%, respectively). Several methods[2] by which the quality assessments of randomised trials could be incorporated into meta-analyses were endorsed by respondents.

The majority of reviewers, methodologists and editors believed that guidelines for assessing the quality of randomised trials included in a meta-analysis would be likely or very likely to increase the rigour and reporting of published meta-analyses (Table 3). Most respondents also believed that such guidelines would likely or very likely make it easier for clinicians to interpret meta-analyses (Table 4).

Current Practice of Quality Assessment by Meta-Analysts

Trial quality was assessed in 114 (48%) of the 240 meta-analyses. The quality of the primary trials was assessed more frequently in the CDSR meta-analyses than in the MAPJ (100% versus 38%, $P < 0.001$]. Fifty-seven (50%) of the 114 meta-analyses in which trial quality was assessed provided data on the reproducibility of the assessments. CDSR meta-analyses evaluated the reproducibility of the assessments more frequently than MAPJ (56% versus 36% respectively; $P = 0.04$). Individual components and scales were the methods most frequently used (46% each) to assess trial quality. Most of the CDSR used individual components to assess

Table 3   Guidelines for assessing the quality of randomised trials included in meta-analyses: potential impact on the rigour and reporting of published meta-analyses?

Respondent	Very likely to increase	Likely to increase	Neutral likely	Very likely	
				To decrease	To decrease
Meta-analyst	21 (17.8)	83 (70.3)	12 (11.0)	0	1 (0.8)
Methodologist	8 (16.0)	34 (68.0)	8 (16.0) 0	0	0
Editor	26 (42.6)	31 (50.8)	4 (6.6)	0	0

The potential impact of guidelines for assessing the quality of randomised trials included in meta-analyses on the rigour and reporting of published meta-analyses is presented here according to views of meta-analysts, methodologists and editors. Data are presented as number of respondents and proportion of the total respondents in each category.
Values in parentheses are percentages.

Table 4   Guidelines for assessing the quality of randomised trials included in meta-analyses: potential impact on the way in which meta-analyses may be interpreted by clinicians

Respondent	Very likely to be easier	Likely to be easier	Neutral likely	Likely to decrease	Very likely to decrease
Meta-analyst	11 (9.2)	61 (51.8)	20 (16.7)	26 (21.7)	2 (1.7)
Methodologist	8 (14.8)	25 (46.3)	12 (22.2)	9 (16.7)	0
Editor	17 (27.4)	30 (48.4)	12 (19.4)	3 (4.8)	0

The potential impact of guidelines for assessing the quality of randomised trials included in meta-analyses on the way in which meta-analyses may be interpreted by clinicians is presented here according to views of meta-analysts, methodologists and editors. Data are presented as number of respondents and proportion of the total respondents in each category.
Values in parentheses are percentages.

trial quality, whilst most MAPJ meta-analyses used scales (Table 5). A total of 21 quality assessment instruments were identified. None of these instruments appeared to have undergone validation following established methodological procedures,[10] and 43% were described for the first time in 1994 and 1995. Eleven of these instruments were not included in a recently published systematic review.[10]

Of the 114 meta-analyses that included assessments of trial quality, only 29 (25%) took such assessments into account during data analyses (Table 5). MAPJ incorporated the quality assessment in the analyses more frequently than CDSR meta-analyses (34% vs. 6% respectively; $P < 0.001$). The two CDSR meta-analyses that incorporated the quality assessments into data analysis used the quality assessments as thresholds. Of the MAPJ meta-analyses, one-third incorporated the quality assessments as thresholds for inclusion or exclusion from the analyses, and one-third incorporated the quality scores in the formulae as weights.

When only the meta-analyses published in 1995 were analysed, most of the patterns outlined above persisted. Twelve of the 39 MAPJ (32%) included assessments of trial quality, and most of them used scales but did not incorporate the assessments into the analyses.

Effects of Quality Assessment on the Results of Meta-Analyses

The overall quality of reporting of randomised trials using a scale assessment was 2.74 (out of five; SD = 1.1), corresponding to 54.8% of the maximum possible value. There were statistically significant differences in the evaluation of the quality of reporting of randomised trials under masked and unmasked conditions. Masked assessment resulted in statistically higher quality scores compared to unmasked assessments; this difference corresponds to 3.8%. All further analyses presented below are based on masked assessments only.

Using a component approach to quality assessment, few randomised trials reported on

Table 5   *Assessment of trial quality in published meta-analyses*

	Meta-analyses (n, %)			
	CDSR	MAPJ (1995)	MAPJ (1977–1995)	Total
Trial quality assessment	36 (100)	12 (32)	78 (38)	114
Method of quality assessment				
Components	33 (92)	1 (8)	20 (26)	53 (46)
Scales	0 (0)	9 (75)	52 (67)	52 (46)
Checklists	0 (0)	1 (3)	3 (4)	3 (3)
Other methods	1 (3)	0 (0)	0 (0)	1 (1)
Not reported	2 (6)	1 (3)	3 (4)	5 (4)
Reproducibility of the assessments	13 (36)	5 (42)	44 (56)	57 (50)
Incorporation of quality assessments into analyses	2 (6)	3 (25)	27 (34)	29 (25)
As a threshold	2	1	9	11
As a weight	0	0	8	8
In a visual plot	0	1	3	3
Other	0	1	7	7

Values in parentheses are percentages.

either the methods used to generate the randomisation schedule (15.0%) or the methods used to conceal the randomisation sequence until the point of randomisation occurred (14.3%). When assessed under masked conditions, compared to unmasked ones, allocation concealment was assessed more frequently (14.3% versus 10.7%) as adequate.

Evaluating the influence that quality assessments of the primary trials have on the results of the meta-analyses is presented in Table 6. A quality score of 2 was utilised, based on empirical evidence, as the threshold value discriminating between low- and high-quality trials.[8,11] Trials with a low quality score ($\leq$2), compared to a high quality one (>2), resulted in a significant increase in the benefits of interventions by 34% (ratio of odds ratios; ROR = 0.66; 95% CI: 0.52, 0.83). The effects of quality assessment on the results of an individual meta-analysis can be seen in Box 2.

The use of quality scores as a quality weight also identified exaggerated effect estimates. Including trials with low quality scores ($\leq$2), compared to a quality weight, resulted in significantly exaggerated treatment effect of 55% (ROR = 0.45; 95% CI: 0.22, 0.91). However, using a sensitivity analysis whereby high-quality trials (score >2) were incorporated into the analysis compared to a quality weight did not produce different treatment effects (see Table 6). Using a quality weight to incorporate estimates of quality also produced less statistical heterogeneity (see Table 6).

We conducted a threshold analysis to determine whether the exaggerated intervention effects reported above, in relation to the quality scores, could be explained by those randomised trials in which allocation concealment was inadequately reported and inadequately carried out, as has been previously suggested.[6] Our analyses (see Table 6) did not result in any meaningful differences in terms of magnitude and direction of bias or statistical significance than those already reported here.

Incorporating estimates of quality based on individual components also detected exaggerated estimates of treatment effect (see Table 6). Clinical trials reporting allocation concealment inadequately, compared to those trials reporting it adequately, produced statistically exaggerated estimates of treatment effects of 37% (ROR = 0.63; 95% CI: 0.45, 0.88).

DEVELOPMENT OF GUIDES FOR ASSESSING THE QUALITY OF RANDOMISED TRIALS INCLUDED IN META-ANALYSIS

Once the three studies described above were conducted and results were available, a conference was held of all the investigators involved with the studies, in Ottawa, Ontario, Canada. Following this conference, monthly teleconferences of investigators were conducted to further develop the evidence into guides. Based on the evidence that resulted from these studies, supplemented with systematically assembled

Table 6   *Relationship between different methods of incorporating quality assessment (threshold, statistical weight, and individual components) into meta-analyses and the resulting estimates (and measures of precision) of treatment effects*

Methods of quality assessment	Ratio of Odds Ratios (95% confidence interval)	Ratio of heterogeneity between trials[§] (P-value from a test of similar degree of heterogeneity between trials)**
Scale		
Low (≤2) versus High (>2)*	0.66 (0.52, 0.83)	1.00♦ (0.51)
Low (≤2) versus Weight[†]	0.45 (0.22, 0.91)	1.77♦ (0.02)
High (>2) versus Weight[†]	0.97 (0.70, 1.33)	1.76♦ (0.006)
Sensitivity analysis		
[excluding trials in which allocation		
concealment is reported adequately]		
Low [≤2] versus High [>2]*	0.73 (0.56, 0.94)	0.82♦ (0.72)
Low [≤2] versus Weight[†]	0.69 (0.55, 0.86)	1.70♦ (0.03)
High [>2] versus Weight[†]	1.16 (0.93, 1.44)	2.08♦ (0.003)
Component randomisation	0.89 (0.67, 1.20)	
Generation[‡]		
Allocation concealment[‡]	0.63 (0.45, 0.88)	
Double-blinding[‡]	1.11 (0.76, 1.63)	

The analysis used the convention that treatment was more effective to prevent an adverse outcome (i.e. a summary odds ratio in each trial of less than 1). Hence a ratio of odds ratios (ROR) of less than 1 indicates an exaggeration of treatment effect. A base model consisted of treatment, trials and the different odds ratios (OR) in each meta-analysis (i.e. interaction term).

*   Allowing for summary ORs to vary according to quality (i.e. quality by treatment interaction) in the base model.
[†] Partial ROR of average treatment effects derived from fitting separate base models.
[‡] Allowing for summary ORs to vary simultaneously according to the components (i.e. component by treatment interactions).
[§] The residual deviance derived from fitting the base model reflects the degree of heterogeneity between trials.
** An approximate F-distribution was assumed for the ratio of residual deviances to compare the heterogeneity between different ways of incorporating quality. ♦ A larger degree of heterogeneity between trials results in a ratio greater than 1.
[††] Sensitivity analysis including trials with allocation concealment reported inadequately.

evidence from the literature,[12,13] guides were formulated and underwent a rigorous review process, and were then revised accordingly by this process.

Should the Quality of Randomised Trials be Assessed?

We have demonstrated that the quality of reports of randomised trials included in meta-analyses was assessed in only 38% of meta-analyses published in peer-reviewed journals. However, our survey of methodologists, journal editors and meta-analysts indicated that 95% or more of respondents believe that quality assessment of randomised trials is very, or somewhat, important. The survey also revealed that 66% of

respondents would be unenthusiastic about publishing a meta-analysis, unless the quality of the primary studies had been assessed.

Strong support for quality assessments comes from studies indicating that several dimensions of study quality can be used to detect bias in treatment estimates (see Table 7).[6,14–17] We recently confirmed Schulz's finding and demonstrated that low-quality randomised trials, compared to high-quality ones, exaggerated the effectiveness of the intervention by 34%, on average (see Table 6).[14] Meta-analysis based on biased randomised trials will also have a similar tendency toward bias (the 'garbage in, garbage out' phenomenon). Therefore, we recommend that the quality of all randomised trials included in a meta-analysis should be assessed.

Box 2   *Effects of quality assessment on results of individual analysis*

Treatment effects to prevent deep vein thrombosis-related death ($n = 5$ randomised trials)	OR [95% CI]
Main analysis	0.53 (0.32, 0.90)
Sensitivity analysis	
Low-quality trials (quality score ≤2; $n = 2$)	0.42 (0.15, 1.17)
Randomised trials	
High-quality trials (quality score >2; $n = 3$)	0.57 (0.30, 1.10)
Randomised trials	
Quality weight ($n = 5$ randomised trials)	0.52 (0.27, 0.98)

Lensing et al. (*Arch. Intern. Med.* 1995; **155**: 601–7) examined the effects of low-molecular weight heparins (LMWH) on several outcomes, including death. Five randomised trials were included in this analysis, resulting in a statistically beneficial effect of LMWH reducing mortality by 47% (OR = 0.53; 95% CI: 0.32, 0.90). Two of the trials scored ≤2, whilst the remaining three scored >2. When quality assessments were incorporated into the analysis, the beneficial effect of LMWH disappeared. Using low-quality trials (score ≤2) the odds ratio was no longer significant (OR = 0.42; 95% CI: 0.15, 1.17), although the point estimate suggests a greater effectiveness of LMWH. Similar results were obtained if only high-quality trials (score >2) were used (OR = 0.57; 95% CI: 0.30, 1.10). Using a quality weight resulted in almost no exaggeration of the point estimate, whilst maintaining the precision of the statistical result (OR = 0.52; 95% CI: 0.27, 0.98).

How should the quality of reports of randomised trials be assessed?

Items for which there is empirical evidence

If quality assessment is performed, the next question becomes how should it be evaluated? Quality assessments should be based on those dimensions of randomised trials that are related to bias in treatment estimates. There is increasing evidence for which dimensions of trial design and conduct affect the estimate of treatment effectiveness. By using 145 trials examining the treatment of myocardial infarction, Chalmers and colleagues demonstrated that trials which were not randomised had a 58.1% difference in case-fatality rates in treatment in comparison to control groups; this compared with a difference of 24.4% in trials that were randomised but not blinded, and an 8.8% difference in trials randomised and blinded (Table 7).[18]

Schulz examined 250 controlled trials from 33 meta-analyses published by the Pregnancy and Childbirth Group of the Cochrane Collaboration. Compared to trials that had adequate allocation concealment, he found that the odds ratio was exaggerated by 41% for inadequately concealed trials, and by 30% for unclearly concealed trials (Table 7). Trials that were not double-blind, compared to those that were, yielded odds ratios exaggerated by 17%.[6] The impact of not using double-blind randomised trials was confirmed in studies by Miller and Colditz.[16,17] Our study showed that inadequately concealed trials generated a 37% increased treatment effect compared to adequately concealed

trials (Table 7).[14] However, there was no significant difference detected in studies that were not double-blinded, or in which there was not adequate description of how the sequence of random numbers were generated.

Khan and colleagues assessed the probability of bias in crossover trials as compared to parallel trials in infertility research that utilised pregnancy as the outcome measure. They found that crossover trials over-estimated the odds ratio by 74% (Table 7). The underlying reason for this bias is that crossover trials will over-estimate the effectiveness of interventions when pregnancy is the outcome because once patients become pregnant they cannot be crossed over to the comparison intervention.[15]

We recommend using primarily evidence based components when assessing the quality of reports of randomised trials. The selection and use of other items cannot be guaranteed to guard against providing erroneous and/or biased information to meta-analysts and the results of meta-analyses. The items for which there are varying degrees of empirical evidence and items that are commonly used, but without such evidence, are summarised in Table 8.

The Use of Scales for Measuring Quality

One attractive feature of using a scale for measuring the quality of randomised trials is that in a scale each item is scored numerically and used to generate an overall quantitative estimate for quality. However, most scales have been developed in an arbitrary fashion with minimal attention to accepted methodological standards of

Table 7 *Summary of empirical evidence relating to quality assessment of randomised trials included in meta-analyses*

Reference	Year of publication	Study design	No. of studies	Disease(s) of interest	Methodological item(s)	Results
Berlin[28]	1997	RCT	5 meta-analyses	Various	Masking of primary studies to reviewers	Masked summary OR (95% CI) = 0.63 (0.57–0.70) and unmasked summary OR (95% CI) = 0.64 (0.57–0.72). Mean quality score for masked reviewers 7.4 and 8.1 for unmasked reviewers (P = 0.036).
Chalmers et al.[18]	1983	Observational	145	Acute myocardial infarction	Blinding/randomisation	Differences in case-fatality rates 8.8% in blinded-randomisation studies, 24.4% in unblinded randomisation studies, and 58.1% in non-randomised studies.
Cho and Bero[26]	1996	Observational	152	Drug studies	Pharmaceutical sponsorship	98% of drug company-sponsored trials were favourable to the drug of interest compared to 79% of those with no drug company sponsorship.
Colditz et al.[16]	1989	Observational	113	Studies in medical journals	Randomisation/double-blinding	Non-randomised trials with sequential assignment had significantly better outcomes for new therapies (P = 0.004). Randomised trials that were not double-blinded trials favoured the new therapy significantly more often (P = 0.02).
Detsky et al.[4]	1992	Observational	8 trials (1 meta-analysis)	TPN in chemotherapy	Incorporating quality into meta-analysis	Four methods of incorporating quality into meta-analyses were demonstrated: 1) Inclusion/exclusion criteria; 2) Quality scores as weights; 3) Plot effect size versus quality score; and 4) Sequential combination of trial results based on quality scores.

Jadad et al.[8]	1996	RCT	36	Pain	Masking of primary studies for quality assessment	Mean quality score was 2.7 in unmasked group compared to 2.3 in masked group (P < 0.01).
Khan et al.[15]	1996	Observational	34	Infertility	Crossover versus parallel study design	Cross-over trials overestimated odds ratio by 74% compared to parallel design (95% CI, 2% to 197%).
Khan et al.[23]	1996	Observational	1 meta-analysis (9 trials)	Infertility	Impact of quality assessment on treatment estimate	The summary odds ratio from all studies was 1.6 (95% CI 0.9–2.6); for low-quality studies 2.6 (95% CI 1.2–5.2) and for high-quality studies 0.5 (0.2–1.5).
Miller et al.[17]	1989	Observational	221	Surgical trials	Randomisation	Significantly greater benefit in non-randomised trials compared to randomised trials.
Moher et al.[2]	1996	Observational	12	Acute ischaemic stroke	Six different quality assessment scales	Significant difference in the quality score and ranking of RCT between the six quality scales.
Moher et al.[14]	1998	RCT for masking; Observational for impact of quality on OR	127	Four disease areas	1) Masking; 2) Impact of quality on treatment estimate; and 3) Methods of incorporating quality assessment into the data analysis	1) Masked quality assessments 2.74 compared to 2.55 for unmasked quality assessment (% difference 0.19; 95% CI 0.06–0.32); 2) Low-quality studies over-estimated benefit by 34%, Inadequately concealed trials over-estimated benefit by 37%; 3) Both high-quality estimates and quality weighted estimates were not exaggerated; however, quality weighted estimates had less heterogeneity and greater precision.
Schulz et al.[6]	1995	Observational	250	Pregnancy and childbirth	Allocation concealment/ double blinding	Odds ratios were exaggerated by 41% for inadequately concealed trials and by 17% for trials that were not double-blinded.

RCT: Randomised controlled trial.

Table 8   *Empirical evidence in clinical trial assessment*

	Items
Empirical evidence	• Allocation concealment • Double-blinding • Type of RCT (parallel or crossover trial)
No empirical evidence, but commonly used	• Sample size

validation and reliability testing.[19,20] In addition, many scales are not truly measuring quality as defined earlier, but rather focusing on extraneous factors more related to generalisability.[2,10]

In fact, through a systematic search of the literature we could find only one scale, initially used for evaluating the pain literature,[8] developed according to accepted methodological principles.[19,20] This scale has been used subsequently to compare trials in different languages and specialty areas.[21,22] It is an interval scale ranging from 0 to 5 (0 = lowest quality; 5 = highest quality) that assesses method of randomisation, double-blinding and handling of withdrawals and drop-outs. Using this scale we have recently shown that low-quality studies exaggerated the odds ratio by 34% compared to high-quality ones (see Table 7).[14] Kahn and colleagues, using this scale in a meta-analysis based on trials conducted in the infertility domain, have recently demonstrated that an estimate based on low-quality trials produced a statistically significant result with treatment, and

that this was not present in trials assessed as high quality.[23]

In our recent assessment of published meta-analyses, nine new scales were identified[24] that had not been previously identified in 1995.[10] None of these newly identified scales had been developed using established methodological standards.[19,20] Moher and colleagues have previously shown that the results of quality assessments depend on how the scales have been developed (see Table 7).[2] We recommend using appropriately developed scales when assessing the quality of reports of randomised trials. There is strong evidence for one scale[8] (see Box 3). The selection and use of less rigorously developed scales for randomised trial quality may lead to erroneous and/or biased information.

Scales Versus Components

Our survey of an international group of methodologists, editors and meta-analysts indicated that between 45% and 62% recommended performing quality assessment through the use of a series of items.[24] There was less support for the use of a scale ranging from 28% of meta-analysts to 38% of editors. We have also found that 92% of systematic reviews published in the CDSR utilised components (e.g. allocation concealment) compared to only 26% of meta-analyses published in paper based peer-reviewed journals.[7] In contrast, none of the reviews in the CDSR used scales for quality assessments compared to 67% of meta-analyses published in paper based peer-reviewed journals.

Box 3   *Scale for measuring the quality of randomised trials*

Please read the article and try to answer the following questions (see attached instructions)
1   Was the study described as randomised (this included the use of words such as randomly, random and randomisation)?
2   Was the study described as double blind?
3   Was there a description of withdrawals and drop-outs?

Scoring the items:
Either give a score of 1 point for each 'yes' or 0 points for each no. There are no in-between marks.
Give 1 additional point if: For question 1, the method to generate the sequence of randomisation was described and it was appropriate (table of random numbers, computer generated, etc.)
and/or: If for question 2 the method of double blinding was described and it was appropriate (identical placebo, active placebo, dummy, etc.)
Deduct 1 point if: For question 1, the method to generate the sequence of randomisation was described and it was inappropriate (patients were allocated alternately, or according to date of birth, hospital number, etc.) and/or: For question 2, the study was described as double blind but the method of blinding was inappropriate (e.g. comparison of tablet versus injection with no double dummy)

This scale, which was originally used to evaluate the likelihood of bias in pain research reports, is the only one found that was developed according to accepted methodological principles.

There is no evidence favouring one particular approach (i.e. component and scale) over the other as regards quality assessment, and in our view using both would be complementary. This is particularly true for the components and scale we advocate using. A limitation of employing the component approach alone is that only a small proportion of articles report adequate allocation concealment; 14% in our study[14] and 32% in a study by Schulz and colleagues.[6] The advantage of the component approach is that it can be tailored to the topic as appropriate and specific, relevant items can be inserted. In addition, as new items are identified through empirical evidence, they can be incorporated easily into study quality assessment. It is important to emphasise that both the scale and component approach led to exaggerated point estimates in our empirical study, and there is no compelling approach to recommend one over the other.

Topic-Specific Quality Assessment

In addition to these generic measures of quality, meta-analysts may include component assessments that are unique to the topic area being explored by the review. Such an approach allows selection of items that are most likely to capture design features important to a given set of trials, and allows omission of elements that do not distinguish among trials with respect to their quality, e.g. blinding in surgical versus medical management. A similar concept has been proposed for quality of life measurement in clinical trials.[25] Respondents to our survey[24] revealed that some thought reliance on universal criteria was considered inappropriate, and that specific items tailored to the meta-analysis question should be utilised. The major disadvantage to topic-specific quality assessment is that they may not always be evidence based. The use of crossover trials in infertility, where pregnancy is the primary outcome, is an example of topic-specific quality assessment (see Table 7).[15] In conditions where patients return to their baseline during a wash-out period, this finding of bias from crossover design would not be anticipated. In the area of pharmaceutical research, Cho and Bero assessed 152 studies examining pharmacotherapy studies in symposia, and found that 98% of these supported by a single drug company favoured the drug of the sponsoring agency compared to only 79% of studies not supported by a single drug company ($P < 0.01$; see Table 7).[26] We recommend using primarily evidence based topic-specific items as part of quality assessment process.

How Should Quality of Reports of Randomised Trials be Incorporated into a Meta-Analysis?

Many meta-analysts incorporate quality at the level of deciding which studies to include in a meta-analysis. Stating that only 'randomised, controlled trials' were included imply that quality has been incorporated in the meta-analysis at the eligibility phase of the review, sometimes referred to as the 'threshold approach' (see Table 7).[4] Other markers for quality, such as blinding, may also be utilised at this stage of the meta-analysis.

One factor that will affect the incorporation of quality assessments of randomised trials into meta-analyses is the number of studies included. If only a few studies are included, then it will be very difficult to do much more than describe their quality. Another factor is whether there is significant heterogeneity based on a test for statistical heterogeneity and a visual inspection of the point estimates.

If there is significant heterogeneity among studies, then it may be helpful to utilise study quality to try to explore this variability.[27] We have explored two methods[14] of incorporating quality assessment into the quantitative analysis: quality weighting and performing a threshold analysis (see Table 6). Quality weighting is a statistical technique whereby studies with lower quality are assigned less influence on the treatment estimate than studies of higher quality.[4] Currently, only 22% of reviewers, 21% of methodologists and 33% of editors endorsed this quality weighting method for incorporating quality.[24]

Threshold analysis, which is one method of sensitivity analysis, involves grouping the studies into different levels of quality (usually low and high), and then examining whether the point estimate varies between the two groups.[4] As compared to quality weighting, significantly more reviewers (63%), methodologists (66%) and editors (43%) supported this method for quality assessment incorporation into meta-analyses.[24] Only 6% of reviews published in CDSR incorporated quality into the analysis, and all of them used the sensitivity analysis method.[24] Our results show that 34% of meta-analyses published in peer-reviewed journals incorporated quality into the analysis and the two leading methods were sensitivity analysis (9%) and quality weighting (8%).[24] Our survey revealed that commonly, quality assessments are made but not utilised to explain variability between studies. In our assessment of published meta-analyses, an overall 48% (114/204) assessed quality, but only 25% (29/114) incorporated quality into the analyses.

There is no strong evidence to support one method over the other. It may be that at present most meta-analysts will find threshold analyses intuitively simpler to perform and that it will be more transparent to the readers. The quality weighting approach is based on the assumption that the scale used for quality weighting is linear and, hence, it is logical to give a study with a score of 5 out of 5 a full quality weight of 1. There appear to be certain conceptual advantages to use of a quality weight rather than a threshold approach. One of these may be that with the use of quality weight all trials can be included rather than a selected sample, as would be common with a threshold approach. In our study the use of quality weighting produced results that were less heterogeneous and maintained greater precision than results from threshold analysis because all studies contributed to the overall estimate (see Table 7)[14] depending on the contribution of their quality scores. Regardless of the method selected, we recommend that all meta-analysts should incorporate an estimate of quality assessment into the quantitative analysis as a 'first-line' sensitivity analysis.

SHOULD THE REPORTS OF RANDOMISED TRIALS BE MASKED WHEN QUALITY IS BEING ASSESSED?

One aspect of quality assessment that may increase the quantity of work in performing a meta-analysis is the masking of individual trials. There is direct evidence that masking does impact on the assessment of quality (see Table 7).[8,14,28] What has not been consistent is the direction of such impact. Both Jadad and colleagues[8] and Berlin and colleagues[28] have shown that masked quality assessments scored lower than those performed under open conditions ($P < 0.01$ and $P = 0.04$, respectively; see Table 7). We on the other hand, found that masked quality assessment resulted in significantly higher scores compared to open assessments, but showed a more normal distribution and greater consistency (see Table 7).[14] In all studies, while the differences were statistically significant, it is not clear whether these are methodologically meaningful differences and whether the magnitude of the difference would be sufficient to make an important difference when quality is being incorporated into the quantitative analyses. Berlin and colleagues randomised reviewers to utilise masked trials versus unmasked trials throughout the systematic review process (see Table 7).[28] They found that, although there were

disagreements between reviewers at the various phases of the review (study selection, quality assessment and data extraction), there was no significant impact on the summary odds ratios for the meta-analyses included in their study. They did not, however, explore the impact of quality assessments on the overall summary estimate.

There is also indirect evidence from the peer-reviewed literature[29–31] that can be used to help inform any recommendation. McNutt and colleagues[29] randomised 127 manuscripts submitted for publication to be assessed under masked or open conditions. The authors reported that masked assessments, compared to open ones, produced statistically higher assessments of quality. Evidence of an effect in a different direction has recently been reported.[30,31] Seventy-four pairs of peer reviewers were randomised to receive a masked or open version of a manuscript, and the quality of peer review was assessed using a validated instrument. The authors reported no statistical differences between both groups in terms of the quality of peer review.[30] Similar results have been reported elsewhere.[31] A prudent next move may be to conduct a systematic review; this is likely to provide insight into the apparent inconsistent results across the trials.

Given the current state of evidence and the effort required to conduct masked quality assessment, strong recommendations are not suggested by available research evidence. However, we recommend that meta-analysts should at least consider this issue and explicitly justify their decision. Further research evidence is needed before making a more definitive recommendation.

Number and Backgrounds of Assessors

At least two individuals should assess the quality of each study included in the meta-analysis, as one reviewer or both may make random or systematic errors. We do not know much about the ideal background and number of quality assessors. When such assessments are performed, we recommend using a measure of agreement, such as kappa (or weighted kappa as appropriate)[32] or intra-class correlation,[33] as appropriate. After completing the quality assessments, these individuals should meet and reach consensus on areas of disagreement; if disagreement persists, then a third party adjudication may be used. These recommendations are not based on empirical evidence, but rather reflect our opinions.

Box 4   *Guidelines for the quality assessment of randomised trials*

- The quality of all randomised trials included in a meta-analysis should be assessed.
- Masked quality assessment should be considered, and meta-analysts should report masking methods used or their reasons for rejecting masking.
- Primarily evidence-based components (e.g. allocation concealment, double-blinding, type of randomised trial) should be used to assess quality. Topic-specific items should be part of the quality assessment process.
- Scales used for assessment should have been appropriately developed and evaluated. A component approach has the advantage that it can be topic-specific. However, there is no compelling evidence to recommend a component approach over a scale approach, or vice versa.
- Meta-analyses should incorporate an estimate of quality assessment into the quantitative analysis as a 'first-line' sensitivity analysis.

These guidelines are a useful tool with which meta-analysts, editors, peer reviewers and readers can deal with issues pertaining to quality assessment of randomised trials including in a meta-analysis.

THE BOTTOM LINE

The greatest potential of meta-analysis lies in its objective methodological engine, which provides the means for information to be prospectively incorporated into a continuum of a large body of evidence, and assessment of study quality plays a crucial role in this process. In addition to helping explore and explain inter-study variability, study quality should assist meta-analysts in making inferences about the robustness of the results of the reviews. If study results are homogeneous but of low quality, then the reviewer should be guarded in making strong inferences based on the results of the meta-analysis, since these results have a higher probability of bias. If results are homogeneous and of high quality, then stronger inferences can be made. Where there is significant heterogeneity, and study quality accounts for this variability, then the point estimate of the high-quality studies should be given stronger emphasis during interpretation of the results, and particularly during the application of these results in the clinical setting.

We undertook to develop these guidelines (Box 4) because the overwhelming majority of meta-analysts (88.1%), methodologists (84%), and editors (93.4%) who responded to our survey[24] indicated that their development would likely or very likely increase the potential impact on the rigour and reporting of meta-analyses.

In Table 7 we have listed the study design used in the cited methodological studies. This table highlights the small amount of empirical evidence on these issues, and the degree of uncertainty behind the proposed guidelines. The studies by Berlin, Jadad and Moher are examples of randomised trials examining the impact of masking assessors to details of potentially relevant primary studies for conducting a meta-analysis.[8,14,28] However, more experimental

---

Table 9   *Check-list for conducting and reporting of quality assessment of randomised trials included in meta-analyses*

---

1   **Does the report include an assessment of trial quality?**
   Report the method of assessment (e.g. scale or component approach) and rationale if no assessment.

2   **Was the assessment completed under masked conditions?**
   If the quality assessment was completed under masked conditions, report how was this achieved (e.g. black marker, computer scanning).

3   **How many assessors completed the assessment and what was their background and area of expertise?**
   If completed by single person, provide the rationale.

4   **Was any measure of inter-observer agreement reported?**
   Report the method used (e.g. weighted kappa or inter-class correlation) and whether consensus was sought.

5   **What instrument did the authors use to assess quality?**
   If the instrument was previously developed, reference it. Report whether or not, the instrument was developed according to standard practice, and whether the included items are evidence based. If the instrument was specifically developed for the meta-analysis, report this.

6   **Were the quality scores incorporated into the quantitative analysis?**
   Report the rationale for or against incorporating quality assessments in the meta-analysis.

---

studies of methodological issues in meta-analyses will help to increase their rigour and thus their usefulness in practice.[34] A useful checklist for meta-analysts, editors, peer reviewers, and readers to assess a meta-analysis for its handling of quality assessment of randomised trials is provided in Table 9.

COMMENT

Most often, assessing the quality of randomised trials means assessing the quality as stated in the report, and not of the actual events that occurred during execution of the trial. With initiatives that attempt to encourage systematic and comprehensive reporting of trials, such as the CONSORT statement,[35] it is expected that the reporting of randomised trials will become more transparent and comprehensive over time. As evidence accumulates in favour of important design features of randomised trials that reduce the probability of bias, the quality of how randomised trials are conducted should improve, particularly if journal editors and funding agencies encourage investigators to conduct and report their work with this evidence in mind.

Whilst strong evidence exists that certain characteristics of the design and execution of randomised trials do impact on the probability of bias, further research is needed to identify other potential aspects influencing the results of randomised trials. Further studies are also needed to clarify the role of masking studies before performing quality assessments, and additionally there is a need for more than one reviewer and different backgrounds and levels of expertise to perform such assessments. Whilst several methods have been described in this chapter for the incorporation of study quality into the results of a meta-analysis, further research in this area is required to determine whether there is any significant advantage of one approach over the other.[4] Additionally, if weighting of studies based on quality assessment proves to be an appropriate method, then software will need to be developed to assist reviewers in this task.

REFERENCES

1. Cook DJ, Guyatt GH, Laupacis A, Sackett DL. Rules of evidence and clinical recommendations of the use of antithrombotic agents. *Chest* 1992; **4**: 102.

2. Moher D, Jadad AR, Tugwell P. Assessing the quality of randomized controlled trials: current issues and future direction. *Int. J. Technol. Assess. Health Care* 1996; **12**: 195–208.

3. Greenland S. Quality scores are useless and potentially misleading. *Am. J. Epidemiol.* 1994; **140**: 300–1.

4. Detsky AS, Naylor CD, O'Rourke K, McGeer AJ, L'Abbe KA. Incorporating variations in the quality of individual randomized trials into meta-analyses. *J. Clin. Epidemiol.* 1992; **45**: 225–65.

5. Chalmers TC, Lau J. Meta-analysis stimulus for changes in clinical trials. *Statist. Methods Med. Res.* 1993; **2**: 161–72.

6. Schulz KF, Chalmers I, Haynes RJ, Altman DG. Empirical evidence of bias: dimensions of methodological quality associated with estimates of treatment effects in controlled trials. *JAMA* 1995; **273**: 408–12.

7. Jadad AR, Cook DJ, Jones A, Klassen T, Moher M, Tugwell P, Moher D. The Cochrane Collaboration: its impact on the methodology and reports of systematic reviews and meta-analyses. *JAMA* 1998; **280**: 278–80.

8. Jadad AR, Moore RA, Carroll D, Jenkinson C, Reynolds DJM, Gavaghan DJ, McQuay HJ. Assessing the quality of reports of randomized clinical trials: is blinding necessary? *Controlled Clinical Trials* 1996; **17**: 1–12.

9. Chalmers TC, Smith H, Blackburn B, Silverman B, Schroeder B, Reitmen D, Ambroz A. Method for assessing the quality of randomized controlled trials. *Controlled Clinical Trials* 1981; **2**: 31–49.

10. Moher D, Jadad AR, Nichol G, Penman M, Tugwell P, Walsh S., Assessing the quality of randomized controlled trials: an annotated bibliography of scales and checklists. *Controlled Clinical Trials* 1995; **16**: 62–73.

11. Pham B, Moher D, Klassen TP. Incorporating quality assessments of randomized controlled trials into meta-analyses: are effect sizes adjusting for quality scores appropriate? Technical Report. Thomas C. Chalmers Centre for Systematic Reviews, 1999.

12. Kunz RA, Oxman AD. The unpredictability paradox: review of empirical comparisons of randomised and non-randomised clinical trials. *Br. Med. J.* 1998; **317**: 1185–90.

13. Kleijnen J, Gotzsche P, Kunz RA, Oxman AD, Chalmers I. So what's so special about randomization? In: Maynard A, Chalmers I (eds). *Non-random reflections on health services research.* London: BMJ publishing group, 1997, pp. 93–106.

14. Moher D, Pham B, Jones A, Cook DJ, Jadad AR, Moher M, Tugwell P, Klassen TP. Does the poor quality of reports of randomized trials exaggerate estimates of intervention effectiveness reported in a meta-analysis? *Lancet* 1998; **352**: 609–13.

15. Khan KS, Daya S, Collins JA, Walter S. Empirical evidence of bias in infertility research: overestimation of treatment effect in cross-over trials using pregnancy as the outcome measure. *Fertil. Steril.* 1996; **65**: 939–45.

16. Colditz GA, Miller JN, Mosteller F. How study design affects outcomes in comparison of therapy. I: Medical. *Stat. Med.* 1989; **8**: 441–5.

17. Miller JN, Colditz GA, Mosteller F. How study design affects outcomes in comparisons of therapy. II: Surgical. *Stat. Med.* 1989; **8**: 455–66.

18. Chalmers TC, Celano P, Sacks HS, Smith H. Bias in treatment assignment in controlled clinical trials. *N. Engl. J. Med.* 1983; **309**: 1358–61.

19. McDowell I, Newell C. *Measuring health: a guide to rating scales and questionnaires*, 1st edn. Oxford: Oxford University Press, 1987.

20. Streiner DL, Norman GR. *Health measurement scales*, 1st edn. Oxford: Oxford University Press, 1989.

21. Moher D, Forin P, Jadad AR, Juni P, Klassen T, Lelorier J, Liberati A, Linde K, Penna A. Completeness of reporting of trials published in languages other than English: implications for conduct and reporting of systematic reviews. *Lancet* 1996; **347**: 363–6.

22. Egger M, Zellweger-Zahner T, Schneider M, Junker C, Lengeler C, Antes G. Language bias in randomised controlled trials published in English and German. *Lancet* 1997; **350**: 326–9.

23. Khan KS, Daya S, Jadad AR. The importance of quality of primary studies in producing unbiased systematic reviews. *Arch. Intern. Med.* 1996; **156**: 661–6.

24. Moher D, Cook DJ, Jadad AR, Tugwell P, Moher M, Jones A, Pham B, and Klassen TP. Assessing the quality of randomized controlled trials: implications for the conduct of meta-analyses. *Health Technology Assessment* 1999; **3**: 1–98.

25. Aaronson NK. Quality of life assessment in clinical trials: methodologic issues. *Controlled Clinical Trials* 1989; **10**: 195S (Supplement).

26. Cho MK, Bero LA. The quality of drug studies published in symposium proceedings. *Ann. Intern. Med.* 1996; **124**: 485–9.

27. Lau J, Ioannidis JPA, Schmid CH. Summing up evidence: one answer is not always enough. *Lancet* 1998; **351**: 123–7.

28. Berlin JA, on behalf of the University of Pennsylvania meta-analysis blinding study group. Does blinding of readers affect the results of meta-analyses? *Lancet* 1997; **350**: 185–6.

29. McNutt RA, Evans AT, Fletcher RH, Fletcher SW. The effects of blinding on the quality of peer review. *JAMA* 1990; **263**: 1371–6.

30. Justice AC, Cho MK, Winker MA, Berlin JA, Rennie D, Berkwits M, Callaham M, Fontanarosa P, Frank E, Goldman D, Goodman S, Pitkin R, Varma R, Waeckerle J. Does masking author identity improve peer review quality? A randomized controlled trial. *JAMA* 1998; **280**: 240–2.

31. VanRooyen S, Godlee F, Evans S, Smith R, Black N. The effect of blinding and unmasking on the quality of peer review: a randomized controlled trial. *JAMA* 1998; **280**: 234–7.

32. Kramer MS, Feinstein AR. The biostatistics of concordance. *Clin. Pharm. Ther.* 1982; **29**: 111–23.

33. Shrout PE, Fleiss JL. Intraclass correlations: uses in assessing rater reliability. *Psychol. Bull.* 1979; **86**: 420–8.

34. Naylor CD. Meta-analysis and the meta-epidemiology of clinical research. *Br. Med. J.* 1997; **315**: 617–19.

35. Begg C, Cho M, Eastwood S, Horton R, Moher D, Olkin I, Pitkin R, Rennie D, Schultz KF, Simel D, Stroup D. Improving the quality of reporting of randomized controlled trials: The CONSORT statement. *JAMA* 1996; **276**: 637–9.

24

Consensus Development Methods, and their Use in Creating Clinical Guidelines

NICK BLACK, MAGGIE MURPHY, DONNA LAMPING,
MARTIN McKEE, COLIN SANDERSON,
JANET ASKHAM and THERESA MARTEAU

SUMMARY

Clinicians regularly make difficult choices about treatment options. Often, there is uncertainty about the value of different options, and practice can vary widely. Although there is debate about the appropriate place of guidelines in clinical practice, guidelines can be seen as one way of assisting clinicians in decision-making. Given the likely diversity of opinion that any group of people may display when considering a topic, methods are needed for organising subjective judgements. Three principal methods (Delphi, nominal group technique, and consensus development conference) exist which share the common objective of synthesising judgements when a state of uncertainty exists.

The objectives of this chapter are to: (i) identify the factors that shape and influence the clinical guidelines that emerge from consensus development methods; (ii) make recommendations about best practice in the use of consensus development methods for producing clinical guidelines; and (iii) to recommend further methodological research for improving the use of consensus development methods as a basis for guideline production.

Consensus development methods may be considered to involve three types of activity: planning, individual judgement, and group interaction. These activities are not necessarily clearly separated or ordered. In addition, five components can be identified: three inputs (questions, participants, information), the process (consensus development method), and the output.

Five electronic databases were searched: Medline (1966–1996), PsychLIT (1974–1996), Social Science Citation Index (1990–1996), ABI inform and Sociofile. From the searches and reference lists of articles, a total of 177 empirical and review articles was selected for review.

An overview of the scientific evidence is presented, followed by a summary of the implications for those wishing to use consensus development methods (and nominal group techniques in particular) to develop clinical guidelines. Finally, the priorities for methodological research to enhance our understanding and as a result, our use of these methods, are outlined.

CONTEXT

Why We Need Consensus Development Methods

Clinicians regularly make difficult choices about treatment options. Often there is uncertainty about the value of different options, and practice can vary widely. Although there is debate about the appropriate place of guidelines in clinical practice, guidelines can be seen as one way of assisting clinicians in decision-making.

In an ideal world, clinical guidelines would be based on evidence derived from rigorously conducted empirical studies. In practice, there are few areas of healthcare where sufficient research based evidence exists or may ever exist.[1] In such situations, the development of guidelines will inevitably have to be based partly or largely on the opinions and experience of clinicians and others with knowledge of the subject at issue.[2,3]

There are two main ways that judgement based guidelines could be devised: have the 'best person' make the judgement, or have a group do it. In theory, the advantages of a group decision are: a wider range of direct knowledge and experience is brought to bear; the interaction between members stimulates consideration of a wide range of options and debate that challenges received ideas and stimulates new ones; idiosyncrasies are filtered out (sometimes wrongly!); and, in terms of influencing the behaviour of others, the group as a whole may carry more weight than any one individual.

Given the likely diversity of opinion that any group of people may display when considering a topic, methods are needed for organising subjective judgements. Although a variety of methods exist (which are described below), they share the common objective of synthesising judgements when a state of uncertainty (differences of opinion) exists.

Our concern is with the use of these methods for developing clinical guidelines, but they have been used for several other purposes in the health sector including forecasting, conflict resolution and prioritisation. Despite their widespread use, consensus development methods have been the subject of relatively little methodological research within the health field.[4] They have, however, been the subject of a considerable amount of investigation elsewhere, in particular in the behavioural sciences, technological and social forecasting literature,[5,6] but this research has had little impact on their application in healthcare.

It is essential to be clear what consensus development is and is not. It is a process for making policy decisions, not a scientific method for creating new knowledge. At its best, consensus development merely makes the best use of available information, be that scientific data or the collective wisdom of the participants. Thus, although it may capture collective knowledge, it is inevitably vulnerable to the possibility of capturing collective ignorance.

The objectives of this chapter are to: (i) identify the factors that shape and influence the clinical guidelines that emerge from consensus development methods; (ii) make recommendations about best practice in the use of consensus development methods for producing clinical guidelines; and (iii) recommend further methodological research for improving the use of consensus development methods as a basis for guideline production.

How Do Individuals and Groups Make Decisions?

Consensus decision-making is a complex process which involves decisions at both individual and group levels. Judgements of appropriateness require people to pay attention to new information, from literature or other group members for example, and they require them to draw on information and experience from memory. They must make judgements about the value of information; they must integrate the various pieces of information; and they must determine how the information relates to the judgement task. They must also provide judgements of the appropriateness of an intervention. This may involve estimating the probabilities of outcomes and assessing values of outcomes. These are largely cognitive aspects of decision-making. As well as these cognitive aspects, there are also motivational aspects. People may be more or less motivated to put effort into the process for example. When the decision-making involves a group of people there are added complexities resulting from social and inter-personal processes. People will try to influence one another for example, and may respond to each other not simply on the basis of the relevant task information provided, but also in terms of the social and personal characteristics of the persons involved.

Research in psychology has been conducted at four levels of analysis: intra-individual, inter-individual (or intra-group), inter-group, and societal. Research on intra-individual processes, generally carried out within cognitive and social-cognitive psychology, examines cognitive processes within individuals. Social psychology focuses on inter-individual and inter-group levels, looking at how individuals and groups interact. The societal level of analysis is generally found in economics, history, and sociology, but also in social psychology. This level focuses on institutional and societal influences on behaviour. Models of behaviour which have been generated from empirical research in social and cognitive psychology are directly relevant to consensus decision-making as follows:

1　Members of a consensus development group are required to draw on information both from their own experience and from new information presented within the group in order to make decisions.

2　How people attend to, organise and remember information helps to understand what information is likely to be used, the impact that it will have, and the possible biases that may operate in decision-making.

3 Attempts to reach consensus will involve the need for some people to change their positions – a process involving persuasion and social influence.
4 Behaviour within and between group members may be influenced by the perceptions of the groups involved: do members of consensus groups see themselves as members of a common group with a common goal, or are subgroup identities more salient, perhaps leading to a conflict of interest between consensus subgroup members?

Why We Need 'Formal' Methods of Consensus Development

It is only since the 1950s that formal consensus development methods have been used in the health sector. This does not mean that collective decisions were not made before then, simply that such decisions emerged through informal methods. Indeed, over the past 40 years the vast majority of collective decisions in healthcare have continued to be based on group meetings, such as committees, which have been largely unstructured with few formal rules or procedures.

Such group discussions, sometimes termed 'free discussion', 'freely interacting' or simply 'consensus' groups involve bringing together a group of people to discuss a problem with the aim of reaching agreement. They are usually not instructed in how to reach a consensus, though they may be given simple instructions such as not to criticise other members' contributions. There may or may not be someone chairing the group. A jury is an example of this type of group.

The case for using formal methods is based on a number of assumptions about decision-making in groups:[7-11]

(a) safety in numbers – several people are less likely to arrive at a wrong decision than a single individual;
(b) authority – a selected group of individuals is more likely to lend some authority to the decision produced;
(c) rationality – decisions are improved by reasoned argument in which assumptions are challenged and members forced to justify their views;
(d) controlled process – by providing a structured process formal methods can eliminate negative aspects of group decision making; and
(e) scientific credibility – formal consensus methods meet the requirements of scientific methods.

Types of Formal Consensus Development Methods

Three main approaches have been used in the health field. In the 1950s the Delphi method was introduced;[12,13] this was followed by the use of the nominal group technique (NGT) in the 1960s,[14] and in 1977 the National Institute of Health in the USA introduced the consensus development conference.[15] The major differences between these methods are described in Table 1 and relate to: (i) whether a mailed questionnaire is used; (ii) whether individuals make separate decisions 'in private' or not, and if so, the degree of anonymity; (iii) whether information on the group's deliberations or interim decisions is fed back to the participants for reconsideration during the process; (iv) whether there is face-to-face contact between group members, and if so, whether it is structured or not; and (v) the method used to aggregate participants' views.

Table 1 *Characteristics of informal and formal consensus development methods*

Consensus development method	Mailed questionnaires	Private decisions elicited	Formal feedback of group choices	Face-to-face contact	Interaction structured	Aggregation method
Informal	No	No	No	Yes	No	Implicit
Delphi method	Yes	Yes	Yes	No	Yes	Explicit
NGT	No	Yes	Yes	Yes	Yes	Explicit
RAND version	Yes	Yes	Yes	Yes	Yes	Explicit
Consensus development conference	No	No	No	Yes	No*	Implicit

* Although there may be no prearranged structure to the group interaction, groups may adopt formal rules, on their own initiative.

One feature common to all the methods, when used as a basis for creating clinical guidelines, is the use of cues. Cues are the dimensions or indications that group members are asked to take into account when making their decisions. For example, if participants were deciding on the appropriate use of a treatment, one of the cues they would need to consider would be the severity of the condition being treated. Others might include age, gender and co-morbidity. Some methods present cues to participants as part of a scenario or vignette – a description of a situation. Participants are presented with a set of scenarios, each describing a different clinical situation, and are asked to decide on the appropriateness of a particular intervention (investigation or treatment) in each.

Delphi method

Participants never meet or interact directly. Instead, they are sent questionnaires and asked to record their views. Commonly, participants are initially asked to suggest the factors or cues that should be considered by the group. Having contributed to drawing up the agenda, the next stage is a questionnaire which seeks their individual views about the items (usually by indicating on a Likert scale) that they and their co-participants have suggested. The responses are collated by the organisers and sent back to participants in summary form, usually indicating the group judgement and the individual's initial judgement. Participants are given the opportunity to revise their judgement in the light of the

group feedback. This process may be repeated a number of times. The judgements of participants are then statistically aggregated, sometimes after weighting for expertise.

Nominal group technique (NGT)

The aim of NGTs is to structure interaction within a group. First, each participant records his or her ideas independently and privately. One idea is collected from each individual in turn and listed in front of the group by the facilitator, continuing until all ideas have been listed. The NGT attempts to structure the interaction that follows by means of a facilitator. Each idea is discussed in turn. Thus, all ideas will be discussed, rather than focusing discussion on only one or two ideas. Individuals then privately record their judgements or vote for options. Further discussion and voting may take place. The individual judgements are aggregated statistically to derive the group judgement.

The most commonly used method for clinical guideline production is a 'modified NGT' developed by the RAND Corporation during the 1970s and 1980s, although the developers referred to it as a 'modified Delphi'. Initially individuals express their views privately via mailed questionnaires. These are fed back to the group. They are then brought together as a group to discuss their views, after which they again privately record their views on a questionnaire (Box 1). An example of the use of this approach is described in Box 2.

Box 1   *The RAND form of a nominal group technique*

A 9-member group of experts first define a set of indications to reflect their concepts of the critical factors (or cues) in decision-making for patients with the condition. The participants are chosen because of their clinical expertise, influence, and geographic location. Furthermore, they may represent academic and community practice and different specialties.

After agreeing on definitions and the structure of the indications (scenarios), the participants rate the indications using a 9-point scale where 1 = extremely inappropriate (risks greatly exceed benefits), 5 = uncertain (benefits and risks about equal), and 9 = extremely appropriate (benefits greatly exceed risks). By appropriate, it is meant that the expected health benefits to an average patient exceed the expected health risks by a sufficiently wide margin that the intervention is worthwhile and it is superior to alternatives (including no intervention).

The final ratings of appropriateness are the result of a two-stage process. The indications are initially rated independently by each participant without discussion or contact with the others. The group then assemble and the collated ratings are presented for discussion. After discussion, each participant independently and confidentially rerates each indication. The median rating is used as the appropriateness score.

To determine agreement and disagreement a statistical definition using the binomial distribution is applied. For a 9-member group, agreement exists when no more than two individuals rate a particular indication outside a 3-point range (ie 1–3, 4–6, 7–9). Disagreement about an indication exists when three or more rate a particular indication 7–9 and another three rate the same indication in the 1–3 range. Other indications are regarded either as equivocal (agreement at the centre of the scale) or as partial agreement.

Based on Bernstein SJ, Laouri M, Hilborne LH et al. 1992. Coronary angiography: a literature review and ratings of appropriateness and necessity. RAND JRA-03.

Box 2   *Developing consensus-based indications for the appropriate use of total hip replacement (THR) in the United Kingdom*[21]

1. The **literature** on THR was reviewed by a medical epidemiologist. One hundred and forty eight articles were identified, encompassing reports on the prevalence of hip arthritis, variations in surgical rates, indications for THR, alternative treatment options, short and long term complications, and long term outcomes.

2. **Cues** to be included in the scenarios were identified by seeking the views of six orthopaedic surgeons. At least one respondent suggested that the following might be relevant: age, sex, severity of hip pain, limitation of mobility, comorbidity, body mass index, arthritis in the knees or spine. The degree of support for each potential cue was determined by mailing the suggestions to the six surgeons. This confirmed the following as relevant: severity of pain and degree of limitation of mobility (categorised by the widely used Charnley Grades), comorbidity (by considering patients with low comorbidity, equivalent to a life expectancy of 5 years or more, medium comorbidity, with a life expectancy of one to five years, and high comorbidity, with a life expectancy of less than a year), body mass index, and the presence or absence of any disability affecting their knees or spine.

3. A **nominal group** was made up of doctors involved in deciding on the appropriateness of THR. Thirty three orthopaedic surgeons and 10 general practitioners working in North East Thames region were approached and of those agreeing to participate, five surgeons and three GPs were selected. They represented a variety of backgrounds – teaching and non-teaching hospitals, urban and rural districts – reflecting the mix of clinicians currently involved in deciding on the use of THR.

4. **Scenarios** were first categorised according to Charnley Grade, then subdivided according to the degree to which a patient was overweight, and the presence or absence of any disability affecting their knees or spine. Finally, the influence of comorbidity was taken into account. Overall, there were 30 different combinations of cues each with three levels of comorbidity, making a total of 90 scenarios to be considered.

5. The two **contextual cues** that the participants considered were (a) if they felt that another form of treatment would be more appropriate as a first line therapy, THR was to be rated as inappropriate, and (b) they should assume the existing resource constraints that they were familiar with in their everyday work in the NHS.

6. Each participant was sent a **questionnaire** with all 90 potential scenarios for THR together with a copy of the literature review. They were asked to rate, independently of one another, the appropriateness of THR for each scenario on a 9-point scale (1 indicated a patient in whom the risks of surgery outweighed any benefits, 5 meant a patient in whom the estimated risks and benefits or surgery were equal, and 9 meant a patient for whom the participant would always recommend surgery, as the benefits clearly outweighed any risks).

7. The participants then met for half a day. At the **meeting** each was given a second copy of the 90 scenarios which included a summary of the initial ratings of all the participants, indicated by the median and the range of ratings, and a reminder of the individual's initial view. Each scenario was discussed in turn. Most of the discussion centred on those indications for which considerable disagreement had been expressed. Cases where the risks were seen as roughly equal to the benefits were also discussed. Following the discussion, participants had an opportunity to reconsider their original rating and alter it if they so wished.

8. In **analysing the results**, the appropriateness of each scenario was assessed along with the extent to which participants agreed or disagreed. The level of agreement and disagreement was classified according to the dispersion of individual ratings. To eliminate any undue influence of outliers, the data were analysed after first discarding the two ratings furthest from the median. Appropriateness was assessed using the median of the ratings. A median of 1–3 was interpreted as the indication being inappropriate, 4–6 as equivocal, and 7–9 as appropriate.

    Participants were defined as being in agreement if their ratings fell within a three-point range disagreement if one rating was in the 1–3 range and one rating in the 7–9 range, and partial agreement if they met neither the agreement nor disagreement definitions.

Consensus development conference

A selected group (of around 10 people) is brought together to reach consensus about an issue. The format involves the participants in an open meeting, possibly over the course of a few days. Evidence is presented by various interest groups or experts who are not members of the decision-making group. The latter then retire to consider the questions in the light of the evidence presented and attempt to reach consensus. Both the open part of the conference and the private group discussion are chaired.

METHODS USED FOR THE REVIEW

Development of a Conceptual Model

To develop a conceptual model to guide and structure this review, we explored relevant material in the health sector, the experiences of members of the review group who had used consensus methods, and drew on psychological theory and research.

Consensus development methods may be considered to involve three types of activity: planning, individual judgement, and group interaction. These activities are not necessarily clearly separated or ordered. In addition, five components can be identified: three inputs (questions, participants, information), the process (consensus development method) and the output. As with the three activities, the components are also interrelated.

By combining these five components and the three activities, a matrix was formed which is shown in Figure 1. Each cell in the matrix describes a component in a particular activity. Brief descriptions of some of the important features of each cell are included in the matrix.

The decision on which methodological issues to focus was based on three criteria:

1 the importance of the particular aspect to consensus decision-making in the health sector;
2 the amount and quality of the literature available on the particular aspect; and
3 the potential for offering practical guidance for those conducting consensus development groups.

Following group discussion, members of the review group indicated which six cells they would give priority (shaded in Figure 1).

Selection of Material to be Reviewed

The amount and type of methodological research on consensus methods used within the health sector is very limited. For example, when consensus groups are compared only a small number of groups (often only two) are used. In addition, many basic issues concerning group decision-making have not been addressed at all.

In contrast, vast amounts of research have been conducted in social and cognitive psychology which address underlying issues involved in consensus development methods, whilst not necessarily directly examining these methods. However, many aspects of these studies (the

	Planning	Individual judgement	Group interaction
Question/s	Selection of topic Selection of cues Comprehensiveness	Influence of cues Question structure Level of detail	Modification of question/s
Participants	Number Type Degree of heterogeneity Selection of individuals	Representation of others Representation of self	Combination of backgrounds
Information provided for participants	Amount Selection Presentation	Read Understand Interpret	Use of information New information Feedback of group view
Method of structuring the interaction	Choice of method Particular brief	Perceptions of process Past experience	Setting Structure of interaction
Output: method of synthesising individual judgements	Type Target audience Aggregation rules	Perceptions of output Acceptance	Production of output

Figure 1 *Matrix representation of the conceptual framework of the review. Shaded cells are those areas on which the review was concentrated.*

approach, subjects, tasks) mean that while the research is relevant, it can only throw an indirect light on consensus development within the health sector. It was necessary, therefore, to glean general ideas and findings from this wider literature rather than pursue specific findings of particular pieces of research which may be of little relevance in the health sector.

The majority of the literature reviewed came from published sources. Most was identified through searches of electronic bibliographic databases, though the reference lists of retrieved articles were also used. Each of the six cells reviewed drew on the results of the principal general search. For some cells, further focused searches were used.

The general criteria for including a paper in the review were that it dealt with a methodological aspect of consensus decision-making and it was relevant to consensus decision-making in the health sector. Five electronic databases were searched: Medline (1966–1996), PsychLIT (1974–1996), Social Science Citation Index (1990–1996), ABI inform, and Sociofile. From the searches and reference lists of articles a total of 177 empirical and review articles were selected for review.

Some Preliminary Considerations

Before starting the review, three fundamental questions had to be considered: what are the objectives of consensus development methods?; how can 'consensus' be defined?; and how can the validity of consensus judgements be determined?

What are the objectives of consensus development methods?

One objective is to arrive at a single statement or set of statements that all participants accept (or at least no one disagrees strongly enough to veto the agreement). Clearly, if participants persist in disagreeing, the consensus statement(s) will have little or no content. Where the process goes through a number of stages, participants have the opportunity to revise their views in the light of discussion and new information. This allows them to identify which aspects of their position are relatively unimportant to them and so can be abandoned.

The other type of objective is to identify any 'central tendency' among the group and the degree of spread of opinion around it. Again the consensus development process may give participants the opportunity to revise their views in the light of discussion and new information.

Thus, on the one hand there is an attempt to facilitate consensus, and on the other hand there

is an attempt to describe the level of agreement. Whilst the first of these is the principal goal when drawing up clinical guidelines, the latter is also of interest. There is value in differentiating between areas of clinical practice in which there is close, moderate or little agreement.

How can 'consensus' be defined?

The answer depends on which of the two objectives is being addressed. When prioritisation is the objective, the output of the consensus method will typically take the form of a rank ordering of a set of alternatives. Each participant's scores or ranks are pooled to arrive at a group ranking.

The production of clinical guidelines generally involves weighing the balance of benefits and risks in order to estimate the parameter, such as the effectiveness of a treatment for a series of different categories of patient.

Technical questions (judgement needed because of insufficient data) need to be distinguished from value questions (judgement needed about competing social goals), because in general they should involve different types of participants. This is an important distinction as there can be no 'correct' answer with value questions, but for technical questions there is a correct, if undiscovered, answer. The distinction between these two types of question is, however, often ignored.

How can the validity of consensus judgements be determined?

How do we ensure that in general we make – or recognise – 'good' judgements? The nature of a 'good' judgement depends critically on the question being asked and, by definition, we can rarely *know* whether any particular judgement is a good one at the time. The best we can do is try to identify a *method* of arriving at judgements that will, on average: (i) produce more good judgements than other methods; or (ii) produce fewer bad judgements than other methods.

Although we might not be able to say at the time whether a particular decision is good or bad, we might – if we can identify a method with these properties – be able to support the use of that method over alternatives. This still leaves us with the problem of how to evaluate whether a method produces good or bad results, and in turn, some way of assessing what a good or bad result is.

There are five possible ways of assessing validity:

1 Comparison with 'gold standard'. Test the method on questions which have correct answers which the participants do not know with any precision. For example, with

almanac questions of the type 'What is the diameter of Jupiter?'

2 Predictive validity. In forecasting it is possible to look at whether the forecast that was made 'came true'.

3 Concurrent validity. If a decision conflicts with research-based evidence, without good reason, we can say that it is invalid.[16]

4 Internal logic. An alternative concurrent approach is to look at the internal logical order of a consensus group's output. In this way, the consistency of the decisions can be determined.[17]

5 Usefulness in terms of commitment and implementation. A good decision-making process might be seen to be one that produces results that are not only correct but also influential. However, this is a difficult definition to defend because whether guidelines are used or not may have little to do with the quality of the decision.

Thus, for clinical guidelines there is no absolute means for judging at the time whether a decision is valid, and thus whether a particular method for producing consensus is valid. This leaves us with the problem of how to evaluate different consensus development methods. Our focus has been to look at the factors which are likely to influence the process of consensus development, and where possible how they might influence the outcome.

FINDINGS

Setting the Tasks or Questions

Judging the appropriate use of investigations and treatments may be based on a few general questions (such as, in what circumstances would you recommend treatment X?) or a more detailed set of subquestions in which hundreds of possible clinical scenarios may be considered. Consensus development conferences usually ask only a few questions. For the Delphi method and the NGT, the task usually involves judgements over a wide range of scenarios.

Do the particular cues included in the question influence judgement?

The particular cues included in a question addressed by consensus development groups influence individual and group judgements.[18] The use of explicit cues in the design may lead participants to ignore or undervalue other cues that they may otherwise have included. This applies both to specific clinical cues and to general contextual cues, such as the level of resources available.[19–22] Table 2 illustrates how the higher overall levels of funding for healthcare in the USA is associated with US physicians' judgement that more clinical situations are appropriate indications for treatment than was true for British physicians. Individuals may not be aware of the importance they attach to specific cues and, when they are aware, the importance they actually attach to a particular cue may differ from the importance they believe they attach to it.[17,23–25] This may lead to difficulties in resolving differences during interaction.

Does the way a question is posed and the level of detail provided influence judgement?

Although research has not been extended to decision-making by consensus development

Table 2 *The impact of a contextual cue (level of resources available): median US and UK group ratings of indications for coronary angiography and for coronary artery bypass grafting (CABG) by appropriateness category*[19]

| US rating category | UK category | | | | | |
| | CABG | | | Coronary angiography | | |
	Appropriate	Equivocal	Inappropriate	Appropriate	Equivocal	Inappropriate
Appropriate	78	86	41	85	69	33
Equivocal	3	63	91	4	25	42
Inappropriate	0	5	113	0	2	40
Total		480			300	

The proportion of scenarios deemed appropriate is higher in the US where health care expenditure is much greater than in the UK.[19]

Note: larger numbers in top right than bottom left of each table indicates lower thresholds for intervening in the US.

groups considering the appropriateness of health-care interventions, it suggests that the way a question is posed may influence judgements about appropriateness.

The level of detail specified in a task affects not only the options participants may consider but also their estimation of probabilities.[26–28] Although research has not been conducted on this issue within consensus judgements of appropriateness, it is possible that judgements derived from general questions may differ from those derived from specific questions. Differences may also occur between appropriateness ratings derived when the starting point is a type of patient and those derived when the starting point is an intervention.

Does the way judgements are elicited influence those judgements?

The answers obtained from a group may be influenced by the way in which the judgement is elicited. Global views on appropriateness do not necessarily reflect participants' probability estimates of different outcomes.[29–31] This is because global views also take values or utilities of different outcomes into account. There is little work on this within consensus decision-making.

Does the level of comprehensiveness or selectivity of the scenarios affect judgement?

Given that groups may experience greater agreement and less disagreement when they are restricted to considering scenarios with which they are familiar, the temptation to be comprehensive by including every theoretically possible scenario may be counter-productive.[32] Also, being selective allows larger numbers of cues to be considered explicitly, which should be an advantage in terms of reliability.

Participants

There are essentially two stages to decisions about who to include as participants in a consensus development group. The first involves questions about the type of participant and the composition of the group. Most writers suggest that consensus development groups should be composed of people who are expert in the appropriate area and who have credibility with the target audience.[15,33,34] This raises the question of what constitutes an expert. Clinicians have clinical expertise, researchers have scientific expertise, and lay people or patients have expertise from having experienced the impact of the condition or intervention. All of these may be required. Once this has been decided, questions about the procedures for selecting, or sampling, individuals need to be considered.

To what extent is a group decision affected by the particular individuals who participate?

Little is known about the representativeness of participants in consensus development groups.[35] Knowledge of the impact of individuals is also limited by a lack of research. Studies that have been performed, listed in Table 3, suggest that the selection of individuals has some, though not a great deal of influence on outcome.[36] Some studies show similarity between similarly composed panels,[1,37] others show differences.[38] Table 4 illustrates this – appropriateness ratings of 82 out of 96 scenarios were the same for two groups, each of which was composed of people with the same disciplinary background. In most studies the number of groups compared is small, and thus the findings are weak. The particular tasks and procedures used also have some shortcomings.

Although the Delphi method has received some attention, very few studies have compared similarly composed groups using a NGT. Thus, any definitive statement about whether similar groups will produce similar results is not possible. The particular application of the method is likely to be an important factor. We do not expect that, as a general class, 'questionnaires' will be equally reliable for all samples of respondents. Rather, we assess the reliability of a particular questionnaire. So too, with consensus instruments; their reliability across samples

Table 3   *Studies that compared groups composed of similar participants*

Author(s)	Participants: subject of consensus method
Kastein et al. (1993)[36]	Mixed (GPs and specialists): abdominal pain + constipation
Duffield (1993)[37]	Nurse managers: competencies
Chassin (1989)[1]	Physicians: appropriate indications for coronary angiography
Pearson et al. (1995)[38]	GPs: sinusitis, dyspepsia
Brown and Redman (1995)[39]	Mixed (doctors): women's health issues
Penna et al. (1997) (pers. comm.)	Mixed (doctors): breast cancer

Table 4   *Ratings of appropriateness by two groups with different participants but from the same background*

	1988 Group		
1984 Group	Appropriate	Equivocal	Inappropriate
Appropriate	59	6	0
Equivocal	2	4	4
Inappropriate	0	2	19

Ratings of 82 out of 96 scenarios were the same for the group convened in 1984 as it was for the 1988 group (Chassin, 1989).[1]

seems highly dependent on the particular application of the method.

What effect does heterogeneity in group composition have on group judgement?

The weight of evidence suggests that heterogeneity in a decision-making group can lead to a better performance than homogeneity.[40] There is, however, some evidence that heterogeneity may have an adverse effect because of conflict that may arise between diverse participants.[41,42] The effect of heterogeneity depends to some extent on the task being undertaken.

Which personal characteristics are important influences on group decisions?

The status of participants affects their degree of influence on the group.[43] In groups of diverse status, those with higher status exert more influence.[44] In more homogeneous groups, group decisions tend to reflect the majority view.[45]

Initial opinions of participants affect the group process. If there is a majority view, this is likely to determine the final decision.[46] If there is an initial consensus, a shift may occur in which the final decision is more extreme.[47] If there is a split view initially, members will tend to move towards one another,[48,49] but this depends on the degree to which those with differing views form cohesive subgroups.[50] The more cohesive the subgroups, the less chance of achieving consensus and the more chance that there may be polarisation.

Do different categories of participants produce different results?

Studies, although few in number, show that differences in group composition may provide different judgements. This issue has been addressed in two ways (Table 5). There have been four studies in which groups of people with different disciplinary composition have been compared, and five studies in which different disciplinary subgroups within a group have been compared. The overall finding is that members of a specialty are more likely to advocate treatments that involve their specialty.[20,36,51–56] Table

Table 5   *Studies that compared (a) groups of different composition, and (b) subgroups of mixed groups*

(a) *Groups of different composition*	
Lomas and Pickard (1987)[57]	Physicians versus patients (communication)
Scott and Black (1991)[51]	Mixed versus surgeons (cholecystectomy)
Leape et al. (1992)[52]	Mixed versus surgeons (carotid endarterectomy)
Coulter et al. (1995)[53]	Mixed versus chiropractics (spinal manipulation)
(b) *Subgroups within mixed groups*	
Park et al. (1986)[54] and	Medical generalists versus medical specialists versus surgeons
Brook et al. (1988)[19]	(coronary artery surgery; cholecystectomy; carotid endarterectomy)
Zadinsky and Boettcher (1992)[56]	Doctors versus nurses (preventability of infant deaths)
Fraser et al. (1993)[20]	Medical generalists versus medical specialists versus surgeons (cholecystectomy)
Kastein et al. (1993)[36]	General practitioners versus specialists (performance criteria for GPs)
Kahan et al. (1996)[55]	Performers versus related area physicians versus primary care physicians (abdominal aortic aneurysm surgery, carotid endarterectomy, cataract surgery, coronary angiography, coronary artery bypass graft, coronary angioplasty).

Table 6   *Comparison of appropriateness of indications according to specialist and to mixed groups. (Specialist groups were more likely to consider a specialised intervention appropriate.)*

Topic	Specialist group (%)	Mixed group (%)
Cholecystectomy[58]		
Agreement	61	67
appropriate	29	13
equivocal	5	4
inappropriate	27	50
Partial agreement	31	18
Disagreement	8	15
Carotid endarterectomy[59]		
appropriate	70	38
equivocal	10	31
inappropriate	19	31
Spinal manipulation[53]		
appropriate	33	9
uncertain	22	37
inappropriate	45	54

6 shows how surgeons are more likely to consider surgery appropriate than would groups composed of surgeons, physicians, and other healthcare professionals. This can be seen in Table 7, which shows that those who perform a procedure tend to rate more scenarios as appropriate for the intervention than do colleagues who do not perform the procedure. This may reflect their greater knowledge of the scientific evidence on the appropriate use of the technique, or their limited perspective on alternative strategies. Even more dramatic contrasts may arise if healthcare professionals are compared with consumers of services.[60] Whatever the explanation, these studies confirm that the composition of groups is important in determining the decision reached.

Does the number of participants matter?

In general, having more group members will increase the reliability of group judgement (Figure 2).[61] However, where the group members interact, large groups may cause coordination problems within the group.[62] Although it is theoretically likely that group size will affect decision-making, the effects are subtle and difficult to detect.[63–66] It seems likely that below about six participants, reliability will decline quite rapidly, while above about 12, improvements in reliability will be subject to diminishing returns.

Information

Participants in consensus development processes may be recruited on the basis that they start with a good knowledge of the research results. Additionally or alternatively, they may contribute relevant experience. They will at least be expected to have sufficient technical background to be able to interpret any additional information, such as a review of research results, that they may be given, and to interact usefully. Thus the scientific aspect of information is generally well provided for. In general, however, information on values is not considered explicitly.

Table 7   *Percentage of indications for six surgical procedures that were rated appropriate by different types of physician*

Procedure	Proportion appropriate*		
	Perform	Related	Primary
Abdominal aortic aneurysm	38	37	29
Coronary angiography	58	45	23
Carotid endarterectomy	34	16	14
Cataract surgery	53	54	40
CABG	47	39	31
Coronary angioplasty	36	42	27

* Those who perform the procedures tend to rate more indications or scenarios as appropriate than do colleagues in the same specialty or primary care physicians (Kahan et al. 1996).[55]
CABG = coronary artery bypass grafting.
Perform = physicians who perform the procedure; Related = physicians in same specialty but do not perform procedure; Primary = primary care physicians.

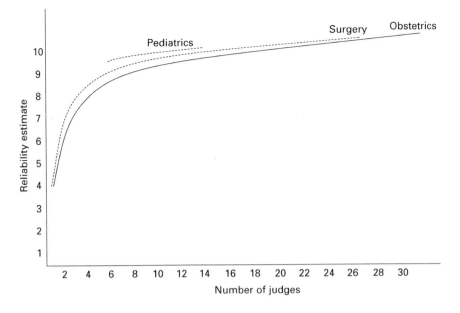

Figure 2   *Change in reliability of group judgement as a function of additional participants for three specialties. (Reliability estimated by applying the Spearman–Brown prophecy formula to the average values of all inter-participant correlations, within a specialty).*[61]

The extraction and synthesis of pertinent information for use by consensus development groups is a major challenge.[15] Without such reviews participants are more likely to rely on their own particular experiences. Anecdotal evidence suggests that when literature reviews have been provided, the evidence was used both in deliberation and in the decisions, making the consensus process easier.[67] The provision of information to participants varies from expert groups which rely on the expertise and knowledge of group members to those which provide a comprehensive synthesis of relevant research.[34] Sometimes it may be decided not to use formal information because the available evidence is so weak.[15]

How does information influence individual decision-making?

The information presented to individuals is an important element in decision-making. Information can influence judgement in a variety of ways. The way information is presented can influence the likelihood of it being used and how it is used.[68] The particular way in which information is framed can also influence judgement.[69–73] This can be seen in Table 8, which reports on the level of support by an English health authority (purchaser) for two policy proposals – the provision of mammography and of cardiac rehabilitation. People tend to be risk averse for losses and risk seeking for gains.[74–76] Individuals' own

Table 8   *Mean score (%) (95% CI) on two health policy issues made by health authority members when same results presented by four different methods*

Method of data presentation	Mammography	Cardiac rehabilitation
Relative risk reduction	79 (76–83); RRR 34%	76 (72–80); RRR 20%
Absolute risk reduction	38 (35–42); ARR 0.06%	56 (53–60); ARR 3%
Proportion of event free patients	38 (34–42); EFP 99.82 v 99.8%	53 (49–57); EFP 84 v 87%
Number needed to treat	51 (47–55); NNT 1592	62 (58–66); NNT 31

Higher score indicates stronger support for purchasing the programme.
The greatest support for both interventions occurred when participants were presented with information on the reduction in relative risk that would be expected. Number needed to treat produced the second greatest level of support. (Fahey et al. 1995)[71]

Table 9   *Change in percentage of agreed upon indications from initial to final ratings using nominal group technique (NGT)*

		Initial ratings	Final ratings	Change
Merrick et al. (1987)[16]	Carotid endarterectomy*	55.6	53.8	−1.8
Chassin (1989)[1]	CABG	23.2	41.9	18.7
Kahan et al. (1996)[55]	Abdominal aortic aneurysm	55	58	3
	Carotid endarterectomy	48	60	12
	Cataract surgery*	16	52	36
	Coronary angiography	38	40	2
	CABG	29	41	12
	Coronary angioplasty	27	40	13
Coulter et al. (1995)[53]	Spinal manipulation			
	Mixed panel	11.8	35.7	23.9
	Chiropractic panel	27.2	63.2	36

* The number of scenarios changed from the first to the second round making comparisons difficult.
CABG = coronary artery bypass grafting.

prior beliefs influence their interpretation of new information.[77] Experts may be better than novices at determining what information is relevant, but only in those areas in which they have expertise.[68,78]

Does the feedback of individual judgements influence group decision-making?

Studies often show a convergence of opinion.[79] Table 9 shows how feedback can have an effect on judgement. Convergence in ratings of appropriateness varies considerably, from slight (only 2–3%) to considerable (36%). The evidence as to whether convergence through feedback leads to improved judgement is slight,[80] and it may be that merely making the judgement again can improve accuracy. There is little research as to what type of feedback is best, though there is some evidence that information on the reasons for divergent views is more useful than simply feeding back the ratings.

How does information influence group decision-making?

The small amount of research on the effects of information on consensus groups suggests that information does affect their decisions.[44] Research on basic group processes suggests that both informational and normative influences are likely to operate in groups.[81] Informational influence is often dominant especially in fact-oriented groups.[82] Confirmatory or supportive information is most likely to be discussed as is information that is shared among group members. Novel information may have the greatest impact on opinion change.[44,48] The more widely information is shared, the more influence it may have.[83,84]

Methods of Structuring the Interaction

During the planning phase, the particular consensus development method to be used needs to be selected. In addition, a detailed description of how the method is to be implemented is needed, given the wide variety of applications reported in the literature. If it does vary from the original application, some justification for this deviation is needed.

Does the choice of consensus development method influence the group's decision?

Formal methods generally perform as well or better than informal methods but it is difficult to tell which of the formal methods is best. The 19 studies that have compared methods are shown in Table 10. The reason why formal techniques are said to work better is because they provide structure to the interaction, though which aspect of the structure is the most important is less well understood.[101–103] Most studies have not examined whether the interaction was actually altered in the ways suggested, and many studies did not operationalise the technique in a consistent way. Hence, there is difficulty in deciding which formal technique performs best. It may well be that the particular operationalisation of the technique and, probably, the particular aspects of the task to which it is applied, affect the relative success of different formal techniques.

Does the setting for group meetings affect the consensus decision?

The environment in which the decision-making session takes place may affect the interaction and satisfaction of participants, and may ultimately have an impact on decision quality. There is little research which actually looks at

Table 10 *Studies comparing methods, categorised by task*

Study	Comparisons	Task	Results
Gustafson et al. (1973)[85]	Informal = e NGT = e-t-e Delphi = e-f-e Staticised = e	Probability estimation	NGT best
Fischer (1981)[86]	Informal = t-e NGT = e-t-e Delphi = e-f-e Staticised = e	Probability estimation	No difference
Brightman et al. (1983)[87]	Informal = t NGT = e-f-t-e	Probability estimation	NGT best
Soon and O'Connor (1991)[88]	Informal = t NGT = e-t-e Staticised = e	Forecasting	No difference
Sneizek (1990)[89]	Informal = e-t Delphi = e-f-e Staticised = e	Forecasting	No difference
Larreche and Moinpour (1983)[90]	Informal = e-t Delphi = e-f-e Staticised = e	Forecasting	Delphi best
Herbert and Yost (1979)[91]	Informal = e-t NGT = e-f-t-e	Ranking	NGT best
Errfmeyer and Lane (1984)[92]	Informal = e-t NGT = e-f-t-e Delphi = e-f-e Structured = e-t	Ranking	Delphi best NGT worst
Nemiroff et al. (1976)[93]	Informal = e-t NGT = e-f-t-e Structured = e-t	Ranking	No difference
Burleson et al. (1984)[94]	Informal = e-t Delphi = e-f-e Staticised = e-e	Ranking	Informal best
Van de Ven and Delbecq (1974)[95]	Informal = t NGT = e-f-t-e Delphi = e-f-e	Idea generation	NGT and Delphi better than informal
White et al. (1980)[96]	Informal = t NGT = e-f-t-e Structured = t	Idea generation	NGT best
Jarboe (1988)[97]	NGT = e-f-t-e Structured = t	Idea generation	NGT best
Miner (1979)[98]	NGT = e-f-t-e? Delphi = e-f-e?	Role play task	No difference
Rohrbaugh (1979)[99]	NGT = e-f-t-e SJA = e-f-t	Judgement policy	No difference
Rohrbaugh (1981)[100]	Delphi = e-f-e SJA = e-f-t	Judgement policy	No difference

t = talk, e = estimate, f = feedback.
Staticised groups are collections of individuals who work independently with no interaction and their views are aggregated statistically.
Social judgement analysis is a form of feedback rather than a comprehensive consensus method.
Structured methods use either a facilitator or instructions to ensure that discussion passes through a series of problem-solving steps in a systematic manner.

this question.[104–106] However, of the many factors which can influence decision-making, the environment is likely to have only a marginal impact except in extreme circumstances.[107]

Do the characteristics of a group facilitator affect the consensus decision?

Although work on leadership suggests that aspects of leader behaviour are important for group decision-making,[108,109] the models of leadership used are often not directly transferable to facilitation.[10] There is little work which examines what a good facilitator is and very little work which looks at the effects of facilitation on group decision-making. However, it is likely that this key role will influence group decision-making.[44,110,111]

Outputs: Methods of Synthesising Individual Judgements

The nature of the outputs of a consensus development process will be determined during its planning, along with decisions as to whom the outputs are aimed. The process of arriving at these decisions will reflect and often help to refine the objectives of the exercise. There may be further revisions when individual judgements are being made in the light of participants' opinions about what they are being asked to do.

In formal consensus development methods individual judgements may remain confidential, aggregation is by explicit methods including some indication of the individuals' degree of agreement, and the group's deliberations are controlled by externally imposed rules. The procedures involved in aggregation fall into two distinct stages. In the first, differential weights may be attached to the contributions of the various participants. (Weights may be fixed for all questions, or vary from one question to another.) In the second, group scores and indices of spread are calculated from each set of participants' assessments, weighted or otherwise.

Is an implicit approach to aggregation of individuals' judgements sufficient?

Voting is only suitable for choosing, ranking or prioritising options rather than assigning specific values to each scenario or statement. Research in this field suggests that the more demanding the rules, the less likely a consensus will be achieved.[112,113] The very act of voting and the timing of a vote can affect the group decision.[114] Voting systems are subject to several paradoxes that might undermine the validity of the outcome.[115,116]

Should the judgements of participants be weighted when using an explicit method?

Although weighting by expertise may seem attractive in theory, the benefits are uneven and difficult to predict.[117] In practice, it is unclear how weights should be assigned to different participants.[118] Inappropriate weights may be worse than no weights.

How should individuals' judgements be aggregated for any one scenario in an explicit method?

The appropriate method of aggregating individual judgements will depend on whether the objective is to identify consensus (rather than a lack of consensus) or the nature and extent of consensus. Use of a frequency distribution avoids arbitrary value judgements. Criteria for choosing a method include robustness, accuracy and fairness. In other contexts, the median and interquartile range have been shown to be robust.[119]

How should consensus be defined in an explicit, quantitative method?

Outcome is partly dependent on the way consensus is defined.[58] Table 11 shows how relaxing the definition of agreement makes little difference to the proportion of scenarios or statements a group agrees about. In contrast, Table 12 shows how relaxing the definition of disagreement has a marked effect on the proportion of scenarios about which a group disagrees. Excluding the judgements of outliers also has a dramatic effect on both levels of agreement and disagreement.[120] Although a number of analytical methods exist, there is no agreed standard.[121,122] Analyses should recognise the difference between reliability and agreement.

IMPLICATIONS AND RECOMMENDATIONS

Although a considerable amount of research has been carried out on consensus development methods,[123] many aspects have not been investigated sufficiently. For the time being at least, advice on those aspects has, therefore, to be based on the user's own commonsense and the experience of those who have used or participated in these methods. To avoid confusion, the extent to which research support for any guidance on good practice is indicated as:

A = clear research evidence;
B = limited supporting research evidence;
C = experienced commonsense judgement.

Table 11   *Impact of different definitions of agreement on the proportion of scenarios about which the group reached agreement (%)*

	Include all ratings		Exclude furthest ratings		Exclude min–max ratings	
	Strict	Relaxed	Strict	Relaxed	Strict	Relaxed
Park et al. (1989)[32]						
Coronary angiography	28	28.7	NA	NA	50	56.3
Endoscopy	25.4	25.4	NA	NA	41.3	41.6
Carotid endarterectomy	40.9	40.9	NA	NA	53.4	53.8
Scott and Black (1991)[51]						
Cholecystectomy						
Mixed panel	45	47	63	67	NA	NA
Surgical panel	35	35	57	61	50	53
Imamura et al. (1997)[21]						
Total hip replacement						
Britain	41.5	41.5	52.8	59.4	48.1	51.9
Japan	23.3	31.7	50.0	68.9	44.2	55.0

Strict = all ratings in one of three predefined ranges 1–3, 4–6, 7–9; Relaxed = all ratings within any 3-point range. NA = no analysis reported.

Table 12   *Impact of different definitions of disagreement on the proportion of scenarios about which the group reached agreement (%)*

	Include all ratings		Exclude furthest ratings		Exclude min–max ratings	
	Strict	Relaxed	Strict	Relaxed	Strict	Relaxed
Park et al. (1989)[32]						
Coronary angiography	2	30	NA	NA	0.3	11
Endoscopy	30.2	48.5	NA	NA	7	28.9
Carotid endarterectomy	14.9	34	NA	NA	2.3	18.1
Scott and Black (1991)[51]						
Cholecystectomy						
Mixed panel	10	31	3	15	NA	NA
Surgical panel	2	26	0	8	0	11
Imamura et al. (1997)[21]						
Total hip replacement						
Britain	0	17	0	1	0	3
Japan	0	25	0	5	0	10

NA = no analysis reported in paper.

B and C should not be regarded as necessarily unsatisfactory, as some aspects of the conduct of consensus development methods are not amenable to scientific study but can be adequately justified on the basis of experience.

Setting the Task(s) or Question(s) to be Addressed

Considerable care must be given to the selection of the cues – the characteristics that influence clinical management, such as the severity of the patient's condition. Participants should be given the opportunity to say which cues they consider important. Doing so may help maintain their participation and help them justify their judgements. Participants' views of the relevant cues can usefully be obtained during a preliminary round of individual open-ended consultations. [C]

Contextual cues (such as whether judgements should assume unlimited healthcare resources or the reality of restricted resources) are as important as those specific to the topic. Participants are likely to make differing assumptions about these cues if they are not specified in the task, so it is important to make them explicit. [B]

The focus of the task may either be ways of managing a particular condition or the indications for using an intervention. If the latter, care needs to be taken as to how other relevant interventions are dealt with because views of the appropriateness of any intervention will depend on whether or not the possibility of using alternative interventions is taken into account. Ambiguity as to whether or not alternatives should be considered can affect group consensus. For example, participants may be instructed either to make their judgements in terms of the intervention under consideration being more or less appropriate than other interventions in general or than some specified intervention(s). [C]

Participants may be asked to provide an overall judgement (for example, treatment is or is not appropriate in a particular scenario) or an attempt can be made to break the judgement down into probability and utility estimates. There are theoretical advantages with the latter, but it is likely to be a more difficult task for some participants (probability estimates are a matter for technical experts, though utility estimates may appropriately involve others, including patients) and it is unclear whether it enhances judgements. [C]

Although including all theoretically possible scenarios will increase the comprehensiveness of the exercise, if many of the scenarios rarely occur in practice, the increased burden on the participants may not be justified by the limited value of the information provided. It is also likely that judgements of scenarios which never or rarely occur are less reliable than judgements of scenarios which more commonly occur in practice [B]. Further, requiring participants to judge what may be seen as numerous irrelevant scenarios may alienate them from the task. [C]

Selecting the Participants

Within defined specialist or professional categories, the selection of the particular individuals is likely to have little impact on the group decision as long as the group is of sufficient size. To enhance the credibility and widespread acceptance of the guidelines, it is advisable that the participants reflect the full range of key characteristics of the population they are intended to influence. The basis for selection should also be seen to be unbiased. [C]

Whether a homogeneous or heterogeneous group (defined in terms of specialist or professional characteristics) is best will in part depend on the purpose of the exercise. If the aim is to define common ground and maximise areas of agreement, then groups should be homogeneous in composition. If, in contrast, the aim is to identify and explore areas of uncertainty, a heterogeneous group is appropriate. [B]

In judgements of clinical appropriateness, the most influential characteristic of participants is their medical speciality. Specialists tend to favour the interventions they are most familiar with. Consensus based guidelines should therefore be interpreted in the context of the specialty composition of the group. [A]

In general, having more group members will increase the reliability of group judgement. However, large groups may cause co-ordination problems. Although it is theoretically likely that group size will affect decision-making, the effects are subtle and difficult to detect. Below about six participants, reliability will decline quite rapidly, while above about 12, improvements in reliability will be subject to diminishing returns. [B]

Choosing and Preparing the Scientific Evidence

Such research-based information as is available should be provided to all participants at an early stage because:

(a) if all members of the group have access to such information it is more likely to be discussed within the group;

(b) providing a literature review to group members before discussion may enhance the perception that the task is research based, which will in turn encourage members to be more reliant on information; and

(c) providing a common starting point may foster group cohesion. [C]

Participants should be encouraged to bring the review and any personal notes to the group sessions as a memory aid. Information presented in the form of articles or abstracts is less easily assimilated than information presented in a synthesised form, such as tables. Presenting information in an easy-to-read and understandable format may mean that participants are more likely to use it. Tabulating the information in a way which increases the salience of the cues to be used for making judgements means that the information is more likely to be processed in this manner. [C]

Those with expertise in judging the quality of scientific research should be involved in conducting any literature review. Organisation of materials by methodologists can highlight those factors which are most relevant to making a judgement, thus making it more likely that judgements will be based on the appropriate information [C]. Grading the quality of studies using a reliable method (such as a standard check-list) may mitigate the biases of the reviewers somewhat, but may not eliminate them. [B]

Structuring the Interaction

Two or three rating rounds are likely to result in some convergence of individual judgements. [A] More than three rounds is likely to have little impact on the level of agreement and to have adverse effects on the response rate. [C]

The status of participants is known to affect their contribution to, and influence within, a group so efforts should be made to mitigate this (for example, by the use of confidential methods for participants to record their views). [B]

If a NGT is being used, a comfortable environment for meetings is likely to be preferred by participants and to be conducive to discussion. In addition, a good facilitator will enhance consensus development and can ensure that the procedure is conducted according to agreed procedures. [C]

Methods of Synthesising Individual Judgements

An implicit approach to aggregating individual judgements may be adequate for establishing broad policy guidelines but more explicit methods based on quantitative analysis are needed to develop detailed, clinical guidelines. [C]

The level of agreement within a group is more dependent on whether or not outliers (individuals with extreme views) are included, than on how agreement is defined (e.g. 'all individual ratings identical' versus 'all within a three-point range'). The exclusion of outliers can have a marked effect on the content of guidelines [A]. If the definition of agreement is too demanding (such as requiring all individuals' ratings to be identical) either no statements will qualify or those that do will be of little interest. [C]

Differential weighting of individual participants' views can only be justified if there is a clear empirical basis, related to the task, for calculating the weights. There is no agreement as to the best method of mathematical aggregation [B]. An indication of the distribution or dispersal of participants' judgements should be reported, and not just the measure of central tendency. In general, the median and the inter-quartile range are more robust to the influence of outliers than the mean and standard deviation. [A]

Some questions are amenable to research because there is an answer. There are also many questions to which there is no answer in terms of what is correct or best. For these questions, however, it may be possible to find out what effect a particular factor has on the process or outcome of consensus development.

As will be apparent, research is needed in many areas of consensus development. Realistically, it will be possible to fund only a limited amount of research on consensus development in the healthcare sector, though relevant studies in other sectors will no doubt continue in parallel. We have, therefore, focused on the five areas of uncertainty which appear to offer the greatest potential benefit for improving our understanding and application of consensus methods.

1 What impact does the framing or presentation of the question have on individual judgement?

For example, to what extent are ratings of appropriateness of one intervention on its own different from ratings of the same intervention in the context of other treatments? Would making other treatments salient affect their ratings?

2 In what form and how inclusive should scenarios be?

Research is needed to compare the ratings obtained using theoretical questions (such as, which age groups of patients would you treat?) with case-based scenarios (in which scenarios of patients of different ages are rated). Does judgement vary by the type of scenario? Are some types of scenario easier to judge than others? Do clinicians draw on different types of information in rating different types of scenarios? Are case-based judgements richer in information than theoretical scenarios? How do clinicians react to making these judgements?

3 How does the extent of heterogeneity of a group affect the process and outcome?

The effects of homogeneous and heterogeneous groups in terms of speciality background needs further investigation. Comparisons have been made between mixed groups and surgeons, but homogeneous groups of non-surgeons (including primary care doctors) have not been investigated. Also, the balance of speciality groups within a panel could be investigated – for example, heterogeneous panels with an equal number of members of each speciality versus panels which include unequal numbers. Analysis of both the processes and outcome within the group is desirable. Do minority views get properly aired? If so, are they eliminated during discussion or by the process of aggregation?

4   What effect does research based information have on individual and on group judgements? Does the effect depend on the amount of information or how it is presented?

This could be examined by studying group interactions or by examining the effect of prompts from the facilitator regarding the information. Studies could compare groups with and without literature reviews, or with the evidence presented in different ways (written, oral presentation, video) to determine if the information is exchanged within groups and whether it affects the outcome. What is the optimal amount of information that should be presented? What techniques can be used to make the information presented more accessible?

5   What effect does the method of feedback of participants' views have on group judgement?

Studies of different ways of providing feedback on group views to individuals are needed. These could examine the effect on outcome, interindividual understanding and discussion within the group. Using a Delphi method, what difference does it make if the feedback is attributed to a named individual or not?

References

1. Chassin M. How do we decide whether an investigation or procedure is appropriate? In: Hopkins A. (ed.). *Appropriate investigation and treatment in clinical practice.* London: Royal College of Physicians, 1989.
2. AHCPR. AHCPR Clinical Practice Guideline Program. Report to Congress. US Department of Health and Human Services, AHCPR, 1995.
3. Mann T. Clinical guidelines. Using clinical guidelines to improve patient care in the NHS. London: Department of Health, 1996.
4. Black NA. Appropriateness of medical care in Europe: a commentary. *Int. J. Qual. Health Care* 1994; **6**: 231–2.
5. Parente FJ, Anderson-Parente JK. Delphi inquiry systems. In: Wright G, Ayton P (eds). *Judgmental Forecasting.* Chichester: Wiley, 1987.
6. Rowe G, Wright G, Bolger F. Delphi: a re-evaluation of research and theory. *Technological Forecasting and Social Change* 1991; **39**: 235–51.
7. Sherif M. An experimental approach to the study of attitudes. *Sociometry* 1937; **1**: 90–8.
8. Asch SE. Studies of independence and conformity: A minority of one against a unanimous majority. *Psychological Monographs* 1956; **70** (9, Whole No. 416).
9. Zajonc RB. Social facilitation. *Science* 1965; **149**: 269–74.
10. Janis I. *Groupthink,* 2nd edn. Boston: Houghton-Mifflin, 1982.
11. Diehl M, Stroebe W. Productivity loss in brainstorming groups: Toward the solution of a riddle. *J. Personality Soc. Psychol.* 1987; **53**: 497–509.
12. Dalkey NC, Helmer O. An experimental application of the Delphi method to the use of experts. *Management Science* 1963; **9**: 458–67.
13. Pill J. The Delphi method: substance, context, a critique and the annotated bibliography. *Socioeconomic Planning Science* 1971; **5**: 57–71.
14. Delbecq A, Van de Ven A. A group process model for problem identification and program planning. *J. Appl. Behav. Sci.* 1971; **7**: 467–92.
15. Fink A, Kosecoff J, Chassin M, Brook RH. Consensus methods: Characteristics and guidelines for use. *Am. J. Public Health* 1984; **74**: 979–83.
16. Merrick NJ, Fink A, Park RE, Brook RH, Kosecoff J, Chassin MR, Solomon DH. Derivation of clinical indications for carotid endarterectomy by an expert panel. *Am. J. Public Health* 1987; **77**: 187–190.
17. Hunter DJW, McKee CM, Sanderson CFB, Black NA. Appropriate indications for prostatectomy in the UK – results of a consensus panel. *J. Epidemiol. Community Health* 1994; **48**: 58–64.
18. Fischoff B, Slovic P, Lichtenstein S. Fault trees: sensitivity to estimated failure probabilities to problem representation. *J. Exp. Psychol. Hum. Percept. Performance* 1978; **4**: 330–44.
19. Brook RH, Kosecoff JB, Park E, Chassin MR, Winslow CM, Hampton JR. Diagnosis and treatment of coronary heart disease: comparison of doctors' attitudes in the USA and the UK. *Lancet* 1988; **i**: 750–3.
20. Fraser GM, Pilpel D, Hollis S, Kosecoff J, Brook RH. Indications for cholecystectomy: the results of a consensus panel approach. *Qual. Ass. Health Care* 1993; **5**: 75–80.
21. Imamura K, Gair R, McKee M, Black N. Appropriateness of total hip replacement in the United Kingdom. *World Hospitals & Health Services* 1997; **32**: 10–14.
22. Bernstein SJ, Hofer TP, Meijler AP, Rigter H. Setting standards for effectiveness: A comparison of expert panels and decision analysis. *Int. J. Qual. Health Care* 1977; **9**: 255–64.
23. Brehmer B, Joyce CRB (eds). *Human Judgement: the SJT view.* Amsterdam: Elsevier, 1988.

24. Brown RL, Brown RL, Edwards JA, Nutz JF. Variation in a medical faculty's decisions to transfuse. Implications for modifying blood product utilization. *Medical Care* 1992; **30**: 1083–93.

25. Evans JStBT, Harries C, Dennis I, Dean J. General practitioners' tacit and stated policies in the prescription of lipid lowering agents. *Br. J. Gen. Pract.* 1995; **45**: 15–18.

26. Tversky A, Koeler DJ. Support theory: a non-extensional representation of subjective probability. *Psychol. Rev.* 1994; **101**: 547–67.

27. Redelmeier DA, Koehler DJ, Liberman V, Tversky A. Probability judgment in medicine: discounting unspecified possibilities. *Medical Decision Making* 1995; **15**: 227–30.

28. Redelmeier DA, Shafir E. Medical decision making in situations that offer multiple alternatives. *JAMA* 1995; **273**: 302–5.

29. Oddone EZ, Samsa G, Matchar DB. Global judgments versus decision-model-facilitated judgments: are experts internally consistent? *Medical Decision Making* 1994; **14**: 19–26.

30. McClellan M, Brook RH. Appropriateness of care – a comparison of global and outcome methods to set standards. *Medical Care* 1992; **30**: 565–86.

31. Silverstein MD, Ballard DJ. Expert panel assessment of appropriateness of abdominal aortic aneurysm surgery: global judgment versus probability estimates. *J. Health Serv. Res. Policy* 1998; **3**: 134–40.

32. Park RE, Fink A, Brook RH, Chassin MR, Kahn KL, Merrick NJ, Kosecoff J, Soloman DH. Physician ratings of appropriate indications for three procedures: theoretical indications vs indications used in practice. *Am. J. Public Health* 1989; **79**: 445–7.

33. Jones, J. & Hunter, D. Consensus methods for medical and health services research. *Br. Med. J.* 1995; **311**: 377–80.

34. Lomas J. Words without action? The production, dissemination, and impact of consensus recommendations. *Annu. Rev. Public Health* 1991; **12**: 41–65.

35. McKee M, Priest P Ginzler M, Black N. How representative are members of expert panels? *Qual. Ass. Health Care* 1991; **3**: 89–94.

36. Kastein MR, Jacobs M, Van der Hell RH, Luttik K, Touw-Otten FWMM. Delphi, the issue of reliability: A qualitative Delphi study in primary health care in the Netherlands. *Technological Forecasting and Social Change* 1993; **44**: 315–23.

37. Duffield C. The Delphi technique: a comparison of results obtained using two expert panels. *International Journal of Nursing Studies* 1993; **30**: 227–37.

38. Pearson SD, Margolis CZ, Davis C, Schreier LK, Sokol HN, Gottlieb LK. Is consensus reproducible? A study of an algorhythmic guidelines development process. *Medical Care* 1995; **33**: 643–60.

39. Brown WJ, Redman S. Setting targets: a three-stage model for determining priorities for health promotion. *Aust. J. Publ. Health* 1995; **19**: 263–9.

40. Jackson SE. Team composition in organizational settings: issues in managing an increasingly diverse work force. In: Worchel S et al. (eds). *Group Processes and Productivity*. London: Sage, 1992.

41. Maznevski ML. Understanding our differences: Performance in decision-making groups with diverse members. *Human Relations* 1994; **47**: 531–52.

42. Guzzo RA, Dickson MW. Teams in organizations: recent research on performance and effectiveness. *Annu. Rev. Psychol.* 1996; **47**: 307–38.

43. Levine JM, Moreland RL. Progress in small group research. *Annu. Rev. Psychol.* 1990; **41**: 585–634.

44. Vinokur A, Burnstein E, Sechrest L, Wortman PM. Group decision making by experts: Field study of panels evaluating medical technologies. *J. Personality Soc. Psychol.* 1985; **49**: 70–84.

45. Kirchler E, Davis JH. The influence of member status differences and task type on group consensus and member position change. *J. Personality Soc. Psychol.* 1986; **51**: 83–91.

46. Davis JH, Kerr NL, Atkin RS, Holt R, Meek D. The decision processes of 6- and 12-person mock juries assigned unanimous and two thirds majority rules. *J. Personality Soc. Psychol.* 1975; **32**: 1–14.

47. Williams S, Taormina RJ. Unanimous versus majority influences on group polarization in business decision making. *J. Soc. Psychol.* 1993; **133**: 199–205.

48. Vinokur A, Burnstein E. Novel argumentation and attitude change: The case of polarization following group discussion. *Eur. J. Soc. Psychol.* 1978; **11**: 127–48.

49. Vinokur A, Burnstein E. The depolarization of attitudes in groups. *J. Personality Soc. Psychol.* 1978; **36**: 872–85.

50. Whitney JC, Smith RA. Effects of group cohesiveness on attitude polarization and the acquisition of knowledge in a strategic planning context. *J. Market. Res.* 1983; **20**: 167–76.

51. Scott EA, Black N. When does consensus exist in expert panels? *J. Public Health Med.* 1991; **13**: 35–9.

52. Leape LL, Freshour MA, Yntema D, Hsiao W. Small group judgment methods for determining resource based relative values. *Medical Care* 1992; **30**: 11 (suppl.) NS28–NS39.

53. Coulter I, Adams A, Shekelle P. Impact of varying panel membership on ratings of appropriateness in consensus panels: a comparison of a multi- and single-disciplinary panel. *Health Services Res.* 1995; **30**: 577–91.

54. Park RE, Fink A Brook RH, Chassin MR, Kahn KL, Merrick NJ, Kosecoff J, Solomon DH. *Physician ratings of appropriate indications for six medical and surgical procedures.* Santa Monica, CA: RAND, R-3280-CWF/HF/PMT/RJW, 1986.

55. Kahan JP, Park RE, Leape LL, et al. Variations by specialty in physician ratings of the appropriateness and necessity of indications for procedures, *Medical Care* 1996; **34**: 512–23.

56. Zadinsky JK, Boettcher JH. Preventability of infant mortality in a rural community. *Nursing Res.* 1992; **41**: 223–7.

57. Lomas J, Pickard L. Patient versus clinician item generation for quality-of-life measures. The case of language-disabled adults. *Med. Care* 1987; **25**: 764–9.

58. Scott EA, Black N. Appropriateness of cholecystectomy in the United Kingdom – a consensus panel approach. *Gut* 1991; **32**: 1066–70.

59. Leape LL, Park RE, Kahan JP, Brook RH. Group judgements of appropriateness: the effect of panel composition. *Qual. Assur. Health Care* 1992; **4**: 151–9.

60. Lomas J, Anderson G, Enkin M, Vayda E, Roberts R, Mackinnon B. The role of evidence in the consensus process: Results from a Canadian consensus exercise. *JAMA* 1988; **259**: 3001–5.

61. Richardson FMacD. Peer review of medical care. *Medical Care* 1972; **10**: 29–39.

62. Shaw ME. *Group Dynamics. The Psychology of Small Group Behavior.* 3rd edn. New York: McGraw-Hill, 1981.

63. McGrath JE. Small group research. *Am. Behav. Scientist* 1978; **21**: 651–74.

64. Nagao DH, Davis JH. Some implications of temporal drift in social parameters. *J. Exp. Soc. Psychol.* 1980; **16**: 479–96.

65. Davis JH. Some compelling intuitions about group consensus decisions, theoretical and empirical research, and interpersonal aggregation phenomena: Selected examples, 1950–1990. *Organizational Behavior and Human Decision Processes* 1992; **52**: 3–38.

66. McGrath JE. *Groups: Interaction and performance.* Englewood Cliffs, NJ: Prentice-Hall, 1984.

67. Jacoby I. Evidence and consensus. *JAMA* 1988; **259**: 3039.

68. Payne JW, Bettman JR, Johnson EJ. Behavioral decision research: A constructive processing perspective. *Annu. Rev. Psychol.* 1992; **43**: 87–131.

69. Bettman JR, Kakkar P. Effects of information presentation format on consumer information acquisition strategies. *J. Consumer Res.* 1977; **3**: 233–40.

70. Jarvenpaa SL. Graphic displays in decision making – the visual salience effect. *J. Behav. Decision Making* 1990; **3**: 247–62.

71. Fahey T, Griffiths S, Peters TJ. Evidence based purchasing: understanding results of clinical trials and systematic review. *Br. Med. J.* 1995; **311**: 1056–60.

72. Laupacis A, Sackett DL, Roberts R. An assessment of clinically useful measures of the consequences of treatment. *N. Engl. J. Med.* 1988; **318**: 1728–33.

73. Bucher HC, Weinbacher M, Gyr K. Influence of method of reporting study results on decision of physicians to prescribe drugs to lower cholesterol concentration. *Br. Med. J.* 1994; **309**: 761–4.

74. Tversky A, Kahneman D. The framing of decisions and the psychology of choice. *Science* 1981; **211**: 453–8.

75. McNeil BJ, Pauker SG, Sox HC, Tversky A. On the elicitation of preferences for alternative therapies. *N. Engl. J. Med.* 1982; **306**: 1259–62.

76. McNeil BJ, Pauker SG, Tversky A. On the framing of medical decisions. In: Bell D, Raiffa H, Tversky A (eds). *Decision making: Descriptive, normative and prescriptive interactions.* Cambridge: Cambridge University Press, 1988.

77. Koehler JJ. The influence of prior beliefs on scientific judgements of evidence quality. *Organizational Behavior and Human Decision Processses* 1993; **56**: 28–55.

78. Shanteau J. How much information does an expert use? Is it relevant? *Acta Psychol.* 1992; **81**: 75–86.

79. Woudenberg F. An evaluation of Delphi. *Technological Forecasting and Social Change* 1991; **40**: 131–50.

80. Gowan JA, McNichols CW. The effects of alternative forms of knowledge representation on decision-making consensus. *Int. J. Man Machine Studies* 1993; **38**: 489–507.

81. Kaplan MF. The influencing process in group decision making. In: Hendrick C (ed). *Review of Personality and Social Psychology, 8, Group Processes.* London: Sage, 1987.

82. Kaplan MF, Miller CE. Group decision making and normative vs. informational influence: Effects of type of issue and assigned decision rule. *J. Personality Soc. Psychol.* 1987; **53**: 306–13.

83. Schittekatte M. Facilitating information exchange in small decision-making groups. *Eur. J. Soc. Psychol.* 1996; **26**: 537–56.

84. Stasser G. Pooling of unshared information during group discussion. In: Worchel S, Wood W, Simpson J (eds). *Group process and productivity.* Newbury Park, CA: Sage, 1992.

85. Gustafson DH, Shukla RK, Delbecq A, Walstre GW. A comparative study of differences in subjective likelihood estimates made by individuals, interacting groups, Delphi groups, and nominal groups. *Organ. Behav. Hum. Performance* 1973; **9**: 280–91.

86. Fischer GW. When oracles fail – a comparison of four procedures for aggregating subjective probability forecasts. *Organ. Behav. Hum. Performance* 1981; **28**: 96–110.

87. Brightman HJ, Lewis DJ, Verhoeven P. Nominal and interacting groups as Bayesian information processors. *Psychol. Rep.* 1983; **53**: 101–2.

88. Soon A, O'Connor M. The effect of group interaction processes on performance in time series extrapolation. *Int. J. Forecasting* 1991; **7**: 141–9.

89. Sniezek JA. A comparison of techniques for judgmental forecasting by groups with common information. *Group Organ. Stud.* 1990; **15**: 5–19.

90. Larreche JC, Moinpour R. Managerial judgement in marketing: the concept of expertise. *J. Marketing Res.* 1983; **20**: 110–21.

91. Herbert TT, Yost EB. A comparison of decision quality under nominal and interacting consensus group formats: the case of the structured problem. *Decis. Sci.* 1979; **10**: 358–70.

92. Erffmeyer RC, Lane IM. Quality and acceptance of an evaluative task: the effects of four group decision-making formats. *Group Organ. Stud.* 1984; **9**: 509–29.

93. Nemiroff RM, Pasmore WA, Ford DL. The effects of the two normative structural interventions on established and ad hoc groups: implications for improving decision making effectiveness. *Decis. Sci.* 1976; **7**: 841–55.

94. Burleson BR, Levin BJ, Samter W. Decision-making procedure and decision quality. *Hum. Commun. Res.* 1984; **10**: 557–74.

95. Van de Ven AH, Delbecq AL. The effectiveness of nominal, Delphi, and interacting group decision making processes. *Acad. Manage. J.* 1974; **17**: 605–21.

96. White SE, Dittrich JE, Lang JR. The effects of group decision-making process and problem-situation complexity on implementation attempts. *Admin. Sci. Q.* 1980; **25**: 428–39.

97. Jarboe SC. A comparison of input-output, process-output, and input-process-output models of small group problem-solving. *Communication Monographs* 1988; **55**: 121–42.

98. Miner FC. A comparative analysis of three diverse group-making approaches. *Acad. Manage. J.* 1979; **22**: 81–93.

99. Rohrbaugh J. Improving the quality of group judgement: social judgement analysis and the Delphi technique. *Organ. Behav. Hum. Performance* 1979; **24**: 73–92.

100. Rohrbaugh J. Improving the quality of group judgement: social judgement analysis and the nominal group technique. *Organ. Behav. Hum. Performance* 1981; **28**: 272–92.

101. Nemiroff RM, King DD. Group decision-making as influenced by consensus and self orientation. *Human Relations* 1975; **28**: 1–21.

102. Hall J, Watson WH. The effects of a normative interaction on group decision-making performance. *Human Relations* 1970; **23**: 299–317.

103. Innami I. The quality of group decisions, group verbal-behavior, and intervention. *Organizational Behavior and Human Decision Processes* 1994; **60**: 409–30.

104. Reagan-Cirincione P, Rohrbaugh J Decision conferencing: A unique approach to the behavioral aggregation of expert judgment. In: Wright G, Bolger F (eds). *Expertise and Decision Support*. New York: Plenum Press, 1992.

105. Argyle M, Dean J. Eye-contact, distance and affiliation. *Sociometry* 1965; **28**: 289–304.

106. Sommer R, Olsen H. The soft classroom. *Environment and Behavior* 1980; **5**: 3–16.

107. Worchel S, Shackelford SL. Groups under stress: the influence of group structure and environment on process and performance. *Personality Soc. Psychol. Bull.* 1991; **17**: 640–7.

108. Flowers ML. A laboratory test of some implications of Janis's groupthink hypothesis. *J. Personality Soc. Psychol.* 1977; **35**: 888–96.

109. Anderson LE, Balzer WK. The effects of timing of leaders opinions on problem solving groups: A field experiment. *Group and Organization Studies* 1991; **16**: 86–101.

110. Wortman PM, Vinokur A, Sechrest L. Do consensus conferences work? A process evaluation of the NIH consensus development program. *J. Health Politics, Policy and Law* 1988; **13**: 469–98.

111. George JF, Dennis AR, Nunamaker JF. An experimental investigation of facilitation in an EMS decision room. *Group Decision and Negotiation* 1992; **1**: 57–70.

112. Davis JH. Group decision and social interaction: A theory of social decision schemes. *Psychol. Rev.* 1973; **80**: 97–125.

113. Davis JH. Group decision and procedural justice. In: Fishbein M (ed.). *Progress in Social Psychology*, Hillsdale, NJ: Erlbaum, 1980.

114. Davis JH, Stasson MF, Parks CD, Hulbert L, Kameda T, Zimmerman SK, Ono K. Quantitative decisions by groups and individuals: voting procedures and monetary awards by mock civil juries. *J. Exp. Soc. Psychol.* 1993; **29**: 326–46.

115. Arrow KJ. *Social Choice and Individual Values*. New Haven: Yale University Press, 1963.

116. Coleman A. *Game Theory and Experimental Games*. Oxford: Pergamon Press, 1982.

117. Flores BE, White EM. Subjective vs objective combining of forecasts: An experiment. *J. Forecasting* 1989; **8**: 331–41.

118. Rowe G. Perspectives on expertise in the aggregation of judgments. In: Wright G, Bolger F. (eds). *Expertise and Decision Support*. New York: Plenum Press, 1992.

119. Huber GP, Delbecq A. Guidelines for combining the judgments of individual memebers in decision conferences. *Academy of Management Journal* 1972; **15**: 161–84.

120. Naylor CD, Basinski A, Baigrie RS, Goldman BS, Lomas J. Placing patients in the queue for coronary revascularization: evidence for practice variations from an expert panel process. *Am. J. Public Health* 1990; **80**: 1246–52.

121. Shrout PE. Analyzing consensus in personality judgments: a variance components approach. *J. Personality* 1993; **61**: 769–88.

122. Kozlowski SWJ, Hattrup K. A disagreement about within-group agreement: disentangling issues of consistency versus consensus. *J. Appl. Psychol.* 1992; **77**: 161–7.

123. Murphy MK, Black NA, Lamping DL, McKee CM, Sanderson CFB, Askham J, Marteau T. Consensus development methods, and their use in clinical guideline development. *Health Technol. Assess.* 1998; **2**(3): 1–88.

Part VI

IDENTIFYING AND FILLING GAPS IN THE EVIDENCE

INTRODUCTION by ANDREW STEVENS

The number of health technologies, including drugs, devices, procedures and settings, is seemingly endless. There are some 10 000 distinguishable diseases in the International Classification of Diseases (ICD-10) coding, each of which is accompanied by at least 10 significant interventions, implying there are some 100 000 existing interventions. To this an ever-expanding annual new intake needs to be added. However, the capacity to identify new technologies as they appear, still less to prioritise them for evaluation, and then evaluate them seems uncomfortably finite. Many healthcare systems now recognise that this gap needs careful managing if they are to avoid the distortion of priorities for healthcare spending. The risks are both distortion due to 'free-for-all' in an uninformed healthcare market, and of distortion due to inappropriate selection in the control of healthcare technologies' availability. In the former circumstance the most heavily promoted new technologies (often, but not always, pharmaceuticals) usurp health budgets whether they are cost-effective or not, and indeed sometimes whether they are effective or not. In the latter circumstance, a selection of some technologies may be evaluated and their diffusion managed, but with no guarantee that this selection reflected a sensible choice. A sensible choice might be one in which priority in evaluation was given to the

most expensive new technologies, affecting the largest numbers, with the greatest degree of uncertainty as to their effectiveness and with the shortest 'window of opportunity' with which to assess them.

Healthcare systems therefore need mechanisms to:

1 identify new and emerging health technologies before they are allowed to diffuse widely into the system. Such a system might also build up an inventory of existing technologies and label them by three of these criteria, i.e. numbers, unit cost and evidence base,

2 select the most important topics for assessment, i.e. both whittling the possibilities down to a manageable number (relative to research capacity wherever it operates), and ensure that expensive research, itself, gives value for money,

3 respond at the appropriate time and with suitable research methods, and

4 operate a system for knowledge dissemination and implementation.

This is not a simple linear progression through four stages, but an iterative process involving stages 2, 3 and 4. This section focuses on the first three stages. The fourth stage including issues of dissemination, including incentives, education guidelines, feedback and peer pressure, is beyond the scope of this book, although a start is made in this area by Black et al.'s review in Chapter 24 on consensus methods in guidelines. Other useful papers include the NHS Centre for Reviews paper on guidelines (1992), on dissemination (1999) and Oxman et al. (1995).[1–3]

As regards the first three stages, this section of the book explores new territory. Robert and colleagues investigate how to scan for new technologies. They note that horizon scanning and early warning are necessary for the managed entry of new technologies into healthcare systems, such that they can be properly evaluated and planned for prior to diffusion. The difficulties confronting horizon scanning concern the breadth of the horizon, the unpredictable pattern of diffusion – many technologies do not follow a simple linear diffusion curve – and the tendency for new technologies to evolve and be used for different indications as they diffuse. Notwithstanding these difficulties, a number of countries have set up early warning systems to accompany their health technology assessment programmes. The methods that such systems use are still in evolution. Using a combination of literature review, survey and case study, the authors conclude on the need for multiple sources in horizon scanning – though particularly the use of key pharmaceutical and medical journals and expert networks.

Harper and colleagues consider the preliminary economic evaluation of health technologies. The process of prioritising health technology assessment projects has two components. The first is to narrow the number of possibilities, and the second is to undertake a preliminary economic evaluation which might inform the value for money of further more expensive research. Harper identifies a number of criteria already in use to do the former, including those used by the health technology assessment programme in the United Kingdom and the Institute of Medicine in the United States. Their main focus, however, is to review attempts to perform preliminary economic evaluation. It is possible to appraise models for such

evaluations using a number of new criteria, including the handling of alternative outcomes, the handling of uncertainty, and the availability of data to feed the model. The authors propose a new model which is being tested on four case studies of publicly funded randomised controlled trials.

Even when new technologies have been identified, priorities have been set and the case for a health technology assessment been shown to be persuasive, the question remains as to when (as well as how) the assessment be undertaken. The problem, identified by Mowatt and colleagues, particularly concerns fast-changing technologies. The argument against early evaluation, is that until a technology has stabilised – for example until surgeons undertaking a new operation have all passed a certain point on the learning curve – the results of the evaluation will not fairly reflect its established use. On the other hand, if an evaluation is undertaken once it has stabilised, the potential for getting clinicians to cooperate with a study will be that much more difficult. Their minds will be made up – equipoise will not be achievable. Mowatt, reviewing the diffusion and development of a number of case studies – laporoscopic cholecystectomy, chorion villus sampling, telemedicine, breast cancer, and gene therapy for cystic fibrosis, favour alertness and early assessment, if necessary undertaken iteratively as the technology evolves.

REFERENCES

1. NHS Centre for Reviews and Dissemination. *Implementing Clinical Practice Guidelines.* Effective Health Care, 1992.
2. NHS Centre for Reviews and Dissemination. Getting evidence into practice. *Effective Health Care* 1999; **5**(1).
3. Oxman A, Thomson M, Davis D, Hayes R. No magic bullets: a systematic review of 102 trials of interventions to improve professional practice. *Can. Med. Assoc. J.* 1995; **153** (10).

25

Identifying New Healthcare Technologies

GLENN ROBERT, ANDREW STEVENS
and JOHN GABBAY

SUMMARY

This chapter explores the most useful sources for identifying new healthcare technologies, and makes recommendations to assist the establishment and operation of an early warning system (EWS) for healthcare innovations.

The introduction of new healthcare technologies can have enormous consequences, both desirable and undesirable, for health services and patients. Early identification of technologies prior to their widespread adoption can enable timely cost–effectiveness evaluations to be undertaken, as well as fulfilling a number of other objectives.

The methods we used comprise: a review of the literature on the methodology of predicting the future of healthcare, a semi-structured telephone enquiry of EWS coordinators from around the world, an international Delphi study about preferred sources for identifying new healthcare technologies, and retrospective case-studies to learn how specific innovations could have been identified prior to their introduction. An understanding of the complex process of adoption and diffusion which underpins the development and use of new healthcare technologies is also required in order to help introduce them rationally.

The overall analysis of the results from the four methods (a form of triangulation) provides a more robust review of the important issues relating to EWS for identifying new healthcare technologies than any single method alone.

A combination of the following information sources (many of which can now be accessed via the Internet) is recommended:

(a) Scanning of 'specialist' medical journals, key medical journals, Food and Drug Administration licensing applications, key pharmaceutical journals, conference abstracts and liaison with pharmaceutical and biotechnology companies to produce a database of potential technologies.
(b) Regular meetings and/or surveys involving sentinel groups of expert health professionals.

The exact form and operation of the EWS (and the sensitivity and specificity, level of detail and timeliness which will be required from the chosen information sources) will ultimately depend upon the healthcare system of which it is a part, and the purposes to which the EWS are to be applied. Important aspects of the operation of an EWS are:

(a) continuity, so that the important monitoring function of an EWS can be performed on those technologies which have a long development phase;
(b) access to experts either through formal committee structures or regular surveys and/or focus meetings;
(c) collaboration with national and international programmes that already exist with the aim of ensuring adequate coverage of all types of technologies and providing sufficient early warning; and
(d) that the EWS should be part of a national programme to allow health technology assessment (HTA) research to be commissioned or run in parallel alongside early clinical trials.

Such an EWS should be evaluated. The overall value of an EWS for HTA purposes should be judged by the extent to which it facilitates timely research based evidence on new technologies. This chapter makes further specific research recommendations.

BACKGROUND

Brief descriptions of the key concepts that are central to this area of study and examined in this chapter are given in the appendix (see pp. 467–70).

Context

Often new technologies (whether drugs, devices, procedures or innovative ways of delivering services) are introduced to a healthcare system in a haphazard and uncontrolled manner, causing unnecessary confusion or expense. Many high-cost, high-profile technologies have diffused rapidly and not always appropriately or in a controlled way.[1] Their diffusion, evaluated or not, is disorganised and occurs at rates that depend on the strengths of various influences[2,3] (for example, pharmaceutical company marketing or clinical enthusiasm for a new surgical technique[4]). This is not surprising given that the key features of the market for healthcare technology include a lack of information, and the separation of technology provision from its financial ramifications.[5]

Concerns are both about effectiveness and the impact of the costs of new technologies in a fixed-budget, publicly funded healthcare system such as the NHS of the United Kingdom. Expensive medical technologies are becoming more frequent relating to expensive capital equipment (for example, a whole-body scanner), highly skilled persons to operate them (for example, renal dialysis) or by their high usage (for example, certain diagnostic tests or drugs). In addition, many new drugs are very expensive, in part at least because of their development cost.

Around 100 new drugs (including major new indications) are introduced each year with increasing policy and expenditure implications. Beta interferon (IFN-β) for multiple sclerosis could cost £400 million per annum in the United Kingdom alone, but at the time of its licensing many questions about its usefulness continued to await a trial with generalisable findings with full assessment of cost and benefit. Research based evidence on cost–effectiveness (not just safety and efficacy) is the only way to establish the appropriateness of uptake of any technology,[6] and earlier identification could have helped to ensure this was available prior to the marketing and introduction of IFN-β.[7] The development of

IFN-β could have been identified in April 1993, or even as early as November 1981.

The introduction of other types of healthcare technologies which have had large implications for the cost and effectiveness of care has also been uncontrolled. Examples include laparoscopic surgery in the early 1990s (which has been termed the 'biggest unaudited free-for-all in the history of surgery'[8]).

The rapid speed with which new healthcare technologies can diffuse, their potential impact, and their increasing numbers mean that there is an urgent need to develop and operate an approach which singles out those health technologies which might have a significant impact on the NHS in the near future.

Response to Date

Many of the technologies in regular use today would have been hard to predict 25 years ago,[9] but there is widespread recognition that a long-term perspective is useful in all aspects of national policy-making. Nevertheless, formal analysis of the future remains a low priority for most national decision-makers,[10] particularly those in the health sector.[11]

Other sectors such as electronics, aviation[12] and agriculture have undertaken extensive studies of technological innovation and diffusion;[13] yet it is in healthcare where major shortcomings in managing technological change have been identified, possibly because of the unusual way in which health technologies diffuse (see below). Such healthcare responses as there have been to date can be classified according to the time span of their perspective and according to whether they are concerned principally with deferment or with encouragement (Figure 1).

An EWS intended to help set priorities for HTA research lies in the upper-left quadrant in Figure 1. It intends to help control and rationalise the adoption and diffusion of technologies that are being promoted by the healthcare industry and professional opinion-leaders.[14] Other than for HTA, an EWS with a short-term perspective may be used by others needing early information on emerging technologies. Commissioners of healthcare are one such group, but there is often too little evidence for their purposes on the categories of people for whom the new intervention will be cost-effective or, for example, on when treatment should be stopped.

Futures studies may also take a longer-term perspective and comprise a more 'cooperative' approach with industry (bottom-left and bottom-right quadrants). For example, futurologists and researchers brought together by British Telecommunications (BT) have tried to look into the

	Technologies that are pushing towards the NHS – plausible futures	Technologies we have to seek – preferable futures
0–5 years (short-term)	*Activity:* EWS *Purpose:* manage and control change	*Activity:* identify unfulfilled technologies/stem unnecessary ones *Purpose:* induce change
5 years + (long-term)	*Activity:* basic science orientated forecasting *Purpose:* long-term planning to anticipate likely developments	*Activity:* predicting desirable futures *Purpose:* design appropriate technologies

Figure 1   *Timescale and purposes of EWS.*

future by combing the literature and talking to leading practitioners. They produced a timetable for major medical and scientific developments over the period 1998–2030.[15] Such initiatives may often be part of national attempts at technology forecasting.

Most of these initiatives are very recent. The longest experience is in the Netherlands which was one of the first countries to identify the potential benefits of HTA.[16,17] Only a very few countries,[18,19] have established programmes for identifying, and monitoring the diffusion of, new and emerging healthcare technologies. A Dutch Steering Committee on Future Health Scenarios (STG) in the Netherlands[18] has been an on-going, iterative process. This has contributed to the healthcare horizon scanning literature, but along with the few other exercises has not been evaluated. There is, therefore, no agreed or empirically proven method of identifying and predicting the likely future impact of new healthcare technologies.

Challenges to Horizon Scanning and Early Warning

A major potential problem for horizon scanning is the unpredictable pattern of healthcare innovation and diffusion.

From the 1970s onwards, studies of biomedical innovation, and of the diffusion of medical technology, have become more frequent, and slowly a base of knowledge is emerging,[20] but the basic mechanisms underlying medical research and development remain largely unknown.[21] The evolution of a new biomedical technology was initially thought of as a series of technical events which is usually described as linear-sequential (known also as the 'science-push' model) (Figure 2).

However, in the 1980s the validity of the linear-sequential model was questioned.[22,23] Its basic limitation was its implication that innovation is much more systematic than it really is, whereas not only research but also the broader environment (as expressed through market forces) influences each stage of the development process.[6] Thus the development and uptake of an innovation is unpredictable and cannot be described in terms of standard processes.[24]

Some healthcare sector research has pointed to the difficulties of identifying the point of innovation.[13] Stocking found that in 22 innovations she studied there was one central person, often a doctor, who had the idea, developed it, and was central in its promotion.[25] This would suggest that knowledge of where such individuals announce their achievements (for example,

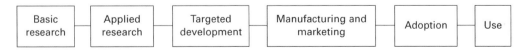

Figure 2   *A linear model of biomedical innovation.*

at conferences) might alert an EWS as to the likely introduction of a new technology.

However, even in the early adoption stage of a technology's diffusion, many uncertainties remain, often concerning either the precise indication or patient group, or both, for which the

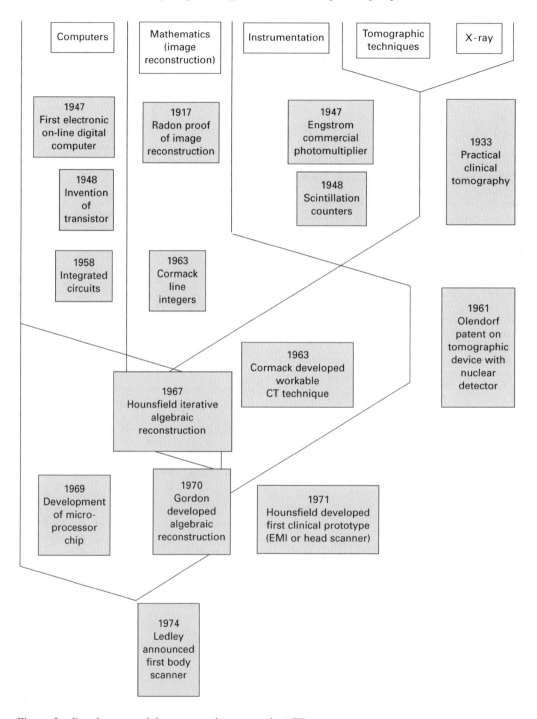

Figure 3   *Development of the computed tomography (CT) scanner.*
Source: Analysis of selected biomedical research programs. Vol 2.
Columbus Ohio: Battelle Columbus Laboratories, 1976.

technology will eventually be used.[24] New healthcare technologies often interact with other technologies in unexpected ways. These interactions frequently cannot be anticipated as the complementary technology may not yet have been invented (for example, day surgery and anaesthetics). Progress in five different biomedical research programmes (X-ray, tomographic techniques, instrumentation, mathematics and computers) were required in order to develop computer tomography (CT) scanners[26] (Figure 3).

Stocking suggests that the important time to assess a new technology is 'at the point when opinion-leaders become interested in it', which is at a very early stage, often before clinical trials data are available.[25] Fineberg likens attempts at assessment 'in this complex of evolution in science, disease, technology and society to standing on shifting ground and aiming at a moving target that is also changing shape'.[27] Assessing the effectiveness and costs of an innovative technology before its introduction and diffusion is therefore problematic.[28,29] Early assessments may not reflect potential capabilities or lower costs, and therefore will be of little use either for the researchers or policy-makers. Later assessments risk being of little use for decision-makers.[30]

Inevitably, earlier warning of a new technology will not be able to provide as precise and detailed information as warnings which come much nearer to the technology's uptake into a healthcare system. This trade-off between level of accuracy and earlier warning may be pertinent when selecting which information sources are to be used as part of an EWS, as some sources will be more likely to provide earlier warning, whilst others will provide greater detail on an already emerging technology.

For prioritising a HTA research programme a major challenge is to forecast which technologies are likely to generate the most policy interest once they are widely used. Some sources will ensure that no important technologies are missed, but the appraisal of such sources will require more resources – much of which will be expended on technologies that come to nothing. They will also need the development of criteria for selecting the technologies most likely to have a large impact. Alternatively, other sources will require less appraisal in order to select the most important technologies, but run the risk of omitting from the research prioritisation exercise technologies which turn out to have large implications for the health service.

Whilst the outputs of an EWS may be aimed at different audiences, the rationale for their existence is the same: 'managed entry' either to help prevent the undesirable consequences of the irrational and haphazard introduction of new healthcare technologies or to promote the adoption of beneficial and cost-effective technologies.

METHODS USED

We used four methods – literature review, telephone survey, Delphi survey and case studies – in order to achieve the stated aims of the project which were: (i) to explore the most useful sources for identifying new healthcare technologies; and (ii) to make recommendations to assist the establishment and operation of an EWS in the UK.

Literature Review

A systematic review was made of the literature on health futures and forecasting in the UK and from healthcare systems overseas to assess information sources which have previously been used to identify new healthcare technologies. The databases searched were: Medline (1966–97), HealthSTAR (1975–97) and ECRI's HTA Information Service database of grey literature in the US (1990–96).

Telephone Survey

A semi-structured telephone survey was carried out of coordinators of existing EWS in six countries (the Netherlands, Sweden, Denmark, France, United Kingdom and Canada) to identify which sources are currently being used, and to inform recommendations on the establishment and operation of an EWS in the UK as part of a national HTA system. The questionnaire focused on the aims, methods and level of support of each of the EWS. The responses have been used to inform the critique of existing EWS.

Delphi Survey

A Delphi study, involving international experts, to assess potential sources for identifying new healthcare technologies, was performed. The content of the three stages of the Delphi study are summarised in Figure 4.

We compiled a list of potential information sources for identifying new healthcare technologies from existing or previous EWS and other

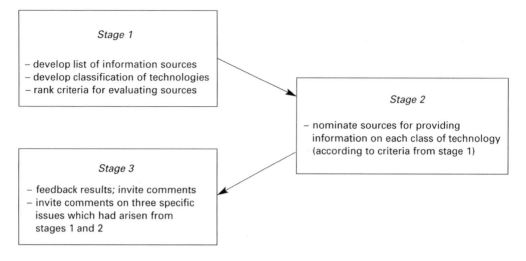

Figure 4   *Content of three-stage Delphi study.*

Table 1   *Information sources on new healthcare technologies*

Baseline list of sources

1   Key medical journals (i.e. *Lancet, British Medical Journal, New England Journal of Medicine*)
2   Key pharmaceutical journals (i.e. *PharmaProjects, Scrip, InPharma*)
3   Key scientific journals (i.e. *Science, Nature*)
4   The financial press and press cuttings generally
5   Patent literature
6   Pharmaceutical companies
7   Private healthcare providers
8   Biotechnology companies
9   Medical engineering companies
10 Sentinel groups of expert health professionals
11 Patient special interest groups
12 Conference/meeting abstracts
13 The results of other countries' horizon scanning exercises (e.g. the Netherlands)

Additional sources suggested by Delphi participants (*n = 31*)
14 Internet (suggested by three respondents)
15 Funding proposals and trial registers in other countries (suggested by two respondents)
16 Stock market analysts/venture capitalists (suggested by two respondents)
17 Newsletters and bulletins from other HTA organisations (suggested by two respondents)
18 Specialist industry sector journals (suggested by two respondents)
19 FDA licensing applications
20 Department of Health Industrial division
21 Science fiction literature
22 Legal cases; product liability/failures
23 Research programme papers
24 Specialist medical journals (defined as those journals which contain early case series/case reports/
    uncontrolled studies which strongly influence early adopters but do not make it into the 'big' journals)
25 Ethical committee applications
26 Drug Information Services

similar initiatives and additional sources were suggested by participants (Table 1). Participants were asked to suggest, using an agreed set of criteria, which information sources would be the most useful for identifying various types of healthcare technology.

Case Studies

The case studies aim to illustrate whether the information sources recommended by the literature review, telephone enquiry and Delphi study would have identified the selected healthcare technologies prior to their initial introduction and early diffusion into the UK's NHS. The sources of data for the case studies were from the literature (books, journals, articles, published and unpublished documents) and discussions with key persons in the relevant industry and within the NHS.

The technologies were: CT scanners, a biosensor (the ExacTech glucose pen), telemedicine, left ventricular assist devices (LVADs), paediatric intensive care units (PICUs), dornase alfa, IFN-β, donepezil and laparoscopic cholecystectomy. We chose these particular case studies in order to ensure examples of each of the broad types of healthcare technology (drugs, devices, settings and procedures). In addition, not all of the case studies are currently emerging examples; using old and contemporary examples provided an opportunity to reflect on the actual diffusion of some of the technologies into the NHS and the benefits that might derive from the operation of an EWS.

RESULTS

Information Sources

Literature review

There were potentially four types of paper to be retrieved on healthcare horizon scanning:

Type I: methodological papers which assessed the processes and information sources by which healthcare technologies could be identified with a short-term perspective, whether set in the context of a national EWS or not.

Type II: scientific attempts at identifying new technologies across a broad spectrum of healthcare, i.e. using formal and empirical methods (but which did not assess those methods).

Type III: discursive pieces (often editorials or polemics) relating to future technological developments in healthcare but without any explicit description of their empirical methods or sources of information.

Type IV: Delphi studies or scenario analyses of future trends in health or healthcare which were concerned not with likely technologies but with preferable 'futures' and/or related to a longer-term perspective than that with which this study is concerned.

The literature review found no type I papers and identified only five type II studies[18,19,31,32,33] (Table 2). Only two national initiatives have been reported on in the peer-reviewed literature (the EWS in the Netherlands and UK[18,19]). Indeed, studies attempting to forecast emerging healthcare technologies are infrequent and, if done at all, are often undertaken 'in-house' and therefore rarely published.[34]

None of these five studies reviewed potential sources of information for identifying new healthcare technologies or used empirical data to justify any suggestions that they have made; no evidence could be found that any retrospective analyses had been carried out on any of the initiatives.[a] Of the three studies[18,31,32] which did provide some discussion around methodological issues such as which sources to use and how to use them, the comments are the authors' subjective views based on experience during their own particular study.

All of the five studies used experts; in one this was part of an ongoing process.[18] Other than experts, the STG project in the Netherlands also used a variety of other sources, such as the published literature, news services, biomedical and bioengineering conference proceedings, and others (for example, *Scrip*). For drugs and devices, additional sources were patent and licensing applications, investigational new drug and investigational device exemption documents released by the FDA in the US, and commercial databases on pharmaceuticals in the development phase. Stevens et al.[19] supplemented expert opinion with the scanning of medical, pharmaceutical and scientific journals and a 'watching brief' on pharmaceuticals going through clinical trials. They also took evidence from other initiatives in the UK [for example, the Changing Medical Practice (CMP) group of the Standing Medical Advisory Committee (SMAC)] and abroad (for example, the work of the Health Council of the Netherlands).

The authors of the five studies have noted that it is inevitable that some of their predictions will be incorrect. Our retrospective analysis suggests that approximately 50% of the predictions made across the five studies have been correct, including the timing of the technology's uptake (for example, drug therapy enhanced by genetic engineering before 1998), 30% have correctly identified what became important technologies but the actual adoption of the technology has been somewhat later than that predicted (for example, microencapsulation of drugs to arrive in 1983–84), or the application of the technology has been different to that predicted, and 20% have been incorrect (for example, artificial blood predicted to arrive in 1983–84).

Table 2 *Scientific attempts at identifying new healthcare technologies*

Study	Main sources	Timescale (years)	Key predictions before 1998 (examples)
Food & Drug Administration, 1981[31]	Experts (postal questionnaire)	Up to 10	Monoclonal antibodies
			Nuclear magnetic resonance imaging
			DNA-produced interferon/antigen
STG, 1987*	1. Experts (Delphi survey and postal questionnaire)	4–15	Magnetic resonance imaging
			Positron emission tomography
	2. Journals		Biosensors
Spiby, 1988[32]	Experts (Delphi survey)	Up to 20	Monoclonal antibodies
			Genetic engineering and gene probes
			Biosensors
Technology Foresight Programme, 1995[33]	Experts (Delphi survey)	Up to 20+	Carbohydrate sequencing
			Visualising molecular structure at atomic level
			Therapies based on non-peptide molecules
Stevens et al. 1997[19]	1. Experts (postal questionnaire)	Up to 5	Magnetic resonance imaging
	2. Journals		Minimally invasive surgery
	3. Pharmaceutical 'watching brief'		Drugs for treatment of refractory schizophrenia

* Summarised in Banta HD, Gelijns AC, Griffioen J, Graaff PJ. An inquiry concerning future health care technology: methods and general results. *Health Policy* 1987; **8**: 251–64; and Banta and Gelijns 1994.[30] These citations relate to the same project undertaken in the Netherlands during the mid-1980s.

Telephone survey

All the systems included in the telephone survey use expert consultation in some form: sometimes through meetings (Netherlands and Sweden), but mostly through telephone contact (Netherlands, Sweden, UK and Canada). Scanning documentary sources is also widely adopted by existing EWS (Table 3). All of the systems scan medical journals, with the majority also scanning conference and meeting abstracts, scientific journals and pharmaceutical journals. Two systems specifically mentioned the Internet as a source of information (Denmark, Canada). Links with other agencies through bulletins and newsletters have also been used (Sweden). Only the UK seems to have specifically maintained a 'watching brief' on drugs going through clinical trials, via formal links with another organisation, although the EWS in the Netherlands has close links both with the Sick Fund Council and the Investigational Medicine programme.

Table 3 *Documentary sources used by existing EWS*

Country	Medical journals	Scientific journals	Pharmaceutical journals	Marketing journals	Internet	Conference abstracts	HTA reports	Other pharm.	News-papers
The Netherlands	✓	✓	✓			✓			
Sweden	✓					✓	✓	✓	✓
United Kingdom	✓	✓						✓	
Denmark	✓	✓	✓		✓				
France	✓	✓		✓		✓			
Canada	✓	✓	✓		✓	✓			

Delphi study

From the responses received, eight information sources could be recommended as forming the minimum of any comprehensive EWS for identifying new healthcare technologies:

1 key pharmaceutical journals,
2 pharmaceutical and biotechnology companies,
3 'specialist' medical journals,
4 principal medical journals,
5 medical engineering companies,
6 private healthcare providers,
7 newsletters and bulletins from other national and regional HTA agencies, and
8 sentinel groups of expert health professionals.

Respondents were most prepared to suggest likely information sources for identifying 'pharmaceuticals' and 'diagnostic strategies'; few were able to recommend particular sources for 'other medical and assistive devices' and 'new professions'.

The costs of collecting information from the various sources must be weighed against the value of the additional information for the specific users.[30] In round 1 of the Delphi study the project team suggested a list of criteria by which each of the potential information sources could be judged, and asked the participants to comment on it. In round 2, participants ranked the criteria in terms of their importance for assessing the potential information sources (1 = least important to 5 = most important). The scores which the 18 respondents gave to each of the suggested criteria for assessing the value of the various possible information sources are presented in Table 4.

It is essential that any source should identify technologies sufficiently early in order for the technology to be evaluated before its widespread diffusion, so 'timeliness' is a vital criterion for any source to meet. This was reflected in the participants' ranking. It is also important that the sources should not be inefficiently labour

intensive to search (as with hand-searching key medical journals), given that only limited resources will be available for this aspect of the identification stage of the HTA process. As highlighted by the responses to the baseline list of sources provided in stage 1 of the survey, participants did not believe that any one source would be able to identify all the different types of new technologies and so 'correlation with other sources' ranked highly, as did the 'objectiveness' of the source, reflecting the desire for a more 'credible evidence base'. Clearly it is important not to miss any items that are likely to have a large expenditure impact on a healthcare system, or are likely to diffuse quickly so sources need to a have a high sensitivity. In the Delphi survey participants ranked specificity as being equally important as sensitivity. Comments showed that participants recognised that any source is likely to identify a large number of false-positives and this would have resource implications for an EWS. In short, the Delphi participants preferred to deal with these false-positives rather than miss something important.

On the specific sources, many respondents commented that, whilst 'principal medical journals' do provide a broad coverage, by the time reports of technologies are appearing in such journals an EWS should already have identified them. Two respondents highlighted the usefulness of the news sections in such journals (for example, the medical progress section in the *New England Journal of Medicine*). 'Scientific journals' were seen as a good source, but one with a long lead-time before the application of the new technology. They could be particularly helpful when innovations or ideas were being transferred from other sectors and into health services. One respondent felt that 'private healthcare providers' and 'patient special interest groups' were more suited to identifying needs for new technology as opposed to predicting which technologies are likely to have an important impact.

Table 4   *Criteria for assessing information sources*

Criteria	Median scores	Modal scores
Timeliness	5	5
Time efficiency	4	4
Agreement with other sources	3	4
Objectiveness	3	4
Sensitivity of source	3	3
Depth of source	3	3
Specificity of source	3	3
Elucidation of likely knock-on effects	3	2
Explicitness of limitations	2	3

Table 5   *Information sources for identifying case studies*

Case study	Information source
CT scanners	Experts, conference/meeting abstracts
Telemedicine	Journals, conference/meeting abstracts, experts
Medisense Exactech pen (biosensor)	FDA, key medical journals
LVADs	Specialist medical journals, FDA
PICUs	Experts, media
Beta Interferon	Specialist medical journals
Dornase alfa	Pharmaceutical/biotechnology companies, key medical journals, conference/meeting abstracts, FDA
Donepezil	Specialist medical journals, FDA
Laparoscopic cholecystectomy	Experts, conferences

Case studies

The case studies provide examples of healthcare technologies that have diffused without having been fully evaluated and/or without adequate consideration of their expenditure and policy implications, and the consequent need for an EWS. They provide a means of validating the results of the other three methods which were adopted to assess information sources for identifying new healthcare technologies (Table 5). However, the retrospective case study findings cannot be regarded as definitive because each source had it been used prospectively might have had an unmanageable yield (low specificity).

In the case of CT scanners, patents appeared to be an important source, but the very small proportion of products for which patents are issued that actually reach the healthcare market makes this source inefficient,[30] and this source was not selected by the respondents to the Delphi survey. Five other case studies (biosensors, LVADs, IFN-β, dornase alfa and donepezil) illustrated that monitoring the regulatory control of drugs and devices in the United States via the FDA would be a useful source.

It is difficult to assess the potential role of pharmaceutical and biotechnology companies and medical engineering companies through retrospective case studies. However, in some cases (telemedicine) there has been a strong technology push from manufacturers, although there has also been a degree of receptiveness on the part of healthcare providers. For example, British Telecommunications (BT) in the UK has developed the CARE project, initiating a series of telemedicine trials designed to gain an insight into the potential impact of telehealth services. In the cases of IFN-β and dornase alfa, pharmaceutical companies were clearly involved in promoting their products directly to clinicians prior to licensing in the UK. Having these clinicians among an expert panel would have provided a few months early warning.

The three drug case studies all revealed that pharmaceutical journals (for example, *Scrip, Hospital Pharmacy, Biotechnology, Drug Therapy, American Pharmacy*) would have provided early warning. In all of the three cases a relatively large number of published studies appeared at key stages of the licensing process, such as at the time of submission of an application to the FDA or announcement of FDA approval, but such events occur relatively late in a drug's development. However, it is problematic to comment on the likely specificity of these sources on the basis of retrospective case studies.

As evidenced by our case studies, journal articles in leading medical journals can provide early warning via:

(a) reports of primary research (for example, a report of a Phase III clinical trial of dornase alfa[35]); or

(b) discursive pieces on the future of a particular technology, such as those type III papers identified by our literature review (for example, *The Lancet* editorial on telemedicine,[36] the *New England Journal of Medicine* editorial on dornase alfa,[37] the *Journal of the American Medical Association* paper on LVADs[38] or series such as the 'medical advances' papers in the *British Medical Journal*); or

(c) news sections which may alert the reader to developments in areas of highly prevalent or serious disease.

Specialist medical journals were helpful in a number of the case-studies (providing particularly early warning in the cases of LVADs, biosensors, IFN-β and donepezil).

In four of the case studies (CT scanning, telemedicine, dornase alfa and laparoscopic cholecystectomy) conferences would have been a useful source as illustrated by Baker's[39] report on the relative importance of sources of information amongst early adopters of CT scanners in the US (Figure 5).

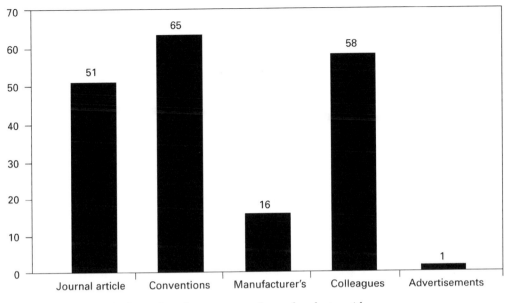

Figure 5   *Sources of information about scanners for early adopters (those ordering scanners 1973–75). Reprinted from* Social Science & Medicine, *vol. 13. Baker S., pp. 155–62, with permission from Elsevier Science.*

Whilst it is problematic to assess retrospectively the benefits of involving experts, six of the nine case studies (biosensors, LVAD technology, telemedicine, dornase alfa, donepezil and laparoscopic surgery) were predicted by one or more of the previous studies identified in the literature review (see page 457). These studies had used experts as their main source of information. Another of the case studies (IFN-β) was briefly referred to in the STG report and used as an exemplar 'new' technology by Stevens et al. in their postal survey.[19] The final two case studies (CT scanning and PICUs) had begun to diffuse before any of the studies were carried out.

Modern day sources such as drug information services could not always be assessed by the retrospective case studies. They are likely to provide helpful corroboration, as indicated by the monograph on dornase alfa produced by the Drug Information Pharmacist's Group.

Many of the information sources which have been identified by the literature review, telephone enquiry, Delphi survey and case studies can be accessed directly via the Internet. For example, many journals are now available on the Internet in some form, and conference reports on specific disease areas can be accessed through various websites.

Popular media coverage may have helped to highlight the likely importance of a number of the case studies, such as LVADs and PICUs, but it seems that such coverage may only appear after the initial introduction of the technology.

Operating an Early Warning System

In 1985 the STG in the Netherlands started a project on future healthcare technologies, in collaboration with WHO Europe. The report recommended a process for identifying new healthcare technologies as shown in Figure 6.[18]

Step 1	Periodical updating through written surveys (open-ended questions in a general letter; future surveys can be more specific; international collaboration is desirable)
Step 2	Work with key informants from different scientific and technological areas of medicine to be sure that technological changes have been identified accurately
Step 3	General screening of the medical literature, and focused literature reviews when a specific subject is identified

Figure 6   *STG process for identifying new healthcare technologies.*[18]

Table 6   *Current national HTA programmes*

Country organisation and start date	Main purpose	Time horizon	Role of experts	Outputs
The Netherlands: Health Council of the Netherlands, 1988	Both national HTA prioritisation and health policy planning	1–2 years before adoption	5–10 experts are used, via postal survey, telephone and meetings, to comment on identified technologies. In addition, nine standing committees (10 members each) are part of the routine operation of the EWS.	50–100 technologies are identified each year, 20 are considered in detail and 10 have reports written or are prioritised for R & D. The results are used to advise the Dutch government on the current level of knowledge and also disseminated to parliament, professional groups and the media. The government uses the results to inform regulatory measures, research decisions and the introduction and adjustment of legislation.
Sweden: 'ALERT': SBU, 1997	Health policy planning	<5 years before adoption	A scientific board of eight members and standing committees in certain fields are used (by telephone and meetings) both to identify technologies initially and to comment on technologies identified by other sources. One or two experts are used to advise on each specific technology.	80 technologies are identified each year, 40 are considered in detail and brief reports of 5–6 pages are written on 30 of these. The reports are published in a database available on the Internet, and in the SBU newsletter.
United Kingdom: University of Southampton (1995–96); University of Birmingham (1997–)	National HTA prioritisation and health policy planning.	<5 years before adoption	Two or three experts used to check on each technology identified by other sources (by telephone)	The EWS directly informs the UKs SGHT, and thus the NHS R & D strategy, of important new healthcare technologies

Denmark: DIHTA, 1997	National HTA prioritisation and health policy planning	1–2 years before adoption	Experts are used both to identify technologies initially and to check on technologies identified by other sources.	Results are fed in to the R & D programme, the health service and industry.
France: ANAES, 1997	National HTA prioritisation and health policy planning	Adoption phase	Use 5–8 experts, who are generally proposed by scientific societies, to check on each technology identified by other sources.	Reports are written on less than 10 technologies each year. The results are disseminated to health policy makers (French Ministry of Health and insurers) and scientific societies, to inform coverage decisions and planning.
Canada: CCOHTA, 1997	Ongoing 1-year pilot project for purpose of health policy planning (planning, budgeting and prioritising for provincial review)	1–2 years before adoption	Use postal surveys and telephone to access experts both to identify technologies initially and to check on technologies identified by other sources. Experts are either nominated by provincial government advisers, or chosen as they are holders of MRC excellence awards or on the basis of their publications. 3–5 experts are used to advise on each specific technology	Identify over 1000 technologies each year, consider 6–12 in detail and write reports on 6–10. Results are published in *Issues in Emerging Health Technologies* newsletter and on Internet. Selective communications are also sent to provincial decision-makers on 'hot' topics.

National HTA organisations have tried to establish an EWS (or at least to systematically identify new healthcare technologies at a given time), and Table 6 summarises the aims and involvement of experts in the six organisations which are currently operating an EWS. Commonly, a small number of experts is used to provide advice on each technology, but in some systems formal committee structures have been established as an integral part of the EWS (the Netherlands, Sweden). In the Netherlands, the EWS incorporates the expertise of the 170 members of the Health Council, as well as the nine standing advisory boards of the Council, each of which have approximately 10 members. The current initiative in Sweden uses a scientific board (with members representing radiology, nursing, physiotherapy, gene technology, oncology, general surgery, general medicine, pharmacology and pharmaco-epidemiology) and standing committees in certain fields. In Canada, experts – who are nominated by provincial government advisers or otherwise identified through Medical Research Council excellence awards and publications – are used via postal surveys and telephone interviews both to identify technologies initially and to comment on technologies identified by other sources (usually, three to five experts are consulted per technology). In addition to the six national initiatives described below, and although the US does not operate a national HTA system as such, there are – or have been – a number of projects undertaken in the US which are similar in scope to an EWS (although not necessarily for the explicit purposes of HTA). Initiatives similar to the EWS in Europe and Canada are undertaken at both the Federal level and within the private sector in the United States by organisations with an interest in the evaluation of healthcare technologies.

The most striking aspect of all these initiatives is, with the exception of the Netherlands, how recently they have been established. It remains to be seen how well established some of the latest initiatives will become.

In the UK there are a number of organisations and initiatives that either explicitly or implicitly have a role in providing early warning of healthcare technologies within the UK.[40] As well as the Forecasting Secretariat to the National Standing Group on Health Technology, which was established in 1995, there are various activities for clinical early warning, such as the Safety and Efficacy Register of New Interventional Procedures (SERNIP) and the CMP subcommittee of the Government's SMAC, which aim to allow time for the preparation of guidelines, or to act as a brake on unjustified expenditure. In addition, there is a well-established network of pharmacists which provides information on new

drugs on a regional and national basis, via the Drug Information Service (DIS) and National Prescribing. Each of these acts as a supply source for the new National Horizon Scanning Centre.

Each of the six national initiatives reported that they are currently disseminating, or are planning to disseminate, detailed information on only a small number of technologies each year, usually 10 to 12. This dissemination is carried out via a wide range of mechanisms and products. This includes providing formal advice to government (the Netherlands) as well as more informal dissemination to politicians (Sweden, France, the Netherlands) and national and provincial health policy-makers (Canada, Sweden, United Kingdom). Two of the initiatives (Canada, Sweden) have Internet sites which provide updated information on the technologies which they have identified and prioritised as being important. Newsletters are used by three of the initiatives (Canada, Sweden, the Netherlands).

The case studies illustrate the benefit of international collaboration. At the international level it would be beneficial to collaborate on definitions, co-ordination, standardisation and communication. In the longer term, there may be a role for a more formal mode of collaboration, perhaps based within the European Community or through INAHTA (International Network of Agencies for Health Technology Assessment).

RECOMMENDATIONS

Recommended Information Sources

One of the key assumptions in our approach has been to assume that different types of technologies will be identified through different, although not necessarily mutually exclusive, information sources. For instance, in the case of procedures that are not product-dependent (for example, arterial operations) the STG relied more heavily on expert opinion, informal documentation of scientific and technological developments, and professional meetings and publications, than on commercial product development databases. A combination of sources will be required in order to ensure that all types of technologies and all important technologies are identified. Using more than one source will provide corroboration, increase the likely accuracy of any predictions, and increase the amount of useful information regarding a new technology.

There were some discrepancies between the information sources which were recommended for identifying new healthcare technologies by

Table 7 *Recommended information sources from each method*

Source	Literature review	Telephone enquiry	Delphi study	Case studies
Primary				
Patients	✗		✗	
FDA licensing	✓		✓	✓✓
Pharmaceutical and biotechnology companies	✗		✓✓	✓
Medical engineering companies	✗		✓✓	
Secondary				
Pharmaceutical journals	✓	✓	✓✓	✓✓
Medical journals	✓	✓✓	✓✓	✓✓
Scientific journals	✓	✓✓	✗	
Specialist medical journals	✓		✓✓	✓
Conferences	✓	✓✓	✓	✓
Experts	✓✓	✓✓	✓✓	✓✓
Patient interest groups	✗		✗	✓
Private healthcare providers	✗		✓✓	
Drug Information Services	✗	✓	✗	✓
Internet	✗	✓	✗	
Media	✓	✓	✗	✓
Tertiary				
Other countries' EWS activities	✓	✓	✓✓	

Key:

Literature review
  ✓✓ = used by all previous studies
  ✓ = used by at least one previous study
  ✗ = not used

Telephone enquiry
  ✓✓ = used by at least 4 of EWS
  ✓ = used by some (1–3) of EWS

Delphi study
  ✓✓ = consensus that this source is a minimum requirement for an EWS
  ✓ = no consensus but from comments received may be useful
  ✗ = not recommended

Case studies
  ✓✓ = in the opinion of the case study reviewer (G.R.) this was the best source for at least one of the case studies
  ✓ = in the opinion of the case study reviewer (G.R.) this source may have been helpful for at least one of the case studies

Blank cells indicate no evidence available as method was not used to assess specific source

previous initiatives (papers from the literature review), the telephone enquiry of existing national EWS, the Delphi study and the retrospective case studies (see Table 7).

The following three information sources were suggested from all four of our methods: key pharmaceutical journals; key medical journals; and experts. It is hardly surprising that experts seem such an important source, and the pertinent question for an EWS is not whether to use experts but how to select and access them. The means of selection is particularly crucial, but the best method for doing so is currently either assumed or arbitrary.

In addition to the three sources above, 'specialist' medical journals, FDA licensing applications, conferences and liaison with pharmaceutical and biotechnology companies were highlighted, with reservations, as being potentially useful, additional information sources.

Therefore, for the purposes of identifying new healthcare technologies we recommend the following approach, using wherever possible resources which are available on the Internet:

(a) scanning of 'specialist' medical journals, key medical journals, FDA licensing applications, key pharmaceutical journals and conference abstracts, and liaison with pharmaceutical and biotechnology companies, to produce a database of potential technologies; and

(b) regular meetings and/or surveys of sentinel groups of expert health professionals in order to review and comment on the technologies identified by the other information sources.

It should be noted that some of the potential sources are changing (for example, HTA agencies and patient special interest groups), and may become capable of playing an increasing role; they should, therefore, be kept under review.

Recommended Methods for Operating an EWS

The results of the literature review and the telephone enquiry suggest that the notion of early warning has only recently emerged from reflections on the nature and utility of health technology assessments. These have emphasised the importance of identifying a new technology as early as possible so that an appropriate evaluation can be initiated at a very early stage.[b] Of the existing national initiatives, the Health Council of the Netherlands – which built on the work of the STG in the mid 1980s – has had the most experience of an EWS. Often it may be possible to make use of existing related schemes or initiatives. However, where such opportunities do not exist specific initiatives are required; even when they do exist, they may require supplementing.

The exact form and operation of the EWS (and the sensitivity and specificity, level of detail and timeliness which will be required from the chosen information sources) will ultimately depend upon the healthcare system of which it is a part and the purposes to which the EWS are to be applied. Important aspects of the operation of an EWS are:

(a) continuity, so that the important monitoring function of an EWS can be performed on those technologies which have a long development phase;

(b) only a relatively small core staffing is required as long as there is access to experts either through formal committee structures or regular surveys and/or focus meetings;

(c) the need for collaboration with national and international programmes that already exist (for example, in the UK collaboration with regional DIS, SERNIP, SMAC-CMP) with the aim of ensuring adequate coverage of all types of technologies and providing sufficient early warning; and

(d) that the EWS should be part of a national programme to allow HTA research to be commissioned or run in parallel alongside early clinical trials.

EWSs for identifying healthcare technologies should not be concerned with making exhaustive, long-term forecasts but with highlighting new and emerging high-impact technologies that are likely to materialise. Wherever possible, the required length of early warning of a new technology is 3 years, although this may vary depending on the type of research that is required (more for a randomised controlled trial, less for a review or modelling exercise) and the technology concerned. Current initiatives are concerned mainly with relatively short time-horizons (i.e. 1–2 years).

One of the key elements in an EWS is a system for contacting and eliciting opinions from experts. Experts can be used both to 'brainstorm' new developments and to filter information from other (documentary) sources.

Having identified new technologies, criteria for selecting those technologies which are in most urgent need of evaluation are needed. The six national EWS used different criteria with which to select which emerging technologies should be highlighted but the following are commonly mentioned:[41]

(a) expected health impact (burden of disease);

(b) efficacy or predicted efficacy of the technology;

(c) type of development (innovativeness, innovation phase, speed of diffusion);

(d) economic consequences (investment cost, total economic impact); and

(e) policy relevance (regulatory decision, research agenda, controversial, ethical concerns).

The value of an EWS to a HTA programme will be determined to a very large extent by the responsiveness of the programme to the outputs of the EWS. An EWS should not aim to provide an exhaustive list of all potential new healthcare technologies, but select the most important technologies and concentrate research planning on these.

Central to the operation of an EWS is the need for consistent methods of updating information; technologies do not suddenly appear with little prior warning, but have been in development for a long time before they begin to diffuse. For example, the bases for the development of telemedicine and LVADs were first conceived in the 1950s and 1960s, respectively.

Often parallel developments in a number of other technological areas are required prior to the full potential of the innovations being able to be realised (for example, CT scanners, tele-medicine, biosensors). This pattern of tech-nological development highlights the need for a 'watchful waiting' approach by an EWS; monitoring technologies at different stages in their innovation, development and adoption. There may often be a progression from reports of discoveries in scientific journals to reports of progress in developing the technologies in specialist journals and then onto key medical journals as the technology is adopted.

CONCLUSIONS

The paucity of empirical evidence means that one must be cautious in deciding which are the most useful sources of information for identify-ing new healthcare technologies and the best methods for operating an EWS. However, EWS are being established simultaneously in a num-ber of countries (often by HTA agencies), and intuitively they would seem to offer obvious benefits.

The relative usefulness of the many available sources of information about new healthcare technologies depends on the particular types of technology under consideration. Additionally, each source has its advantages and disadvantages, and some provide earlier (and often, as a con-sequence, less certain) warning of new tech-nologies than others. Each will also provide information about different aspects of a technol-ogy and its likely impact, and some sources will provide more detail than others. Thus the choice of information sources which feed into an EWS may be influenced by the choice between:

(a) earlier warning of a potential technology with little certainty of its likely impact in terms of its precise application and timing of introduction (examples include confer-ence abstracts and, perhaps, pharmaceut-ical and biotechnology companies); and

(b) very clear and precise information of a specific technology but relatively late warn-ing (i.e. shortly before introduction of the new healthcare technology) to the health system (examples include key medical journals and FDA licensing).

Our conclusions and recommendations are based on the results of four separate methods which approached the two study questions from differ-ent perspectives; each of these provided some-what different findings, which emphasises the importance of a multi-faceted approach. We adopted this approach as there is no single best method, and each has disadvantages: the litera-ture review revealed very few relevant studies, the EWS co-ordinators who participated in the telephone enquiry are developing their systems by trial and error, the opinions of the partici-pants in the Delphi study are necessarily sub-jective and open to bias, and the case studies are historical exemplars only. However, the overall analysis of the results from the four methods (a form of triangulation) provides a more robust review of the important issues relating to EWS for identifying new healthcare technologies than any single method alone.

Given the lack of empirical evidence on the practical value of an EWS it is important that any new initiative be evaluated and monitored. Our findings would support further research on:

1 Prospectively recording the information sources used to identify new technologies in order that their accuracy can be assessed at a later date when the value of the output from the EWS is known.

2 Undertaking detailed prospective case studies of new healthcare technologies to map the diffusion processes of technologies and to assess information sources for identifying them prior to their introduction into health services.

3 Estimating the likely 'payback' from pro-viding early warning of new healthcare technologies.

4 Determining how much early warning is required for: (i) strategic policy decision making (e.g. HTA research prioritisation); and (ii) day-to-day operational management decisions, which will include determin-ing what is the most appropriate balance between length of early warning and the level of certainty as to the likelihood of the importance of the new technology.

ACKNOWLEDGEMENTS

We are particularly grateful to all the partici-pants in the international Delphi study, the co-ordinators of EWS who responded to our tele-phone enquiry, the respondents to our e-mail survey of ISTAHC members, to Professor Tom Walley (University of Liverpool), Professor Duncan Colin-Jones (Portsmouth) for providing a retrospective analysis of the accuracy of earlier initiatives, to David Hands of the South and West Drug Information Centre (Southampton), to Deborah Anthony at the Wessex Institute for Health Research and Development for her assistance with the case studies on biosensors and telemedicine, to Graham Mowatt and colleagues for assistance with the case studies on laparoscopic cholecystectomy and telemedicine, and to Dr Pamela Akerman for assistance with the paediatric intensive care case study.

NOTES

a. Personal communication, Professor D. Banta and Dr J. Spiby, April 1998. Banta noted that the predictions in the STG report, whilst being 'globally' accurate, would have 'problems with timing and focus', citing that the study did not pick up minimally invasive surgery, although endoscopes and microsurgery were mentioned.

b. Blume S. 'Early warning in the light of theories of technological change', European Workshop: Scanning the horizon for emerging health technologies, Copenhagen, 12–13 September 1997.

REFERENCES

1. Dent THS, Hawke S. Too soon to market. *Br. Med. J.* 1997; **315**: 1248–9.
2. Whitted GS. Medical technology diffusion and its effects on the modern hospital. *HCM Review* 1981; Spring: 45–54.
3. Rutten FFH, Reiser SJ (eds.). *The Economics of Medical Technology.* Proceedings of an International Conference on Economics of Medical Technology, 1988.
4. Freiman MP. The rate of adoption of new procedures among physicians. The impact of specialty and practice characteristics. *Medical Care* 1985; **23**: 939–45.
5. Abel Smith B. The marketplace for medical technology. In: *The Economics of Medical Technology.* Proceedings of an International Conference on Economics of Medical Technology, 1988.
6. Peckham M. Towards research based health care. In: Newsom-Davis J, Weatherall D (eds). *Health policy and technological innovation.* London: The Royal Society, 1994.
7. Smith L, McClenahan J. *Management of the introduction of Betaseron. A Developmental Evaluation.* London: Kings Fund, 1997.
8. Cuschieri A. Whither minimal access surgery: tribulations and expectations. *Am. J. Surg.* 1995; **169**: 9–19.
9. Newsome-Davis J, Weatherall D (eds). *Health policy and technological innovation.* London: The Royal Society, 1994.
10. Hadridge P, Hodgson T. *The Hemingford Scenarios: Alternative futures for health and health care.* Oxford & Anglia Regional Health Authority, September 1994.
11. Garrett MJ. A way through the maze. What futurists do and how they do it. *Futures* 1993: 254–74.
12. Chen K, Jarboe K, Wolfe J. Long-range scenario construction for technology assessment. *Technological Forecasting and Social Change* 1981; **20**: 27–40.
13. Rogers EM. *Diffusion of innovations*, 4th edn. New York: Free Press, Macmillan, 1995.
14. Vallance P. Separate R&D budget is needed for monitoring effects of new drugs. *Br. Med. J.* 1998; **316**: 939.
15. Researchers try crystal ball gazing to predict future. *Br. Med. J.* 1996; **313**: 706.
16. Szczepura A, Kankaanpaa J (eds.). *Assessment of health care technologies. Case studies, key concepts and strategic issues.* Cambridge: John Wiley & Sons, 1996.
17. Borst-Eilers E. Assessing hospital technology in the Netherlands. *Br. Med. J.* 1993; **306**: 226.
18. Scenario Commission on Future Health Care Technology. *Anticipating and assessing health care technology. Volume 1: General Considerations and Policy Conclusions.* The Netherlands: Martinus Nijhoff Publishers, 1987.
19. Stevens A, Robert G, Gabbay J. Identifying new health care technologies in the United Kingdom. *Int. J. Technol. Assess. Health Care* 1997; **13**: 59–67.
20. Bonair A, Perrson J. Innovation and diffusion of health care technologies. In: Szczepura A, Kankaanpaa J (eds). *Assessment of Health Care Technologies. Case studies, key concepts and strategic issues.* Cambridge: John Wiley & Sons, 1996.
21. Battista RN. Innovation and diffusion of health-related technologies. A conceptual framework. *Int. J. Tech. Assess. Health Care* 1989; **5**: 227–48.
22. Gelijns A, Rosenberg N. The dynamics of technological change in medicine. *Health Affairs* 1994: 28–46.
23. Smith R. The roots of innovation. *Br. Med. J.* 1987; **295**: 1335–8.
24. Luiten AL. The birth and development of an innovation: the case of magnetic resonance imaging. In: Rutten FFH, Reiser SJ (eds). *The Economics of Medical Technology. Proceedings of an International Conference on Economics of Medical Technology.* Berlin: Springer-Verlag, 1988.
25. Stocking B (ed.) *Expensive health technologies.* Oxford: Oxford University Press, 1988.
26. Battelle. *Analysis of selected biomedical research programs. Vol. 2.* Columbus Ohio: Battelle Columbus Laboratories, 1976.
27. Fineberg HV. Effects of clinical evaluation on the diffusion of medical technology. In: *Institute of*

Medicine. Assessing medical technologies. Washington DC: National Academy Press, 1985.

28. Greer AL. Medical technology: assessment, adoption and utilization. *J. Med. Syst.* 1981; **5**: 129–45.

29. Foote SB. *Managing the Medical Arms Race. Innovation and Public Policy in the Medical Devices Industry.* Berkeley: University of California Press, 1992.

30. Banta HD, Gelijns AC. The future and healthcare technology: implications of a system for early identification. *WHO Statist. Q.* 1994; **47**: 140–8.

31. Food & Drug Administration. *Forecast of emerging technologies.* US Dept of Health & Human Services, June 1981.

32. Spiby J. Advances in medical technology over the next 20 years. *Community Medicine* 1988; **10**: 273–8.

33. Technology Foresight Programme, Health & Life Sciences Panel. *Notes on the Delphi survey.* Companion paper B to the Health & Life Sciences Panel report. Office of Science & Technology, London: HMSO, 1995.

34. Spiby J. *Future and emerging medical technology. A study to investigate advances in medical technology in the United Kingdom.* Submission to Membership of the Faculty of Community Medicine, 1987.

35. Fuchs HJ, Borowitz DS, Christiansen DH et al. Effect of aerosolized recombinant human Dnase on exacerbations of respiratory symptoms and on pulmonary function in patients with cystic fibrosis. *N. Engl. J. Med.* 1994; **331**: 637–42.

36. Telemedicine: fad or future? *Lancet* 1995; **345**: 73–4.

37. Davis PB. Evolution of therapy for cystic fibrosis. *N. Engl. J. Med.* 1994; **331**: 672–3.

38. Berger RL, McCormick JR, Stetz JD et al. Successful use of a paracoroperal left ventricular assist device in men. *JAMA* 1980; **243**: 46–9.

39. Baker SR. The diffusion of high technology medical innovation: the computed tomography scanner example. *Soc. Sci. Med.* 1979; **13**: 155–62.

40. Stevens A, Packer C, Robert G. Early warning of new health care technologies in the United Kingdom. *Int. J. Technol. Assess. Health Care* 1998; **14**: 680–6.

41. Carlsson P, Jorgensen T (eds). *European workshop: scanning the horizon for emerging health technologies.* Copenhagen, September, 1997.

42. Bezold C. The future of health futures. *Futures* 1995; **27**: 921–5.

43. NHS Executive. *Report of the NHS Health Technology Assessment Programme 1996.* London: HMSO, June, 1996.

44. Rosen R. *Introducing new medical technologies: what role for purchasers?* Membership of the Faculty of Public Health Medicine Part II Examination, 1995.

45. Gelijns AC, Thier SO. Medical technology development: an introduction to the innovation-evaluation nexus. In: Gelijns AC (ed.). *Medical innovation at the crossroads. Vol. I: Modern methods of clinical investigation.* Washington DC: National Academy Press, 1990.

46. Warner KE. The need for some innovative concepts of innovation: an examination of research on the diffusion of innovations. *Policy Sciences* 1974; **5**: 433–51.

Appendix

Definitions

Futures studies and futurology

Futures is an extremely wide field, and futures studies fulfil many, and quite different, purposes.[11,42] Figure 7 sets the scope of this chapter in the context of the discipline of futurology. This chapter is concerned principally with new healthcare technologies in the short term, and making plausible predictions as to which are likely to be important and introduced into a healthcare system:

New and emerging healthcare technologies

Healthcare technology 'encompasses all methods used by health professionals to promote health, prevent and treat disease, and improve rehabilitation and long-term care. It includes the activities of the full range of healthcare professionals, and the use of equipment, pharmaceutical and healthcare procedures generally'.[43] *New* healthcare technologies are those which are only just about to be introduced, or have only recently been introduced, to clinical practice[44] (including new applications of existing technologies). *Emerging* technologies are earlier in the pre-adoption phase, for example pharmaceuticals in Phase II and III trials.

Thus, new and emerging technologies comprise those technologies in the applied research stage, about the time of initial clinical testing, and those past the stage of clinical trials but not yet in widespread use. They may include technologies localised to a few centres, and as a general rule tend to be relatively unevaluated.

Innovation

An *innovation* is an idea, practice or object that is perceived as new by an individual or other unit of adoption.[13] Technological innovation in medicine covers the wide range of events that includes the

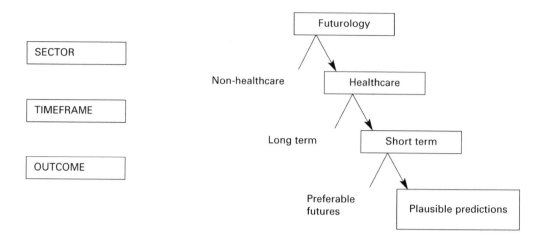

Figure 7 *Focus of this chapter within the context of 'futures' research.*

discovery or invention, development and dissemination of a new healthcare technology.[45]

Diffusion

Diffusion is the process, whether planned or spontaneous, by which an innovation is dispersed over time among the members of a 'social system' (healthcare system).[13] The study of diffusion is concerned with three phenomena:[46]

1 the speed of diffusion;
2 its extent (what percentage of potential adopters ever adopt the innovation); and
3 patterns of diffusion (including patterns of spread over time, place and persons).

Early warning systems (EWS)

The aim of an *early warning system* in the healthcare sector is to identify potential healthcare technologies expected to diffuse into that sector in the years (typically 0–5 years) to follow. An early technology assessment and other preparatory work (guideline prepara-

tion, budgetary planning) can then be performed if needed.

Primary, secondary and tertiary information sources

Primary information sources are those close to the point of innovation (for example, patents, licensing applications to the Food and Drug Administration (FDA) in the United States or pharmaceutical and biotechnology companies). *Secondary* sources are those 'designed' for other purposes, such as general clinical expertise; this is a wide group including conference abstracts, the published literature and patient special interest groups). *Tertiary* sources are concerned with early warning/horizon scanning as one of their principal functions (i.e. other EWS or horizon-scanning initiatives).

There is some overlap between these categories (for example, experts at the cutting edge of research may also act as 'primary' information sources), but the classification highlights the important trade-off between earlier warning and greater accuracy.

26

Timing of Assessment of Fast-Changing Health Technologies

GRAHAM MOWATT, ADRIAN M. GRANT,
D. JANE BOWER, JOHN A. BREBNER,
JOHN A. CAIRNS and LORNA McKEE

Summary

The assessment of fast-changing technologies presents a dilemma to health services. Early assessment may under- or over-estimate the real value of the technology, while assessment after the technology has become more stable may be methodologically so weak or so late as to have little if any impact on adoption and use.

The study reported here aimed to provide insights into factors influencing the timing of assessment of fast-changing health technologies. Whilst observations were made about health technology assessment (HTA) in general, the perspective was based on the situation in the United Kingdom.

A series of literature searches was undertaken in an attempt to identify papers focusing on, firstly, general principles involved in the timing of HTAs, and secondly, assessments of six specific medical applications. Reported assessments of laparoscopic cholecystectomy, chorion villus sampling, teleradiology, teledermatology, diagnosis of genetic susceptibility to breast cancer, and gene therapy for cystic fibrosis were analysed in order to try to identify factors which influenced their timing. The applications were selected to allow meaningful comparisons between a range of technologies, of various ages and at various stages of evaluation. A study of the publication trends of the six applications was also undertaken in an attempt to identify points in the development of a technology that could be used as indicators to initiate an assessment.

We identified the special challenges of evaluating fast-changing technologies, reviewed what others have said about them, and illustrated through the six case studies some of the difficulties involved. Many of these difficulties reflect external pressures that are not directly related to healthcare innovation and evaluation. The best timing of evaluation is problematic. The danger of leaving evaluation too late is that it then becomes impossible or irrelevant. This argues for alertness to the evolution of the technology under consideration and also for earlier assessment. Whilst fast-changing technologies are no different from other, more stable, technologies in many respects, the particular difficulty relates to the likely stability of the technology at a particular time, and hence the reliability of any evaluation undertaken. There are persuasive arguments for waiting until the period when opinion leaders are considering the technology, before initiating an evaluation. There is also a strong case for randomisation of the 'first patient' to receive a new treatment.

There is no easy formula for the evaluation of fast-changing technologies. A culture of vigilance and alertness should lead to prompt, early and iterative evaluation.

Introduction

Healthcare is in a state of flux. The health technologies used today differ from those of the past, and will differ from those that will be used in the future. Whilst health technology assessment (HTA) seeks to inform and influence this evolution to encourage the adoption of effective and safe forms of healthcare, it is only one, still relatively weak, factor influencing this process. Much more often, changes occur for other reasons, such as political, social, economic and commercial pressures. The instability in health technologies that results commonly causes difficulties for HTA, even undermining it. By the time a formal assessment has been completed, the technology may have changed so much that the results are considered to be irrelevant to current practice. These issues and the ways they may best be addressed are the focus of this chapter. Given that all technology is subject to change, albeit at markedly varying rates, there is no simple definition of 'fast-change'. We have chosen to use the term to characterise a technology whose time-scale of development is so quick as to jeopardise the value of any HTA.

The most obvious reason for fast-change is developments in the technology itself. Sometimes such change is step-wise, reflecting occasional fundamental alterations in the technology; at other times it is categorised by multiple small changes giving the appearance of a smooth change over time. A particular example of the latter type of change is the learning associated with a new technology, such as a surgical technique, that requires operator skill. The term 'learning curve' is commonly used to describe this. Whilst it is such changes in the technology itself which are the focus of this chapter, it is important to recognise that other types of 'fast-changes' may occur, which are independent of the technology itself. For example, there may be rapid changes in the types of healthcare problem to which the technology is applied, or in alternative approaches to healthcare and parallel types of management, or in the costs of the technology.

Whatever the reason for fast-change, such developments raise questions about the value of any evaluation performed prior to a significant change. Whilst the impact of such changes will always be a matter of opinion, it ranges from such fundamental change that the performance of the technology has obviously altered, through to subtle or minor change such that the technology is essentially unchanged, from an assessment point of view.

Change tends to be most rapid during the early life of new technology. Taken at face value it may therefore seem most sensible to wait for stability before any formal assessment is undertaken. Indeed, this is a commonly adopted position. Proponents of new technologies often argue that to evaluate a new method before it is stable is to put it to an unfair test. The difficulty

is that once stability has been identified, these same proponents are no longer willing to conduct rigorous evaluation (such as through a randomised trial) because by then they are convinced, rightly or wrongly, of the value of the new technology. This problem is exacerbated by the fact that technology change often occurs in an unpredictable way, such that stability is only recognisable in retrospect some significant time after it has actually occurred. The consequence of waiting for stability is therefore that any health technology assessment performed is commonly not sufficiently rigorous to be really useful, or is too late to inform diffusion. This then is the dilemma for evaluating fast-changing technologies: early assessment may lead to a distorted evaluation which under-values (or over-values) the technology; on the other hand, late assessment may be methodologically so weak (and so late) that it has little if any impact on the technology's adoption and use.

It was against this backdrop that we conducted a systematic review of research on these issues, drawing on detailed case studies of six specific health technologies to inform the review.[1] After describing the methods of our research in the next section, we go on to summarise our findings, before drawing their implications together in the final section of the chapter. Whilst observations are made about HTA in general, our perspective was based on the situation in the United Kingdom.

METHODS

A series of literature searches was undertaken in an attempt to identify papers focusing on, firstly, general principles involved in the timing of HTAs, and secondly, reported assessments of six specific medical applications. Reported assessments of laparoscopic cholecystectomy, chorion villus sampling, teleradiology, teledermatology, diagnosis of genetic susceptibility to breast cancer, and gene therapy for cystic fibrosis (Table 1) were analysed in order to try to identify factors which influenced the timing of those assessments.

The generic technologies and applications were selected to allow meaningful comparisons between a range of technologies, of various ages and at various stages of evaluation, so as to provide insights into the problems of how and when to assess new and fast-changing technologies. The technologies chosen allowed comparison between those that were unregulated/ highly regulated, those with a low/high media profile, those that were commercially driven/ publicly funded, those that were diagnostic/

Table 1 *Medical applications reviewed, and their generic technologies*

Generic technology	Application
Karyotyping	Chorion villus sampling
Minimal access surgery	Cholecystectomy
Genetic manipulation	Gene therapy (cystic fibrosis)
	Diagnosis of genetic susceptibility to breast cancer
Videoconferencing (telemedicine)	Radiology
	Dermatology

therapeutic, and those that were invasive/non-invasive.

Systematic searches for papers on the timing of HTA and on each of the six medical applications were made primarily on the electronic databases Medline and EMBASE. Other databases searched included the Cochrane Library, PROMT (national and international business journals and newspapers), System for Information on Grey Literature in Europe (SIGLE), and the Index of Scientific and Technical Proceedings. Reference lists of important papers identified were hand-searched. The following journals were also hand-searched during 1996: *Bandolier, British Medical Journal, Controlled Clinical Trials, Evidence Based Medicine, Health Service Journal, International Journal of Technology Assessment in Health Care, Journal of Health Services Research and Policy, The Lancet,* and *Quality in Health Care.* Key individuals were also interviewed.

Literature-based indicators may provide useful information on the activity around a technology.[2,3] Therefore, in addition to carrying out literature searches, the publication trends of the six applications were also analysed. Using data from a Medline search, these trends were displayed graphically in an attempt to relate the patterns generated to events in the development and diffusion of the technologies, with the aim of identifying key points in time that could be used as indicators to trigger assessment.

WHEN TO ASSESS

General Principles

Initially, attempts were made to implement a search strategy specific enough to retrieve papers solely on the timing of HTA, but this proved unproductive. Therefore, a more sensitive search strategy was devised and papers were sought on HTA at a broad level, with the intention of analysing these for any information included on

timing. The Medline search (1966–96) retrieved 1477 references in total, but in order to keep numbers at a manageable level was restricted to the period 1991–96, resulting in 605 references. The EMBASE search from 1980–96 retrieved 260 references. The titles (and abstracts where available) of references retrieved by the searches were scanned, and those concerned with the principles of HTA (176) obtained and analysed for any information on timing of assessment. Searches carried out on the other electronic databases were unsuccessful in retrieving references on timing of assessment.

The literature on the timing of HTA does not appear to be extensive; of the 176 papers concerning HTA in general which were obtained and analysed, 47 contained some mention of timing. No papers were identified which focused solely on the issue of timing; where timing was mentioned, comments were of a general rather than specific nature and within the context of a broad-ranging discussion on HTA.

There was a broad consensus that new health technologies should be evaluated before they were allowed to diffuse, unevaluated, into clinical practice.[4] In addition to safety, effectiveness and cost issues, ethical issues should also be addressed.[5] To be regarded as successful, assessments had to be done early enough to affect decision-making.[6] There was a perception that the results of evaluations were generally available too late, when decisions on adoption had already been taken and the technology had diffused into practice.[7,8]

Several authors proposed the idea of an identifiable point in time at which an evaluation should be undertaken, as opposed to being merely 'early'. The importance of the 'critical point' was such that if evaluations were undertaken too early they would be largely forgotten, whereas if they were undertaken too late, they would be of little value.[9] This raised the issue of timing of evaluation of fast-changing technologies, in the context of determining when they were sufficiently stable for this to be done.

Stocking maintained that the first group to adopt an idea would be the innovators involved in designing the new procedure or technology.[10] This in itself, however, does not lead to widespread adoption. Stocking argued that it was only when the opinion leaders of the relevant group of clinicians began to take up the idea that the majority of clinicians would follow. The important period for initiating an evaluation was the time when the opinion leaders were still considering the new technology.[10] During this phase there was clearly an emerging technology, but it had not yet diffused out of control. Therefore the period when opinion leaders were considering the technology might also signal the time when it had become sufficiently stable to be evaluated.

There was also agreement that assessment should be an iterative process rather than a one-off study.[9,11,12] This raised the possibility of the existence of a number of critical points to guide first and subsequent evaluations. Policy-making often depended on understanding the implications of a new technology at several points in its diffusion.[13] A change in the nature of the condition, expanded professional knowledge, a shift in clinical practice, or publication of a new, conflicting assessment were some of the factors that might trigger a decision to re-assess.[14] Assessment could also be linked to the life cycle of a technology, starting with prospective assessment of an emerging technology, assessment of the technology in practice, then later assessments as it changed, was used for new indications, or to decide whether it should be replaced or abandoned.[13,15]

The issues outlined above underline the complex environment in which health technologies are developed and applied. One of the key requirements of rigorous assessment that is influenced by rapid environmental change is that of 'equipoise', defined by Lilford and Jackson as a situation in which there is no preference between the treatment options to be compared.[16] They argued that randomised controlled trials (RCTs) were only ethical under conditions of equipoise.[16] One of the implications of equipoise was that, practically and ethically, the period during which rigorous RCTs could be undertaken might be brief since the length of time during which a clinician had no preference between the treatment options to be compared was likely to be short.

Some authors have argued for randomisation of the first patient to receive a new treatment, as opposed to delaying until randomisation could be carried out with no further changes to the treatment in question.[17] Chalmers maintained that physicians could never undertake a controlled trial if they were consciously enthusiastic about one of the procedures.[17] Chalmers' argument was that where surgical procedures had been tested by trials, such trials had been preceded by many consecutive series of patients receiving the technique in which it might have been slowly modified. He maintained that it was unethical to wait until the technique had been modified before evaluating it. This was because physicians would be asking certain patients to give up their right to the standard accepted therapy in favour of a procedure not yet sufficiently developed to justify comparing it with that standard therapy. Chalmers argued that it would be more ethical to randomise from the beginning and explain to patients that they had an equal chance of receiving whichever was the more beneficial therapy.[17]

Other authors, however, have drawn attention to the fact that during the initial stages the practitioner's skills and expertise with a procedure were still evolving, with the result that the risks and benefits associated with it might change considerably.[18] Gelijns stated that in view of this 'learning curve' phenomenon, the initial assessment of a new procedure would probably need to involve non-experimental studies.[18] She argued that such early reporting of clinical experience might form the basis for the design of subsequent RCTs or otherwise well-controlled trials to determine a procedure's safety and efficacy.[18]

Diffusion and Development of Health Technologies

If the pattern of development and diffusion of health technologies could be predicted, this information would be useful in helping to inform the decision of when to initiate an evaluation. However, other than for highly regulated technologies such as pharmaceuticals, this process does not generally follow a simple linear progression. A more complex model in which clear transition points can no longer be easily identified has now largely replaced the earlier, conventional view that technologies had a simple, consistent pattern of development and diffusion. In addition, the same technology might also be modified in different ways by different adopters, without rigorous evaluation taking place. Health technology development is now generally seen as an iterative process, with evolving scientific knowledge interacting with market demand to generate a particular pattern of innovation.[18,19]

The introduction into healthcare of technologies already developed for other purposes, in different sectors, further complicates this situation. A high percentage of new medical devices are not generated from biomedical research but emerge through the transfer of technologies developed outwith the healthcare sector.[4] One example of this process is that of adapting videoconferencing for 'telemedicine' applications. In such cases, not only the early phases but also much of the later development of the technology is unknown to organisations responsible for clinical evaluation. Thus the course that emerging, 'fast-changing' technologies take is unpredictable; they are able to evolve independently of any health service constraints.

The way in which healthcare is organised and delivered may also impact on the innovation process. Traditionally, the developers of new health technologies looked upon physicians as their primary customer base. More recently, however, other groups such as policy-makers, hospital managers, patients, the general public and regulators have begun to be seen as significant stakeholders in the demand for technology.[20]

Following adoption, development does not suddenly come to an end. Adoption of a technology may be the start of a long-term process of modification and redesign, based on the experiences of the technology's new-found users. Health technologies therefore may continue to evolve for some time after their initial introduction into practice. This raises the difficult question of when exactly is the best time to evaluate a 'fast-changing' health technology, bearing in mind that the eventual results of an evaluation may be made irrelevant by developments in the technology since the evaluation was initiated.

The Case Studies

Systematic reviews of reported assessments of the following six medical applications were undertaken in an attempt to clarify factors which had influenced the timing of those assessments, and which might prove relevant to the wider debate on timing. The search strategy aimed to identify RCTs, major observational studies, systematic reviews and also other overviews of the literature. Titles (and abstracts where available) of papers retrieved by the searches were scanned and those that met the above criteria were obtained and analysed.

Laparoscopic cholecystectomy

Laparoscopic cholecystectomy (LC) is a form of minimal access surgery (MAS) for removing the gallbladder. Since its introduction, the procedure has diffused rapidly into routine clinical practice. Factors influencing the rate of diffusion include technological 'push' from instrumentation manufacturers, and the 'pull' of demand, both from health professionals and patients.

At the time LC was first introduced there was no requirement for surgeons to undergo specialised training before adopting it. This situation for new surgical procedures contrasted markedly with that governing the introduction of new drugs. New drugs had to conform to strict, centrally imposed regulations, which required rigorous testing in animals according to strict experimental designs, followed by carefully controlled testing in humans with appropriate protocols and follow-up observation. In contrast, no formal government regulatory system existed for the development and evaluation of clinical procedures; their development had traditionally taken place in the context of clinical autonomy and the relationship of trust between physician and patient, with evaluation depending to a great extent on professional self-regulation.[18] This had led to a situation where the potential safety, efficacy and effectiveness of many surgical procedures had not been evaluated systematically during their development, allowing a 'tidal wave' of new healthcare technologies to diffuse through healthcare systems before proper evaluation was undertaken.[21]

This was the case with LC, where diffusion was not preceded by adequate evaluation of the technique, and much of the reported assessments consist of uncontrolled, descriptive studies.[22] Searches of Medline and EMBASE identified 496 and 194 papers respectively. There has been no large-scale RCT of laparoscopic versus open cholecystectomy (OC). A few small RCTs have been undertaken of LC versus OC.[23-26] There have been a similar number of RCTs of laparoscopic versus mini-cholecystectomy (MC).[27-30] The observational studies and RCTs of LC versus OC generally reported a longer operating time, shorter hospital stay, less postoperative pain, faster return to normal activity, and a much smaller scar. Whilst early RCTs of LC versus MC found in favour of LC, later RCTs concluded that LC offered no clear advantage over MC. A systematic review of the effectiveness and safety of LC reported that the most serious complication was an increased likelihood of injury to the bile duct, and one of the review's recommendations was that surgeons should not be encouraged to replace MC with LC.[31]

Evaluating LC posed several major problems. There were difficulties associated with varying levels of surgical skill. For example, a lack of skill due to being at an early point on the 'learning curve' might result in poor performance by surgeons. As early as 1990 it was being argued that LC should be confined to specialised centres that would participate in prospective studies.[32] However this call was not heeded. Training issues were eventually addressed by a Working Group on the Implications of MAS for the NHS.[33] Another problem was that MAS technologies were potentially fast-changing, which was partly a function of the parallel development of similar technology for non-medical applications. One of the features of the 'assessment' part of HTA, as defined by the NHS Executive, was that a health technology should be sufficiently stable before it was evaluated.[34] The value of an RCT would be diminished if, midway through the study, clinicians felt that the procedure should be altered in some way to reflect new and important developments.[35]

Media reports of the apparent benefits of LC increased public awareness of the procedure and led to patients requesting it in preference to OC. It was argued that patient demand, fostered by press reports, was the most important factor in facilitating the diffusion of minimal access therapies such as LC.[36] This led to problems with patient recruitment to RCTs. Given the apparent benefits of the procedure, it became difficult to persuade patients to enter a clinical trial where they had an equal chance of receiving the conventional form of therapy.[35] However it could be argued that for this situation to have arisen in the first place, patients were not being fully informed about the potential risks involved in undergoing the LC procedure. It was in such circumstances of patient-led demand, where MAS procedures were diffusing rapidly, that RCTs were most needed to evaluate the benefits and risks involved.

The long-term implications of LC also needed to be taken into account when considering how to evaluate MAS technologies. RCTs would have had to be large in patient numbers and based on a long period of follow-up in order to detect important, but rare, adverse events. The cost and logistical difficulties involved generally inhibited such trials from taking place.[35]

As early as 1991 voices were being raised that the obvious benefits of LC rendered an RCT unethical,[37] and by 1993 it was being argued that the opportunity to conduct a large-scale controlled trial had passed.[38] With hindsight, systematic evaluation of LC should have started from the earliest stages of its introduction. The reasons for this not being the case included that there was no consensus to withhold new techniques until properly evaluated, neither was there centralised control to prevent diffusion of unevaluated techniques. Media reports fuelled initial demand for the new treatment, and favourable clinical audit during the 'learning curve' period led to ethical objections to undertaking RCTs, despite a lack of reliable evidence about rare or longer-term outcomes.

Chorion villus sampling

Chorion villus sampling (CVS) and amniocentesis are the most common methods of prenatal diagnosis of chromosomal abnormalities. CVS involves retrieving cells for chromosomal analysis from the developing placenta, and was originally performed at about 9 weeks gestation in the first trimester of pregnancy, with a diagnosis available around 2 weeks later. CVS can be undertaken either transabdominally or transcervically. Amniocentesis involves transabdominal sampling of fetal cells from the amniotic fluid which surrounds the fetus and is usually performed at about 16 weeks gestation in the second trimester of pregnancy, with a diagnosis available around 3 weeks later.

CVS was established in 1982 as a method for prenatal diagnosis,[39] and has been used clinically since early 1984.[40] Transabdominal CVS was introduced by Smidt-Jensen et al. in 1984.[41]

Searches of Medline and EMBASE identified 209 and 34 papers, respectively. Three major RCTs have been undertaken comparing first-trimester CVS with second-trimester amniocentesis, with the aim of measuring pregnancy outcome, antenatal complications and diagnostic accuracy. These included a Canadian trial from 1984–88,[42] a Danish trial from 1985–90,[43] and a European multi-centre trial from 1985–89.[44] In a large US trial from 1985–86 randomisation was attempted but then abandoned because of patient reluctance to be randomised to the amniocentesis arm.[45] A prerequisite for clinicians taking part in the three major RCTs and in the large US study was that they should have undertaken the procedure a number of times prior to the commencement of the trials.

The Canadian study was initiated in 1984 to ensure that CVS was not introduced before its risks and safety had been assessed.[42] The reason given for undertaking the Danish trial in 1985 was that, since CVS was a recent technical innovation, it was important to test the procedure critically before it was used routinely.[43] The MRC European trial was initiated in the same year because of the emergence of CVS as an alternative to amniocentesis; although CVS allowed earlier diagnosis, its safety and diagnostic accuracy were unknown.[44]

A Cochrane systematic review of CVS compared with amniocentesis for prenatal diagnosis described the three major RCTs as being of generally good quality.[46] The review concluded that second-trimester amniocentesis was safer than CVS, and therefore the benefits of earlier diagnosis by CVS had to be set against its greater risks. If earlier diagnosis was required, then transabdominal CVS was seen as being preferable to the transcervical approach.

The Canadian trial was remarkable in that CVS was only available in Canada to women who participated in the study. Women who were eligible, but declined to take part, frequently cited physician influence in helping them reach a decision.[47] Some women, who initially took part and were allocated to the amniocentesis arm, found this unacceptable and subsequently travelled to the USA to obtain CVS.[48]

The possibility of a causal link between CVS and limb defects was first reported in 1991,[49] though none of the three major RCTs had identified such a link. A number of other studies produced conflicting results, with some arguing in favour of a link,[50,51] whilst others argued against.[39,52,53]

A number of factors appear to have influenced when and how evaluations have been carried out. Reports of the RCTs indicated that there was a perceived need to ascertain the safety, efficacy and diagnostic accuracy of CVS. Clinical experience in using the technique was regarded as an important factor in its safety and success. The ability to conduct successful RCTs was dependent on factors such as patient and physician preferences, and the extent to which CVS was available outwith the confines of an RCT.

Teleradiology and teledermatology

Telemedicine can be defined as the use of transmitted images, voice and other data to permit consultation, education and integration in medicine over a distance. Such systems can be used to deliver, for example, radiology and dermatology services to patients who are located in a different place from the specialist radiologist or dermatologist.

Searches of Medline and EMBASE for teleradiology identified 158 and 100 papers respectively, and for teledermatology 10 and five papers respectively. A search on the bibliography of the Telemedicine Information Exchange on the internet identified 231 papers on teleradiology, and 21 on teledermatology. Although telemedicine has been around since the 1950s, the early programmes failed to meet physician and patient expectations and were not cost-effective. When external funding was withdrawn the projects came to an end and popular interest declined. A cycle of technological development continued approximately every decade, resulting in renewed activity followed by a waning of interest when expectations were not realised. From around 1990 there has been a resurgence

of interest, mainly due to factors such as further technological advances, reduced costs, an emphasis by healthcare programmes on improving efficiency, and a demand by rural patients and physicians for equal access to high-quality healthcare.

The main driving force in telemedicine appears to have been developments in communications technology.[54] The latest resurgence in interest was at least partly due to technology providers keen to expand their markets. By funding telemedicine research in medical organisations and academic institutions, telecommunications companies have succeeded in stimulating interest among the medical community and the general public alike, thereby generating new markets for their products.[55]

Legal issues have also influenced the development of telemedicine, especially in the United States, where most activity has taken place. Were litigation to be successful, this might lead to reduced funding of projects and restrict future telemedicine development. US physicians are licensed by state, which raises questions over their professional status if they undertake interstate remote diagnosis of a patient. The issue of professional status also extends to international programmes, where the patient is located in a different country from the telemedicine consultant.

Reported assessments of teleradiology and teledermatology systems have been primarily descriptive. Factors which appear to have influenced the timing of these projects include the technology-driven, as opposed to needs-based, nature of telemedicine development in general. Projects have mainly focused on technical feasibility, not clinical efficacy or cost–effectiveness, and taken place during periods when commercial providers have made funding available. The short time scale and limited funding of many projects would have made it difficult to implement RCTs. In addition, telemedicine projects have generally served sparsely populated areas, resulting in insufficient patient numbers to provide statistically reliable data.

Diagnosis of genetic susceptibility to breast cancer

There are around 25 000 new cases of breast cancer in the UK each year, with up to 10% having an inherited basis. Mutations of the breast cancer genes *BRCA*1 and *BRCA*2 may account for at least 80% of families with a history of breast cancer. Genetic tests can determine whether an individual is predisposed to develop a disease such as breast cancer.

Searches of Medline and EMBASE identified 81 and 47 papers, respectively. Evaluation of genetic diagnosis for predisposition to breast cancer is still at an early stage. In the United States in 1994 the National Center for Human Genome Research (NCHGR), along with the National Cancer Institute, the National Institute of Nursing Research, and the National Institute of Mental Health, jointly awarded more than $2.5 million to research groups to answer some of the questions surrounding genetic testing. A major European Union-funded project, integrating several European centres and co-ordinated by the University of Aberdeen, UK, was in its early stages. The aims of the project included documentation and evaluation of clinical services, management of familial breast cancer and preparation of guidelines.

Genetic testing has raised a number of ethical, legal and social issues, and these concerns have been widely covered by the media. The usefulness of providing a test for *BRCA*1 and *BRCA*2 for the general population remains controversial. These two forms of genetic predisposition account for less than 10% of all breast cancers. In the event of a positive result, there is no clear action to take which would effectively prevent the disease from developing. In addition, some women who test positive for *BRCA*1 or *BRCA*2 will not go on to develop breast cancer. Also, a negative test result does not guarantee that breast cancer will not occur. Notification of test results, both positive and negative, can cause psychological distress. In addition, individuals who opt for genetic testing may inadvertently leave themselves open to insurance and employment discrimination. Even while it was being argued that genetic testing should remain in the research setting until these issues were resolved, commercial organisations were in the process of developing commercial diagnostic testing services to identify mutations of *BRCA*1 and *BRCA*2.

Gene therapy for cystic fibrosis

Cystic fibrosis (CF) is one of the most common lethal hereditary disorders, occurring once in approximately every 2500 births. The disease is caused by a chromosomal abnormality, which results in the creation of abnormally thick mucus. Individuals who have CF tend to suffer from chronic lung infections, and lung damage is the usual cause of premature death, with few patients surviving much beyond 30 years of age. Gene therapy involves replacing the defective gene with a copy of a normal gene.

Searches of Medline and EMBASE identified 248 and 355 references, respectively. There have been a small number of evaluations of gene

therapy for cystic fibrosis.[56–59] These were Phase I studies involving a small number of patients. Most of the US studies have used adenovirus-mediated gene transfer, while a liposome-mediated vector was the method of preference in Europe. The studies generally reported a temporary improvement in function, followed by a return to pre-treatment levels. By mid 1996 there were five protocols in Europe, and 11 in the United States, for studies involving gene therapy for cystic fibrosis.

Regulation of gene therapy is still evolving. The Medicines Control Agency (MCA) is the statutory body in the UK responsible for all aspects of medicinal products for human use. Assessment of protocols by this agency is currently a prerequisite of all gene therapy trials in the UK. In the United States, the Recombinant DNA Advisory Committee (RAC) exists to develop and oversee the application of guidelines for different types of genetic manipulation. The US and European regulators are imposing a similar regime as that applied to pharmaceuticals, while considering the ethical issues raised by the invasive use of genetic technologies.

Gene therapy is a high-risk undertaking with no products on the market, and no guarantees of commercial success. A number of large pharmaceutical companies have made investments in the technology, and many biotechnology companies have also made major commitments. Most of the biotechnology companies are relatively small, the research is labour-intensive, and costs are high. There is an expectation that gene therapy will eventually realise a commercial return, and there will be pressure from this sector to translate research findings into marketable products at the earliest opportunity.

Genetic technology in medicine has been receiving wide coverage in the media in recent years, with gene therapy one of the applications attracting much interest. However, concern has been expressed that over-optimistic media reports on gene therapy might lead patients to make potentially life-threatening decisions based on false expectations.[60]

Little information was provided in published reports about when trials were undertaken or reasons for timing. One major factor that might affect timing was that gene therapy development was being controlled much like that of a drug, with a strict, centralised, regulatory process through which clinical protocols had to pass before receiving approval. Thus, although technical capability might be determining the point at which trials were planned, the evolving regulatory processes were deciding the actual dates at which they would be implemented.

Lessons From the Case Studies

The six medical applications illustrated various difficulties of evaluating health technologies that were developing and changing, and the lessons to be learned. Laparoscopic cholecystectomy was a classic example of the problems involved in evaluating a fast-changing surgical technique. LC demonstrated the importance of distinguishing the process of using a technology from its outcome, and of finding methods when evaluating that took into account learning effects and differing levels of underlying skill. Learning issues have since been addressed.[61]

Chorion villus sampling exemplified a technology where step-wise changes of uncertain significance were taking place, demonstrated by the shift away from the transcervical to the transabdominal approach. CVS also illustrated the challenge in health technology assessment of identifying rare but serious adverse effects and relating them to the technology. CVS demonstrated the value of RCTs that straddle changes in the technology. The RCTs allowed the impact of the differences to be evaluated, but also highlighted the fact that these kinds of study design may not be the most appropriate for long-term safety and monitoring issues.

Teleradiology and teledermatology were examples of technologies developed originally for purposes other than healthcare. They demonstrated constantly changing technical performance, such that image quality continued to improve significantly during the course of trials; telemedicine developments were primarily technology-driven applications trying to find a place in healthcare.

Diagnosis of genetic susceptibility to breast cancer illustrated the development of tests that were thought to be inherently beneficial, before a policy was established for their management and for handling the wider ethical and societal issues. The technology involved was also originally developed for a different purpose, that of gene mapping. Its application to genetic risk assessment was unpredictable in terms of benefits and risks. There was, nevertheless, an increasing public perception of and demand for this technology.

Gene therapy for cystic fibrosis showed a technology at a very early stage of development that eventually could have profound implications in terms of benefits, risks, and the ethical issues raised. Gene therapy demonstrated the challenge of evaluating emerging technologies by choosing the right research methods at the appropriate time, how regulation affected this process, and also the challenging ethical and societal issues that can be presented by an emerging (and changing) technology.

PUBLICATION TRENDS ANALYSIS

Our starting assumption was that the publication trends associated with a technology might in some way be related to its rate of development and diffusion. Therefore, we analysed the publication trends for the six medical applications to establish whether there might be identifiable 'critical' points in time that could be used as indicators to initiate an evaluation, particularly in the context of a fast-changing technology becoming sufficiently stable to allow assessment to take place.

We searched Medline from 1970–95, using exploded MeSH terms combined with textword terms for each of the six applications. The total numbers of references retrieved for each application were then subdivided by year of publication and plotted on graphs (x-axis = year of publication; y-axis = number of references). Numbers given are for all references retrieved on each application, not just reports of clinical trials.

Figure 1 shows the publication trends for all six medical applications. Whilst the numbers of references per year for LC and CVS appear to have peaked and are now declining, those for the remaining four applications, although far fewer in number, continue to increase. It can be seen that LC has generated a far higher number of references over a much shorter period of time that CVS. This may indicate the level of interest generated by the technology, or the amount of controversy surrounding it.

The decline in the annual numbers of references for LC and CVS suggests that these health technologies have reached a reduced level of activity in terms of research and evaluation. This may be because they are now perceived by healthcare professionals as having been sufficiently well evaluated to resolve any remaining uncertainty over their safety and effectiveness. The graph suggests that the remaining four applications have not yet reached this situation; their annual numbers of publications, although by comparison low, continue to increase.

Figure 2 shows the annual number of references, represented by columns, for LC for the period 1989–1995. The principal RCTs, represented by horizontal lines, are also included; these compare laparoscopic versus open cholecystectomy (LC-OC) and laparoscopic versus mini-cholecystectomy (LC-MC). (In both Figures 2 and 3 the horizontal lines of the RCTs relate to the x-axis only.)

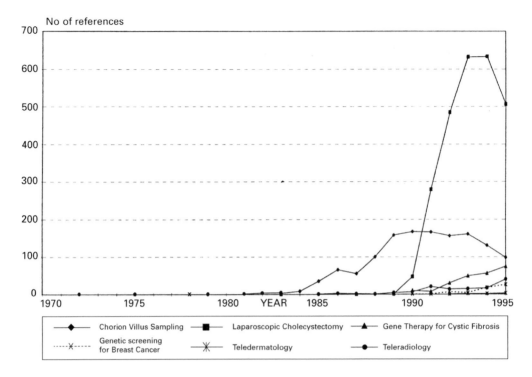

Figure 1   *Medline references: six medical applications.*

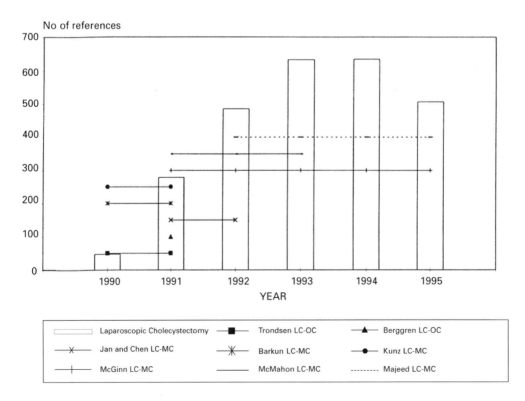

Figure 2   *Laparoscopic cholecystectomy: Medline references, major clinical trials.*

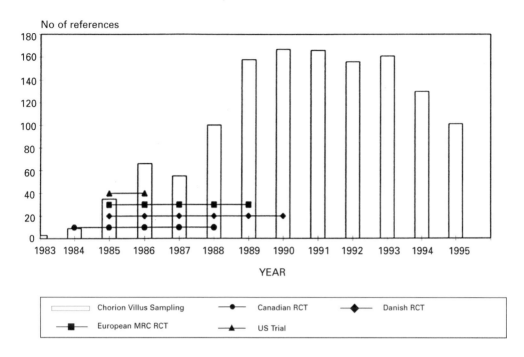

Figure 3   *Chorion villus sampling: Medline references, major clinical trials.*

One reference appeared in 1989. This was followed by a dramatic increase in numbers over the next few years, peaking at over 600 references each year for 1993 and 1994. A decline in numbers began to appear in 1995. Over a relatively short period of time a significant amount of publishing activity was generated on the subject of LC. The fact that trials were being initiated during the period to 1992 demonstrated the existence of continuing uncertainty over LC, and also that it was still feasible to undertake RCTs (even if small-scale) during this time.

Figure 3 shows the annual number of references, represented by columns, for CVS for the period 1983–1995. The principal clinical trials, represented by horizontal lines, are also included; these compare CVS with amniocentesis. The first references to CVS appeared in 1983, with numbers on the whole steadily increasing until reaching a plateau over the period 1989–1993, followed by a decline in 1994–1995. All the large trials in Figure 3 were initiated by the end of 1985.

Information from the publication trends for LC (Figure 2) and CVS (Figure 3) does suggest that there may be a narrow and relatively early 'window of opportunity' when it is possible to initiate an RCT of a new procedure. This

'window' may open from around the time that the first papers on a new procedure appear in the clinical literature; it may close when coverage in the clinical literature and the wider media leads to reduced uncertainty about the procedure's safety and effectiveness.

However, the publication trends analysis covered too few applications and was too crude to give a clear indication as to whether this might be an approach that would yield useful indicator points to trigger HTAs. In addition, the applications other than LC and CVS had such a limited literature (for example teledermatology) that the absolute numbers of publications were too small to be meaningful. The retrospective nature of this type of analysis renders it less useful than if it could be applied prospectively, so that the information was then available when most needed. It should also be borne in mind that some databases are more 'immediate' than others in the length of time taken to incorporate new bibliographic references. For example, Internet databases such as the Telemedicine Information Exchange may reflect a more 'real-time' picture of publication trends than conventional databases such as Medline and EMBASE. They may therefore be more useful for monitoring technology development with a view to timing evaluation.

CONCLUDING COMMENTS

We have identified the special challenges of evaluating fast-changing technologies, reviewed what others have said about them, and illustrated some of the difficulties through the six case studies. Arguably, the biggest issue is the best timing of evaluation. In important respects, fast-changing technologies are no different from other more stable technologies in this regard; for example, efficacy studies should precede studies of effectiveness, which in turn should come before long-term surveillance. The difficulty relates to the likely stability of the technology at a particular time, and hence the reliability of any evaluation then conducted.

There are clear dangers of leaving evaluation too late – it then becomes impossible or irrelevant – and this argues for alertness to the issue and earlier assessment. (If it later proves to have been too early, the evaluation can still be repeated.) There were striking differences between CVS and LC in this respect. The relatively early start to the CVS trials allowed not only more reliable evaluation but also useful description of the transition in technique. In contrast, large trials of LC were never mounted successfully because it proved too late when attempts were eventually made. We were attracted by the suggestion that the period when opinion leaders were considering a technology might indicate the best time for evaluation,[10] because in the context of changing technology it might also signal relative stability. The proposal to randomise the first patient is also attractive,[17] partly because there are ethical issues about how a new technology should first be used, but also because study of the early experience has the potential to describe not only later effectiveness, but also the process of 'learning' before the technology reaches a steady state. In another project funded by the NHS R&D HTA Programme we have found that statistical methods used to address 'learning curve' issues in HTA have been simplistic in comparison with other areas such as psychology and manufacturing, where learning is also an issue. Improved HTA methods to describe and then allow for learning effects would be very helpful for the evaluation of fast-changing technologies by reassuring innovators that the evaluation would not be biased by early 'poor' performance.

Many of the difficulties reflect external pressures not directly related to healthcare innovation and evaluation. Powerful commercial and political pressures may run counter to HTA. HTA may be viewed as a delay to marketing, and so be unpopular with innovators and manufacturers. Indeed, continuous technology change may prove to be advantageous commercially, if it can be used as an excuse to avoid formal evaluation. The need to move quickly to evaluate a new technology may be particularly urgent if the technology arrives ready for use after development outside healthcare; telemedicine and genetic testing are examples of this. Pressure to diffuse a technology may also reflect over-optimistic claims from innovators, the media, and hence potential patients. The need to maintain open-minded uncertainty and avoid unrealistic expectations is clear, but often discounted. The unexpected association of serious limb abnormalities with CVS is one illustration of the potential for innovation to cause unanticipated harm, and it is salutary how the use of CVS has so decreased since this link was made. We think that the importance of resisting pressures for rapid unevaluated dissemination and implementation may justify more powerful regulation such that the requirements for non-drug technologies are closer to those applied to drugs.

In short, there is no easy formula for the evaluation of fast-changing technologies. We would argue for a culture of vigilance and alertness leading to prompt, early and iterative evaluation.

REFERENCES

1. Mowatt G, Bower DJ, Brebner JA, Cairns JA, Grant AM, McKee, L. When and how to assess fast-changing technologies: a comparative study of medical applications of four generic technologies. *Health Technol. Assess.* 1997; **1**(14).

2. Edwards KL, Gordon TJ. *Characterisations of innovations introduced on the US market since 1992*. Glastonbury, Connecticut: Futures Group, 1984.

3. Coombs R, Narandren P, Richards A. A literature-based innovation output indicator. *Research Policy* 1996; **25**: 403–13.

4. Gelijns A, Rosenberg N. The dynamics of technological change in medicine. *Health Aff.* 1994; **13**: 28–46.

5. Department of Health. *Assessing the effects of health technologies: principles, practice, proposals*. London: Department of Health, 1992.

6. Banta HD. Dutch committee assesses the future of health technology. *Dimensions in Health Service* 1986; **63**: 17–20.

7. Feeny D, Guyatt G, Tugwell P. *Health care technology: effectiveness, efficiency and public policy*. Canada: Institute for Research on Public Policy, 1986.

8. Luce BR, Brown RE. The use of technology assessment by hospitals, health maintenance

organizations, and third-party payers in the United States. *Int. J. Technol. Assess. Health Care* 1995; **11**: 79–92.

9. Banta HD, Andreasen PB. The political dimension in health care technology assessment programs. *Int. J. Technol. Assess. Health Care* 1990; **6**: 115–23.

10. Stocking B. Factors influencing the effectiveness of mechanisms to control medical technology. In: Stocking B (ed.). *Expensive health technologies.* Oxford: OUP, 1988.

11. Franklin C. Basic concepts and fundamental issues in technology assessment. *Intensive Care Med.* 1993; **19**: 117–21.

12. Advisory Council on Science and Technology. *A report on medical research and health.* London: HMSO, 1993.

13. Banta HD, Thacker SB. The case for reassessment of health care technology. Once is not enough. *JAMA* 1990; **264**: 235–40.

14. Donaldson MS, Sox HC. *Setting priorities for health technology assessment.* Washington: National Academy Press, 1992.

15. Steering Committee on Future Health Scenarios. *Anticipating and assessing health care technology.* Dordrecht: Martinus Nijhoff, 1987.

16. Lilford RJ, Jackson J. Equipoise and the ethics of randomization. *J. R. Soc. Med.* 1995; **88**: 552–9.

17. Chalmers TC. Randomization of the first patient. *Med. Clin. North Am.* 1975; **59**: 1035–8.

18. Gelijns AC. *Modern methods of clinical investigation.* Washington: National Academy Press, 1990.

19. Deber RB. Translating technology assessment into policy. Conceptual issues and tough choices. *Int. J. Technol. Assess. Health Care* 1992; **8**: 131–7.

20. Bower DJ. Innovation in health care: developments in NHS trusts. *J. Manage. Med.* 1994; **8**: 54–61.

21. Sheldon TA, Faulkner A. Vetting new technologies: those whose efficacy and safety have not been established will now be registered and evaluated. *Br. Med. J.* 1996; **313**: 508.

22. Pearson VAH. *Minimal access surgery: a review.* Bristol: Health Care Evaluation Unit, Department of Epidemiology and Public Health Medicine, University of Bristol, 1994.

23. Barkun JS, Barkun AN, Sampalis JS, et al. Randomised controlled trial of laparoscopic versus mini cholecystectomy. The McGill Gallstone Treatment Group. *Lancet* 1992; **340**: 1116–19.

24. Trondsen E, Reiertsen O, Andersen OK, Kjaersgaard P. Laparoscopic and open cholecystectomy. A prospective, randomized study. *Eur. J. Surg.* 1993; **159**: 217–21.

25. Jan YY, Chen MF. [Laparoscopic versus open cholecystectomy: a prospective randomized study]. *J. Formos. Med. Assoc.* 1993; **92**(Suppl. 4): S243–9.

26. Berggren U, Gordh T, Grama D, Haglund U, Rastad J, Arvidsson D. Laparoscopic versus open cholecystectomy: hospitalization, sick leave, analgesia and trauma responses. *Br. J. Surg.* 1994; **81**: 1362–5.

27. Kunz R, Orth K, Vogel J, et al. [Laparoscopic cholecystectomy versus mini-lap-cholecystectomy. Results of a prospective, randomized study]. *Chirurg* 1992; **63**: 291–5.

28. McMahon AJ, Russell IT, Baxter JN, et al. Laparoscopic versus minilaparotomy cholecystectomy: a randomised trial. *Lancet* 1994; **343**: 135–8.

29. McGinn FP, Miles AJG, Uglow M, Ozmen M, Terzi C, Humby M. Randomized trial of laparoscopic cholecystectomy and minicholecystectomy. *Br. J. Surg.* 1995; **82**: 1374–7.

30. Majeed AW, Troy G, Nicholl JP, et al. Randomised, prospective, single-blind comparison of laparoscopic versus small-incision cholecystectomy. *Lancet* 1996; **347**: 989–94.

31. Downs SH, Black NA, Devlin HB, Royston CMS, Russell RCG. Systematic review of the effectiveness and safety of laparoscopic cholecystectomy. *Ann. R. Coll. Surg. Engl.* 1996; **78**: 235–323.

32. Cuschieri A, Berci G, McSherry CK. Laparoscopic cholecystectomy. *Am. J. Surg.* 1990; **159**: 273.

33. Cuschieri A. *Minimal access surgery: implications for the NHS.* Report from a Working Group chaired by Professor Alfred Cuschieri. Edinburgh: HMSO, 1994.

34. NHS Executive. *Report of the NHS Health Technology Assessment Programme.* London: NHS Executive, 1996.

35. Sculpher M. *A snip at the price? A review of the economics of minimal access surgery.* Uxbridge: Brunel University, 1993.

36. Banta HD. Minimally invasive therapy in five European countries: diffusion, effectiveness and cost-effectiveness. *Health Policy* 1993; **23**: 1–178.

37. Neugebauer E, Troidl H, Spangenberger W, Dietrich A, Lefering R. Conventional versus laparoscopic cholecystectomy and the randomised controlled trial. *Br. J. Surg.* 1991; **78**: 150–4.

38. Macintyre IMC, Wilson RG. Laparoscopic cholecystectomy. *Br. J. Surg.* 1993; **80**: 552–9.

39. Froster UG, Jackson L. Limb defects and chorionic villus sampling: results from an international registry, 1992–94. *Lancet* 1996; **347**: 489–94.

40. Jackson LG, Zachary JM, Fowler SE, et al. A randomized comparison of transcervical and transabdominal chorionic-villus sampling. The U.S. National Institute of Child Health and Human Development Chorionic-Villus Sampling and Amniocentesis Study Group. *N. Engl. J. Med.* 1992; **327**: 594–8.

41. Schemmer G, Johnson A. Genetic amniocentesis and chorionic villus sampling. *Obstet. Gynecol. Clin. North Am.* 1993; **20**: 497–521.

42. Lippman A, Tomkins DJ, Shime J, Hamerton JL. Canadian multicentre randomized clinical trial of chorion villus sampling and amniocentesis. Final report. *Prenat. Diagn.* 1992; **12**: 385–408.

43. Smidt-Jensen S, Permin M, Philip J, et al. Randomised comparison of amniocentesis and transabdominal and transcervical chorionic villus sampling. *Lancet* 1992; **340**: 1237–44.

44. MRC Working Party on the Evaluation of Chorion Villus Sampling. Medical Research Council European Trial of chorion villus sampling. *Lancet* 1991; **337**: 1491–9.

45. Rhoads GG, Jackson LG, Schlesselman SE, et al. The safety and efficacy of chorionic villus sampling for early prenatal diagnosis of cytogenetic abnormalities. *N. Engl. J. Med.* 1989; **320**: 609–17.

46. Alfirevic Z, Gosden C, Neilson JP. Chorion villus sampling versus amniocentesis for prenatal diagnosis (Cochrane Review). In: *The Cochrane Library, 1995*. Oxford: Update Software.

47. Fahy MJ, Lippman A. Prenatal diagnosis and the Canadian Collaborative Randomized Trial of chorionic villi sampling: the physician's view. *Am. J. Med. Genet.* 1988; **31**: 953–61.

48. Hamerton JL. Chorionic villus sampling vs amniocentesis. *Lancet* 1989; **1**: 678.

49. Firth HV, Boyd PA, Chamberlain P, MacKenzie IZ, Lindenbaum RH, Huson SM. Severe limb abnormalities after chorion villus sampling at 56–66 days' gestation. *Lancet* 1991; **337**: 762–3.

50. Mastroiacovo P, Botto LD, Cavalcanti DP, et al. Limb anomalies following chorionic villus sampling: a registry based case-control study. *Am. J. Med. Genet.* 1992; **44**: 856–64.

51. Olney RS, Khoury MJ, Alo CJ, et al. Increased risk for transverse digital deficiency after chorionic villus sampling: results of the United States Multistate Case-Control Study, 1988–1992. *Teratology* 1995; **51**: 20–9.

52. Kaplan P, Normandin J Jr, Wilson GN, Plauchu H, Lippman A, Vekemans M. Malformations and minor anomalies in children whose mothers had prenatal diagnosis: comparison between CVS and amniocentesis. *Am. J. Med. Genet.* 1990; **37**: 366–70.

53. Brambati B. Chorionic villus sampling. *Curr. Opin. Obstet. Gynecol.* 1995; **7**: 109–16.

54. McLaren P, Ball CJ. Telemedicine: lessons remain unheeded. *Br. Med. J.* 1995; **310**: 1390–1.

55. Coles SFS. *Telemedicine: the rise of digital healthcare*. London: FT Pharmaceuticals and Healthcare Publishing, 1995.

56. Zabner J, Couture LA, Gregory RJ, Graham SM, Smith AE, Welsh MJ. Adenovirus-mediated gene transfer transiently corrects the chloride transport defect in nasal epithelia of patients with cystic fibrosis. *Cell* 1993; **75**: 207–16.

57. Crystal RG, McElvaney NG, Rosenfeld MA, et al. Administration of an adenovirus containing the human CFTR cDNA to the respiratory tract of individuals with cystic fibrosis. *Nature Genet.* 1994; **8**(1): 42–51.

58. Knowles MR, Hohneker KW, Zhou Z, et al. A controlled study of adenoviral-vector-mediated gene transfer in the nasal epithelium of patients with cystic fibrosis. *N. Engl. J. Med.* 1995; **333**: 823–31.

59. Caplen NJ, Alton EW, Middleton PG, et al. Liposome-mediated CFTR gene transfer to the nasal epithelium of patients with cystic fibrosis. *Nature Med.* 1995; **1**: 39–46.

60. Touchette N. Gene therapy: not ready for prime time. *Nature Med.* 1996; **2**: 7–8.

61. Border P. *Minimal access ('keyhole') surgery and its implications*. London: Parliamentary Office of Science and Technology, 1995.

27

Preliminary Economic Evaluation of Health Technologies

GARETH HARPER, JOY TOWNSEND
and MARTIN BUXTON

SUMMARY

This chapter presents a review of the existing methodologies for prioritising health technology assessment projects. It sets out criteria for appraising models based on the EUR-ASSESS project guidelines and the priorities of the UK National Health Service Research and Development Health Technology Assessment (HTA) Programme. Most HTA organisations currently employ criteria based systems for prioritisation which do not include the specific cost–effectiveness calculations which are the main subject of this review. The literature reviewed here includes models that allow an a priori quantitative assessment of likely payback to HTA. Seven major models were selected as appropriate, and each was appraised against 13 criteria, including whether the model explicitly considered alternative outcomes, the counterfactual and the costs and benefits of implementation, and whether it was transparent and flexible to adjust to different scales of research. Models that seem most appropriate for funding bodies to use are identified. The chapter discusses issues of how to deal with uncertainty, operationalising a model, resource requirements, the timing of costs and benefits, and the likely impact on practitioners' behaviour. It takes the view that if the ultimate purpose of applied HTA is to improve healthcare, it is insufficient to see the outcome in terms of the reduction of uncertainty alone, but needs to include the implications of the resultant likely use of the technology.

INTRODUCTION

This chapter appraises models for prioritising health technology assessment (HTA) projects, and assesses criteria currently used to prioritise proposed assessments. Conclusions are drawn from the review and used to recommend a model to assess the expected costs and benefits from HTA projects that can be used to prioritise research or appraise a specific research proposal.

Any organisation funding HTA is faced with the problem of prioritisation. The continuing development of healthcare technologies has increased the supply for potential assessment, and the move towards evidence based healthcare has increased the demand for assessments in terms of effectiveness and cost–effectiveness to inform and influence practice. However, just as resources for providing new technologies are limited, so are resources for their assessment, and some form of prioritisation is necessary. Funding bodies frequently consider likely costs and benefits in general terms, but rarely attempt to estimate systematically the cost–effectiveness of undertaking a research project. If such estimates were available, HTA funding organisations could use the calculations to aid funding decisions.

The increased demand for evidence to inform practice and decision-making has resulted in the rapid growth of HTA programmes, and of assessments proposed for funding. The funds available limit the number of technologies that can be evaluated: in 1997, approximately 1800 topics were proposed as candidates for assessment under the UK National Health Service R&D HTA programme; only 2% secured research funds in that funding cycle.[1] HTA organisations need to assess the potential returns to the proposed research to allocate limited research funds efficiently. The concept of cost–effectiveness needs to be applied to the choice of trials, as well as to the use of the technologies themselves.

HTA organisations such as the National Health Service R&D HTA programme and the Medical Research Council in the UK currently employ a criteria-based system for the prioritisation of research projects.[1,2] However, these systems do not include an explicit calculation of the cost–effectiveness of undertaking the research. The panels assessing research proposals are given a check-list of criteria (for example, would the project lead to a reduction in uncertainty, are the costs justified, are the objectives clearly stated) against which research proposals are judged.

The EUR-ASSESS project (an international group designed to stimulate and co-ordinate developments in HTA in Europe and to improve decision-making concerning adoption and use of health technology) produced a set of guidelines for the prioritisation of HTA projects.[3] These guidelines suggest that

(a) it should be clear to all involved in an HTA programme how priorities are identified;
(b) there should be agreement regarding the approach, method and criteria for assessment between those responsible for priority setting;
(c) the approach should reflect the goals of the programme and the resources available;
(d) the aim of the priority setting process should be to ensure that the priorities reflect the likely costs and benefits of the possible assessments;
(e) where possible, the method for priority setting should allow possible assessments to be rated in a systematic way against explicit criteria;
(f) information on priorities should be shared between those responsible for HTA programmes; and
(g) the processes and outcomes of priority setting should be evaluated to assess whether, and if so how, it has affected the topics assessed.

These guidelines have been considered in developing a set of criteria for assessing the literature below. The Institute of Medicine (IoM) in the USA has developed a more formalised methodology which assigns values and weights to seven criteria in order to achieve a global score,[4] with which the proposed research topics and projects can be prioritised.

These criteria-based systems are inherently sensitive to the interpretation of the criteria by the panel members. Implicit within the decisions concerning research proposals are judgements based upon potentially incomplete or inaccurate information and opinion. Due to the nature of these processes, there is no way of controlling for the potential variation in interpretation. It is for this reason that a number of researchers have undertaken the task of developing a systematic, quantitative model to assess research proposals, to work alongside the conventional process of scientific peer review.

METHODS

Search strategies were developed for use with Medline, HealthSTAR and BIDS SSCI. These search strategies were designed for maximum retrieval, using both index terms and free text searches. Once titles had been selected, papers were selected according to whether or not the article contained a proposed theoretical model for relating the costs (at whatever level) of undertaking a health services research project with any form of projected benefits of health services research. This selection was undertaken by two of the authors (G.H. and J.T.). In addition, more general papers concerning the payback to research, whilst not explicitly relating the costs of the research to the payback, were also considered for providing the context for the discussion below. The selected articles were collected and their models appraised using the following criteria, adapted from earlier work by the authors.[5]

Appraisal Criteria

These were as follows:

1 Does the proposed model state its aims? In particular, is it concerned with identifying technologies for assessment or for prioritising individual trials, or both?
2 Does the proposed model consider the alternative outcomes of a trial, and the inherent uncertainty surrounding the outcomes in a probabilistic framework?
3 Can the model be used within an iterative economic evaluation framework, using data from earlier stages and also informing later stages?
4 Does the process appear transparent and easily interpretable by a research funding body and potential funding applicants?

5 Does the model consider the counterfactual – what would happen if the trial were not to be funded?

6 Does the model consider the likely implementation of the intervention following the reporting of the trial's conclusions?

7 Is there a data source for the model to be operationalised?

8 Are other forms of payback to the research considered? If so, how? In particular, are weights assigned to a range of potential benefits to research?

9 How is the uncertainty and subjectivity inherent in the data collection and modelling process considered?

10 How efficient is the process likely to be? In particular, will the process itself consume resources (researchers time, costs of data collection), and will the outcome be useful to research-funding bodies?

11 Is the process flexible to adjust to different scales of research?

12 Can the model accommodate alternative outcome measures of the trial, if necessary?

13 Can the model accommodate the analysis of particular subgroups of patients?

LITERATURE REVIEW

Seven major studies were selected as appropriate from the articles identified in the literature search. The selection criterion was that the article contained a proposed model or a quantitative example of assessing the benefits of a research project in relation to the proposed costs. Methods which simply rated a proposed HTA against a set of criteria were excluded. The selected articles were:

- Claxton K, Posnett J. An economic approach to clinical trial design and research priority-setting. *Health Economics* 1996; **5**: 513–24.
- Detsky AS. Using economic analysis to determine the resource consequences of choices made in planning clinical trials. *Journal of Chronic Diseases* 1985; **38**: 753–65.
- Drummond MF, Davies LM, Ferris III FL. Assessing the costs and benefits of Medical Research: the Diabetic Retinopathy Study. *Social Science and Medicine* 1992; **34**: 973–81.
- Eddy DM. Selecting technologies for assessment. *International Journal of Technology Assessment in Health Care* 1989; **5**: 485–501.
- Phelps CE, Parente ST. Priority setting in medical technology and medical practice

assessment. *Medical Care* 1990; **28**: 703–23; ISSN: 0025-7079.
- Thompson MS. Decision-analytic determination of study size. The case of Electronic Fetal Monitoring. *Medical Decision Making* 1981; **1**: 165–79.
- Townsend J, Buxton M. Cost effectiveness scenario analysis for a proposed trial of hormone replacement therapy. *Health Policy* 1997; **39**: 181–94.

Each of these studies will be described briefly and then systematically appraised using the criteria above.

In the paper by Thompson,[7] the optimal sample size of a trial is estimated using decision analysis. The aim of the model is to identify the break-even sample size of a proposed trial, by valuing benefit of reduced mortality in terms of estimated life earnings, with the cost of the trial containing a fixed component plus a variable component per subject. Thompson applied the methodology to a trial for electronic fetal monitoring of low-risk babies.

The Detsky[8] model is based on the prior distribution of the risk reduction of the intervention under consideration and the effect of a trial (with a given power and significance level) on the distribution of this risk reduction. By combining this effect with, for example, the number of people currently dying per year when treated with the traditional therapy, Detsky produced a measure of effectiveness of a clinical trial. By relating this to the cost of the trial, Detsky was able to estimate a cost–effectiveness ratio of the research. Detsky's model assumed 100% implementation following the conclusion of the trial.

Eddy[9] developed the Technology Assessment Priority Setting-System (TAPSS) which models the effect of a range of factors on a single research outcome measure. These factors include the number of potential candidates for the intervention under evaluation, the probability that the assessment will arrive at a particular result, the implementation following that result, and the number likely to receive the technology. By adjusting these parameters, TAPSS can systematically account for any variation in the key variables, and in the inevitable uncertainty that exists around the estimation of some of these variables. Repeating the exercise for other possible outcomes and combining these probabilistically into a single figure can determine the effects on more than one outcome. The TAPSS model forms the basis for the development of a number of later models.

Phelps and Parente[6] developed a model to account for unexplained variation in medical expenditure in counties in New York State,

Table 1 *Appraisal of the seven major studies*

	Claxton and Posnett (1996)[11]	Detsky (1985)[8]	Drummond et al. (1992)[10]	Eddy (1989)[9]	Phelps and Parente (1990)[6]	Thompson (1981)[7]	Townsend and Buxton (1997)[12]
Does the proposed model state its aims? In particular, is it concerned with identifying technologies for assessment or for prioritising individual trials, or both?	The model's aim is to ensure that a trial design is efficient. The objective is to promote consistency in decision-making and priority setting between research and service provision.	The procedure aims to demonstrate that 'economic principles can be used to make explicit the consequences of planning or management decisions ...' The model relates the cost of the trial (but not the treatment) to the sample size and the clinically important difference identified in the trial. The aim is to consider the marginal productivity of research funding, when expanding or contracting trial sizes.	The objective is to 'develop and test a methodology for assessing the social costs and benefits of research.' It is designed to consider prospectively whether a research project should be funded.	The model developed was 'a simple framework and quantitative method for estimating the value of assessing different technologies.' It considers a proposed assessment and evaluates how it will affect health and economic outcomes. The assessment can be compared between different proposed assessments.	To account for unexplained variation in medical expenditure between New York counties and thus to estimate an implicit value of assessing the technology.	To estimate the optimal sample size of a trial using decision analysis.	To develop a methodology for the ex ante evaluation of a proposed technology assessment, comparing the costs and benefits following an assessment's conclusion with the likely practice in the absence of the assessment.
Does the proposed model consider the alternative outcomes of a trial?	The model compares the cost of a trial with the expected net benefits for different sample sizes. The alternative outcomes are incorporated in the determination of the expected benefits.	To calculate the power of the trial, the model uses an expected level of risk reduction, taking all possible risk reductions (−100% to +100%) into account, by weighting them with the probability that each of these outcomes will occur.	The model is constructed using a decision-theoretic approach, with the alternative outcomes of the trial represented by the probabilities assigned to the different events and through sensitivity analysis applied to these probabilities.	Yes, the alternative conclusions of the assessment are reflected in the range of Delta results selected for the assessment. For each Delta result (the result of an assessment that can potentially change the use of a technology) a probability needs to be estimated that reflects the likelihood that the assessment will reach that Delta result.	No.	Yes – net gain or loss of life.	Alternative outcomes are considered explicitly, with positive, negative and inconclusive outcomes defined in terms of varying health gains (or losses) and weighted with the probabilities of the trial reaching those outcomes.

Can the model be used within an iterative economic evaluation framework, using data from earlier stages and also informing later stages?	The calculation of the expected value of sample information (EVSI) and the expected value of perfect information (EVPI) may be of little value in the later stages of economic evaluation.	Unlikely. Calculation of effectiveness depends on the change in the risk reduction following the trial, which may be of little value to the researchers. However, the marginal approach would be of value should further funds be requested by the researchers	Yes. The cost-effectiveness analysis is in terms of the effectiveness measure of the trial (vision years gained). Such information can inform the full evaluation.	Potentially yes, as the detailed claculations involved in the TAPSS model would be of benefit in identifying important sub-groups for specific analyses during later stages of the assessment.	No, it is a highly specific macro type model.	Yes.
Does the process appear transparent and easily interpretable by a research funding body and potential funding applicants?	It is a highly theoretical model, using techniques and concepts that may mean little to potential research applicants.	The concept of the prior distribution of the risk reduction is highly subjective, and the implications of such may not be fully understood.	The decision-analytic approach clearly shows the processes of the evaluation, the assumptions made and what adjustments have been made.	Uncertain, as the model involves the interaction between a number of factors. The means of calculation may not be particularly transparent.	It is a broad field methodology and the strong assumptions between methodology and interpretation mean it is not really transparent.	Probably, although dependent on prior distribution.
Does the model consider the counterfactual – what would happen if the trial were not to be funded?	Not explicitly.	No.	Yes.	No.	The methodology centres on local practice moving directly to current average, but it is not incremental.	No.
Does the model consider the likely implementation of the intervention following the reporting of the trial's conclusions?	Not explicitly.	No.	Yes.	Yes.	No, it is implied to be perfect.	Yes.

Table 1 *Continued*

	Claxton and Posnett (1996)[11]	Detsky (1985)[8]	Drummond et al. (1992)[10]	Eddy (1989)[9]	Phelps and Parente (1990)[6]	Thompson (1981)[7]	Townsend and Buxton (1997)[12]
Is there a data source for the model to be operationalised?	Theoretical model, with no example used.	Published literature.	Published literature and expert opinion.	Estimated by author.	Published literature and estimates based on existing US state data.	Expert opinion and published literature. Benefits calculated from published estimates of lifetime earnings.	Published literature.
Are other forms of payback to the research considered? If so, how? In particular, are weights assigned to a range of potential benefits to research?	The benefits are based on patient utilities, converted into population benefits. Other forms of payback are not explicitly considered.	No.	No. Health gains only.	No, but model can be re-estimated using other outcomes.	No.	No.	No.
Can and how is the uncertainty and subjectivity inherent in the data collection and modelling process considered?	Not explicitly, although the EVPI can be re-calculated, with adjustments in the probabilistic framework.	Yes, through sensitivity analysis around the prior distribution of the risk reduction and the power curve.	Yes, through sensitivity analysis in calculating the cost-effectiveness ratios.	The model could be re-calculated using different values for the variables.	No.	Could be incorporated into the decision-theoretic framework.	Yes, through adjusting the proportion of people receiving treatment following a trial's conclusion.
How efficient is the process likely to be? In particular, will the process itself	Uncertain.	Process is relatively simple, but subject to the interpretation of the prior distribution.	Modelling exercise would be relatively straightforward.	The data required to calculate results either requires estimation or resource-intensive collection,	Interesting approach, but the categories are probably too broad to be useful and	Dependent on prior distribution and strong assumptions, but would be usable.	If data or informed opinion, is available, then yes.

consume resources (researchers' time, costs of data collection), and will the outcome be used?	effective in changing practice.		for example, a trial.			Yes.	
Is the process flexible to adjust to different scales of research?	Uncertain – not applied to data.	Yes – the model was applied retrospectively to a number of trials ranging in costs from $78 000–$150 000.	Yes, although the application was to the NEI Diabetic Retinopathy Study, the cost of which was $10.5 million. For an application to a smaller trial, the sensitivity analysis would need to be more precise.	No.	Unlikely, as data on small trials will be unavailable to the extent required by the TAPSS model.	Potentially more applicable to big trials, such as the proposed HRT to which the model is applied in the article. Implementation following trial outcomes will require precise sensitivity analysis for smaller trials.
Can the model accommodate alternative outcome measures of the trial, if necessary?	It can accommodate a number of patient based outcomes, as the effectiveness is based around patients' utilities. However, it may be difficult to include other forms of benefits from research.	Difficult, as effectiveness is based on change in risk reduction, requiring one health related outcome.	Use of QALYSs is possible, which combine a number of health related outcomes. However, other forms of benefits may be difficult to use in the model.	Yes, but the model would need to be re-calculated, and the results combined with some (arbitrary) weighting procedure.	No – potential benefits are based on the assumed welfare losses from deviation from current average practice.	In a limited way if they can be translated into monetary terms to feed into the break-even equation.	Yes, application can use QALYs, combining a number of health outcomes. However, other forms of benefits may be difficult to use in the model.
Can the model accommodate the analysis of particular subgroups of patients?	Not explicitly considered, but would be possible.	Not explicitly considered, but would be possible.	Yes, within the decision-analysis framework.	Yes.	No, it is relevant to average county practice.		Not explicitly considered, but would be possible.

which estimates an implied value of assessing the technology. The model assumes that any variation in expenditure not explained by demographic or socio-economic factors is due to uncertainty about the outcome of the intervention. The model operates under the assumptions that the 'correct' level of expenditure is approximated by the adjusted mean level of expenditure and that the elasticity of demand for all health technologies is 0.15. These factors are combined to determine the welfare losses associated with the unexplained variation in expenditure. These welfare losses are then compared across Diagnosis Related Groups (DRGs) to identify the highest payoff from potential research spending. The analysis is focused at a technology rather than a research proposal level, and is limited by the fact that a DRG may require more than one particular technology.

Drummond et al.[10] used a decision analytical model to assess the economic returns from a piece of applied research. The model was applied retrospectively to the Diabetic Retinopathy Study, which was funded by the National Eye Institute from 1972–1981. Adjustments to the probabilities within the decision tree (the relative probabilities of whether a patient has diabetic retinopathy before and after the trial) and also to the extent of the population who might benefit from the intervention following the trial, the benefits they might receive and the costs of implementation ensure that uncertainty surrounding the modelling processes is sufficiently covered.

Claxton and Posnett[11] used a Bayesian concept of the value of information within their model. Their model used the expected value of perfect information (EVPI) and the expected value of sample information (EVSI), expressed in monetary units, in two 'hurdles' designed to assess first the technologies for assessment and then the specific research proposals. Firstly, the EVPI is used to assess whether a reduction in the uncertainty surrounding a technology area would be valuable. The criteria set by Claxton and Posnett is that the EVPI must exceed the fixed costs of the research. Secondly, to ensure the design of the trial is cost-effective when conducted at the optimal scale, the trial design must clear a second 'hurdle', namely that the expected net benefits of the research (ENBR) is greater than zero, at the optimal sample size.

Townsend and Buxton[12] developed a decision analysis model applied to an example of a proposed trial of the long-term use of hormone replacement therapy (HRT). The authors were able to draw upon detailed empirical data and published estimates of the long-term benefit of HRT, but recognised that for other technologies, such detail might not be available. Where it is

not, the authors argue that expert opinion can be used to provide estimates of the gaps and to provide the necessary data. Three trial outcomes (positive, negative and inconclusive) were identified, and changes in the long-term use of HRT were predicted for each outcome scenario, together with the net effects of these changes in terms of discounted streams of costs and benefits.

APPRAISAL OF THE STUDIES

The seven major studies identified from the literature search are appraised in Table 1.

Commentary

Certain issues arise from the review. Although a number of papers consider the process by which research funds are allocated, very few actually propose a systematic model to determine whether a research proposal is likely to be a cost-effective investment. Only seven such models are identified above and are reviewed according to the criteria listed.

Aims of the models, their methods and levels of information

The criteria used to assess the models are based on how practical they are in terms of effectiveness and efficiency. In general, the models had similar aims, namely to assess the 'value' of undertaking a particular piece of health services research or health technology assessment, although the method used vary in each case. The predominant methods used are variants of a decision–analysis approach, with the costs and benefits for each trial outcome (and subsequent implementation pattern) combined probabilistically. Such an approach has the advantages that the benefits of the research are clearly defined in terms of the health outcomes of the trial's effect on practice. The models that require a calculation of the expected value of information have two major problems. The level of information available before the trial needs to be combined into a prior distribution, for example of the perceived mortality risk reduction of undergoing a surgical procedure. Also, some models attempt to convert the increased value of information into financial terms, and the problems of this have long been recognised. As Buxton and Hanney argue, such problems are 'probably no more readily soluble for research payback assessment than for the assessment of the interventions themselves'.[13]

Staged approach

A major test of the efficiency of a model is likely to be the ease with which the model could fit into an HTA funding organisation's existing processes of funding allocation. Sculpher et al. described the possibility of using economic evaluation iteratively as part of the HTA process,[14] possibly with earlier preliminary analysis being used to inform later decisions, for example in identifying subgroups on which the full evaluation might concentrate. Data collected for analysis at an earlier stage might be used productively at a later stage. For example, that collected to assess whether the technology requires assessment might be used to assess a specific trial. The earlier stages of the iterative process involve the prioritisation of technologies. Buxton and Hanney[13] described a three-stage approach to the prioritisation in terms of estimating the payback from research. The first two stages (theoretical potential payback and expected potential payback) consider topics or technologies, whilst the third stage (likely realisable payback) considers specific research proposals designed to reduce specific elements of uncertainty surrounding the technology that had been identified in the previous two stages. Our review throws doubts on whether the more theoretical models have the requisite characteristics to satisfy this overall three-stage approach.

Dealing with uncertainty

It is the existence of uncertainty that prompts the initial demand for some form of HTA. The nature of the uncertainty is most appropriately investigated at the technology stage, to see whether the existence of this uncertainty is detrimental and if ameliorated, whether net benefits might accrue. The extent of the uncertainty is important, and the greater the number of 'unknowns', the higher will be the likely cost of the necessary specific research projects. The cost of a specific proposal will depend upon *what* it is we are uncertain about. Uncertainty may surround the cost of a particular intervention, the effectiveness of a particular intervention, or both the costs and the effectiveness. Identification of the nature and extent of the uncertainty will influence both the research proposal and the full evaluation stages. There will be uncertainty also and some degree of subjectivity about implementation – how the research results will influence practice. This will depend on the effectiveness of existing means of dissemination of information amongst practitioners, commissioners and policy-makers, and on the professional

and institutional rigidities. There will also be uncertainty surrounding the data used and the models reviewed could be recalculated, with sensitivity analysis for this.

Models such as those of Drummond et al. and Townsend and Buxton, that use direct health outcomes within a probabilistic, decision–analysis framework, and clear measures of the proportion of the population likely to benefit from the intervention following the trial's conclusion, are likely to be able to handle uncertainty more systematically. With models that use a more 'theoretical' approach, such as those of Claxton and Posnett and Phelps and Parente, it may be more difficult to handle the uncertainty that surrounds variables such as the extent of implementation and the variation of the effect of size in different subgroups of the population. In our context, the major criteria of the efficiency of the model is how likely it will be able to influence decisions made by a research-funding organisation. This may raise problems for models using concepts that may appear abstract to potential funding applicants.

The incremental effects of a trial: considering the counterfactual

To consider the incremental effects of the trial on subsequent practice, a model needs to include what practice would be were the trial not funded. It may not be sufficient to assume that current practice continues. The incremental effects of the trial relating to changes in practice need to be explicitly accounted for in terms of health gains. A trial that finds in favour of an intervention that would have been introduced or continued in use anyway, but would not have prevented its adoption had it found against the intervention is clearly unnecessary. Few models satisfy the necessary criteria of explicitly calculating the incremental costs and benefits of a trial.

The likely impact on practitioners' behaviour

We take the view that, given the ultimate purpose of HTA is improved healthcare, the outcomes need to include the implications of the resultant likely use of the technology, and so it would be insufficient for outcomes to be in terms of the reduction of uncertainty alone. That is, an assessment's health-related benefits must consider the extent to which an assessment's conclusions will affect health service practitioners' subsequent behaviour. A number of models, including those of Detsky and Phelps and Parente assume full implementation of the intervention following the report of a trial's findings. This is unlikely: organisational barriers, ineffective information dissemination and poor management of change are likely to operate at varying levels, and prevent or delay the immediate adoption of the more effective or cost-effective technology or intervention in some organisations. A more realistic model would allow some means of assessing the extent of the likely adoption of the more cost-effective technology, perhaps through the use of expert opinion.

Non-health benefits

A conflict arises between the multi-dimensional nature of payback from health services research and the need for a precise quantitative model. Buxton and Hanney[15] have identified five different categories of potential benefits from health services research: knowledge benefits; benefits to future research; political and administrative benefits; health benefits; and broader economic benefits. According to their objectives and sources of funding, HTA organisations may place different emphases on these, and it is possible to argue that a model designed to prioritise research projects should relate these potential benefits from research directly to the resource implications of undertaking the research. As stated earlier, such a model would require estimates of the relative importance of each form of benefit. For some HTA programmes, it is clear that the prime motivation is to improve the cost–effectiveness of the health system. Any other form of benefit or payback, albeit important, would be considered secondary. Therefore, preliminary cost–effectiveness studies using 'equation-based models' to evaluate a research proposal have understandably concentrated on the health benefits, to reduce subjectivity in terms of weighting alternative forms of payback from research. Other forms of benefits however should not be ignored, and whereas the majority of applications of the models concentrate upon the health benefits, minor modifications of models such as TAPSS would allow other forms of payback to be assessed and non-health benefits could and should be considered alongside the model.

Resource requirements to operationalise the model

Central to all of these considerations is the availability of data required to operationalise a model. A number of models rely on existing published data. Frequently, given the inherent uncertainty, the requisite data may not be available and a surrogate alternative such as using expert opinion may be necessary. Data requirements of a model may be demanding or too costly for a modelling exercise to be efficient. Sheldon[16] described modelling as 'a way of representing the complexity of the real world in a more simple and comprehensible form'. However, if the model itself requires data collection that is likely to consume significant resources – as might be the case with the TAPSS model – the cost of the preliminary modelling exercise might begin to approach the costs of undertaking the assessment itself, in which case, the efficiency of the model and its usefulness to HTA funding organisations comes into question.

A model that requires a wide range of variables and considers more than one outcome may appear attractive, but the data requirements might be too great for it to run effectively, especially where little research has been undertaken previously.

The timing of the costs and benefits of the technology

The timing of the costs and benefits relating to the HTA will affect its overall cost–effectiveness. It is unlikely that the payback, and the costs of changes in implementation, will occur immediately after the trial. All the models considered above are able to incorporate appropriate discounting; however, a number of the applications on which the models were tested did not, but rather assumed immediate implementation. Related to this is the potential lifespan of a technology. If a particular technology or pharmaceutical considered for assessment is expected to be superseded shortly by a rival, which is at an earlier stage of development, then the 'shelf-life' of the technology being considered for assessment might be relatively short, and a substantial investment in the assessment may not be efficient. The benefits of the research over a given time period needs therefore to be adjusted for varying 'shelf-life'. The value of an assessment may also be reduced or negated if results of a similar or related assessment of the same technology is impending.

DEVELOPMENT

This section presents a new model as a response to the problems and strengths identified in the literature review. The model developed maintains the multi-stage approach to the preliminary economic evaluation of health technologies as identified by Buxton and Hanney,[13] recognises how these stages connect together and how data and information from previous stages may assist a later stage. This general model is represented in Figure 1. The specific quantitative component concentrates on the stage of whether a specific HTA proposal should be funded, following the earlier and equally important stage, namely assessing whether any uncertainty exists, and if so in which area. Data are needed to decide whether there is uncertainty about the cost and/or effectiveness of an intervention, and whether this uncertainty reasonably prevents informed adoption or rejection of the technology. If it is concluded that a reduction in uncertainty would, given a particular outcome and the necessary resources, lead to a beneficial change in practice or policy, then a trial should be considered. Following the submission of specific research proposals, the expected incremental cost–effectiveness ratio of the research proposal could be determined using Equation (1). This ratio could be subject to sensitivity analysis to allow for the uncertainty and subjectivity around the inputs to the model. The results of the application of the model could then be incorporated into a report for the research-funding organisation, which could weigh this 'expected incremental cost–effectiveness ratio' together with other considerations about whether the research project should be funded or not.

Figure 1 sets out the full model for the ex ante evaluation of likely payback to a health technology assessment (PATHS model), from the generation of ideas for assessment (incorporating ideas such as horizon scanning), through to the rejection or funding of a specific research proposal.

The quantitative model set out in Equation (1) is designed to answer the question towards the end of the algorithm, namely whether a *specific* research proposal should be funded. The model as set out below is based on three alternative potential broad outcomes to the trial, although this can be adapted according to the needs of specific research proposals. The three broad potential outcomes include a 'favourable' conclusion, an 'unfavourable' conclusion, and an 'inconclusive' outcome. Each of these conclusions will have an associated level of benefits (or disbenefits) and a level of costs depending on the outcome and effect on implementation; there will also be an associated probability that the trial will come to that conclusion. The expected incremental cost–effectiveness ratio (EICER) can be derived using the following equation:

Equation (1)

$$EICER = \frac{C_T + p_1(C_1 - C_C) + p_2(C_2 - C_C) + p_3(C_3 - C_C)}{p_1(B_1 - B_{C_1}) + p_2(B_2 - B_{C_2}) + p_3(B_3 - B_{C_3})}$$

where: C_T = cost of the trial (trial outcome identifier (n): 1 = Favourable to intervention; 2 = Unfavourable to intervention; 3 = Inconclusive result); C_n = cost associated with likely practice, given trial outcome n; C_C = cost associated with likely practice if trial did not occur; B_n = benefits associated with likely practice given trial outcome n; B_{C_n} = benefits associated with likely practice if trial did not take place, given the outcome of the trial, if the trial did take place; and p_n = probability that trial will produce outcome n.

The EICER is designed as a tool for HTA funding bodies to assess potential returns from proposed research. By comparing the expected cost–effectiveness ratio of one or a series of research proposals within the same area and the cost and effects of continuing with the current provision, a funding body would be in a position to allocate limited research funds to projects likely to provide the most efficient returns to research. It compares a range of alternative implementation patterns following the trial's conclusion, against the likely practice in the absence of the trial within a probabilistic framework. It measures the effectiveness of the trial in terms of the primary outcome measure of the research proposal itself. It can use existing published data, or expert opinion if necessary, but does not require an expensive process of data collection. It is a relatively straightforward model to operationalise, and should be relatively transparent. Also, it can easily be re-calculated using alternative values for the net costs and benefits for each scenario, and for adjusting the probabilities associated with each trial outcome. By adjusting the net benefits accordingly, the extent of the implementation can be adjusted. This reflects the view that an HTA proposal is not solely concerned with how much it will reduce uncertainty, but that its value depends upon the assessment's likely impact upon practice within the health sector.

Data for the Model

Where empirical data required are not available for use within the model, relevant expert opinion would be used to provide estimates. The choice of experts would depend on the nature of the proposed trial under analysis, in particular the level of intervention, but usually a range of expertise would be used to triangulate the estimates.

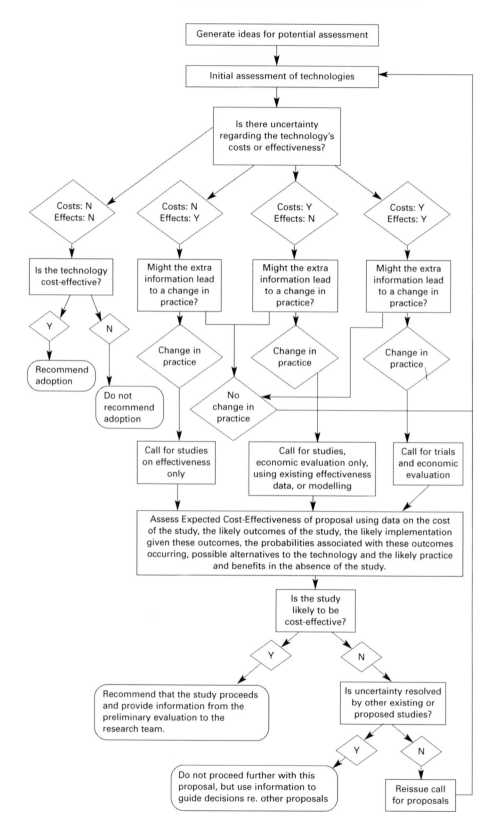

The information needed to operationalise the above model would be:

(a) the likely development of policy or practice, in the absence of the trial;

(b) the likely implementation of the experimental intervention following the reporting of the trial results, given alternative scenarios for the results:
  - the extent to which the technology or service might be adopted;
  - how existing policy might affect the level of implementation; and
  - whether the technology or service would be introduced for all potential candidates, or whether it would be targeted at specific groups.

(c) how other relevant services might be affected following the adoption or change in practice of the experimental intervention;

(d) whether the outcomes used within the trial are appropriate, whether they are likely to influence future policy and/or practice and whether there are any alternative outcome measures that might be more appropriate;

(e) whether the expert considers there are threshold levels for costs, effectiveness or cost–effectiveness, that might trigger adoption of the experimental intervention; and

(f) the probabilities that the overall outcome of the trial will be positive, negative or inconclusive.

CONCLUSIONS

This chapter has considered a range of characteristics that a quantitative model for the prioritisation of HTA projects needs to portray. There is often a trade-off between the 'completeness' of the model (and therefore the resource implications of the modelling exercise) and the ease of operationalising the model. A balance needs to be struck between these two factors. The models presented here do not replace the existing processes of research prioritisation, but would be complementary to the process of peer review and criteria-based approaches that consider also benefits that are not applicable to direct quantification. A model therefore needs to fit within the existing processes and be able to use earlier analyses within an iterative framework.

Transparency is an essential characteristic of an acceptable model. Potential applicants need to know how their proposal is to be assessed.

Highly theoretical models using abstract methods to determine the benefits of the research, are unlikely to demonstrate this transparency.

The models based on a decision analysis framework in which the cost–effectiveness of the research is expressed in terms of the health intervention appeared to be the most transparent. These models tend to rely on published data to inform the process, and providing that a competent literature search is undertaken, such data (costs and health-related benefits) should be accessible and translation of health benefits into monetary form is not necessary. By the nature of the problem, there will be information required that will not be available, but which might best be obtained by appropriate use of expert opinion, for example through Delphi groups.

Use of a range of expert opinion would help to obviate bias, and sensitivity analysis is relatively straightforward in models based upon decision analysis theory, as the costs, benefits and probabilities of each arm can be easily adjusted. On the other hand, models in which the benefits are difficult to disentangle may not be easily adjusted by sensitivity analysis to account for uncertainty.

With these considerations in mind we developed our model, aiming to include the various necessary characteristics identified, and attempting to strike a balance between the issues of rigour, transparency and resource requirements. Ideally to test this model it would be used prospectively on a number of randomly selected trials, and the predicted outcomes compared with a number of trials which had been funded but not subjected to the analysis. However, such an evaluation would be lengthy and difficult to undertake. As a realistic approximation therefore we are currently testing and evaluating the model on four case studies of four publicly funded randomised trials, identified by the authors in liaison with the UK NHS R&D HTA programme and the Medical Research Council. These case studies are running concurrently with the preliminary modelling exercise and are being evaluated prior to completion, and the evaluation compared with what professionals think the reported results imply for future use of the technology. On completion of the project we hope to provide a practical guide to HTA organisations, particularly on quantitative assessment that can be used as an adjunct to prioritise research or to appraise specific research proposals.

Figure 1 (opposite) *Model of ex ante evaluation of likely payback to a health technology assessment (PATHS model).*

References

1. NHS Executive. National Co-Ordinating Centre for Health Technology Assessment. The Annual Report of the NHS Health Technology Assessment programme 1997. Identifying questions, finding answers. NHS Executive, 1997.
2. Medical Research Council. *Developing High Quality Proposals in Health Services Research*, 1994.
3. Henshall C, Oortwijn W, Stevens A, Granados A, Banta D. Priority setting for health technology assessment. Theoretical considerations and practical approaches. A paper produced by the priority setting subgroup of the EUR-ASSESS project. *Int. J. Technol. Assess. Health Care* 1997; **13**: 144–85.
4. Donaldson MS, Sox HC (eds). *Setting Priorities for Health Technology Assessment. A Model Process*. Washington D.C.: National Academy Press, 1992.
5. Harper G, Townsend J, Buxton M. The preliminary appraisal of health technologies: a discussion. *Int. J. Technol. Assess. Health Care* 1998; **14**: 652–62.
6. Phelps CE, Parente ST. Priority setting in medical technology and medical practice assessment. *Med. Care* 1990; **28**: 703–23. [Published erratum appears in *Med. Care* 1992; **30**: 744–51.]
7. Thompson MS. Decision-analytic determination of study size. The case of electronic fetal monitoring. *Medical Decision Making* 1981; **1**: 165–79.
8. Detsky AS. Using economic analysis to determine the resource consequences of choices made in planning clinical trials. *J. Chron. Dis.* 1985; **38**: 753–65.
9. Eddy DM. Selecting technologies for assessment. *Int. J. Technol. Assess. Health Care* 1989; **5**: 485–501.
10. Drummond MF, Davies LM, Ferris III FL. Assessing the costs and benefits of medical research: the Diabetic Retinopathy Study. *Soc. Sci. Med.* 1992; **34**: 973–81.
11. Claxton K, Posnett J. An economic approach to clinical trial design and research priority-setting. *Health Economics* 1996; **5**: 513–24.
12. Townsend J, Buxton M. Cost effectiveness scenario analysis for a proposed trial of hormone replacement therapy. *Health Policy* 1997; **39**: 181–94.
13. Buxton M, Hanney S. *Assessing payback from Department of Health Research and Development: Preliminary Report. Vol. 1: The Main Report*. Brunel University: HERG, 1994.
14. Sculpher MS, Drummond MF, Buxton M. The iterative use of economic evaluation as part of the process of health technology assessment. *J. Health Services Res. Policy* 1997; **2**: 26–30.
15. Buxton M, Hanney S. How can payback from health services research be assessed? *J. Health Services Res. Policy* 1996; **1**: 35–43.
16. Towse A, Drummond M (eds). *The Pros and Cons of Modelling in Economic Evaluation*. Office of Health Economics, Briefing No. 33, London: OHE, 1997.

Index